高等教育出版社　中國・北京

Higher Education Press, Beijing, China

3
方　剂　学

	中　文	英　文
主　编	蔡剑前	徐象才
	孔繁芝	
副主编	张盛新	路玉滨
编　者	潘青海	韩　玫
	于建军	欧阳勤
	尤　可	
	于淑芬	
审　校	白永波	

PHARMACOLOGY OF TRADITIONAL CHINESE MEDICAL FORMULAE

	English	Chinese
Chief Editors	Xu Xiangcai	Cai Jianqian
Deputy Chief Editors	Zhang Shengxin	Kong Fanzhi
	Lu Yubin	
Editors	Han Mei	Pan Qinghai
	Ouyang Qin	Yu Jianjun
		You Ke
		Yu Shufen
Reviser		Bai Yongbo

The Leading Commission of Compilation and Translation
编译领导委员会

Honorary Director 名誉主任委员	Hu Ximing 胡熙明		
Honorary Deputy Directors 名誉副主任委员	Zhang Qiwen 张奇文	Wang Lei 王镭	
Director 主任委员	Zou Jilong 邹积隆		
Deputy Director 副主任委员	Wei Jiwu 隗继武		
Members 委员 (以姓氏笔划为序)	Wan Deguang 万德光	Wang Yongyan 王永炎	Wang Maoze 王懋泽
	Wei Guikang 韦贵康	Cong Chunyu 丛春雨	Liu Zhongben 刘中本
	Sun Guojie 孙国杰	Yan Shiyun 严世芸	Qiu Dewen 邱德文
	Shang Chichang 尚炽昌	Xiang Ping 项平	Zhao Yisen 赵以森
	Gao Jinliang 高金亮	Cheng Yichun 程益春	Ge Linyi 葛琳仪
	Cai Jianqian 蔡剑前	Zhai Weimin 翟维敏	
Advisers 顾问	Dong Jianhua 董建华	Huang Xiaokai 黄孝楷	Geng Jianting 耿鉴庭
	Zhou Fengwu 周凤梧	Zhou Ciqing 周次清	Chen Keji 陈可冀

The Commission of Compilation and Translation
编译委员会

Director 主任委员	Xu Xiangcai 徐象才

Preface

I am delighted to learn that THE ENGLISH—CHINESE ENCYCLOPEDIA OF PRACTICAL TRADITIONAL CHINESE MEDICINE will soon come into the world.

TCM has experienced many vicissitudes of times but has remained evergreen. It has made great contributions not only to the power and prosperity of our Chinese nation but to the enrichment and improvement of world medicine. Unfortunately, differences in nations, states and languages have slowed down its spreading and flowing outside China. At present, however, an upsurge in learning, researching and applying Traditional Chinese Medicine (TCM) is unfolding. In order to maximize the effect of this upsurge and to lead TCM, one of the brilliant cultural heritages of the Chinese nation, to the world for it to expand and bring benefit to the people of all nations, Mr. Xu Xiangcai called intellectuals of noble aspirations and high intelligence together from Shandong and many other provinces in China and took charge of the work of both compilation and translation of THE ENGLISH—CHINESE ENCYCLOPEDIA OF PRACTICAL TRADITIONAL CHINESE MEDICINE. With great pleasure, the medical staff both at home and abroad will hail the appearance of this encyclopedia.

I believe that the day when the world's medicine is fully

developed will be the day when TCM has spread throughout the world.

I am pleased to give it my preface.

Prof. Dr. Hu Ximing
Deputy Ministerof the Ministry of Public Health of the People's Republic of China,
Director General of the State Administrative Bureau of Traditional Chinese Medicine and Pharmacology,
President of the World Federation of Acupuncture —Moxibustion Societies,
Member of China Association of Science & Technology,
Deputy President of All—China Association of Traditional Chinese Medicine,
President of China Acupuncture & Moxibustion Society.

December, 1989

Preface

The Chinese nation has been through a long, arduous course of struggling against diseases and has developed its own traditional medicine—Traditional Chinese Medicine and Pharmacology (TCMP). TCMP has a unique, comprehensive, scientific system including both theories and clinical practice. Some thousand years since its beginnings, not only has it been well preserved but also continuously developed. It has special advantages, such as remarkable curative effects and few side effects. Hence it is an effective means by which people prevent and treat diseases and keep themselves strong and healthy.

All achievements attained by any nation in the development of medicine are the public wealth of all mankind. They should not be confined within a single country. What is more, the need to set them free to flow throughout the world as quickly and precisely as possible is greater than that of any other kind of science. During my more than thirty years of being engaged in Traditional Chinese Medicine(TCM), I have been looking forward to the day when TCMP will have spread all over the world and made its contributions to the elimination of diseases of all mankind. However it is to be deeply regretted that the pace of TCMP in extending outside China has been unsatisfactory due to the major difficulties in expressing its concepts in foreign languages.

Mr. Xu Xiangcai, a teacher of Shandong College of TCM, has sponsored and taken charge of the work of compilation and

translation of The English—Chinese Encyclopedia of Practical
Traditional Chinese Medicine—an extensive series. This work is a
great project, a large—scale scientific research, a courageous effort
and a novel creation. I deeply esteem Mr. Xu Xiangcai and his
compilers and translators, who have been working day and night
for such a long time, for their hard labor and for their firm and
indomitable will displayed in overcoming one difficulty after another, and for their great success achieved in this way. As a leader
in the circles of TCM, I am duty—bound to do my best to support
them.

I believe this encyclopedia will be certain to find its position
both in the history of Chinese medicine and in the history of
world science and technology.

Mr. Zhang Qiwen

Member of the Standing Committee of
All—China Association of TCM,
Deputy Head of the Health Department
of Shandong Province.

March, 1990

Publisher's Preface

Traditional Chinese Medicine(TCM) is one of China's great cultural heritages. Since the founding of the People's Republic of China in 1949, guided by the farsighted TCM policy of the Chinese Communist Party and the Chinese government, the treasure house of the theories of TCM has been continuously explored and the plentiful literature researched and compiled. As a result, great success has been achieved. Today there has appeared a world—wide upsurge in the studying and researching of TCM. To promote even more vigorous development of this trend in order that TCM may better serve all mankind, efforts are required to further it throughout the world. To bring this about, the language barriers must be overcome as soon as possible in order that TCM can be accurately expressed in foreign languages.

Thus the compilation and translation of a series of English—Chinese books of basic knowledge of TCM has become of great urgency to serve the needs of medical and educational circles both inside and outside China.

In recent years, at the request of the health departments, satisfactory achievements have been made in researching the expression of TCM in English. Based on the investigation into the history and current state of the research work mentioned above, the English—Chinese Encyclopedia of Practical TCM has been published to meet the needs of extending the knowledge of TCM around the world.

The encyclopedia consists of twenty—one volumes, each dealing with a particular branch of TCM. In the process of compilation, the distinguishing features of TCM have been given close attention and great efforts have been made to ensure that the content is scientific, practical, comprehensive and concise. The chief writers of the Chinese manuscripts include professors or associate professors with at least twenty years of practical clinical and / or teaching experience in TCM. The Chinese manuscript of each volume has been checked and approved by a specialist of the relevant branch of TCM. The team of the translators and revisers of the English versions consists of TCM specialists with a good command of English professional medical translators, and teachers of English from TCM colleges or universities. At a symposium to standardize the English versions, scholars from twenty—two colleges or universities, research institutes of TCM or other health institutes probed the question of how to express TCM in English more comprehensively, systematically and accurately, and discussed and deliberated in detail the English versions of some volumes in order to upgrade the English versions of the whole series. The English version of each volume has been re—examined and then given a final checking.

Obviously this encyclopedia will provide extensive reading material of TCM English for senior students in colleges of TCM in China and will also greatly benefit foreigners studying TCM.

The assiduous efforts of compiling and translating this encyclopedia have been supported by the responsible leaders of the State Education Commission of the People's Republic of China, the State Administrative Bureau of TCM and Pharmacy, and the Education Commission and Health Department of Shandong

Province. Under the direction of the Higher Education Department of the State Education Commission, the leading board of compilation and translation of this encyclopedia was set up. The leaders of many colleges of TCM and pharmaceutical factories of TCM have also given assistance.

We hope that this encyclopedia will bring about a good effect on enhancing the teaching of TCM English at the colleges of TCM in China, on cultivating skills in medical circles in exchanging ideas of TCM with patients in English, and on giving an impetus to the study of TCM outside China.

Higher Education Press
March, 1990

Foreword

The English—Chinese Encyclopedia of Practical Traditional Chinese Medicine is an extensive series of twenty—one volumes. Based on the fundamental theories of traditional Chinese medicine(TCM) and with emphasis on the clinical practice of TCM, it is a semi—advanced English—Chinese academic works which is quite comprehensive, systematic, concise, practical and easy to read. It caters mainly to the following readers: senior students of colleges of TCM, young and middle—aged teachers of colleges of TCM, young and middle—aged physicians of hospitals of TCM, personnel of scientific research institutions of TCM, teachers giving correspondence courses in TCM to foreigners, TCM personnel going abroad in the capacity of lecturers or physicians, those trained in Western medicine but wishing to study TCM, and foreigners coming to China to learn TCM or to take refresher courses in TCM.

Because Traditional Chinese Medicine and Pharmacology is unique to our Chinese nation, putting TCM into English has been the crux of the compilation and translation of this encyclopedia. Owing to the fact that no one can be proficient both in the theories of Traditional Chinese Medicine and Pharmacology and the clinical practice of every branch of TCM, as well as in English, to ensure that the English versions express accurately the inherent meanings of TCM, collective translation measures have been taken. That is, teachers of English familiar with TCM, professional medical translators, teachers or physicians of TCM and even teachers of palaeography with a strong command of English were all invited together to co—translate the Chinese manuscripts and, then, to co—deliberate and discuss the English versions. Finally English—speaking foreigners studying TCM or teaching English in China were asked to polish the English versions. In this way, the skills of the above translators and foreigners were merged to ensure the quality of the English versions. However, even using this method, the uncertainty that the English versions will be wholly accepted still remains. As for the Chinese manuscripts, they do reflect the essence, and give a general picture, of traditional Chinese medicine and pharmacology. It is not asserted, though, that they are perfect, I whole—heartedly look forward to any criticisms or opinions from readers in order to make improvements to future editions.

More than 200 people have taken part in the activities of compiling, translating and revising this encyclopedia. They come from twenty—eight institutions in all parts of China. Among these institutions, there are fifteen colleges of TCM:Shandong, Beijing, Shanghai, Tianjin, Nanjing, Zhejiang, Anhui, Henan, Hubei, Guangxi, Guiyang, Gansu, Chengdu, Shanxi and Changchun, and scientific research centers of TCM such as China Academy of TCM and Shandong Scientific Research Institute of TCM.

The Education Commission of Shandong province has included the compilation and translation of this encyclopedia in its scientific research projects and allocated funds accordingly. The Health Department of Shandong Province has also given financial aid together with a number of pharmaceutical factories of TCM. The subsidization from Jinan Pharmaceutical Factory of

TCM provided the impetus for the work of compilation and translation to get under way.

The success of compiling and translating this encyclopedia is not only the fruit of the collective labor of all the compilers, translators and revisers but also the result of the support of the responsible leaders of the relevant leading institutions. As the encyclopedia is going to be published, I express my heartfelt thanks to all the compilers. translators and revisers for their sincere cooperation, and to the specialists, professors, leaders at all levels and pharmaceutical factories of TCM for their warm support.

It is my most profound wish that the publication of this encyclopedia will take its role in cultivating talented persons of TCM having a very good command of TCM English and in extending, rapidly, comprehensive knowledge of TCM to all corners of the globe.

Chief　Editor　　Xu Xiangcai

Shandong College of TCM

March, 1990

Contents

Notes

Part One   General Statement

Part Two   Detailed Statement

4　Prescriptions for Removing Heat ································· 95

14   Prescriptions for Treating Wind Syndromes ················· 328

15   Prescriptions for Treating Dryness Syndromes ················· 348

Notes

"Pharmacology of Traditional Chinese Medical Formulae" is the third volume of " ENGLISH−CHINESE ENCY− CLOPEDIA OF PRACTICAL TRADITIONAL CHINESE MEDICINE".

This volume consists of two parts: Part 1 and Part 2. Part 1, General Statement, introduces the basic knowledge of pharmacology of traditional Chinese medical formulae such as " relationship between medical formulae and therapeutic methods","commonly used therapeutic methods", "classification of medical formulae","principles of composing formulae","usage of different dosage forms", etc. Part 2, Detailed Statement, deals with not only the source, ingredients, administration, explanation, effect, indications and case study of each of 233 fundamental and commonly used prescriptions, but also the modern−pharmacological−research fruits of some of the prescriptions. The prescriptions introduced are classified as 21 kinds such as "diaphoretic","purgation", "mediation","removing heat", etc.

Including both the experience of Chinese forefathers and the successful administration in clinical practice, and written in the form of entries, this book is characterized by "concentration of main points" ,"concision and easily−reading ", "integration of theories and practice"and "strong practicality". So it is suitable for all kinds of physicians and medical students both in and out- side China.

Associate Prof. Wu Zhenghe from Shandong University once helped proofread part of the Latin names of Chinese medicines. Liu Qiang, Cao Huilai, Zhang Zhe, Guo Jing, Kong Jian, etc. also helped to check part of the English terms of traditional Chinese medicine.

The Editor

Part One
General Statement

1　Pharmacology of Traditional Chinese Medical Formulae

Pharmacology of Traditional Chinese Medical Formulae is a subject expounding and researching the laws of compatibility of medicines in a prescription and the application of these laws in clinical practice. It is one of the basic subjects concerning every clinical branch of traditional Chinese medicine (TCM).

2　Relationship between Medical Formulae and Therapeutic Methods

Medical formulae are inseparably related to therapeutic methods. As a component part of the theory of "pathogenesis, method, prescription and medicine", the former is the key means by which the latter is embodied and fulfilled, while the latter is the guiding principle of making up the former. The relationship between these two may be demonstrated through the following example. When exterior syndrome of excess type due to wind–cold pathogens marked by chilly sensation, fever, headache, general pain, dyspnea without sweating, thin and whitish tongue coating is treated, once the therapeutic method of relieving the exterior syndrome with drugs pungent in flavor and warm in property is defined, the prescription of *Mahuang Tang* is prescribed which embodies the principles of the established therapeutic method.

3 Commonly Used Therapeutic Methods

The therapeutic methods of TCM are manifold. Many were recorded in the book *Huang Di Nei Jing* as early as in the Warring States Period(475—221B. C.). By the final stage of the Han Dynasty, Zhan Zhongjing, an outstanding physician, had put forward through summarization a complete set of TCM methods to diagnose and treat a disease through an overall differentiation and analysis of its cause, nature, etc. and its relationship with other factors, enriching and developing the theories on which therapeutic methods are based and the ways that they are carried out. From then on, the outstanding physicians through the ages continued to classify many therapeutic methods according to the different features in their own clinical practice. Among those, Cheng Zhongling in the Qing Dynasty put forward eight therapeutic methods such as diaphoresis, mediation, purgation, resolution, emesis, heat—clearing, warming and tonification, which are concise and clinically practical. And they have continued to be the commonly used methods till the present.

4 Diaphoresis

Diaphoresis is a therapeutic method to promote perspiration so as to circulate *Qi* and blood, to regulate *Ying* and *Wei* and to expel exopathogens through the exterior of the body by means of facilitating the flow of the lung—*Qi* , promoting the circulation of *Ying* and *Wei,* dilating the striae between the skin and flesh, etc.

It is mainly used to treat exterior syndromes caused by any of the six exopathogens. It may also be used when rashes tend not to erupt at the early stage of measles, when swelling due to edema above the lumbar region is severe, when skin and external diseases with the exterior syndrome marked by fever and chills are at their early stages, when pathogenic factors going from the interior to the exterior need to be expelled from the body or when the exterior syndrome complicated by the interior one is to be first eliminated.

Because syndromes may be of cold type or heat type, pathogenic factors may be more than one, and the constitution of a patient may be weak or strong, diaphoretic method is accordingly classified into two major categories: the pungent warm type and the pungent cool type. Additionally, it may be used in combination with the methods of tonification, resolution, etc.

5　Emesis

Emesis is a therapeutic method to eliminate phlegm, stagnated food and toxic substances retained in the throat, thorax and gastric cavity by inducing vomiting. It is used when phlegm is accumulated in the throat or stagnated in the thorax, when food is retained in the gastric cavity or when toxic substances taken by accident remain in the stomach. This method does have certain curative effects. But when it is used, damage will be done to vital$-Qi$ by the vomiting induced by the irritation to the throat and gastric cavity. Patients generally find this method repulsive. So it is rarely used by physicians of the later ages except when an emergency case whose disease location is in the upper body necessitates urgent vomiting of the pathogenic factor of excess type.

6 Purgation

Purgation is a therapeutic method to expel from the lower orifices (the urethral opening and anus) stagnated food, stercoroma, heat of excess type, accumulation of cold type, blood stasis, stagnated phlegm and water retained in the stomach and intestines so as to eliminate disease. It is used to treat the syndrome of excessiveness of both pathogen and vital–Qi, caused by the retention of stercoroma due to constipation resulting from accumulated heat, phlegm, water and blood stasis retained in the stomach and intestines.

As a syndrome may be of cold type or heat type, vital–Qi may be deficient or excessive, and more than one pathogenic factor may be involved, the following different types of purgation may be performed: cold, warm, moist, hydragogue, combining reinforcement with elimination and in conjunction with other therapeutic methods.

7 Mediation

Mediation is a therapeutic method to eliminate pathogenic factors by means of regulation and adjustment. It involves regulating the state of the interior, relieving exterior syndrome, coordinating *Yin* and *Yang* of the body and adjusting the functions of *Zang* and *Fu* organs. It is used when the following syndromes are treated: the semi–exterior and semi–interior type marked by the pathogen of febrile disease attacking *Shao Yang* channel and the type marked by incoordination between the liver and the spleen, or the liver and the stomach, or *Qi* and blood, or *Ying* and *Wei*. Among the methods of mediative type are the one to relieve the syndromes in *Shao Yang* channel and the one to coordinate the liver and the spleen or the liver and the stomach, which are frequently used in clinical practice.

8   Warming Method

Warming method is a therapeutic method to treat interior cold syndromes by warming *Yang*, expelling cold pathogens, recuperating *Yang*, and clearing and activating the channels and collaterals to adjust the flow of *Qi* and blood. It is used when exopathogenic cold directly invades the interior, when drugs impair *Yang—Qi* or when cold pathogens originate from the interior due to the deficiency of the kidney—*Yang*. This method works through warming the middle—*Jiao* to dispel cold, recuperating depleted *Yang* to rescue the patient from collapse, and warming the channels to dispel cold. Because cold is usually accompanied by deficiency, warming method is often used in combination with tonification.

9   Heat—clearing Method

Heat—clearing method is a therapeutic method to treat internal heat syndrome by clearing away heat pathogens. It is often used to treat epidemic febrile disease. Due to the fact that internal heat may be in the *Qi*—system, the *Ying*—system, the blood system or *Zang* and *Fu*, and the excess of it may develop into toxins, the way that this method works differs as follows: clearing heat from the *Qi*—system, dispelling heat from the *Ying*—system, clearing away heat from both the *Qi*—system and the blood system, removing heat and toxic materials, and eliminating heat from *Zang* and *Fu* organs.

Because heat pathogen tends to consume body fluids, and the excess of it may even damage *Qi,* drugs with the action of clearing away heat are often administered together with those with the action of promoting the production of body fluids and invigorating *Qi.* Both the heat—clearing method and that of nourishing *Yin* should be used when heat impairs *Yin* at the final stage of epidemic febrile disease or when heat is retained in the interior due to the deficiency of *Yin* resulting from prolonged disease.

10   Resolution

Resolution is a therapeutic method to resolve gradually visible masses developed due to the accumulations of *Qi,* blood, phlegm, food, water or worms by promoting digestion and disintegrating masses and swelling. In a broad sense, methods of removing phlegm, eliminating dampness, expelling worms, regulating the flow of *Qi* and treating blood disorders all belong in the method of resolution. But now resolution is generally limited to promoting digestion to remove stagnated food, and disintegrating masses and swelling. It is often used to treat such syndromes as food retention and masses or the like due to the stagnation of *Qi* and blood.

11　Tonification

Tonification is a therapeutic method to nourish, replenish and restore *Qi*, blood, *Yin, Yang, Zang* or *Fu* organs of the body when any of them is deficient or impaired. It functions through replenishing *Qi*, blood, *Yin* or *Yang* to make them balanced. The purpose of strengthening the body resistance to eliminate pathogenic factors may be reached through using the method of tonification to reinforce vital–*Qi* when it is too deficient and weak to resist pathogenic factors or to expel residual pathogens.

Because deficienciness and weaknesses may differ, tonifying methods are also different as follows: invigorating *Yin, Yang* and *Qi*, enriching blood, and tonifying the heart, liver, spleen, lung or the kidney. But those which are often used are invigorating *Qi*, blood, *Yin* or *Yang* or both *Yin* and *Yang*, or both *Qi* and blood.

12　Classification of Medical Formulae

There are a number of ways to classify medical formulae, among which the following are the main ones: "seven formulae"; " ten kinds of prescription" ; classification " according to syndromes", "clinical branches", "*Zang* and *Fu* " or "therapeutic methods"; and " synthetical" classification. Being first found in the book *Huang Di Nei Jing,* the classification of " seven formulae" is mainly based on the condition, location, seriousness of illness, the number of drugs, etc., classifying medical formulae as the following seven: strong, mild, slow–acting, quick–acting, with ingredients odd in number, with ingredients even in number and compound. Coming from Xu Zhicai, a well–known physician (493–592) in the Northern and Southern Dynasties, the classification of "ten kinds of prescription" classifies medical formulae according to the actions of drugs as the following ten: dispelling, obstruction–removing, tonifying, purgative, mild, strong, lubricant, astringent, dry, and moisture, It was Zhao Ji, a well–known physician in the Song Dynasty, who began to call this method as "ten kinds of prescription". The representative books which classify medical formulae according to syndromes are *Wu Shi Er Bing Fang, Tai Ping Sheng Hui Fang, Pu Ji Fang* etc. The bood *Fu Ren Ying Er Fang* is among the representative books which classify medical formulae "according to clinical branches". Those which classify medical formulae" according to *Zang* and *Fu* " are *Qian Jin Bei Ji Yao Fang, Wai Tai Mi Yao, San Yin Bing Zheng Ji Yi Fang Lun,* etc. The method of classifying medical formulae "according to syndromes" is found in the book *Jing Yue Quan Shu Gu Fang Ba Zhen* (a chapter of the book *Jing Yue Quan Shu)*. The book *Yi Fang Kao* written by Wang Ang in the Qing Dynasty classifies medical formulae synthetically as the following twenty–two: tonification and nourishment, diaphoresis, emesis, purgation, dispelling the interior pathogens through the body superficies, mediation, regulating the flow of *Qi,* treating blood disorders, expelling pathogenic wind, dispelling pathogenic cold, clearing away summer–heat, diuresis, moistening dryness, purging intense heat, removing phlegm, promoting digestion, astringency, parasiticide, improving acuity of vision, treating skin and external diseases, treating female disorders and first aid. This kind of classification not only deals with therapeutic methods and etiology but also involves clinical branches, making the concepts clear and being suitable for clinical use. Today the method of classification of Wang's is the most frequently used for reference. According to the method of classification in the textbooks of TCM specialities of TCM colleges, the second part of this volume will introduce concisely the twenty-two kinds of medical formulae in the order of diaphoresis, purgation, mediation, removing heat, clearing away summer-heat, warming up the interior, expelling pathogenic factors from both the interior and exterior of the body, tonification, tranquilization, inducing resuscitation, astringency, regulating the flow of *Qi,* treating blood disorders, treating wind syndrome, treating dryness syndrome, eliminating dampness, removing phlegm, promoting digestion, parasiticide, emesis and treating skin and external disorders, in order that the readers may study, grasp and practise them.

13 Composition of a Formula

According to the experience obtained in treating a disease with special drugs in a simple prescription, the principle of diagnosis and treatment based on overall differentiation and analysis of a disease, and the needs of therapeutic methods, the composition of a formulae is fulfilled by mixing the ingredients together organically. It aims at, firstly, enhancing or synthesizing the actions of the drugs to improve the curative effects, secondly, administering different drugs according to the variation of syndromes to widen the range of treatment and thirdly, restricting the toxicity or intensity of the drugs to eliminate the side effects on the human body.

14　Principle of Composing Formulae

The principles were concluded and known in brief in ancient times, as *Jun Chen Zuo Shi,* but in modern times they are known as *Zhu Fu Zuo Shi.* The terms of *Jun* (monarch)*Chen* (minister)*Zuo* (adjuvant)*Shi* (conductance) mean the different roles played by different ingredients of a prescription in their actions. They are concrete and vivid description of the principles of composing formulae.

The monarch drug in a prescription is the principal ingredient which produces the leading action in treating the cause or the main symptoms of a disease. The minister drug is that which strengthens the action of the monarch drug, helps treat the cause or the main symptoms of a disease, and takes a leading role in treating the accompanying disease cause or symptoms. The adjuvant drug is that which cooperates with the monarch and ministerial drugs to reinforce the curative effects. It functions directly in treating secondary symptoms, eliminating or reducing the toxicity of the monarch and ministerial drugs, or restricting their intensity. When serious diseases due to excessive pathogenic factors make patients incapable of taking the monarch drug, the adjuvant drug, whose property and flavor are opposite to those of the monarch drug but whose action is complementary to that of the monarch drug, is cooperately administered. The conductant drug is that which directs the actions of all the other drugs in a prescription to the affected channel, or tempers their actions.

15　Variations in Composition

There are principles to follow for composing formulae and set prescriptions to be prescribed according to the therapeutic methods. In clinical practice, however, set prescriptions should be modified according to the condition of a disease, the constitution and age of a patient, and the climatic and other favorable or unfavorable environmental factors. Generally speaking, the modification of a set prescription takes place in three ways: to add or omit one ingredient or more, to increase or decrease the amount of one ingredient or more, or to change for another dosage form.

16　Modification of Ingredients

In clinical practice, one drug or more are to be added to, or omitted from, a set prescription according to the particular condition of a disease in order to make the prescription more suitable for treating the disease. The addition and omission of one drug or more to and from a set prescription may bring three variations to it .

(1)Under the condition in which the principal drug of the prescription and the main symptoms of the disease remain the same, assistant drugs are added to or omitted from a set prescription according to different secondary or accompanying symptoms, so as to meet the need of treating the corresponding symptoms of the disease. For instance, the indication of *Guizhi Tang* is the exterior syndrome of "deficiency" due to wind—cold marked by fever, aversion to wind—cold, headache and floating slow pulse. But when the syndrome is accompanied by dyspnea and cough, *Hou Po* (Cortex Magnoliae Officinalis) and *Xing Ren* (Semen Armeniacae Amarum) are added to *Guizhi Tang* to form *Guizhi Jia Houpo Xingzi Tang*, whose indication includes lowering the adverse flow of the lung—*Qi* to relieve asthma. When the syndrome is accompanied by running pulse and fullness in the chest resulting from erroneous administration of purgatives, *Shao Yao* (Radix Paeoniae Alba) cool in nature and *Yin*—soft in property is omitted from *Guizhi Tang* to form *Guizhi Qu Shaoyao Tang*, which can promote the upward and outward movement of *Yang—Qi* to remove fullness in the chest and expel pathogenic factors from the muscles and skin.

(2)The addition or omission of one ingredient or more to or from a set prescription changes the principal drug and the indication for the others. The name of the prescription is accordingly changed. For example, when *Sheng Jiang* (Rhizoma Zingiberis Recens) is omitted from, and *Dang Gui* (Radix Angelicae Sinensis), *Xi Xin(Herba Asari)* and *Tong Cao* (Medulla Tetrapanacis) are added to, *Guizhi Tang*, the principal drug of this prescription becomes *Dang Gui* (Radix Angelicae Sinensis) and *Shao Yao* (Radix Paeoniae Alba), and its name changes to *Danggui Sini Tang*. Its indication becomes the syndrome due to the invasion of Jueyin channel by cold marked by cold limbs and thready indistinct pulse.

(3)The Principal drug of a prescription remains the same, but the compatible ones are changed, and what is more, the indication is also changed, For instance, *Huang Lian* (Rhizoma Coptidis) bitter in taste, cold in nature and functioning in clearing away heat, and *Wu Zhu Yu* (Fructus Evodiae) pungent in flavor, warm in nature and functioning in lowering the adverse flow of

Qi are compound to form *Zuo Jin Wan,* whose indication is distending pain in the chest and hypochondrium due to the depressed fire in the liver channel. But when *Huang Lian* (Rhizoma Coptidis) is mixed with *Mu Xiang* (Radix Aucklandiae) with the action of promothing the circulation of *Qi* and relieving pain, *Xiang Lian Wan* is formed whose indication is dysentery due to damp—heat pathogen.

17　Modification of Dose

The principal drug, the indication and the potency of a prescription become different and the treatment range of this prescription is widened when the ingredients remain the same but their doses are altered. The modification of the doses of the drugs in a prescription may result in the following three kinds of changes:

(1)The principal drug and the indication of a prescription are varied. For example, Both the prescriptions *Xiao Chengqi Tang* and *Houpo Sanwu Tang* contain *Da Huang* (Radix et Rhizoma Rhei), *Zhi Shi* (Fructus Aurantii Immaturus) and *Hou Po* (Cortex Magnoliae Officinalis). The former contains 12g of *Da Huang,* 9g of *Zhi Shi* and 6g of *Hou Po:* the latter, 12 g of *Da Huang,* 15 g of *Zhi Shi* and 24 g of *Hou Po*. The ratio of *Hou Po* in them is 1：4. The dose of *Da Huang* in them appears to be equal. But because the decoction of the former is taken twice, while that of the latter, 3 times, the dose of *Da Huang* in the former is , in fact, greater than that of the latter. Therefore, the principal drug in the former is *Da Huang;* but in the latter, *Hou Po* becomes the principal drug. Obviously, it is the variation of drug dose that leads to the change of the principal drug. Such variations bring about the change of indication. *Xiao Chengqi Tang* (the former) is indicated for excess syndrome of *Yangming Fu* organ whose pathogenesis is the accumulation of gastrointestinal heat, while *Houpo Sanwu Tang* (the latter) is indicated for constipation and pain due to abdominal distention whose pathogenesis is the stagnation of *Qi*.

(2)The potency of a prescription is altered. For instance, both the prescriptions *Sini Tang* and *Tongmai Sini Tang* contain *Fu Zi* (Radix Aconiti Lateralis Preparata), *Gan Jiang* (Rhizoma Zingiberis Recens) and *Zhi Gan Cao* (Radix Glycyrrhizae Preparata). Because the former contains less *Gan Jiang* and *Fu Zi* than the latter, its function is different from the latter's. The former functions in recuperating depleted *Yang* and rescuing a patient from collapse, and is used to treat the syndrome due to the excess of *Yin* and the deficiency of *Yang* marked by cold limbs, aversion to cold, lying with the legs drawn up, diarrhea and faint thready pulse or deep slow thready weak pulse. The latter, however, functions in recuperating depleted *Yang* and driving away *Yin,* and rescuing a patient from collapse through promoting blood circulation, and is used to treat the syndrome due to *Yang* retained in the exterior because of *Yin*—excess in the interior marked by cold limbs, no aversion to cold, diarrhea with undigested food in stools and extremely faint pulse.

(3)The treatment range of the prescription is widened. For example, with retention of *Gui Zhi* (Ramulus Cinnamomi) as the principal drug, the prescription *Guizhi Jia Shaoyao Tang,* in which the dose of *Shao Yao* (Radix Paeoniae Alba) has been doubled so as to relieve spasm and pain, is used to treat the syndrome, which is the indication of the prescription *Guizhi Tang,* accompanied by intermittent pain due to abdominal distention.

18 Dosage Forms of Formulae

Pharmaceutical preparations may come in different forms processed in accordance with the different needs of treating various diseases in clinical practice with Chinese herbal medicines (CHM) in order that the potencies of drugs are given full play. The dosage forms of CHM derive from the experience accumulated by the outstanding physicians medical expert through the ages in their long struggle against diseases. For instance, such dosage forms as decoction, pill, powder, herb paste and spirit were recorded in the thirteen prescriptions of the book *Huang Di Nei Jing*. Later on, dosage forms continued to be developed, there appearing such new ones as drink, distillate, lozenge, cake, roll, thread, smoking, fumigation, washing, ear—dropping, enema, nasal—dropping and vaginal suppository. Today, to meet the needs of various clinical branches, good traditional processes of CHM preparations have been used together with modern ones, and many new dosage forms have been developed such as injection, tablet, syrup, extract, liquid extract, adhesive plaster, and powder preparation to be taken after being infused in water.

19 Modification of Dosage Form

According to the condition of a disease, the dosage form of a prescription may be altered, which will bring about changes in its therapeutic effects. For instance, the prescription *Lizhong Wan* consists of *Gan Jiang* (Rhizoma Zingiberis) 90 g, *Bai Zhu* (Rhizoma Atractylodis Macrocephalae) 90 g,*Ren Shen* (Radix

Ginseng) 90 g and *Gan Cao* (Radix Glycyrrhizae) 90 g. It is in the form of honeyed boluses, each of which is as big as a yolk, prescribed to treat deficient. cold—syndrome of the middle—*Jiao* marked by incessant loose stools, vomiting, abdominal pain, pale tongue with whitish coating, and deep slow weak pulse. When the obstruction of *Qi* in the chest due to *Yang*—deficiency of the upper—*Jiao* marked by choking sensation in the precordial region, fullness in the chest, attack of the heart by *Qi* from under the hypochondrium, cold limbs, shortness of breath, languor and deep thready pulse is treated, the four ingredients of the prescription, each weighing 9 g, are decocted in water for oral use, the decoction being taken 3 times. Thus, different dosage forms of the same prescription are used to treat different diseases with different locations and degrees of seriousness, with pills where slow action of the prescription is required but decoction where quick action is required.

20 Decoction

All the drugs in a prescription are steeped in an appropriate amount of water, the content being boiled for a specific period of time, after which the solid material is removed, thus obtaining the medical solution which is called decoction. By and large, decoctions such as *Mahuang Tang* and *Da Chengqi Tang* are for oral administration. Decoction is characterized by being absorbed quickly, exerting its potency presently, being easy to modify so that it may meet, more comprehensively and flexibly, the needs of individual patients and the peculiarity of various syndromes. So it has been the most widely—used dosage form in the clinical practice of TCM.

21 Powder

Drugs in a prescription are ground into very wellmixed dry powder which is for oral administration or for external application. That for oral administration is finer, smaller in dose and may be taken directly with water. *Qili San* is such an example. However, there is also coarse powder. Before being applied, it is boiled in water, the coarse powder being removed and the solution is obtained for oral administration. *Xiangsu San* is such an example. Powder for external use is usually applied externally and topically on a sore or on the affected part of the body. *Shengji San* and *Jinhuang San* are such examples. There is also powder for eye—dropping or laryngeal insufflation. *Bing Peng San* is such an example. Being easy to carry and take, not prone to deterioration, being absorbed quickly and processed simply and with less medicinal material are the characteristics of such powders.

22 Pill

Drugs in a prescription are ground into fine powder. The powder is mixed with such excipients as honey, water, rice flour paste, wheat flour paste, spirit, vinegar or decoction into round solid dosages——pills, Smaller in size and easy to take, carry and preserve, pills are absorbed slowly and have persistent potency. This dosage form is a commonly used one which is suitable for chronic diseases or diseases of weakness. *Guipi Wan* and *Renshen Yang—rong Wan* are such examples. There are pills, too, for first aid. *Angong Niuhuang Wan* and *Suhexiang Wan* are such examples. Containing drugs aromatic in flavor, they cannot be heated or boiled. Some drugs with toxic or intense potencies are processed into pills in order that their actions may be given a slow play.

Pills which are common in clinical practice are honeyed pills, water—paste pills, paste pills and concentrated pills. Honeyed pills are soft and moist in nature, slow in acting and have the action of rectifying taste, tonifying and nourishing, thus being suitable for the treatment of chronic diseases. Being small in size, easy to swallow and being absorbed quickly, water—paste pills are used to treat many kinds of diseases. Paste pills are absorbed slowly within the body after being swallowed, which may give a full play to drug effects and reduce the irritation produced by strongly irritant drugs. to the gastrointestinal tract. For this reason, it is preferable to process drugs with great toxicity and irritative effects into paste pills. Concentrated pills are small in size and dose, easy to swallow, and contain more efficacious elements. Various kinds of disease may be treated with concentrated pills.

23 Herb Paste

Herb paste is a dosage formed by concentrating drugs by way of decocting them in water or vegetable oil. It is for oral administration or external use. Those for oral administration are liquid extract, extract and soft extract. Those for external use are softer paste and harder paste.

The effective elements of 1 ml of liquid extract are equal to those of 1 g of medicinal material, higher than those of tincture. The side effects of the solvent content are small and so is the dose administered *Gancao Liujingao* and *Yimucao Liujingao* are such examples. Extract is semi—solid, high in concentration, and small in volume and applied dose. The active principles of 1 g of extract are equal to those of 2—5 g of medicinal material. It contains no solvent, has no side effects of it, and is usually used for processing tablets or pills. *Maodongqing Jingao* is such an example. Dry fine powder, such as *Zizhucao Jingao* and *Longdancao Jingao,* is called dry extract, which may be taken diretly with water or put into capsules for oral administration. Soft extract, small in volume and easy to take, contains great amount of honey or sugar and tastes sweet. With plenty of nutrients, it has the action of moistening and tonifying, being suitable for debilitated patients suffering from persistent diseases. *Shen Qi Gao* and *Piba Gao* are such examples. Soft plaster is a preparation for external use. It is semi—solid and sticky at normal temperature. Coated on the skin or the mucous membrane, it will be softened or melted gradually, with its active elements being absorbed slowly. It is suitable for the sore, carbuncle, swelling and furuncle of surgery, *Sanhuang San Ruangao* and *Chuanxinlian Ruangao* are such examples. Plaster (adhesive plaster) is solid at normal temperature, but melts at 36—37℃. Easy to use, carry and preserve, it may play a role in topical or general treatment and in mechanical protection after being applied externally. It is used to treat such syndromes as traumatic injury, arthralgia due to pathogenic wind—dampness, skin and external diseases, etc. *Fengshi Dieda Zhitong Gao* and *Goupi Gao* are such examples.

24 Dan

Dan usually means a compound preparation which is produced by heating and sublimating minerals containing mercury, sulfur, etc. The applied dose of it is small but has great potency. Although it may be administered for both oral and external use, it is, in general, used for external application in surgery. *Hongsheng Dan* and *Baijiang Dan* as such examples. It is customary to call some precious drugs or dosage forms of some drugs with special actions as *Dan*. So *Dan* does not have a fixed dosage form. For example, *Heixi Dan* is in pill form, while *Zhibao Dan,* in bolus form. They and their like are usually for oral administration.

25 Spirit

Spirits, including those made with yellow rice or millet, are used as solvent. The drugs are usually soaked or boiled in spirit, after which the solid material is removed, thus obtaining the medicated spirit. Medicated spirit is usually administered to tonify and nourish the weak body, to relieve pain due to pathogenic wind—dampness and to treat traumatic injury. *Shiquan Dabu Jiu* and *Fengshi Yaojiu* are such examples.

26 Moxibustion

Chinese mugwort leaves are pounded until floss—like. The floss is twisted into moxa— sticks, moxa—roll or moxa—cone. One end is lit and held at a certain distance from the skin of some acupoints or an affected part of the body to cause the subject to experience a warm or painful sensation for preventive or thrapeutic purpose. Moxibustion is such a dosage form for external use.

27 Powder to Be Infused

Drugs are refined into thick paste, to which is added an appropriate amount of sugar powder and other supplementary materials such as starch, flour of Chinese yam or dextrin. The content is stirred until it is even and rubbed into small round pieces. The pieces are riddled with a riddle whose mesh number is 10−12 and made into small granules. The granules are dried at temperatures of 4−60℃. When dried, they are sifted again with a sieve whose mesh number is 8−14. They are, then, mixed evenly and put in plastic sacks to protect them from dampness. Powder to be infused is at last obtained. Powder taken after being infused in boiling water is quick in action, small in volume, light, convenient to carry and take, and suitable to treat various kinds of diseases. *Kelu Chongji* and *Ganmao Chongji* are such examples.

28 Method of Decocting Drugs

The correct method of decocting drugs may ensure complete utilization of the actions of drugs. For decocting, it is preferable to use an earthenware pot rather than ones made of tin or iron in case drugs should precipitate, the solubility of drugs should descend and side effects should come about. Water for decocting is usually running or distilled water or fresh well water which should be pure and clean unless a special type of water is required in the prescription. The level of water in the pot should be about three centimetres higher than that of the drugs. The fire or source of heat should be adjusted according to whether strong or mild heat is required. In general, the mixture is first boiled strongly and, then, simmered.

The procedure in decocting is as follows. The drugs are placed in a container (pot), to which cold water is then added, ensuring that the water level covers the drugs. The pot should be heated only after thorough soaking of the drugs in order that the active elements may be readily decocted out. In the course of decocting, be sure to keep the pot covered in order to minimize the loss of aromatic and volatile elements. In the process of boiling, it should be ensured that the heat is not too strong so as to prevent the loss of the decoction. However, drugs aromatic in nature or for relieving exterior syndrome and clearing away heat are to be decocted with strong heat in case the potencies of the drugs should be volatilized through prolonged boiling and thus the effects of them, lowered or changed. Tonic drugs rich in fat or drugs for nourishing blood and invigorating *Qi* should be decocted on mild heat for a longer period so as to decoct the active elements out completely. If drugs are burned due to improper decocting, they should be discarded, not decocted again in fresh water or taken. Special methods of decocting should be noted in the prescription. Drugs of shell and mineral type are to be broken up and then decocted, for they are too hard. Taking *Gui Ban* (Colla carapacis Plastri Testudinis), *Bie Jia* (Carapax Trionycis), *Dai Zhe Shi* (Ochra Haematitum) *Shi Jue Ming* (Concha Haliotidis), *Sheng Mu Li* (Concha Ostreae), *Sheng Long Gu* (Os Draconis Fossilia), *Sheng Shi Gao* (Gypsum Fibrosum) as examples, they should be boiled for 10—20 minutes before adding the other ingredients. Aromatic drugs, such as *Bo Re* (Herba

Menthae), *Sha Ren* (Fructus Amomi), etc., are to be added to the mixture only for the final five minutes of decocting so that their active elements, which are easy to volatilize, are held up. Some drugs, such as *Chi Shi Zhi* (Halloysitum Rubrum), *Hua Shi Fen* (Pulvis Talci), *Xuan Fu Hua* (Flos Inulae), etc., should be wrapped in thin cloth when being decocted, so as to decrease the perssimal irritation produced by the particles to the gastrointestinal tract and throat as well as to decrease the turbidity of the decoction containing them. The active elements of certain precious drugs will be absorbed when they are decocted together with others. Such drugs should be decocted separately. For example, *Ren Shen* (Radix Ginseng) in a prescription should be cut into small pieces and stewed alone for over an hour. Gelatin, such as E Jiao (Colla Corii Asini), *Lu Jiao Jiao* (Colla Cornus Cervi), *Yi Tang* (Saccharum Granorum), etc., are highly sticky and easy to dissolve. When being decocted with others, they tend to stick to the pot and be burned, and to attach to others to influence their effectiveness. Thus, when being used, they should be separately dissolved in boiling water or in decoction which is being warmed with gentle heat. Powder, *Dan,* pill, natural juice as well as some aromatic or precious drugs, such as *Niu Huang* (Calculus Bovis), *She Xiang* (Moschus), *Chen Xiang Mo* (Lignum Aquilariae Resinatum), *Tian San Qi* (Radix Notoginseng), etc., are to be taken following their infusion.

29   Method of Taking Medicine

The method of taking medicine includes two aspects: time and way.

(1)Time: In general, about one hour before a meal is the proper time. Those which irritate the gastrointestinal tract should be taken after a meal. Tonifying and nourishing drugs are to be taken on an empty stomach. Antimalaria drugs should be taken two hours before the disease's relapse. Sedatives are taken before sleep. Medicines for emergency cases are taken when needed. Patients with chronic disease must take pill or powder or soft extract or medicated wine on time.

(2)Way: Usually the decoction of the prescribed dose is divided into two or three portions, one portion being taken each time, one dose daily. A patient whose disease's condition is critical takes the whole decoction at a draught. A patient whose disease has the symptoms of hiccup, vomiting and difficulty in swallowing takes small portions of the decoction frequently throughout the day. To enhance the potencies of drugs, two doses may be taken daily according to the needs of the disease's condition. The decoction is better taken warm. After taking decoction for relieving exterior syndromes, the patient should cover himself with something to avoid wind and to sweat a little. When heat syndrome is treated with drugs cold in natute, the decoction is to be taken hot. When a patient has cold syndrome complicated by heat syndrome, vomiting may result after the decoction is taken. Under this condition, the first priority is to recognize the property of the mixed syndromes. If the cold syndrome is accompanied by a pseudo—heat syndrome, the hot natured decoction is to be taken cold. If the heat syndrome is accompanied by a pseudo—cold syndrome, the cold—natured decoction is to be taken hot. A patient who vomits after taking decoction may add a little ginger juice to it or chew a little tangerine peel before taking it, or use fresh ginger to rub his tongue, or take the decoction cold or in many small portions. Give decoction to a comatose patient with difficulty in swallowing by nasal feeding. Take medicines with toxic or intense nature in small amount in the beginning and raise the amount gradually. Once the effects appear, stop administering them. Over dosage is strictly forbidden in case poisoning should occur.

Part Two
Detailed Statement

1 Diaphoretic Prescriptions

1.1 Diaphoretic Prescriptions

Prescriptions mainly consisting of diaphoretics; having the action of inducing diaphoresis, expelling pathogenic factors from the muscles and skin and promoting eruption; and used to treat exterior syndromes are all known as "diaphoretic prescription". Diaphoretic prescriptions may be chosen to treat syndromes caused by the invasion of any of the six pathogenic factors into the muscles and skin and marked by aversion to cold, fever, headache, pantalgia and floating pulse, and such diseases at their early stages and with exterior syndrome as measles, skin and external disorders, edema, etc. Because the six pathogenic factors are different in the nature of cold or warmth and the constitutions of patients are different in the type of deficiency or excess, diaphoretic prescriptions are accordingly classfied as the following three kinds according to their different indications: those composed of drugs pungent in flavor and warm in nature and used to treat exterior syndrome of cold type, those composed of drugs pungent in flavor and cold in nature and used to treat exterior syndrome of heat type and those having the action of strengthening body resistance to relieve exterior syndrome resulting from the affection of pathogens due to general deficiency of Qi.

Diaphoretic prescriptions are mainly made up of drugs pungent in flavor and having the action of dispersing. The time of decocting should not be prolonged. After taking any of them, the patient should protect himself from exposure to wind or cold, and should keep himself warm to the point of mild sweating but avoiding over sweating. In hot weather of in the case of an old or very young or debilitated patient, the dosage administered should be small. The exterior syndrome accompanied by an interior syndrome is treated by means of relieving both the exterior and interior syndromes simultaneously or relieving the exterior one first and the interior one second. Diaphoretic prescriptions are contraindicated for isolated interior syndromes. In the course of taking this kind of medicine, patients must obstain from eating raw, cold and heavy food.

1.2 Diaphoretic Prescriptions Composed of Drugs Pungent in Flavor and Warm in Nature

This kind of prescriptions mainly consist of drugs pungent in flavor, warm in nature and acting to relieve exterior syndrome. Their indication is the exterior syndrome due to the effect of exogenous wind—cold pathogens and marked by aversion to cold, fever, rigidity of nape with headache, stiffness in the nape, soreness and pain in the limbs, no thirst, sweating or not, thin and whitish tongue coating and superficial tense or slow pulse. Drugs, such as *Ma Huang* (Herba Ephedrae), *Gui Zhi* (Ramulus Cinnamomi), *Jing Jie* (Herba Schizonepetae), *Fang Feng* (Radix Saposhinkoviae), *Su Ye* (Folium Perillae), etc., are commonly used in diaphoretic prescriptions composed of drugs pungent in flavor and warm in nature, whose representatives are *Mahuang Tang* (Ephedra Decoction), *Guizhi Tang* (Cinnamon Twig Decoction), *Xiao Qinglong Tang* (Minor Decoction of Green Dragon), *Jiuwei Qianghuo Tang* (Notoptreygium Decoction of Nine Ingredients), etc.

1.3   The Prescription of *Mahuang Tang*

Name: Ephedra Decoction

Source: The book *Shang Han Lun*

Ingredients:

Ma Huang (Herba Ephedrae) 6 g, *Gui Zhi* (Ramulus Cinnamomi) 4 g, *Xing Ren* (Semen Armeniacae Amarum) 9 g, *Zhi Gan Cao* (Radix Glycyrrhizae Preparata) 3 g.

Explanation:

Ma Huang: The principal drug, being pungent and bitter in flavor and warm in nature, relieving superficies syndrome by means of diaphoresis, facilitating the flow of the lung–*Qi* to stop asthma.

Gui Zhi: Expelling pathogenic factors from the muscles and skin by means of diaphoresis, warming the channels to expel pathogenic cold, assisting *Ma Huang* in inducing diaphoresis to relieve exterior syndrome, relieving pain in the limbs.

Xing Ren: Promoting the flow of the lung—*Qi,* aiding *Ma Huang* in relieving asthma.

Zhi Gan Cao: Tempering the actions of all the other ingredients.

Effect: Relieving exterior syndrome by means of diaphoresis, facilitating the flow of the lung—*Qi* to relieve asthma.

Indications: Exterior syndrome of excess type due to wind—cold pathogens, marked by aversion to cold, fever, asthma without sweating, headache, general pain, whitish thin tongue coating and superficial tense pulse; including such diseases with the above symptoms as common cold, influenza, bronchitis, bronchial asthma, etc.

Administration:Decocted in water for oral dose to be taken twice.

Contraindication: Syndromes with *Qi*,blood or body fluid deficiency (because this decoction is powerful).

Case Study: *Mahuang Tang* was clinically administered to treat influenza spreading among young miners and marked by severe chills,high fever,headache,general pain,stuffy and running nose, no sweat and floating tense pulse.2—3 doses, on the whole, induced diaphoresis and abated the fever, curing the patients.

The modification of *Mahuang Tang* and *Siwu Tang* was prescribed to treat 10 cases of children's psoriasis,each of whom took 4—49 doses,19 on an average. 2 cases were cured, 5 basically cured, 2 were remarkably improved and 1 improved.

1.4   The Prescription of *Guizhi Tang*

Name: Cinnamon Twig Decoction

Source: The book *Shang Han Lun*

Ingredients:

Gui Zhi (Ramulus Cinnamomi) 9 g, *Bai Shao* (Radix Paeoniae Alba) 9 g, *Zhi Gan Cao* (Radix Glycyrrhizae Preparata) 6 g, *Sheng Jiang* (Rhizoma Zingiberis Recens) 9 g, *Da Zao* (Fructus Jujubae) 3 dates.

Explanation:

Gui Zhi: The principal drug, being pungent and sweet in flavor and warm in nature, expelling pathogenic factors from the muscles and skin by means of diaphoresis, warming the channels to dispel pathogenic cold.

Bai Shao: Replenishing *Yin* and astringing *Ying*, uniting *Gui Zhi* to take a role in regulating *Ying* and *Wei*.

Sheng Jiang: Being pungent in flavor and warm in nature, assisting *Gui Zhi* in expelling pathogenic factors from the muscles and skin, warming the stomach to prevent vomiting.

Da Zao: Being sweet in flavor and neutral in nature, supplementing *Qi* and strengthening the middle–*Jiao*, nourishing the spleen, promoting the production of body fluids.

Zhi Gan Cao: Supplementing *Qi* and regulating the stomach, together with *Gui Zhi* aiding in expelling the pathogenic factors from the muscles and skin, together with *Shao Yao* replenishing *Yin*, tempering the actions of all the other ingredients.

Effect: Expelling pathogenic factors from muscles and skin by means of diaphoresis, regulating *Ying* and *Wei*.

Indications: Exterior syndrome of deficiency type due to windcold pathogens, marked by headache, fever, aversion to wind after sweating, retching with sounds from the nose, nausea, no thirst, whitish tongue coating and floating slow pulse; including such diseases with the above symptoms as common cold, rheumatic arthritis, heart disease, nephritis, etc.

Administration: Decocted in water for oral dose to be taken 3 times, followed by the taking of thin gruel or boiled water.

Contraindication: Raw or cold or greasy food

Case Study: A case whose symptoms and signs were fever of more than 20 days (38 ℃), sweating, lassitude, anorexia, dizziness, no thirst, whitish tongue coating and superficial pulse was treated with *Guizhi Tang,* with one dose abating the fever.

20 cases of allergic rhinitis were treated with *Guizhi Tang* plus:

Ting Li Zi (Semen Lepidii seu Descurainiae), *Chan Tui* (Periostracum Cicadae). 14 cases were cured, 2 cases were not improved, 4 cases relapsed, each of whom took 2—14 doses.

1.5 The Prescription of *Jiuwei Qianghuo Tang*

Name: Notopt erygium Decoction of Nine Ingredients
Source: The book *Ci Shi Nan Zhi*
Ingredients:

Qiang Huo (Rhizoma seu Radix Notopterygii) 5 g, *Fang Feng* (Radix Saposhinkoviae) 5 g, *Cang Zhu* (Rhizoma Atractylodis) 5 g, *Xi Xin* (Herba Asari) 1 g, *Chuan Xiong* (Rhizoma Chuangxiong) 3 g, *Bai Zhi* (Radix Angelicae Dahuricae) 3 g, *Sheng Di* (Radix Rehmanniae)3 g, *Huang Qin* (Radix Scutellariae) 3 g, *Gan Cao* (Radix Glycyrrhizae) 3 g.

Explanation:

Qiang Huo: The principal drug, being pungent and bitter in flavor and warm in nature, going up to disperse wind—cold—dampness pathogens in the exterior.

Fang Feng and *Cang Zhu:* Inducing diaphoresis to remove dampness and assisting *Qiang Huo* in relieving exterior syndrome.

Xi Xin, Chuan Xiong and *Bai Zhi:* Dispersing windcold pathogens, relieving arthralgia due to pathogenic dampness, promoting the flow of *Qi* and blood.

Huang Qin: Expelling the pathogenic heat from the *Qi* system.

Sheng Di: Dispelling the pathogenic heat from the blood system, removing pathogenic heat of accompanying syndrome, restricting the dryness resulting from the pungency and warmth of other drugs.

Gan Cao: Tempering the actions of all the other ingredients.

Effect: Inducing diaphoresis to remove pathogenic dampness and expelling, simultaneously, pathogenic heat in the interior.

Indications: Syndrome due to the effect of exogenous wind—cold—dampness pathogens and internal heat, marked by chills, fever, absence of sweating, headache, stiff nape, soreness and pain of the limbs, thirst with bitter taste; including such diseases with the above symptoms as common cold, influenza, rheumatic arthritis, etc.

Administration: Decocted in water for oral dose to be taken twice.

Case Study: 120 cases of common cold marked by chills, low fever, headache and soreness and pain of the limbs were treated with modified *Jiuwei Qianghuo Tang,* to which 112 cases (93.33%) were sensitive.

152 cases of acute urticaria were also treated with modified

Jiuwei Qianghuo Tang whose main ingredients were as follows:

Qiang Huo (Rhizoma seu Radix Notopterygii) 10 g, *Fang Feng* (Radix Saposhinkoviae) 6 g, *Chao Cang Zhu* (Rhizoma Atractylodis parched) 6 g, *Xi Xin* (Herba Asari) 1.5 g, *Chuan Xiong* (Rhizoma Chuanxiong) 6 g, *Bai Zhi* (Radix Angelicae Dahuricae) 6 g, *Sheng Di* (Radix Rehmanniae) 10 g, *Chao Huang Qin* (Radix Scutellariae parched) 6 g, *Gan Cao* (Radix Glycyrrhizae) 6 g, *Sheng Jiang* (Rhizoma Zingiberis Recens) 2 pieces, *Cong Bai* (Bulbus Allii Fistulosi) 3 pieces.

Cases of wind—cold type were susceptible to it, and so were cases of wind—heat type complicated by dampness pathogen. Among 152 cases treated, 119 were cured with each taking 3 doses, 15 with 5, 10 with 7.6 cases who suffered from frequent relapses were improved with each taking 10 doses; in 2 cases there was no improvement.

1.6   The Prescription of *Xiao Qinglong Tang*

Name: Minor Decoction of Green Dragon

Source: The book *Shang Han Lun*

Ingredients:

Ma Huang (Herba Ephedrae) 9 g, *Shao Yao* (Radix Paeoniae) 9 g, *Xi Xin* (Herba Asari) 9 g, *Gan Jiang* (Rhizoma Zingiberis) 9 g, *Zhi Gan Cao* (Radix Glycyrrhizae Preparata) 9 g, *Gui Zhi* (Ramulus Cinnamomi) 9 g, *Wu Wei Zi* (Fructus Schisandrae) 9 g, *Ban Xia* (Rhizoma Pinelliae) 9 g.

Explanation:

Ma Huang and *Gui Zhi:* The principal drugs, inducing diaphoresis to relieve exterior syndrome, facilitating the flow of the lung–*Qi* to relieve asthma.

Gan Jiang and *Xi Xin:* Warming the lung to reduce watery phlegm, assisting *Ma Huang* and *Gui Zhi* in relieving exterior syndrome.

Wu Wei Zi: Astringing *Qi*.

Shao Yao: Nourishing blood.

Ban Xia: Lowering the adverse flow of *Qi* by means of removing phlegm and regulating the stomach.

Zhi Gan Cao: Supplementing *Qi* and regulating the stomach, tempering the actions of all the other ingredients.

Effect: Inducing diaphoresis to reduce watery phlegm, relieving cough and asthma.

Indications: Syndrome due to the stagnation of wind–cold pathogens in the exterior and water retention in the interior, marked by aversion to cold, fever, no sweat, dyspnea, cough, profuse thin sputum, difficulty in lying down, or general pain and heavy sensation, swelling of face and limbs, whitish slippery tongue coating and floating pulse; including such diseases with the above symptoms as chronic bronchitis, bronchial asthma, senile emphysema, etc.

Administration: Decocted in water for oral dose to be taken 3 times

Contraindication: Drugs in this prescription are pungent in flavor and dry in nature, so this prescription is contraindicated for syndromes marked by cough without sputum or with yellowish thick sputum and dryness of the mouth and throat.

Case Study: 6 cases of intractable allergic bronchitis, a syndrome due to exogenous cold pathogen and interior water retention which had been unsuccessfully treated with aminophylline, salbutamol, prednisone and dexamethasone, were treated with heavy dosage of *Xiao Qinglong Tang,* whose main ingredients were as follows:

Zhi Ma huang (Herba Ephedrae Preparata) 15 g, *Gui Zhi* (Ramulus Cinnamomi) 9 g, *Wu Wei Zi* (Fructus Schisandrae) 9 g, *Gan Jiang* (Rhizoma Zingiberis) 9 g, *Zhi Ban Xia* (Rhizoma Pinelliae Preparata) 30 g, *Bai Shao* (Radix Paeoniae Alba) 30 g, *Xi Xin* (Herba Asari) 6—9 g, *Gan Cao* (Radix Glycyrrhizae) 9—15 g.

Within 0.5—2 hours after one dose was taken by each of them, wheeze in their lungs was greatly lowered or nearly eliminated. After 2—3 doses were taken, the condition of their disease tended to be stable. Treatment was carried on with smaller and smaller dosage, the signs of the disease disappeared with the asthma being basically controlled in 6 cases.

Xiao Qinglong Tang plus:

Zhu ling (Polyporus), *Fu Ling* (Poria), *Ze Xie* (Rhizoma Alismatis), *Fu Zi* (Radix Aconiti Lateralis Preparata), *Kuan Dong* (Flos Farfarae), *Bai Zhu* (Rhizoma Atractylodis Macrocephalae). was applied to treat cases who had been suffering for many years from general edema, fullness sensation in the chest, asthma, pale tongue proper with white coating and wiry slippery pulse. More than 30 doses were taken by each of them and they were cured.

In an experiment, the decotion of modified *Xiao Qinglong Tang* was injected into an anaesthetized cat that had suffered from bronchospasm, showing obvious action of antibronchial spasm.

1.7　The Prescription of *Daqinglong Tang*

Name: Major Green Dragon Decoction

Source: The book *Shang Han Lun*

Ingredients:

Ma Huang (Herba Ephedrae) 12 g, *Gui Zhi* (Ramulus Cinnamomi) 4 g, *Zhi Gan Cao* (Radix Glycyrrhizae Preparata) 5 g, *Xing Ren* (Semen Armeniacae Amarum) 6 g, *Shi Gao* (Gypsum Fibrosum) 12 g, *Sheng Jiang* (Rhizoma Zingiberis Recens) 9 g, *Da Zao* (Fructus Jujubae) 3 dates.

Explanation:

Ma Huang: The principal drug , being pungent and bitter in flavor and warm in nature, expelling wind—cold pathogens.

Gui Zhi: Expelling the pathogenic factors from the muscles and skin, aiding *Ma Huang* in inducing diaphoresis.

Shi Gao: Being pungent in flavor and cold in nature, clearing away the interior heat and assisting *Ma Huang* in expelling exogenous pathogenic factors.

Xing Ren: Moistening the lung to arrest cough.

Sheng Jiang and *Da Zao:* Promoting diaphoresis, reinforcing *Qi* of the middle—*Jiao*.

Gan Cao: Regulating the stomach, tempering the actions of all the other ingredients.

Effect: Relieving exterior syndrome by means of diaphoresis, clearing away heat and restlessness.

Indications: Exterior excess syndrome due to wind—cold pathogens and pathogenic heat in the interior, marked by severe chills, high fever, general pain, restlessness without sweat and floating tense pulse; including such diseases with the above symptoms as bad cold, acute bronchitis, bronchopneumonia, lobar pneumonia, etc.

Administration: Decocted in water for oral dose to be taken 3 times

Contraindication: The administration of this prescription should be ceased once the case would begin to sweat, as its effects in inducing diaphoresis are extremely strong. And it must not be used in treating cases with exterior syndrome of deficiency type marked by spontaneous perspiration.

Case Study: One case, whose disorder was due to the effect of exopathogens and marked by chills, high fever (39.5℃), restlessness without sweat, cough, headache, general aching, whitish thin tongue coating and floating rapid pulse, was treated with *Da Qinglong Tang*. The chills and fever were both abated after one dose was taken. After two doses, the case was cured.

1.8 Diaphoretic Prescriptions Composed of Drugs Pungent in Flavor and Cold in Nature

This kind of prescriptions are mainly made up of drugs pungent in flavor, cold in nature and having the action of relieving exterior syndrome. Their indication is the exterior syndrome due to the effect of exogenous wind—heat pathogens, marked by fever, sweat, slight aversion to wind and cold, headache, thirst, sore throat or cough, whitish thin or slightly yellowish tongue coating and floating rapid pulse. Drugs, such as *Bo He* (Herba Menthae), *Niu Bang Zi* (Fructus Arctii), *Sang Ye* (Folium Mori), *Ju Hua* (Flos Chrysanthemi), *Ge Gen* (Radix Puerariae), etc., are common in the prescriptions, whose representatives are *Sang Ju Yin, Yinqiao San, Ma Xing Shi Gan Tang*, etc.

1.9　The Prescription of *Sang Ju Yin*

Name: Decoction of Mulberry Leaf and Chrysanthemum

Source: The book *Wen Bing Tiao Bian*

Ingredients:

Sang Ye (Folium Mori) 7.5 g, *Ju Hua*(Flos Chrysanthemi) 3 g, *Xing Ren* (Semen Armeniacae Amarum) 6 g, *Lian Qiao* (Fructus Forsythiae) 5 g, *Bo He* (Herba Menthae) 2.5 g, *Jie Geng* (Radix Platycodi) 6 g, *Gan Cao* (Radix Glycyrrhizae) 2.5 g, *Wei Gen* (Rhizoma Phragmitis) 6 g.

Explanation:

Sang Ye: The principal drug, being sweet and bitter in flavor and cold in nature, clearing away heat from the lung–collaterals.

Ju Hua: The other principal drug, being pungent sweet and bitter in flavor and slightly cold in nature, dispelling wind–heat from the upper–*Jiao*.

Bo He: Aiding in dispelling wind–heat from the upper–*Jiao*.

Jie Geng and *Xing Ren:* Promoting the dispersing function of the lung to arrest cough with one ascending and the other descending the lung–*Qi*.

Lian Qiao: Expelling heat from above the diaphragm.

Wei Gen: Clearing away heat, promoting the production of body fluids, relieving thirst.

Gan Cao: Tempering the actions of all the other ingredients.

Effect: Dispelling wind, removing heat, promoting the dispersing function of the lung to arrest cough.

Indications: Wind-warm syndrome in the initial stage, marked by cough, low fever and mild thirst; including such diseases with the above symptoms as influenza, acute bronchitis, acute tonsillitis, epidemic conjunctivitis, etc.

Administration: Decocted in water for oral dose to be taken twice.

Case Study: 50 cases of influenza marked by aversion to cold, fever, headache, stuffy running nose, cough, poor appetite, etc., were climicall treated with modified *Sang Ju Yin*. Among 86.5% of the patients, the fever was abated completely and the general symptoms became mild 2 days later. Most of the cases were cured within 4 days.

Modified *Sang Ju Yin* was also prescribed to treat 11 cases of chin cough, the course of which averaged 18.6 days with the shortest duration being 10 days and the longest 34 days. Each of them was cured by taking 8-14 doses, averaging 10.2 doses.

1.10　The Prescription of *Yinqiao San*

Name: Powder of Lonicera and Forsythia

Source: The book *Wen Bing Tiao Bian*

Ingredients:

Lian Qiao (Fructus Forsythiae) 9 g, *Yin Hua*(Flos Lonicerae) 9 g, *Jie Geng*(Radix Platycodi) 6 g, *Bo He* (Herba Menthae) 6 g, *Zhu Ye* (Herba Lophatheri) 4 g, *Gan Cao* (Radix Glycyrrhizae) 5 g, *Jing Jie* (Spica Schizonepetae) 5 g, *Dan Dou Chi*(Semen Sojae Preparatum) 5 g, *Niu Bang Zi* (Fructus Arctii) 9 g, *Wei Gen* (Rhizoma Phragmitis) 18 g.

Explanation:

Yin Hua: The principal drug, being sweet in flavor and cold in nature, mildly promoting the dispersing function of the lung, clearing away heat and toxic material.

Lian Qiao: The other principal drug, being bitter in flavor and slightly cold in nature, mildly relieving the exterior syndrome, clearing away heat and toxic material.

Jing Jie Sui and *Dou Chi:* Being pungent in flavor and warm in nature, aiding *Yin Hua* and *Lian Qiao* in driving out exterior pathogens by means of relaxing the muscles and skin.

Niu Bang Zi and *Jie Geng:* Facilitating the flow of the lung–*Qi* to do good to the throat.

Gan Cao: Clearing away heat and toxic material.

Zhu Ye: Removing the heat in the upper–*Jiao*.

Wei Gen: Clearing away heat, promoting the production of body fluids.

Effect: Dispelling pathogenic factors in the superficies, clearing away heat and toxic material.

Indications: Exterior syndrome of wind–heat type in the initial stage of febrile disease, marked by fever, slightly aversion to wind–cold, thirst, reddened tongue with whitish thin coating and floating rapid pulse; including such diseases with the above symptoms as measles, influenza, acute suppurative tonsillitis, encephalitis B, parotitis, etc.

Administration: Decocted in water for oral dose to be taken twice (made into powder originally)

Case Study: 25 cases of acute upper respiratory infection marked by chills, fever, headache, general aching, sore throat, whitish thin tongue coating and floating rapid pulse, among which 2 were complicated by pregnancy, and 1 by heart failure due to rheumatic heart disease, were clinically treated with *Yinqiao San* packed in sacks, each of which contained 2 g of it and infused in boiling water in a cup with cover for 3—5 minutes for oral use. 2—4 sacks were taken each time, three times a day. 23 (90.2%) cases were cured. Their fever subsized within 8—72 hours, averaging 35 hours.

Modified *Yinqiao San* was administered to treat 400 cases of fulminant severe rubella. 395 were cured, each taking 2—5 doses. The rest 5 were unimproved, their rubella having been complicated by parotitis or periodontitis or meningitis or myocarditis.

1.11   The Prescription of *Ma Xing Shi Gan Tang*

Name: Decoction of Ephedra, Apricot Kernel, Gypsum and Licorice

Source: The book *Shang Han Lun*

Ingredients:

Ma Huang (Herba Ephedrae) 5 g, *Xing Ren* (Semen Armeniacae Amarum) 9 g, *Zhi Gan Cao* (Radix Glycyrrhizae Preparata) 6 g, *Shi Gao* (Gypsum Fibrosum) 18 g.

Explanation:

Ma Huang: The principal drug, being pungent and bitter in flavor and warm in nature, facilitating the flow of the lung—*Qi* to relieve asthma.

Shi Gao: Being pungent and sweet in flavor and very cold in nature, facilitating the flow of the lung—*Qi* to clear away the lung—heat and preventing the other drugs warm in nature from producing heat, with its dose as two times as that of *Ma Huang*.

Xing Ren: Discending the lung—*Qi,* assisting *Ma Huang* and

Shi Gao in removing heat from the lung to relieve asthma.

Zhi Gan Cao: Invigorating *Qi* and regulating the stomach, uniting *Shi Gao* to promote the production of body fluids to quench thirst, regulating the cold or warm nature and ascending or descending actions of the other ingredients.

Effect: Dispersing superficial pathogens, removing heat from the lung to relieve asthma.

Indications: Syndrome due to the attack of wind—heat on the lung or stagnated wind—cold which has turned into heat and stayed in the lung, marked by fever, cough, shortness of breath, nasal flare, thirst with or without sweat, whitish thin or yellowish tongue coating and slippery rapid pulse; including such diseases with the above symptoms as acute tracheitis, lobar pneumonia, infantile bronchopneumonia, scarlet fever, urticaria, chronic tracheitis, bronchial asthma, etc.

Administration: Decocted in water for oral dose to be taken twice.

Case Study: 178 cases of children's syndrome of dyspnea and cough due to the lung affection were clinically treated with modified *Ma Xing Shi Gan Tang*, whose main ingredients were as follows:

Cong Bai (Bulbus Allii Fistulosi), *Dou Chi* (Semen Sojae Preparatum), *Ma Huang* (Herba Ephedrae), *Shi Gao* (Gypsum Fibrosum), *Gan Cao,*(Radix Glycyrrhizae), *Sang Bai Pi* (Cortex Mori), *Zhe Bei Mu* (Bulbus Fritillariae Thunbergii), *Chuan Po* (Cortex Magnoliae Officinalis), *Gua Lou* (Fructus Trichosanthis), *Lian Qiao* (Fructus Forsythiae), *Chi Xiao Dou* (Semen Phaseoli).

149 cases (83.7%) were cured, 20(11.2%) improved, 9 (5.1%) unimproved.

Ma Xing Shi Gan Tang was administered to treat 30 cases of infantile pneumonia marked by fever, dyspnea, cough, sore throat, etc. 26 cases were cured, 1 remarkedly improved, 3 improved, the effective rate being 100%.

1.12 The prescription of *Shengma Gegen Tang*

Name: Decoction of Cimicifuge and Pueraria
Source: The book *Yan Shi Xiao Er Fang Lun*
Ingredients:

Sheng Ma (Rhizoma Cimicifugae) 3 g, *Ge Gen* (Radix Puerariae) 3 g, *Shao Yao* (Radix Paeoniae Alba) 6 g, *Zhi Gan Cao* (Radix Glycyrrhizae Preparata) 3 g.

Explanation: *Sheng Ma:* The principal drug, being pungent and sweet in flavor and slightly cold in nature, expelling pathogenic factors from the muscles and skin, promoting eruption, removing toxic substances.

Ge Gen: Assisting *Sheng Ma* in promoting eruption and expelling exo—pathogens, aiding in the production of body fluids.

Shao Yao: Regulating the nutrient system, dispelling pathogenic heat.

Zhi Gan Cao: Invigorating *Qi*, removing toxic substances.

Effect: Expelling pathogenic factors from the muscles and skin, promoting eruption.

Indications: Onset of measles without skin eruption or with poor skin eruption, marked by fever, aversion to wind, headache, general pain, sneeze, cough, blood—shot eyes, watery eyes, thirst, reddened tongue with dry coating and floating rapid pulse; including such diseases with the above symptoms as measles, rubella, drug rash, allergic purpura, etc.

Administration: Decocted in water for oral dose to be taken 3 times

Case Study: 20 cases of herpes zoster manifested as severe itching and pain and intermittent exudate in the affected part, complicated by chills, fever, insomnia, were clinically treated with *Shengma Gegen Tang* plus *Zi Cao* (Radix Arnebiae). All the 20 cases were rapidly cured.

Modified *Shengma Gegen Tang* was also used to treat 162 cases of psoriasis, with 77 cured, 76 improved and 9 unimproved.

1.13 The Prescription of *Chai Ge Jieji Tang*

Name: Bupleurum and Pueraria Decoction for Dispelling Pathogenic Factors from Superficial Muscles.

Source: The book *Shang Han Liu Shu*

Ingredients:

Chai Hu (Radix Bupleuri) 6 g, *Ge Gen* (Radix Puerariae) 9 g, *Gan Cao* (Radix Glycyrrhizae) 3g, *Huang Qin* (Radix Scutellariae) 6 g, *Qiang Huo* (Rhizoma seu Radix Notopterygii) 3g, *Bai Zhi* (Radix Angelicae Dahuricae) 3 g, *Shao Yao* (Radix Paeoniae Alba) 6 g, *Jie Geng* (Radix Platycodi) 3 g, *Sheng Jiang* (Rhizoma Zingiberis Recens) 3 pieces, *Da Zao* (Fructus Jujubae) 2 dates, *Shi Gao* (Gypsum Fibrosum) 5 g.

Explanation:

Ge Gen: One of the two principal drugs, being pungent and sweet in flavor and cold in nature, expelling pathogenic factors from the muscles and skin, clearing away heat.

Chai Hu: The other principal drug, being bitter and pungent in flavor and slightly cold in nature, expelling pathogenic factors from the muscles and skin, removing heat.

Qiang Huo and *Bai Zhi:* Aiding *Chai Hu* and *Ge Gen* in expelling pathogenic factors from the muscles and skin, relieving pains.

Huang Qin and *Shi Gao:* Clearing away accumulated heat.

Jie Geng: Facilitating the flow of the lung–*Qi*.

Shao Yao and *Gan Cao:* Regulating nutritive *Qi*, dispersing heat.

Sheng Jiang and *Da Zao:* Regulating nutritive *Qi* and defensive *Qi*.

Effect: Expelling pathogenic factors from the muscles and skin, clearing away heat.

Indications: Syndrome due to exogenous wind–cold which has stagnated and turned into heat, marked by chills with a milder tendency, fever with a higher tendency, no sweat, headache, eyes aching, dry nose, restlessness, insomnia, orbital aching and floating slightly full pulse; including such diseases with the above symptoms as influenza, prosopalgia, periodontitis, etc.

Administration: Decocted in water for oral dose to be taken twice.

Case Study: *Chai Ge Jieji Tang* was administered in clinical practice to treat 62 cases of infantile viral infection of upper respiratory tract marked by high fever. The patients'age ranged from 3 month to 13 years old and their body temperature from 38℃ to over 40℃. In 13 cases, increased bronchovascular shadows were shown on X–ray examination. The treatment result was that 56 cases were improved.

1.14　Prescriptions for Strengthening Body Resistance and Relieving Exterior Syndrome

Prescriptions for strengthening body resistance and relieving exterior syndrome are made up of drugs having the action of strengthening body resistance and drugs of relieving exterior syndrome. Their indication is exterior syndrome due to general deficiency of the vital *Qi* and the simultaneous effect of exogenous pathogens, marked by lassitude, sweating, thirst, aversion to wind and cold, and floating, feeble or deep pulse. The common drugs used to strengthen body resistance are *Ren Shen* (Radix Ginseng), *Yu Zhu* (Rhizoma Polygonati Odorati), *Fu Zi* (Radix Aconiti Lateralis Preparata) which are compatible with such drugs used to relieve exterior syndrome as *Qiang Huo* (Rhizoma seu Radix Notopterygii) and *Cong Bai* (Bulbus Allii Fistulosi) in this kind of prescriptions, whose representatives are *Baidu San, Mahuang Xixing Fuzi Tang, Jiajian Weirui Tang*, etc..

1.15　The Prescription of *Baidu San*

Name: Antiphlogistic Powder
Source: The book *Xiao Er Yao Zheng Zhi Jue*
Ingredients:

Chai Hu (Radix Bupleuri) 9 g, *Qian Hu* (Radix Peucedani) 9g, *Chuan Xiong* (Rhizoma Chuanxiong) 9 g, *Zhi Qiao* (Fructus Aurantii) 9 g, *Qiang Huo* (Rhizoma seu Radix Notopterygii) 9 g, *Du Huo* (Radix Angelicae Pubescentis) 9 g, *Fu Ling* (Poria) 9 g, *Jie Geng* (Radix Platycodi) 9 g, *Ren Shen* (Radix Ginseng) 9 g, *Gan Cao* (Radix Glycyrrhizae) 4.5 g, *Sheng Jiang* (Rhizoma Zingiberis Recens) 3 g, *Bo He* (Herba Menthae) 3 g.

Explanation:

Qiang Huo and *Du Huo*: The principal drugs, being pungent and bitter in flavor and warm in nature, removing wind, cold and dampness pathogens from the whole body.

Chuan Xiong: Promoting the circulation of blood, dispersing pathogenic wind.

Chai Hu: Being pungent in flavor and dispersing in nature, expelling the pathogens from the muscles and skin, aiding *Qiang Huo* and *Du Huo* in driving away exo-pathogens, relieving pain.

Zhi Qiao: Descending *Qi*.

Jie Geng: Promoting the flow of the lung-*Qi*.

Qian Hu: Removing phlegm.

Fu Ling: Eliminating dampness.

Gan Cao: Tempering the actions of all the other ingredients, invigorating *Qi*, regulating the stomach.

Sheng Jiang and *Bo He:* Expelling wind pathogen.

Ren Shen: Invigorating *Qi* to expel pathogens.

Effect: Relieving exterior syndrome by invigorating *Qi*, expelling pathogenic wind-dampness.

Indications: Syndrome caused by the effect of exogenous wind-cold-dampness pathogens because of the deficiency of vital *Qi*, marked by chills, high fever, stiff nape, pain of the limbs, no sweating, stuffy nose with deep voice, cough with sputum, fullness sensation in the chest, whitish and greasy tongue coating and floating feeble pulse; including such diseases with the above symptoms as influenza, measles, rheumatic arthritis, dysentery, etc.

Administration: Decocted in water for oral dose to be taken twice

Case Study: *Baidu San* was clinically administered to treat 2 cases of dysentery——a syndrome due to the effect of exogenous pathogens of summer–dampness, wind and cold and the stagnation of raw and cold food in the interior, marked by chills, high fever without sweat, mild distending pain in the chest and abdomen, bloody and mucous stools, tenesmus, 20 to 30 times of bowel movements within a 24–hour period, whitish and moistening tongue coating and floating tense pulse. Either of the patients began to perspire after taking one dose, with the exterior syndrome relieved and the times of diarrhea reduced. They were both cured after two further doses were taken by either of them.

Modified *Baidu San* was also used to treat two cases of rabies. One dose made the symptoms and signs less serious, and two doses, the cases cured, without any side effects.

1.16 The Prescription of *Mahuang Xixin Fuzi Tang*

Name: Decoction of Ephedra, Asarum and Aconite

Source; The book *Shang Han Lun*

Ingredients:

Ma Huang (Herba Ephedrae) 6g, *Xi Xin* (Herba Asari) 6g, *Fu Zi* (Radix Aconiti Lateralis Preparata) 9g.

Explanation:

Ma Huang: Relieving exterior syndrome, dispelling cold pathogen.

Fu Zi: Warming up the channels and supporting Yang–*Qi*.

Xi Xin: Assisting *Ma Huang* in relieving exterior syndrome, aiding *Fu Zi* in warming up the channels.

Effect: Restoring *Yang*, expelling pathogenic factors from the superficies.

Indications: Syndrome due to the effect of exogenous wind−cold pathogens and *Yang* insufficiency, marked by chills, low fever and deep pulse; including such diseases with the above symptoms as chronic bronchitis, chronic nephritis, rheumatic arthritis, rheumatoid arthritis, etc.

Administration: Decocted in water for oral dose to be taken 3 times

Case Study: *Mahuang Xixin Fuzi Tang* was clinically administered to treat more than 30 cases of prolonged cough−a syndrome caused by the effect of exogenous wind−cold pathogens and *Yang* insufficiency, and satisfactory curative effects were achieved.

Modification of this prescription was prescribed to treat one case of lethargy−a syndrome belonging to the insufficiency of the heart−*Yang* and marked by dizziness, distending sensation of the head, lassitude, difficulty in waking up in the morning, enlarged tongue with thin coating and thready slow pulse. Remarkable curative effects were obtained after 9 doses were taken.

1.17   The Prescription of *Jiajian Weirui Tang*

Name: Modified Decoction of Fragrant Solomonseal
Source: The book *Chong Ding Tong Su Shang Han Lun*
Ingredients: *Wei Rui* (Rhizoma Polygonati Odorati) 9 g, *Cong Bai* (Bulbus Allii Fistulosi) 6 g, *Jie Geng* (Radix Platycodi) 5g, *Bai Wei* (Radix Cynanchi Atrati) 3 g, *Dan Dou Chi* (Semen Sojae Preparatum) 12 g, *Bo He* (Herba Menthae) 5 g, *Zhi Gan*

Cao (Radix Glycyrrhizae Preparata) 2 g, *Hong Zao* (Fructus Jujubae) 2 dates.

Explanation:

Wei Rui: The principal drug, being sweet in flavor and slightly cold in nature, nourishing *Yin,* moistening the lung, aiding in the production of body fluids.

Cong Bai, Dou Chi, Bo He and *Jie Geng:* Relieving exterior syndrome, facilitating the flow of the lung *Qi,* relieving cough, benefiting the throat.

Bai Wei: Removing heat from blood to relieve restlessness and thirst.

Gan Cao and *Da Zao:* Being sweet in flavor, helping to moisten and nourish the spleen.

Effect: Nourishing *Yin* to clear away heat, inducing diaphoresis to relieve exterior syndrome.

Indications: Syndrome due to the effect of exopathogens with the deficiency of *Yin,* marked by headache, fever with little or no sweat, slightly aversion to wind—cold, cough, restlessness, thirst, dry throat, reddened tongue and rapid pulse; including such diseases with the above symptoms as common cold, sicca syndrome, etc.

Administration: Decocted in water for oral dose to be taken twice.

2　Purgative Prescriptions

2.1　Purgative Prescriptions

Prescriptions mainly consisting of purgative drugs and having the action of relaxing the bowels, removing stagnancy in the stomach and intestines clearing away heat of excess type eliminating water retention and getting rid of accumulation of cold are all known as "purgative prescriptions". Because the constitutions of patients are different in the type of deficiency or excess and the syndromes are caused by different accumulations of heat, cold, dryness or water, purgative prescriptions are accordingly classified as the following five kinds according to their different indications: those composed of drugs cold in nature and used to treat the excess syndrome due to accumulation of heat in the interior, those composed of drugs warm in nature and used to treat the excess syndrome due to accumulation of cold in the interior, those for moistening the intestines to induce laxation and used to treat constipation due to general deficiency of Qi, those for reducing fluid retention and used to treat the interior excess syndrome due to water retention, and those for both reinforcement and purgation and used to treat constipation due to interior excess complicated by the deficiency of vital-Qi.

Purgative prescriptions are established for the purpose of treating interior excess syndrome. It isn't advisable to use them when an interior syndrome hasn't become excessive and the exterior syndrome hasn't been relieved. When the exterior syndrome hasn't been relieved but an interior excess syndrome has formed, the exterior syndrome should be first relieved or both the exterior and interior ones are relieved together. When constipation is treated in those who are infirm with age, in those who have just given birth and are suffering from blood deficiency or in those who have just recovered from diseases and have had their body fluid impaired, purgative prescriptions should be cautiously used. This kind of constipation may be treated, if necessary, in either of the two ways: reinforcement and purgation in combination or purgation followed by reinforcement. Purgative prescriptions should not be further used once their effects have been achieved, for they have the side effects of comsuming and impairing the stomach−Qi. People should not eat heavy or indigestible food so soon after recovering from diseases lest the stomach−Qi be re−impaired.

2.2 Purgative Prescriptions Composed of Drugs Cold in Nature

This kind of prescriptions are those mainly composed of drugs cold in nature and suitable for the treatment of the excess syndrome due to accumulation of heat in the interior and marked by constipation, fullness or distention or pain in the abdomen, or even tidal fever, yellowish tongue coating and replete pulse. The commonly used drugs in these prescriptions are *Da Huang* (Radix et Rhizoma Rhei), *Mang Xiao* (Natrii Sulfas), etc.. The representative prescriptions are *Dachengqi Tang* and *Daxianxiong Tang*.

2.3　The Prescription of *Dachengqi Tang*

Name: Potent Purgative Decoction

Source: The book *Shang Han Lun*

Ingredients:

Da Huang (Radix et Rhizoma Rhei) 12 g, *Hou Po* (Cortex Magnoliae Officinalis) 15 g, *Zhi Shi* (Fructus Aurantii Immaturus) 15 g, *Mang Xiao* (Natrii Sulfas) 9 g.

Explanation: *Da Huang:* The principal drug, being bitter in flavor and cold in nature, purging heat to relax the bowels, removing stagnancy in the stomach and intestines.

Mang Xiao: Being salty in flavor and cold in nature, purging heat, softening hard masses, moistening dryness.

Hou Po and *Zhi Shi:* Promoting the circulation of *Qi* to resolve masses, relieving fullness and distention, assisting *Mang Xiao* and *Da Huang* in eliminating stagnancy to remove accumulation of heat.

Effect: Drastically eliminating heat accumulation and relieving constipation.

Indications: Excess syndrome due to interior heat, marked by constipation, frequent farting, fullness and distention in the gastric and abdominal region, tenderness with hard sensation in the abdomen, or even tidal fever, delirium, persistent sweating in the soles and palms, dry and yellowish tongue coating with prickles or dry black fissure tongue coating, and deep forceful pulse, or marked by green watery stools, pain in the abdomen or around the umbilicus, palpable masses in the abdomen, dry mouth and tongue, and slippery forceful pulse; including such diseases with the above symptoms as acute simple intestinal obstruction, cohesive intestinal obstruction, ascaris intestinal obstruction, acute cholecystitis, acute appendicitis, acute bacillary dysentery, toxic dysentery, schizophrenia, etc.

Contraindication: Because of its drastic action, this prescription should not be prescribed for pregnant women. The administration of it should be stopped once its effectiveness appears.

Administration: Decocted in water for oral dose to be taken twice, *Da Huang* and *Mang Xiao* should be decocted for a shorter time in order to keep their purgative action.

Case Study: Modified *Dachengqi Tang* was clinically prescribed to treat heat syndrome of excess type in acute and serious diseases. For example, 12 cases of jaundice were treated with *Dachengqi Tang* plus:

Huang Bai (Cortex Phellodendri), *Zhi Zi* (Fructus Gardeniae), *Jin Qian Cao* (Herba Lysimachiae), *Chuan Lian Zi* (Fructus Toosendan).

5 days later, 7 cases were cured and 2 improved. 15 cases of acute appendicitis were treated with *Dachengqi Tang* plus:

Pu Gong Ying(Herba Taraxaci), *Jin Yin Hua* (Flos Lonicerae), *San Ye Gui Zhen Cao* (Herba Bidentis).

3—5 days later, 13 cases were cured. 36 cases of dysentery due to damp—heat pathogens were treated with *Dachengqi Tang* plus:

Huang Lian (Rhizoma Coptidis), *Bai Shao* (Radix Paeoniae Alba).

29 cases were cured, 5 improved and 2 unimproved.

Dachengqi Tang minus:

Hou Po (Cortex Magnoliae Officinalis), but plus:

Shan Zha (Fructus Crataegi), *Hong Teng* (Caulis Sargentodoxae).

Bai Jiang Cao (Herba Patriniae)
was prescribed to treat 56 cases of acute pancreatitis manifested as severe tender pain in the upper abdomen which refers to the hypochondrium nausea, vomiting, eructation with fetid odour, abdominal distention, fever, greasy or yellowish tongue coating, and small taut slippery pulse. The result was that 54 cases were cured; in the rest 2 cases, the signs were relieved and then disappeared. The relapse took place only in 3 cases.

2.4   The Prescription of *Daxianxiong Tang*

Name: Major Decoction for Removing Phlegm—heat from the chest

Source: The book *Shang Han Lun*

Ingredients:

Da Huang (Radix et Rhizoma Rhei) 10 g, *Mang Xiao* (Natrii Sulfas) 10 g, *Gan Sui* (Radix Kansui) 1 g.

Explanation:

Gan Sui: One of the principal drugs, being bitter in flavor and cold in nature, purging water retention, clearing away heat, resolving masses.

Da Huang: The other principal drug, being good at sweeping out pathogenic heat by relaxing the bowels, purging together with *Gan Sui* pathogens due to water—heat accumulation.

Mang Xiao: Dispelling heat, softening masses, aiding *Gan Sui* and *Da Huang* in removing accumulations.

Effect: Purging heat, removing water retention, resolving masses.

Indications: Syndrome due to water and pathogenic heat retained in the chest and abdomen, marked by 5 / 6—day—absence of laxation, hard and full sensation and tenderness in the whole abdomen, mild hectic fever in the afternoon, or shortness of breath, severe vexation, dry tongue with thirst, and deep tense forceful pulse; including such diseases with the above symptoms as exudative pleurisy, intestinal obstruction, peritonitis, etc.

Administration: Decoct *Da Huang*, melt *Mang Xiao* and infuse the powder of *Gan Sui* in water for oral dose to be taken twice.

Contraindication: This prescription should not be prescribed for treating patients with weak constitution or those who have just recovered from disease and are intolerant of purgation. It should not be further administered once its effectiveness has been achieved.

Case Study: *Daxianxiong Tang* was clinically prescribed to treat 6 cases of tuberculous exudative pleurisy manifested as fever, chest pain, shortness of breath, restlessness, headache and aversion to cold. Thoracic exudate was found, small amount in 4 cases, at the level of the 5th rib in 1, at the 3rd in 1. The prescription used was as follows:

Da Huang (Radix et Rhizoma Rhei) 9 g, *Mang Xiao* (Natrii Sulfas) 9 g, *Gan Sui* (Radix Kansui) 3 g.
which was decocted in water for oral use. The small amount of thoracic exudate in the 4 cases disappeared after 1—3 doses were taken by each of them. The thoracic exudate in the other 2 cases also disappeared after 6—9 doses were taken by either of them. Simultaneously, other symptoms went away.

20 cases of acute pancreatitis, a combined disorder of *Taiyang* and *Yangming* channels, were treated with the modifica-

tion of *Daxianxiong Tang* and *Dachengqi Tang*. Fasting, fluid transfusion and antibiotics were not advocated in the course of treatment. After the decoction was taken, the abdominal pain began to be relieved in 2—48 hours, averaging 19.5 hours; began to completely disappear in 24—96 hours, averaging 68 hours.

2.5 Purgative Prescriptions Composed of Drugs Warm in Nature

This kind of prescriptions are those mainly made up of drugs with the action of purging and warming the interior of the body. Their indication is cold accumulation of excess type in the *Zang—Fu* organs, a syndrome marked by constipation, fullness and distention in the gastric and abdominal region, abdominal pain which will be relieved by warming, cool or even cold extremities, deep tense pulse, etc. In these prescriptions, purgative drugs such as *Da Huang* (Radix et Rhizoma Rhei) and *Ba Dou* (Fructus Crotonis) are usually prescribed together with drugs having the action of warming the interior of the body such as *Fu Zi* (Radix Aconiti Lateralis Preparata) and *Gan Jiang* (Rhizoma Zingiberis). The representative prescriptions are *Dahuang Fuzi Tang* and *San wu Beiji Wan*.

2.6 The Prescription of *Dahuang Fuzi Tang*

Name: Decoction of Rhubarb and Mankshood
Source: The book *Jin Gui Yao Lue*
Ingredients:

Da Huang (Radix et Rhizoma Rhei) 9 g, *Pao Fu Zi* (Radix Aconiti Lateralis Preparata) 9 g, *Xi Xin* (Herba Asari) 3 g.

Explanation:

Fu Zi: The principal drug, being pungent and sweet in flavor and extreme heat in nature, warming up *Yang—Qi,* dispelling pathogenic cold.

Xi Xin: Expelling pathogenic cold, resolving masses.

Da Huang: Relaxing the bowels to sweep away the stagnancy of food or other pathogenic factors.

Effect: Warming up *Yang—Qi* dispelling pathogenic cold resolving masses, eliminating accumulation.

Indications: Syndrome due to cold accumulation of excess type in the interior, marked by abdominal pain, constipation, pain in the hypochondrium, fever, cold limbs, whitish greasy tongue coating and wiry tense pulse; including such diseases with the above symptoms as chronic dysentery uremia, ulcerative colitis, acute intestinal obstruction, etc.

Administration: Decocted in water for oral dose to be taken 3 times. Because this prescription is intended to purge warmly, the dosage of *Da Huang* should be smaller than that of *Fu Zi.*

Case Study: Modified *Dahuang Fuzi Tang* was clinically used to treat 1 case of biliary ascariasis, a syndrome due to cold accumulation of excess type in the interior and *Yang* insufficiency, marked by sudden onset of pain in the hypochondriac region, paroxysmal colicky pain in the right hypochondrium which radiates to the back and the right shoulder, profuse cold sweat, cold limbs, no vomiting and thirst, 2—day—absence of laxation, pale and enlarged tongue with whitish coating and deep tense pulse. The ingredients were as follows:

Da Huang (Radix et Rhizoma Rhei) 10 g, *Fu Zi* (Radix Aconiti Lateralis Preparata) 30 g, *Xi Xin* (Herba Asari) 5 g, *Wu*

Mei (Fructus Mume) 40 g, *Bing Lang* (Semen Arecae) 30 g.

All the above were decocted in water with *Fu Zi* decocted first. The decoction of one dose was taken at a draught and the pain was eliminated.

Dahuang Fuzi Tang was used to treat 1 case of allergic purpura, 1 case of refractory eczema, 1 case of drug allergic purpura and 1 case of infectious eczema. All the 4 disorders are included in the syndrome due to cold accumulation of excess type in the interior, marked by cold limbs, aversion to cold, clear and diluted urine, dry stools and tense pulse. Remarkable curative effects was achieved and all the 4 cases were cured.

2.7   The Prescription of *Wenpi Tang*

Name: Decoction for Warming the Spleen

Source: The book *Bei Ji Qian Jin Yao Fang*

Ingredients:

Da Huang (Radix et Rhizoma Rhei) 12 g, *Fu Zi* (Radix Aconiti Lateralis Preparata) 9 g, *Gan Jiang* (Rhizoma Zingiberis) 6 g, *Ren Shen* (Radix Ginseng) 9 g, *Gan Cao* (Radix Glycyrrhizae) 3 g.

Explanation:

Ren Shen : One of the two principal drugs, being sweet and slightly bitter in flavor and neutral in nature, invigorating the spleen, replenishing *Qi*.

Gan Jiang: The other principal drug, being pungent in flavor and warm in nature, warming up the spleen to dispel cold.

Fu Zi: Assisting *Gan Jiang* in warming up *Yang—Qi,* dispelling pathogenic cold.

Da Huang: Eliminating accumulation due to pathogenic factors.

Gan Cao: Invigorating *Qi,* regulating the stomach, tempering the actions of all the other ingredients.

Effect: Warming up the spleen—*Yang,* purging cold accumulation.

Indications: Syndrome due to insufficiency of the spleen—*Yang* and stagnation of pathogenic cold, marked by constipation resulting from accumulation of cold pathogens, or protracted dysentery with purulent and bloody stools, abdominal pain, cool extremities, whitish slippery tongue coating and deep wiry pulse; including such diseases with the above symptoms as chronic dysentery, ulcerative colitis, ascariasis and ascites due to cirrhosis.

Administration: Decocted in water for oral dose to be taken 3 times.

Case Study: *Wenpi Tang* was clinically prescribed to treat 1 case of ascites due to cirrhosis, 1 case of infantile indigestion and 2 cases of ascariasis, all the disorders being included in the syndrome due to *Yang*—deficiency of the spleen and stomach and stagnation resulting from cold accumulation, marked by abdominal pain and constipation. Satisfactory curative effects were achieved in all the 4 cases.

Modified *Wenpi Tang* was used to treat 1 case of dysentery, a syndrome due to cold—damp in the spleen and stomach and stagnancy in the gastrointestinal tract, which was complicated by exterior symptom and marked by purulent stools with white and red mucous, 6—7 times of laxation each day, colicky pain in the lower abdomen, tenesmus, whitish tongue coating, moderate slow pulse in the right and thready uneven pulse in the left. 7 doses cured the case.

2.8   The Prescription of *Sanwu Beiji Wan*

Name: Pill of Three Drugs for Emergency

Source: The book *Jin Gui Yao Lue*

Ingredients:

Da Huang (Radix et Rhizoma Rhei) 30g, *Gan Jiang* (Rhizoma Zingiberis) 30 g, *Ba Dou* (Fructus Crotonis) with its oil removed 30 g.

Explanation:

Ba Dou: The principal drug, being pungent in flavor and hot in nature, drastically purging cold accumulation.

Gan Jiang: Warming up *Yang−Qi,* assisting *Ba Dou* in removing cold pathogens.

Da Huang: Eliminating pathogenic stagnancy in the gastrointestinal tract, restricting the toxicity of *Ba Dou.*

Effect: Eliminating cold accumulation

Indications: Syndrome due to cold accumulation of excess type, marked by sudden prickly distending pain in the gastrointestinal region, shortness of breath, trismus, constipation, whitish tongue coating and deep tense pulse; including such diseases with the above symptoms as food poisoning, acute simple intestinal obstruction, etc.

Contraindication: This prescription is a drastic one with purgative action. *Ba Dou* in it should be cautiously prescribed, because it has great toxicity and strong irritation to the gastrointestinal tract. When sudden and acute abdominal pain is treated in pragnant women or in those infirm with age or due to pathogenic summer—heat, this prescription is not allowed to be prescribed. Cool rice gruel can be taken to alleviate persistent diarrhea which might be brought about by taking this medicine.

Administration: Ground into powder, 0.6—1.5 g of the powder is taken each time. If no bowel movements result after this dosage is taken, the second taking is preferable according to the need of disease condition. (Originally, this medicine was also in the form of honeyed boluses.)

Case Study: *Sanwu Beiji Wan* (put in capsules) was clinically used to treat 35 cases of intestinal obstruction, whose course ranged from 1 hour to 3 days, averaging 10 hours. About 30 minutes later after the medicine was taken, active bowel sound appeared; 1—3 hours later, laxation occurred. The treatment result was: 27 cases were cured, of which 5 were the syndrome of cold nature, 22, warm nature; the rest 8 didn't respond to this medicine and were treated with surgical operation thereafter.

Experiments have shown that *Sanwu Beiji Wan* has an evident action of Strengthening the contraction of the intestinal tract, which often varies with the drug concentration.

2.9 Prescriptions for Moistening the Intestines to Cause Laxation

This kind of prescriptions are mainly composed of drugs with lubricant nature and purgative action. They are indicated for the syndrome of constipation due to weakness of the body, marked by dry stools which is difficulty to discharge. In these prescriptions, such drugs with lubricant nature as *Ma Zi Ren*

(Fructus Cannabis), *Xing Ren* (Semen Armeniacae Amarum) and *Shao Yao* (Radix Paeoniae) are usually compatible with purgative drugs such as *Da Huang* (Radix et Rhizoma Rhei). The representative prescriptions are *Maziren Wan* and *Jichuan Jian*.

2.10   The prescription of *Maziren Wan*

Name: Hemp Fruit Pill

Source: The book *Shang Han Lun*

Ingredients: *Ma Zi Ren* (Fructus Cannabis) 500 g, *Shao Yao* (Radix Paeoniae) 250g, *Zhi Shi* (Fructus Aurantii Immaturus) 250 g, *Da Huang* (Radix et Rhizoma Rhei) 500 g, *Hou Po* (Cortex Magnoliae Officinalis) 250 g, *Xing Ren* (Semen Armeniacae Amarum) 250 g.

Explanation:

Ma Zi Ren: The principal drug, being sweet in flavor and neutral in nature, moistening the bowels to relieve constipation.

Xing Ren: Keeping the adverse flow of the lung—*Qi* downwards, lubricating the intestines.

Shao Yao: Nourishing *Yin,* regulating the interior of the body.

Da Huang: Promoting laxation, purging heat.

Zhi Shi and *Hou Po:* Keeping the adverse flow of *Qi* downwards to relieve stagnancy.

Feng Mi: Moistening dryness to induce bowel movements.

Effect: Moistening the intestines, purging heat, removing stagnation of *Qi,* inducing bowel movements.

Indications: Syndrome due to dryness—heat in the gastrointestine and shortage of fluids, marked by dry stools and frequent urination; including such diseases with the above symptoms as habitula constipation, constipation due to hemorrhoid, etc.

Administration: Ground into powder and mixed with honey into pills. 9 g of the pills is taken each time, twice daily; or decocted in water for the decoction with the dosage of the ingredients adequately reduced according to their proportions.

Contraindication: This prescription is contraindicated for pragnant women and constipation due to blood deficiency and shortage of body fluid.

Case Study: Modified *Maziren Tang* was clinically used to treat 47 cases of ascaris in testinal obstruction. The abdominal pain was usually relieved 1—2 hours later after the first decoction was taken; 6—12 hours later, worms, usually in ascaris balls, were discharged with feces. Following that, the symptoms and signs disappeared completely. No toxic reaction and side—effects were seen in the course of treatment.

Maziren Wan was used to prevent 500 cases from suffering from pain and bleeding due to dry stools, which was likely to appear during the first bowel movement after anal operations. If the feces were softened and in the form of strip while they were being easily discharged after *Maziren Wan* had been taken, the effectiveness was considered to have been achieved. If the feces were still dry and laxation took place one time 2—3 days after *Maziren Wan* had been taken, the ineffectiveness was considered to result. The effectiveness was seen in 497 cases (95.8%). Among the ineffective cases, 16 were patients suffering from habitual constipation.

2.11 The Prescription of *Jichuan Jian*

Name: Decoction of *Jichuan Jian*

Source: The book *Jing Yue Quan Shu*

Ingredients:

Dang Gui (Radix Angelicae Sinensis) 12 g, *Niu Xi* (Radix Achyranthis Bidentatae) 6 g, *Rou Cong Rong* (Herba Cistanches) 7.5 g, *Ze Xie* (Rhizoma Alismatis) 4.5 g, *Sheng Ma* (Rhizoma Cimicifugae) 2 g, *Zhi Qiao* (Fructus Aurantii) 3 g.

Explanation:

Rou Cong Rong: The principal drug, being sweet and salty in flavor and warm in nature, warming up the kidney, replenishing vital-essence, moistening the intestines to defecate.

Dang Gui: Nourishing and regulating blood, relaxing the bowel to relieve constipation.

Niu Xi: Invigorating the kidney to strengthen the loins, tending to go downward.

Zhi Qiao: Making stagnated *Qi* in the intestines go downwards, aiding in relaxing the bowels.

Ze Xie: Tending to go downwards to promote the discharging of turbidity in the kidney.

Sheng Ma: Ascending the clear *Yang* so as to descend the turbid *Yin*.

Effect: Warming up the kidney, replenishing vital essence, lubricating the intestines to induce defecation.

Indications: Syndrome of constipation due to deficiency of the kidney, marked by constipation, clear and dilute urine, dizziness and vertigo, and soreness and weakness of the loins and knees; including such diseases with the above symptoms as constipation due to infirmity with age, tuberculosis or tumor.

Administration: Decocted in water for oral dose to be taken twice

2.12 Prescriptions for Reducing Water Retention

This kind of prescriptions are mainly made up of drugs with the action of eliminating retained fluids. They are indicated for the syndrome of excess type due to water retention in the interior, marked by edema, abdominal swelling, oppressed sensation in the chest, pain in the hypochondrium caused by cough or spitting, headache, dizziness, slippery tongue coating and deep wiry pulse. The commonly used drugs in these prescriptions are *Yuan Hua* (Flos Genkwa), *Gan Sui* (Radix Kansui), *Da Ji* (Radix Cirsii Japonici), *Qian Niu Zi* (Semen Pharbitidis), etc. The representatives are *Shizao Tang, Zhouche Wan*, etc.

2.13 The Prescription of *Shizao Tang*

Name: Ten—date Decoction

Source: The book *Shang Han Lun*

Ingredients(with the same dose):

Yuan Hua (Flos Genkwa), *Gan Sui* (Radix Kansui), *Da Ji* (Radix seu Herba Cirsii Japonici) and *Da Zao* (Fructus Jujubae) 10 dates.

Explanation:

Gan Sui: Being bitter in flavor and cold in nature, removing retained water in the channels.

Da Ji: Being bitter in flavor and cold in nature, purging water retained in *Zang—Fu* organs.

Yuan Hua: Being pungent in flavor and warm in nature, eliminating retained water and phlegm from the hypochondrium.

Da Zao: Replenishing *Qi,* protecting the stomach, alleviating the drastic action and toxicity of all the other ingredients to prevent impairment of vital *Qi* due to purgation.

Effect: Eliminating water retention drastically

Indications: Syndrome due to retention of excessive fluids in the interior, marked by pain in the hypochondriac region caused by cough and expectoration, fullness and rigidity in the epigastrium, nausea, shortness of breath, headache, dizziness, or difficulty in breathing due to chest pain referring to the back, deep wiry pulse, or marked by general edema which is especially severe below the loins, dyspnea and fullness due to abdominal distention, and difficulty in urination and defecation; including such diseases with the above symptoms as exudative pleuritis, tuberculous peritonitis, ascites due to cirrhosis and chronic nephritis, etc.

Contraindication: This prescription should be cautiously prescribed for the debilitated or pregnant women.

Administration: *Yuan Hua, Gan Sui* and *Da Ji* are ground into powder, *Da Zao* is decocted for the decoction. 1.5—3 g of the powder is infused with adequate amount of the decoction and taken on an empty stomach in the morning, 1 time daily. Because this prescription is a drastic one for eliminating retained water, the administration of it should start with smaller dose (1.5g). Persistent diarrhea, if occurring after it is taken, may be stopped through taking cool and thin gruel or drinking cold boiled water.

Case Study: 51 cases of exudative pleuritis were clinically

treated with *Shizao Tang* which consisted of the same dose of:

Yuan Hua (Flos Genkwa), *Gan Sui* (Radix Kansui), *Da Ji* (Raidx seu Herba Cirsii Japonici) and *Da Zao* (Fructus Jujubae) 10–15 dates.

Yuan Hua, Gan Sui and Da Ji were ground into powder and *Da Zao* was decocted in water for the decoction. 3 g of the powder was infused with adequate amount of *Da Zao* decoction and taken on an empty stomach in the morning, 1 time every other day. 4–6 doses were taken altogether. The result was: The hydrothorax was reduced within 11 days in 96% of the cases, disappeared completely within 20 days in 88.2%. The length for the hydrothorax to vanish averaged 16.2 days. Chest pain remained in a few cases after their hydrothorax was absorbed.

5 cases of ascites due to cirrhosis were treated with *Shizao Wan*. 1.5–6 g of it was taken with *Dazao* decoction on an empty stomach in the morning, 1 time daily. or 12 g of it was taken with *Dazao* decoction, twice daily. The result was: The ascites in all the cases was reduced to some extent.

2.14   The Prescription of *Zhouche Wan*

Name: Pill for Relieving Ascites

Source: The book *Jing Yue Quan Shu*

Ingredients:

Qian Niu Zi (Semen Pharbitidis) 120 g, *Gan Sui* (Radix Kansui) 30 g, *Yuan Hua* (Flos Genkwa) 30 g, *Da Ji* (Radix Cirsii Japonici) 30 g, *Da Huang* (Radix et Rhizoma Rhei) 60 g, *Qing Pi* (Pericarpium Citri Reticulatae Viride) 15 g, *Chen Pi* (Pericarpium Citri Reticulatae) 15 g, *Mu Xiang* (Radix Aucklandiae) 15 g, *Bing*

Lang (Semen Arecae) 15 g, *Qing Fen* (Calomelas) 3 g.

Explanation:

Yuan Hua, Gan Sui and *Da Ji:* The principal drugs, eliminating retained water in the thoracic and abdominal cavities and the channels.

Da Huang and *Qian Niu Zi:* Sweeping away retained water and heat in the stomach and intestines.

Qing Pi: Relieving the depressed liver to remove the stagnancy of *Qi.*

Chen Pi: Regulating the lung and spleen to free the flow of *Qi* along the diaphragm.

Bing Lang: Leading *Qi* to flow downwards, inducing diuresis to resolve masses.

Mu Xiang: Dredging the 3 *Jiao* to remove stagnancy, promoting the flow of *Qi* and the distribution of body fluids to relieve edema.

Qing Fen: Eliminating retained water, relaxing the bowels, assisting the other ingredients in relieving edema and inducing laxation.

Effect: Eliminating retained water drastically, promoting the flow of *Qi* to resolve masses.

Indications: Syndrome due to stagnation of *Qi* resulting from accumulation of water and heat in the interior, marked by edema and distention due to it, thirst, rough breathing, hard feeling in the abdomen, dysuria, constipation, and deep rapid forceful pulse; including such disease with the above symptoms as ascites due to cirrhosis.

Contraindication: Because of its drastic purgation, this prescription is contraindicated for pregnant women as well as patients whose vital *Qi* is deficient.

Administration: *Gan Sui* is wrapped in flour paste and baked, *Da Ji* is parched with vinegar, and then they are ground into powder together with all the other ingredients. Finally, the powder is made into pills. 3−6 g of the pills is taken with warm boiled water on an empty stomach in the morning, 1 time daily.

Qing Fen, Yuan Hua, Gan Sui and *Da Ji* have strong toxicity, be sure not to take them in large dosage or for longer time for fear that poisoning result.

Case Study: *Zhouche Wan* was clinically used to treat case of amenorrhea due to ascariasis manifested as 3−year−impregnability after marriage, edema occurring 2 years ago followed by abdominal distention, amenorrhea, polyphagia, loose stools, oliguria, desiring for eating salt particles, intermittent salivation, heavy sensation of the limbs, lassitude, and pale lips with pimples on the inner surface. 1.5 g of *Zhouche Wan* was taken on an empty stomach in the morning. 2 hours later, nausea and vomiting and abdominal colic were observed; 3 hours later, large amount of water and worms were discharged through the anus, the ascites being remarkably relieved. In the morning after the next, another 1.5 g was taken and the same thing happened, the ascites being completely relieved.

2.15 The Prescription of *Shu Zao Yinzi*

Name: Decoction for Diuresis

Source: The book *Ji Sheng Fang*

Ingredients:

Ze Xie (Rhizoma Alismatis) 12 g, *Chi Xiao Dou* (Semen

Phaseoli) 15 g, *Shang Lu* (Radix Phytolaccae) 6 g, *Qiang Huo* (Rhizoma Seu Radix Notopterygii) 9 g,

Da Fu Pi (Pericarpium Arecae) 15 g,

Jiao Mu (Semen Zanthoxyli) 9 g,

Mu Tong (Caulis Akebiae) 12 g,

Qin Jiao (Radix Gentianae Macrophyllae) 9 g,

Bing Lang (Semen Arecae) 9 g,

Fu Ling Pi (Cortex Poriae) 30 g,

Sheng Jiang Pi (Cortex Zingiberis Recens) 4.5 g.

Explanation:

Shang Lu: The principal drug, being bitter and pungent in flavor and neutral in nature, purging retained water, inducing laxation and diuresis.

Bing Lang and *Da Fu Pi:* Promoting the circulation of *Qi* to eliminate retained water.

Fu Ling Pi, Ze Xie, Mu Tong, Jiao Mu and *Chi Xiao Dou:* Inducing laxation and diuresis to remove retained water in the interior.

Qiang Huo, Qin Jiao and *Sheng Jiang Pi:* Tending to give their potency full play in the skin, expelling pathogenic wind through the superficies of the body, removing retained water in the superficies through the muscles.

Effect: Purging retained water by inducing bowel movements and diuresis, expelling wind pathogens through the superficies of the body.

Indications: Syndrome due to excessive water retention both in the exterior and in the interior, marked by general edema, asthma, thirst, and difficulty in defecation and urination; including such diseases with the above symptoms as acute nephritis, nephrotic syndrome, etc.

Administration: Decocted in water for oral dose to be taken twice (used in the form of powder originally)

2.16 Prescriptions for Both Reinforcement and Purgation

This kind of prescriptions are mainly composed of drugs with the action of purgation of tonification. They are indicated for the syndrome due to pathogenic accumulation of excess type and insufficiency of vital *Qi* in the interior, marked by constipation, lassitude, shortness of breath, dry mouth and throat, etc. Purgative drugs such as *Da Huang* (Radix et Rhizoma Rhei) and *Mang Xiao*(Natrii Sulfas) are usually compatible with tonifying drugs such as *Ren Shen*(Radix Ginseng), *Dang Gui* (Radix Angelicae Sinensis) and *Sheng Di* (Radix Rehmanniae) in these prescriptions, whose representatives are *Xinjia Huanglong Tang*, *Zengye Chengqi Tang*, etc.

2.17 The Prescription of *Xinjia Huanglong Tang*

Name: Decoction of Yellow Dragon with Supplement
Source: The book *Wen Bing Tiao Bian*.
Ingredients:
Sheng Di (Radix Rehmanniae) 15 g, *Gan Cao* (Radix Glycyrrhizae) 6 g, *Ren Shen* (Radix Ginseng) 4.5g, *Da Huang* (Radix et Rhizoma Rhei) 9 g, *Mang Xiao*(Natrii Sulfas) 3 g, *Xuan Shen* (Radix Scrophulariae) 15 g, *Mai Dong* (Radix Ophiopogonis) 15 g, *Dang Gui* (Radix Angelicae Sinensis) 4.5 g, *Hai Shen* (sea cucumber) 2 pieces, *Jiang Zhi* (ginger juice) 6

spoons.

Explanation:

Da Huang and *Mang Xiao*: The principal drugs, purging heat, inducing bowel movements, softening masses, moistening dryness.

Xuan Shen, Sheng Di, Mai Dong and *Hai Shen*: Nourishing *Yin*, promoting the production of body fluids.

Ren Shen, Gan Cao and *Dang Gui*: Invigorating *Qi*, enriching blood.

Effect: Nourishing *Yin*, replenishing *Qi*, resolving masses, purging heat.

Indications: Syndrome due to heat accumulation of excess type in the interior and deficiency of both *Qi* and *Yin*, marked by constipation, severe fullness and distention in the abdomen, lassitude, weak breathing, dry mouth and throat, crack of lips, dry tongue with yellow or black fissured coating; including such disorders with the above symptoms as constipation in tumor and constipation in tuberculosis.

Administration: Decocted in water for oral dose to be taken 3 times. But *Ren Shen* is decocted isolatedly.

2.18 The Prescription of *Zengye Chengqi Tang*

Name: Purgative Decoction for Increasing Fluid and Sustaining *Qi*.

Source: The book *Wen Bing Tiao Bian*

Ingredients:

Xuan Shen (Radix Scrophulariae) 30 g, *Mai Dong* (Radix Ophiopogonis) 25 g, *Sheng Di* (Radix Rehmanniae) 25 g, *Da*

Huang (Radix et Rhizoma Rhei) 9 g, *Mang Xiao* (Natrii Sulfas) 5g.

Explanation:

Da Huang: The principal drug, being bitter in flavor and cold in nature, purging heat, inducing bowel movements.

Sheng Di and *Mai Dong*: Nourishing *Yin*, promoting the production of body fluids, lubricating the bowels to cause defecation.

Mang Xiao: Resolving masses, removing pathogenic dryness.

Effect: Nourishing *Yin*, promoting the production of body fluids, inducing bowel movements to purge heat.

Indications: Syndrome of constipation due to accumulation of pathogenic heat and exhaustion of body fluids, marked by dry stools, crimson tongue with little coating and thready rapid pulse; including constipation due to hemorrhoid, liver abscess or tumor with the above symptoms.

Administration: Decocted in water for oral dose to be taken twice

Case Study: Modified *Zengye Chengqi Tang* was clinically used to treat 1 case of sporadic viral encephalitis, marked by unconsciousness, delirium, restlessness, aphasia, deviation of the mouth to the left, frequent convulsion of the extremities, 6—day absence of laxation, incontinence of dark scanty urine, reddened tongue with yellowish and dry coating, and wiry slippery pulse. Remarkable effectiveness was seen after 10 doses were taken.

75 cases of epidemic hemorrhagic fever in the oliguric stage were treated with modified *Zengye Chengqi Tang* whose ingredients were as follows:

Sheng Di (Radix Rehmanniae) 30 g, *Xuan Shen* (Radix

Scrophulariae) 30 g, *Mai Dong* (Radix Ophiopogonis) 30 g, *Shui Niu Jiao(Cornu Bubali)* 30 g, *Chi Shao* (Radix Paeoniae Rubra) 15 g, *Dan Pi* (Cortex Moutan) 15 g, *Da Huang* (Radix et Rhizoma Rhei) 30 g, *Mang Xiao* (Natrii Sulfas) 30 g.

Da Huang was steeped in boiled water and *Mang Xiao* was infused with boiling water. They were taken with the decoction of all the other ingredients. Nasal feeding or retention—enema was given to those who could not take the decoction orally. 12 g of *Hou Po* (Cortex Magnoliae Officinalis) and *Zhi Shi*(Fructus Aurantii Immaturus) with the same dosage of 12 g was added in case of enteroparalysis, 15 g of *Hua Fen* (Radix Trichosanthis) in case of too much thirst 12 g of *Zhu Ru* (Caulis Bambusae in Taeniam) in case of vomiting, 9 g of *Shi Di* (Calyx Kaki) in case of hiccup, and *Angong Niuhuang Wan* in case of unconsciousness and delirium due to transmission of pathogenic heat direcly to the pericardium. The treatment result was that among the 75 cases, 73 were cured but the other 2 died.

3 Mediation Prescriptions

3.1 Mediation Prescriptions

Mediation prescriptions are composed in the following way. Exterior—syndrome—relieving drugs are compatible with interior—disorder—alleviating ones, pathogen—eliminating drugs are used together with vital—*Qi*—Strengthening ones, stagnated—liver—*Qi*—dispersing drugs are administered together with spleen—invigorating ones, drugs pungent in flavor and warm in nature are coordinated with those bitter in flavor and cold in nature, and drugs with tonifying action are harmonized with drugs warm or cool in nature. This kind of prescriptions function in mediating the two aspects of a syndrome, removing the stagnated *Qi*, freeing the flow of *Qi*, and promoting the coordination of *Zang—Fu* organs. They are classified as the following three kinds: those of mediating *Shaoyang* channels to treat *Shaoyang* diseases, those of regulating the liver and spleen to promote the coordination between them, and those of mediating the intestine and stomach to treat the disorders due to the incoordination between them.

Mediation prescriptions should not be prescribed when pathogens have been found not to be in the half interior or the half exterior, or when deficiency is more severe than excess and vice versa. Wrong administration of any of them will lose the opportunity to treat a disease timely, making it chronic and hard—healing and even bringing the pathogens into the interior or deriving other syndromes.

3.2 Prescriptions for Mediating *Shaoyang* Channel

This kind of prescriptions are mainly made up of drugs with the action of mediating *Shaoyang* channel. They are indicated for the syndrome due to pathogens in the Gallbladder Channel of Foot—Shaoyang, marked by bitter taste in the mouth, dry throat, dizziness, alternative episodes of chills and fever, full sensation in the chest and hypochondrium, restlessness with strong disire for vomiting, languor, loss of appetite, and taut pulse. *Chai Hu* (Radix Bupleuri) and *Qing Hao* (Herba Artemisiae Annuae) are usually compatible with *Huang Qin* (Radix Scutellariae) in these prescriptions, whose represen tatives are *Xiao Chaihu Tang, Hao Qin Qingdan Tang*, etc.

3.3 The Prescription of *Xiao Chaihu Tang*

Name:Minor Decoction of Bupleurum

Source:The book *Shang Han Lun*

Ingredients:

Chai Hu (Radix Bupleuri)12 g,*Huang Qin* (Radix Scutellariae)9 g,*Ren Shen* (Radix Ginseng)6 g,*Ban Xia* (Rhizoma Pinelliae)9 g,*Zhi Gan Cao* (Radix Glycyrrhizae Preparata)5 g, *Sheng Jiang* (Rhizoma Zingiberis Recens)9 g,*Da Zao* (Fructus Jujubae)4 dates.

Explanation:*Chai Hu:*The principal drug, being bitter and pungent in flavor and slightly cold in nature, tending to distribute so as to disperse pathogenic factors from the superficies of the body.

Huang Qin: Being bitter in taste and cold in nature, being adept in removing pathogenic heat in *Shaoyang* channel.

Ban Xia: Regulating the function of the stomach to promote the descending of the stomach—*Qi*, resolving masses, relieving fullness.

Ren Shen, Gan Cao, Sheng Jiang and *Da Zao:* Invigorating the stomach—*Qi*, promoting the production of body fluid, coordinating *Ying* and *Wei*.

Effect: Mediating Shaoyang channel

Indications: Syndrome due to the attack of exogenous pathogens on *Shaoyang* channel and the struggle between pathogens and vital *Qi*, marked by bitter taste in the mouth, dry throat, dizziness, alternate attacks of chills and fever, fullness and discomfort in the chest and hypochondrium, languor, loss of appetite, restlessness with strong disire for vomiting, thin whitish tongue coating, and taut pulse; including such diseases with the above symptoms as chronic cholecystitis, chronic hepatitis, chronic pelvic inflammation, exudative pleurisy and fever due to cold in the menstrual period.

Administration: Decocted in water for oral dose to be taken twice

Case Study: Modified *Xiao Chaihu Tang* was used to treat 86 cases of high fever. Of all the cases, 36 were due to infection of the respiratory system, 20 due to infection of billiary tract, 9 due to infection of the urinary system, 4 due to postpartum infection, 2 due to hematosepsis, 3 due to hepatitis, 2 due to encephalitis B, 2 due to typhoid fever, 5 due to parotitis and 3 due to bacilary dysentery. The courses of the diseases ranged from 1—30 days, averaging 15 days. The fever due to them subsided within 1—5 days, averaging 3 days.

1 case of strabismus due to the invasion of wind—heat pathogen into Shaoyang channel, marked by one year disease duration, hypopsia with the two pupils tilting to the left at an angle of 50—60 °, pale and reddish tongue with thin whitish coating, and taut thready pulse, was treated with modified *Xiao Chaihu Tang*, whose ingredients were as follows:

Chai Hu (Radix Bupleuri)18 g, *Huang Qin* (Radix Scutellariae)12 g,*Ban Xia* (Rhizoma Pinelliae)12 g, *Dang Shen* (Radix Codonopsis)9 g,*Gan Cao* (Radix Glycyrrhizae)9 g, *Ju Hua* (Flos Chrysanthemi)30 g,*Huang Qi* (Radix Astragali)20 g, *Dang Gui* (Radix Angelicae Sinensis)12 g,*Shan Yu Rou* (Fructus Corni)12 g, *Bai Shao* (Radix Paeoniae Alba)15 g,*Sheng Jiang* (Rhizoma Zingiberis Recens)5 g, *Da zao* (Fructus Jujubae) 5 dates.

The case was cured by taking the decoction every day for a month.

3.4 The Prescription of *Hao Qin Qingdan Tang*

Name: Sweet Wormwood and Scutellaria Decoction for Clearing Damp—heat from Gallbladder

Source: The book *Chong Ding Tong Su Shang Han Lun*

Ingredients:

Qing Hao (Herba Artemisiae Annuae)6 g, *Zhu Ru* (Caulis Bambusae in Taeniam)9 g,*Xian Ban Xia* (Rhizoma Pinelliae)5 g, *Chi Fu Ling* (Poria Rubra)9 g,*Huang Qin* (Radix Scutellariae)6 g, *Zhi Qiao* (Fructus Aurantii)5 g,*Chen Pi* (Pericarpium Citri Reticulatae)5 g,*Biyu San* composed of *Hua Shi* (Talcum), *Gan Cao* (Radix Glycyrrhizae) and *Qing Dai* (Indigo Naturalis)9 g.

Explanation:

Qing Hao: The principal drug, being bitter and pungent in flavor and cold in nature, clearing away pathogenic heat in *Shaoyang* channel.

Huang Qin: The principal drug, being bitter in flavor and cold in nature, removing the pathogenic heat in the gallbladder.

Zhu Ru and *Ban Xia:* Eliminating heat and resolving phlegm.

Chen Pi and *Zhi Qiao:* Smoothing the chest and diaphram, regulating the stomach to cause the adverse flow of *Qi* to go downwards.

Chi Fu Ling and *Biyusan:* Clearing away heat and promoting diuresis,

Effect: Removing heat in the gallbladder, promoting diuresis regulating the stomach and resolving phlegm.

Indications: Syndrome due to damp—heat and phlegm retained in *Shaoyang* channel,marked by alternate attacks of chills and fever with the former being milder than the latter as that in malaria, bitter taste in the mouth, fullness in the stomach, regurgitation of sour and bitter watery fluid or vomiting of yellow thick saliva, and even nausea, hiccup, distending pain in the chest and hypochondrium region, reddened tongue with whitish greasy coating , and rapid pulse with the right slippery and the left taut; including such diseases with the above symptoms as acute cholecystitis, acute gastritis, acute hepatitis, chronic pancreatitis, etc.

Administration: Decocted in water for oral dose to be taken twice Case Study: *Hao Qin Qingdan Tang* was clinically used to treat 13 cases of leptospirosis manifested as fever, headache, general soreness, pain in the gastrocnemius muscle, conjunctival congestion, swelling and pain in the lymph nodes. 1 dose taken, the fever was abated in 2 cases; 2—4 doses taken, the body temperature was returned to normal in 11 cases; 2—6 doses taken, the rest symptoms vanished.

48 cases of cholecystitis were treated with modified *Hao Qin Qingdan Tang* which was composed of:

Qing Hao (Herba Artemisiae Annuae) 10 g, *Huang Qin* (Radix Scutellariae)15 g,*Zhi Qiao* (Fructus Aurantii)9 g, *Zhu Ru* (Caulis Bambusae in Taeniam)9 g,*Ban Xia* (Rhizoma Pinelliae)10 g, *Chen Pi* (Pericarpium Citri Reticulatae)6 g,*Fu Ling* (Poria)15 g, *Hua Shi* (Talcum)30 g, *Gan Cao* (Radix Glycyrrhizae)5 g,*Qing Dai* (Indigo Naturalis) 0.2 g, *Chai Hu* (Radix Bupleuri)10 g, *Da Huang* (Radix et Rhizoma Rhei)6 g, *Long Dan Cao* (Radix Gentianae)10 g, *Che Qian Zi* (Semen Plantaginis)10 g,*Yin Chen* (Herba Artemisiae Scopariae)20 g.

(*Qing Dai* was wrapped in cloth when decocted). The effectiveness was seen in 40 cases,6 cases were improved , and there were no effects in 2 cases.

3.5　The Prescription of *Chaihu Dayuan Yin*

Name:　Bupleurum　Decoction　for　Eliminating Phlegm—dampness in Pleuro—diaphragmatic Interspace

Source: The book *Chong Ding Tong Su Shang Han Lun*

Ingredients:

Chai Hu (Radix Bupleuri)5 g, *Zhi Qiao* (Fructus Aurantii)5 g,*Huan Po* (Cortex Magnoliae Officinalis) 5 g, *Qing Pi* (Pericarpium Citri Reticulatae Viride) 5 g,*Zhi Gan Cao* (Radix Glycyrrhizae Preparata) 2 g, *Huang Qin* (Radix Scutellariae)

5 g,*Jie Geng* (Radix Platycodi) 3 g, *Cao Guo* (Fructus Tsaoko) 2 g,*Bing Lang* (Semen Arecae) 6 g, *He Ye Geng* (Petiolus Nelumbinis) 12 g.

Explanation:*Chai Hu:* The principal drug, being bitter and pungent in flavor and slightly cold in nature, promoting the out—going of exopathogens in the half interior.

Huang Qin: The principal drug, purging the stagnated heat.

Zhi Qiao and *Jie Geng:* Activating the *Qi* in the upper—*Jiao* with the former ascending and the latter descending.

Huan Po and *Cao Guo:* Being pungent in taste and drastic in nature, eliminating turbidity , drying dampness , resolving phlegm, regulating the *Qi* of the middle—*Jiao*.

Qing Pi and *Bing Lang:* Letting *Qi* go downwards to relieve its stagnation, removing phlegm and stagnated food, promoting the flow of *Qi* of the lower—*Jiao*.

He Ye Geng: Being good at promoting the flow of *Qi*, relieving the choking sensation in the chest.

Zhi Gan Cao: Invigorating *Qi*, regulating the stomach, tempering the actions of all the other ingredients.

Effect: Drying dampness and resolving phlegm,eliminating pathogenic factors from pleurodiaphragmatic interspace.

Indications: Syndrome due to phlegm—dampness stagnated in pleuro—diaphragmatic interspace, marked by fullness in the chest and hypochondrium, restlessness, burning sensation in the heart, dizziness, greasy mouth cavity, difficulty in expectoration, onset of alternative chills and fever as that in malaria every other day, thick rough tongue coating, and taut slippery pulse; including such diseases with the above symptoms as malaria, infection of the biliary system ,etc.

Administration:Decocted in water for oral dose to be taken twice

3.6   Prescriptions for Regulating the Liver and Spleen

This kind of prescriptions are mainly composed of drugs with the action of regulating the function of the liver and spleen. They are indicated for the syndrome due to stagnation of the liver—*Qi,* which affects the spleen and stomach, or the dysfunction of the spleen in transportation , which results in failure of the liver in governing normal flow of *Qi;* marked by fullness in the chest and pain in the hypochondriac region, distending pain in the gastrointestinal region, loss of appetite , loose stools, and even alternate attacks of chills and fever. *Chai Hu* (Radix Bupleuri), *Bai Shao* (Radix Paeoniae Alba), *Bai Zhu*(Rhizoma Atractylodis Macrocephalae), *Gan Cao* (Radix Glycyrrhizae),etc. are the commonly used drugs in these prescriptions, whose representatives are *Sini San, Xiaoyao San, Tongxie Yaofang,*etc.

3.7   The prescription of *Sini San*

Name: Powder for Treating Cold Limbs

Source: The book *Shang Han Lun*

Ingredients:

Zhi Gan Cao (Radix Glycyrrhizae Preparata) 6 g, *Zhi Shi* (Fructus Aurantii Immaturus) 6 g, *Chai Hu* (Radix Bupleuri) 6 g, *Shao Yao* (Radix Paeoniae Alba) 9 g.

Explanation:

Chai Hu: The principal drug, being bitter and pungent in

flavor and slightly cold in nature, smoothing the liver and regulating the circulation of Qi, clearing away pathogenic heat from the interior by inducing diaphoresis.

Zhi Shi: Making Qi flow downwards to relieve its stagnancy.

Shao Yao: Replenishing *Yin* to nourish blood, combining *Chai Hu* to disperse the depressed liver−Qi and regulate the spleen.

Gan Cao: Replenishing Qi to regulate the stomach, getting together with *Bai Shao* to relieve spasm and pain, tempering the actions of all the other drugs.

Effect: Letting out pathogens and promoting the circulation of Qi,relieving the depressed liver−Qi and regulating the spleen.

Indications: Cold limbs due to stagnation of *Yang*−Qi in the interior or syndrome due to the incoordination between the liver and the spleen, marked by cold limbs or pain in the chest and abdomen, or loose stools,and wiry pluse; including such diseases with the above symptoms as chronic hepatitis, chronic cholecystitis, gastroduodenal ulcer, intercostal neuralgia, etc.

Administration: Decocted in water for oral dose to be taken twice (Taken as a powder originally)

Case Study: *Sini San* plus *Qing Pi* (Pericarpium Citri Reticulatae Viride) was clinically used to treat 15 cases of acute mastitis. All the cases were cured, among whom 4 were cured, each with 1 dose, 10 each with 2, and 1 with 3, 1 dose being taken daily.

30 cases of heterotypic hyperplasia of gastric mucosa , a morbid condition due to stagnation of the liver−Qi and failure of descending of the stomach−Qi , were treated with modified *Sini San* ,whose ingredients were as follows:

Chai Hu (Radix Bupleuri) 10 g, *Zhi Shi* (Fructus Aurantii Immaturus) 10 g,*Chi Shao* (Radix Paeoniae Rubra) 10 g, *Bai Shao* (Radix Paeoniae Alba) 10 g,*Zhi Gan Cao* (Radix Glycyrrhizae Preparata) 5 g, *Zhi Ban Xia* (Rhizoma Pinelliae Preparata) 10 g,*Chen Pi* (Pericarpium Citri Reticulatae) 6 g.

The gastroscopy made after 3-6 months of treatment showed effectiveness in 25 cases, improvement in 3 and unimprovement in 2 , the effective rate being 93.3%.

3.8   The Prescription of *Chaihu Shugan San*

Name: Bupleurum Powder for Relieving Liver—*Qi*

Source: The book *Jing Yue Quan Shu*

Ingredients:

Chai Hu (Radix Bupleuri) 9 g, *Chen Pi* (Pericarpium Citri Reticulatae) 9 g,*Chuan Xiong* (Rhizoma Chuanxiong) 6 g, *Xiang Fu* (Rhizoma Cyperi) 10 g,*Zhi Qiao* (Fructus Aurantii) 9 g, *Shao Yao* (Radix Paeoniae) 10 g,*Gan Cao* (Radix Glycyrrhizae) 4.5 g.

Explanation:

Chai Hu: The principal drug, being bitter and pungent in taste and slightly cold in nature , soothing the liver to regulate the circulation of *Qi*.

Shao Yao and *Chuan Xiong:* Regulating the flow of blood , nourishing the liver,relieving pain.

Chen Pi: Promoting the circulation of *Qi*, strengthening the stomach.

Xiang Fu and *Zhi Qiao:* Soothing the liver, regulating the circulation of *Qi*.

Gan Cao : Tempering the actions of all the other ingredients, coordinating with *Shao Yao* to exert the action of relieving spasm and pain.

Effect: Soothing the liver to promote the circulation of *Qi*, regulating blood flow to alleviate pain.

Indications:

Syndrome due to stagnation of the liver—*Qi*, marked by hypochondriac pain, fullness and distention in the chest and abdomen, alternate chills and fever, whitish tongue coating, and taut pulse; including such diseases with the above symptoms as chronic gastritis, chronic hepatitis, intercostal neuralgia, etc.

Administration: Decocted in water for oral dose to be taken twice (Taken as a powder originally)

Case Study: 1 case of Gilles dela Tourette's syndrome, a syndrome due to disorders of movement of *Qi* resulting from stagnation of the liver—*Qi* and marked by emotional depression occurred ten days ago and followed by the next day's paroxysmal retching, sound in the throat, tapir mouth and bent legs, all of which gradually became more serious and frequent episode, attacking once about every ten minutes but not in sleep, reddish face, anorexia, dry stools, reddened tongue with yellowish greasy coating, and wiry slippery pulse , was treated with modified *Chaihu Shugan Tang*, whose ingredients were as follows:

Chai Hu (Radix Bupleuri) 10 g, *Zhi Qiao* (Fructus Aurantii) 10 g, *Xiang Fu* (Rhizoma Cyperi) 15 g, *Chuan Xiong* (Rhizoma Chuanxiong) 15 g, *Yu Jin* (Radix Curcumae) 15 g, *Bai Shao* (Radix Paeoniae Alba) 15 g, *Lu Hui* (Aloe) 15 g, *Xuan Fu Hua* (Flos Inulae) 25 g, *Dai Zhe Shi* (Haematitum) 20 g, *Long Gu* (Os Draconis Fossilia) 15 g, *Mu Li* (Concha Ostreae) 15 g, *Gan Cao* (Radix Glycyrrhizae) 15 g.

The case was cured by taking ten doses.

80 cases of internal injury of the thorax were treated with modified *Chaihu Shugan Tang*, whose main ingredients were as follows:

Chai Hu (Radix Bupleuri) 9 g, *Chi Shao* (Radix Paeoniae Rubra) 9 g, *Bai Shao* (Radix Paeoniae Alba) 9 g, *Xiang Fu* (Rhizoma Cyperi) 9 g, *Chuan Xiong* (Rhizoma Chuanxiong) 9 g, *Zhi Qiao* (Fructus Aurantii) 6 g, *Chen Pi* (Pericarpium Citri Reticulatae) 6 g, *Gan Cao* (Radix Glycyrrhizae) 6 g.

In case of *Qi* damaged, *Hou Po* (Cortex Magnoliae Officinalis) and *Mu Xiang* (Radix Aucklandiae) were added; blood injured, *Dan Shen*(Radix Salviae Miltiorrhizae), *Hong Hua* (Flos Carthami) and *Ju Luo* (Retinervus Citri Reticulatae Fructus); injury in the chest ,*Jie Geng* (Radix Platycodi)   and *Xie Bai* (Bulbus Allii Macrostemi); damage under the xiphoid process, *Ding Xiang* (Flos Caryophylli) and *Rou Gui* (Cortex Cinnamomi); severe pain, *Ru Xiang* (Resina Oliboni) and *Mo Yao* (Myrrha);severe dyspnea and cough, *Hou Po* (Cortex Magnoliae Officinalis) and *Xing Ren* (Semen Armeniacae Amarum); and constipation, *Gua Lou Ren* (Semen Trichosanthis) and *Sheng Da Huang* (Radix et Rhizoma Rhei). The treatment result was that all the 80 cases were cured.

3.9   The Prescription of *Xiaoyao San*

Name : Ease Powder

Source: The book *Tai Ping Hui Min He Ji Ju Fang*

Ingredients:

Chai Hu (Radix Bupleuri) 9 g, *Dang Gui* (Radix Angelicae Sinensis) 9 g, *Bai Shao* (Radix Paeoniae Alba) 9 g, *Bai Zhu* (Rhizoma Atractylodis Macrocephalae) 9 g, *Fu Ling* (Poria) 9 g,

Zhi Gan Cao (Radix Glycyrrhizae Preparata) 4.5 g,*Sheng Jiang* (Rhizoma Zingiberis Recens) 6 g, *Bo He* (Herba Menthae) 3 g.

Explanation:

*Chai Hu:*The principal drug, being bitter and pungent in flavor and slightly cold in nature , soothing the liver to promote the circulation of *Qi*.

Dang Gui and *Bai Shao:* Nourishing blood, tonifying the liver.

Bai Zhu and *Fu Ling:* Strengthening the spleen, replenishing *Qi*.

Bo He: Assisting *Chai Hu* in soothing the liver and promoting the circulation of *Qi*.

Sheng Jiang: Warming up the stomach, regulating the middle—*Jiao*.

Zhi Gan Cao: Replenishing *Qi* and strengthening the middle—*Jiao*, getting together with *Bai Shao* to check the hyperactivity of the liver.

Effect: Soothing the liver and promoting the circulation of *Qi*, invigorating the spleen and nourishing blood.

Indications: Syndrome due to stagnation of the liver—*Qi* ,deficiency of blood and failure of the spleen in transportation, marked by pain in the hypochondriac region, alternate attacks of chills and fever , headache, dizziness, dry mouth and throat, lassitude, poor appetite, or irregular menstruation, distention of the breast, pale reddish tongue, and deficient and wiry pulse; including such diseases with the above symptoms as chronic hepatitis, irregular menstruation, chronic gastritis, etc.

Administration: Decocted in water for oral dose to be taken twice (Taken in the form of powder originally)

Case Study: Modified *Xiaoyao San* was clinically used to treat 253 cases of anicteric hepatitis, manifested as distending pain in the hypochondriac region, hepatosplenomegaly,lassitude, weak limbs , anorexia , irregular bowel movements, palpitation, shortness of breath, insomnia, dreamfulness, soreness of the back and loins, and frequent chills and fever. The liver function tests after the treatment showed that 36 cases were cured, 139 improved, the general effective rate being 68.9%.

160 cases of leukorrhagia were treated with modified *Xiaoyao San,* whose main ingredients were as follows:

Chai Hu (Radix Bupleuri), *Dang Gui* (Radix Angelicae Sinensis), *Bai Shao*(Radix Paeoniae Alba), *Bai Zhu* (Rhizoma Atractylodis Macrocephalae), *Fu Ling* (Poria), *Yin Hua* (Flos Lonicerae), *Guan Zhong* (Rhizoma Dryopteris Crassirhizomae).

The result was : Among the 71 cases with whitish vaginal discharge, 48 were cured, 17 remarkably improved, and 6 improved ; of the 89 cases with yellowish vaginal discharge, 60 were cured, 20 noticeably improved, and 9 improved. Most cases each took 4—8 doses.

Better curative effects will be achieved if this prescription is used to treat leukorrhagia due to salpingitis , but a case who has had a long disease duration will be cured only by taking 10—20 doses. If this prescription is used to treat leukorrhagia due to artificial abortion, effectiveness will be found after 3—5 doses are taken.

3.10   The Prescription of *Tongxie Yaofang*

Name: Prescription of Importance for Diarrhea with Pain
Source: The book *Jing Yue Quan Shu*

Ingredients:

Bai Zhu(Rhizoma Atractylodis Macrocephalae) 12 g, *Bai Shao* (Radix Paeoniae Alba) 9 g,*Chen Pi* (Pericarpium Citri Reticulatae) 6 g, *Fang Feng* (Radix Saposhinkoviae) 9 g.

Explanation:

Bai Zhu: One of the principal drugs, being bitter and sweet in flavor and warm in nature , strengthening the spleen to dry pathogenic dampness.

*Bai Shao :*The other principal drug, being bitter and sour in flavor and slightly cold in nature, nourishing the liver to relieve pain.

Chen Pi : Regulating the middle—*Jiao* to remove pathogenic dampness.

*Fang Feng :*Dispersing the liver—*Qi* and regulating the spleen.

Effect: Replenishing the spleen—*Qi* and dispersing the liver—*Qi*

Indications: Syndrome due to stagnation of the liver—*Qi* and deficiency of the spleen, marked by bowel sound, abdominal pain, loose stools, retention of abdominal pain after laxation, thin whitish tongue coating, and taut slow pulse; including such diseases with the above symptoms as allergic colitis, acute enteritis, etc.

Administration: Decocted in water for oral dose to be taken twice (Taken as a powder dose originally)

Case Study: Modified *Tongxie Yaofang* was clinically used to treat 60 cases of acute enteritis , whose disease duration averaged 1—2 days with 4 days as the longest, whose clinical manifestations were as follows: bowel sound, abdominal pain, frequent bowel movements, watery stools in 39 cases, stools of thin gruel—like in 17 cases, pus and bloody stools in 4 cases, rectal tenesmus in 5 cases,fever in 8 cases. All the subjects were adults and all the diagnoses were established through microscopic stools. The treatment result was that most of the subjects were cured , each with 1—2 doses, no side effects being seen ,the curative rate being 90%, and the effective rate being 98%.

187 Cases of enteric irritable syndrome were treated with the prescription of *Tongxie Yaofang* in combination with the prescription of *Sishen Wan* , of which the main ingredients were:

Chai Hu (Radix Bupleuri) 15 g, *Bai Shao* (Radix Paeoniae Alba) 20 g,*Fang Feng* (Radix saposhinkoviae) 15 g, *Rou Kou* (Semen Myristicae) 20 g,*Gu Zhi* (Fructus Psoraleae) 20 g, *Wu Wei Zi* (Fructus Schisandrae) 15 g,*Bai Zhu* (Rhizoma Atractylodis Macrocephalae) 15 g, *Chen Pi* (Pericarpium Citri Reticulatae) 15 g.

One course of treatment involved 7 days and there was an interval of 3 days between 2 courses. 54 cases covered 1 course of treatment ; 87, 2; 36, 3; and 10, 4. The subjects were at the age of 15—78. Their disease duration averaged3 months —26 years, within 10 years in 114 cases. The result was: 128 (68.4%) cases were cured; 41 (21.9%) , improved; 18 (9.7%), unimproved. The effectiveness was seen in 169 cases , in whom the duration for the symptoms such as diarrhea and abdominal pain to disappear averaged 6.8 days. 1 year of follow—up survey was given to 95 cases, among whom 82 (86%) didn't see any relapse of the symptoms, 13 cases who had suffered from a relapse were retreated with the same prescription, curative effects being obtained in 11 cases.

3.11 Prescriptions for Regulating the Intestines and Stomach

This kind of prescriptions are mainly composed of drugs with the action of regulating the function of the intestines and stomach. They are indicated for the syndrome due to the attack of pathogens on the gastrointestine and the combination of heat pathogen with cold one, marked by fullness in the epigastric region, nausea, vomiting, distending pain in the abdomen, bowel sound and loose stools. Drugs such as *Gan Jiang* (Rhizoma Zingiberis), *Huang Qin* (Radix Scutellariae), *Huang Lian* (Rhizoma Coptidis) and *Ban Xia* (Rhizoma Pinelliae)are commonly used in these prescriptions, whose representatives are *Banxia Xiexin Tang*, etc. .

3.12 The Prescription of *Banxia Xiexin Tang*

Name: Pinellia Decoction for Purging Stomach Fire

Source: The book *Shang Han Lun*

Ingredients:

Ban Xia (Rhizoma Pinelliae) 9 g, *Huang Qin* (Radix Scutellariae) 6 g,*Gan Jiang* (Rhizoma Zingiberis) 6 g, *Ren Shen* (Radix Ginseng) 6 g,*Zhi Gan Cao* (Radix Glycyrrhizae Preparata) 6 g, *Huang Lian* (Rhizoma Coptidis) 3 g,*Da Zao* (Fructus Jujubae) 4 dates.

Explanation:

Ban Xia : The principal drug, being pungent in flavor and warm in nature,dispersing accumulation of pathogens, letting the adverse flow of the stomach−*Qi* go downwards to arrest vomiting.

Gan Jiang: Being pungent in flavor and warm in nature, dispelling pathogenic cold.

Huang Qin and *Huang Lian :* Purging pathogenic cold.

Ren Shen and *Da Zao:* Replenishing the *Qi* of the middle—*Jiao.*

Gan Cao : Invigorating the spleen and stomach, tempering the actions of all the other ingredients.

Effect: Letting the upward adverse flow of the stomach—*Qi* go downwards to regulate the function of the stomach, dispersing the accumulation of pathogens to relieve distention.

Indications: Syndrome due to the accumulation of pathogenic cold and heat in the gastro intestines, marked by epigastric fullness without painful sensation,or retching or vomiting , bowel sound, loose stools, thin yellowish greasy tongue coating , and taut rapid pulse; including such diseases with the above symptoms as chronic gastitis, gastroduodenal ulcer, gastroneurosis and chronic enteritis.

Administration: Decocted in water for oral dose to be taken twice

Case Study : 41 cases of cardiaspasm, a syndrome due to phlegm stagnancy and blood stasis in the stomach, which results from the accumulation of pathogenic cold and heat, were clinically treated with modified *Banxia XiexinTang,* whose main ingredients were as follows:

Fa *Ban Xia* (Rhizoma Pinelliae Preparata) 10 g, *Huang Qin* (Radix Scutellariae) 10 g,*Gan Cao* (Radix Glycyrrhizae) 10 g, *Dang Shen* (Radix Codonopsis) 10 g,*Xuan Fu Hua* (Flos Inulae) 10 g, *Huang Lian* (Rhizoma Coptidis) 5 g,*Gan Jiang* (Rhizoma Zingiberis) 5 g, *Dai Zhe Shi* (Haematitum) 30 g,*Da Zao* (Fructus

Jujubae) 30 g.

5–30 doses were taken by each of the cases, averaging 10–20 doses. The result was that 29 cases were cured, 8 remarkably improved, 4 unimproved.

Modified *Banxia Xiexin Tang* was used to treat 48 cases of bleeding due to gastraduodenal ulcer, of which the duration was 2–6 years. In case of hematemesis, *Pao Jiang* (Rhizoma Zingiberis Preparata) was substituted for *Gan Jiang* (Rhizona Zingiberis) and 10 g of *Xiao Ji* (Herba Cirsii) was added. In case the test of occult blood in stool be positive , *Gan Jiang* and 10 g of *E Jiao* (Colla Corii Asini) were administered. In case of abdominal pain, 10 g of *Yan Hu Suo* (Rhizoma Corydalis) was added. The result was that 3 doses led to hemostasis in 31 cases, 5 in 15, and 10 in 2.

4 Prescriptions for Removing Heat

4.1 Prescriptions for Removing Heat

Prescriptions mainly composed of drugs with the action of removing heat, used to clear away pathogenic heat, purge fire pathogen ,eliminate heat from blood , remove toxic material, nourish *Yin* and expel heat from the superficies of the body , and suitable for the treatment of the syndrome due to the heat in the interior are all known as prescriptions for removing heat. Warm , heat and fire are different in degree, but they are the same in property. That is, over warm becomes heat and over heat becomes fire. Therefore, syndromes due to interior heat caused by pathogen of warm , heat or fire may all be treated with prescriptions for removing heat . Syndrome due to interior heat may come from *Qi* system, blood system or *Zang—Fu* organs, so prescriptions for removing heat are classified as the following six kinds: prescriptions for clearing away heat in *Qi* system, suitable for the treatment of the syndrome due to excessive heat in *Qi* system; prescriptions for clearing away heat in *Ying* system and blood system, suitable for the syndrome due to excessive heat in *Ying* and blood systems; prescriptions for clearing away heat and toxic material, suitable for the syndrome due to excessive heat and fire—toxin; prescriptions for clearing away heat from both *Qi* and blood systems, suitable for the syndrome due to intense heat in both *Qi* and blood systems; prescriptions for clearing away heat in *Zang—Fu* organs, suitable for the syndrome due to intense heat in *Zang—Fu* organs; and prescriptions for clearing away heat of deficiency type,suitable for the syndrome due to excessive heat resulting from *Yin* deficiency.

Prescriptions for removing heat are usually administered when exterior syndrome has been relieved but heat in the interior is running wild, or when internal heat is excessive but hasn't become accumulated. When pathogenic heat is in the exterior,the exterior syndrome should be first relieved. When internal heat has been accumulated,purgation should be performed. When exterior syndrome hasn't been relieved but pathogenic heat has appeared in the interior, both the exterior and interior syndromes should be relieved at the same time. Removing heat from blood system when heat is, in fact, in *Qi* system will lead pathogenic factors to the interior, while removing heat from *Qi* system when heat is ,in fact, in blood system will make pathogenic heat in blood system hard to eliminate. Before prescriptions for removing heat are prescribed, the deficient or excess nature of a heat syndrome should be identified, knowing that heat is in *Zang* or in *Fu,* and being sure not to mistaken a false heat syndrome for a true one . Prolonged taking of drugs bitter in flavor and cold in nature with the action of nourishing *Yin* will impair the stomach or injure the *Yang* of the middle—Jiao . When necessary, drugs with the action of enlivening and regulating the stomach are used coordinately. Sometimes, drugs warm and heat in nature are added to those cold and cool in property, which is called as "using corrigent". But under this condition the dose of drugs warm and heat in nature administered should be smaller.

4.2　Prescriptions for Removing Heat in Qi System

This kind of prescriptions are mainly made up of drugs with the action of clearing away heat in Qi system. They are indicated for the syndrome due to intense heat in Qi system which has impaired body fluids. or the syndrome due to intense heat in both Qi and Yin systems,marked by high fever , polydipsia , profuse sweating, aversion to heat, full large pulse, or fever, profuse sweat, restlessness, fullness in the chest, dry mouth,reddened tongue, etc. .lThe commonly used drugs in these prescriptions are *Shi Gao* (Gypsum Fibrosum), *Zhi Mu* (Rhizoma Anemarrhenae), *Zhu Ye* (Herba Lophatheri)and *Zhi Zi* (Fructus Gardeniae), which are usually compatible with drugs with the action of replenishing Qi to promote the production of body fluids such as *Ren Shen* (Radix Genseng), *Mai Dong* (Radix Ophiopogonis), etc. , for heat tends to impair body fluids. The representative prescriptions are *Baihu Tang, Zhuye Shigao Tang* , etc.

4.3　The Prescription of *Baihu Tang*

Name: White Tiger Decoction

Source: The book *Shang Han Lun*

Ingredients:

Shi Gao (Gypsum Fibrosum) 30 g, *Zhi Mu* (Rhizoma Anemarrhenae) 9 g,*Zhi Gan Cao* (Radix Glycyrrhizae Preparata) 3 g, *Jing Mi* (Semen Oryzae Sativae) 9 g.

Explanation:

Shi Gao: The principal drug , being pungent and sweet in flavor and very cold in nature, purging heat in the lung and stomach, eliminating vexation.

Zhi Mu : Purging heat in the lung and stomach, being moisture in nature to moisten dryness.

Gan Cao and *Jing Mi:* Benifiting the stomach , protecting body fluids from being impaired, letting prescriptions very cold in nature not injure the spleen and stomach.

Effect: Removing heat and promoting the production of body fluids

Indications: Syndrome due to intense heat in *Yangming Qi* system, manifested as high fever, flushed face, extreme thirst and strong desire for drink, perspiration and aversion to heat , full large forceful pulse or slippery rapid pulse;including such diseases with the above symptoms as acute or chronic febrile infective diseases, diabetes, heatstroke, diab acute conjunctivitis , etc.

Administration: Decocted in water for oral dose to be taken twice

Case Study: 40 cases (16 were mild, 11 were usual, 10 were severe, and 3 were critical .) of epidemic hemorrhagic fever, which is considered in TCM as a syndrome due to the impairment of body fluid caused by the dryness transformed from epidemic febrile pathogens and due to exhaustion of *Yin* fluid , marked by high fever , being apt to lead to coma and delirium , skin eruption, haematemesis , convulsion due to stirring—up wind, were clinically treated with modified *Baihu Tang,* whose main ingredients were:

Shi Gao (Gypsum Fibrosum) 30—300 g, *Zhi Mu* (Rhizoma Anemarrhenae) 12 g,*Gan Cao* (Radix Glycyrrhizae) 10 g, *Jing Mi* (Semen Oryzae Sativae) 10 g.

In the stage of fever , drugs added were *Shuang Hua* (Flos

Lonicerae), *Lian Qiao* (Fructus Forsythiae) and *Ban Lan Gen* (Radix Isatidis). In the stage of hypotension, such drugs were added as *Ren Shen* (Radix Ginseng), *Mai Dong*(Radix Ophiopogonis), *Wu Wei Zi* (Fructus Schisandrae)and *Dan Shen* (Radix Salviae Miltiorrhiae). In the stage of oliguria , *Jing Mi* (Semen Oryzae Sativae)was omitted and *Xuan Shen* (Radix Scrophulariae), *Sheng Di* (Radix Rehmanniae),*Tian Dong* (Radix Asparagi), *Da Huang* (Radix et Rhizoma Rhei) and *Mang Xiao* (Natrii Sulfas) were added . In the stage of polyuria, drugs added were *Sheng Di* (Radix Rehmanniae), *Shan Yao* (Rhizoma Dioscoreae), *Mai Dong* (Radix Ophiopogonis),*Wu Wei Zi* (Fructus Schisandrae), *Tu Si Zi* (Semen Cuscutae) and *Dang Shen* (Radix Codonopsis). In the stage of restoration, modified *Zhuye Shigao Tang* was prescribed instead. The result was that all the cases were cured within 6—15 days.

21 cases of diabetes were treated with modified *Baihu Tang* and proved prescriptions. The main ingredients of the prescription prescribed were:

Shi Gao (Gypsum Fibrosum) 30—120 g, *Zhi Mu* (Rhizoma Anemarrhenae) 15 g,*Yuan Shen* (Radix Scrophulariae) 30 g, *Shan Yao* (Rhizoma Dioscoreae) 30 g,*Shi Hu* (Herba Dendrobii) 15 g, *Tian Dong* (Radix Asparagi) 15 g,*Hua Fen* (Radix Trichosathis) 15 g, *Lu Gen* (Rhizoma Phragmitis) 30 g,*Gan Cao* (Radix Glycyrrhizae) 3—6 g.

After 3—6 doses ware taken by each of the cases, thirst was obviously relieved and the amount of drink was apparently reduced and both of them were even returned to normal. Then proved prescription was used. Its ingredients were:

Qian Shi (Semen Euryales) 30 g, *Bai Bian Dou* (Semen

Lablab Album) 30 g, *Yi Zhi Ren* (Fructus Alpiniae Oxyphyllae) 30 g, *Yi Yi Ren* (Semen Coicis) 30 g,1 cock (Remove the feather and internal organs and then wash it clean.).

The above 4 ingredients were put into the body cavity of the cock which was closed by sewing. The cock was placed in an earthware pot and heated until the flesh of it was well done . The well—done flesh was eaten and the decoction, even with the dregs, was taken in adequate amount, 1 cock daily or every 2 days. 3—5 cocks taken, 1 dose was prescribed every week or every 10 days in order to consolidate the curative effects.

4.4   The Prescription of *Zhuye Shigao Tang*

Name: Lophatherum and Gypsum Decoction

Source: The book *Shang Han Lun*

Ingredients:

Zhu Ye (Herba Lophatheri) 15 g, *Shi Gao* (Gypsum Fibrosum) 30 g, *Ban Xia* (Rhizoma Pinelliae) 9 g, *Mai Dong* (Radix Ophiopogonis) 15 g, *Ren Shen* (Radix Ginseng) 5 g, *Gan Cao* (Radix Glycyrrhizae) 3 g *Jing Mi* (Semen Oryzae Sativae) 15 g.

Explanation:

Zhu Ye: The principal drug, being sweet and tasteless in flavor and cold in nature, clearing away heat and relieving restlessness.

Shi Gao: The other principal drug, being pungent and sweet in taste and very cold in nature, removing heat and restlessness.

Ren Shen: Replenishing *Qi*.

Mai Dong: Nourishing *Yin*, promoting the production of body fluids.

Ban Xia: Letting the upward adverse flow of the stomach—*Qi* go downwards to arrest vomiting.

Gan Cao and *Jing Mi:* Benefiting and regulating the stomach.

Effect: Clearing away heat and promoting the production of body fluids, replenishing *Qi* and regulating the stomach.

Indications: Syndrome due to lingering fever in the later stage of febrile diseases, marked by fever, profuse sweating, distress in the chest ,nausea due to the adverse flow of *Qi*,dry mouth with desire for drinking , or insomnia due to vexation, reddened tongue with little coating, and weak rapid pulse; including such diseases with the above symptoms as influenza, infant heat stroke syndrome, etc.

Administration: Decocted in water for oral dose to be taken twice

Case Study: *Zhuye Shigao Tang* was clinically used to treat 1 case of fever due to staphylococcus aureus hematosepsis, a syndrome in the later stage of an epidemic febrile disease, in which the pathogens had retreated but the fever was lingering. The case had been treated with antibiotics and *Huanglian Jiedu Tang*. But the treatment failed and the fever remained, varying from 38–39℃ . Treated with modified *Zhuye Shigao Tang,* the case was cured.

1 case of aphtha of pregnancy, 1 case of dyspnea with cough and 1 case of headache were treated with *Zhuye Shigao Tang.* They were all cured.

4.5　The Prescription of *Zhizi Chi Tang*

Name: Decoction of Capejasmine and Phellodendron
Source: The book *Shang Han Lun*

Ingredients: *Zhi Zi* (Fructus Gardeniae) 9 g, *Dan Dou Chi* (Semen Sojae Preparatum) 9 g.

Explanation:

Zhi Zi: The principal drug, being bitter in flavor and cold in nature, purging pathogenic heat.

Dou Chi: Relieving restlessness and assisting *Zhi Zi* in removing heat.

Effect: Clearing away pathogenic heat to relieve restlessness.

Indications: Syndrome due to mild attack of exogenous heat on *Qi* system or lingering fever in the later stage of a disease, marked by fever, fullness in the chest, mania, insomnia due to fidget even with the body turning over in bed again and again reddish tongue with slightly yellowish coating , and rapid pulse; including such diseases with the above symptoms as neurosism, chronic cholecystitis, coronary heart diseases, etc.

Administration: Decocted in water for oral dose to be taken twice

4.6 Prescriptions for Clearing Heat in *Ying* and Blood Systems

This kind of prescriptions are mainly composed of drugs with the action of clearing away heat from both *Ying* and blood systems. They are indicated for the syndrome due to the invasion of pathogenic heat into *Ying* or blood system, marked by fever, dysphoria, thirst or no thirst, coma and delirium, haematemesis, skin eruption, deep red tongue, and rapid pulse. The representative prescriptions are *Qingying Tang, xijiao Dihuang Tang,* etc., in which the common drugs are *Sheng Di* (Radix Rehmanniae), *Xuan Shen* (Radix Scrophulariae), *Dan Pi* (Cortex Moutan), *Chi*

Shao (Radix Paeoniae Rubra) and *Xi Jiao* (Cornu Rhinoceri).

4.7 The Prescription of *Qingying Tang*

Name: Decoction for Clearing Heat in the *Ying* System
Source: The book *Wen Bing Tiao Bian*
Ingredients:

Xi Jiao (Cornu Rhinocerotis) 2 g, *Sheng Di* (Radix Rehmanniae) 15 g, *Yuan Shen* (Radix Scrophulariae) 9 g, *Zhu Ye Xin* (Leaves bud of Herba Lophatheri) 3 g, *Mai Dong* (Radix Ophiopogonis) 9 g, *Dan Shen* (Radix Salviae Miltiorrhizae) 6 g, *Huang Lian* (Rhizoma Coptidis) 5 g, *Yin Hua* (Flos Lonicerae) 9 g, *Lian Qiao* (Fructus Forsythiae) 6 g.

Explanation:

Xi Jiao: One of the principal drugs, being salty in flavor and cold in nature, clearing heat from both *Ying* and blood systems.

Sheng Di: The other principal drug, being sweet and bitter in taste and cold in nature, removing heat from both *Ying* and blood systems.

Yuan Shen and *Mai Dong:* Nourishing *Yin*, dispersing heat pathogens.

Yin Hua, Lian Qiao, Huang Lian and *Zhu Ye:* Promoting the dispersion of pathogens through removing heat and toxic material.

Dan Shen: Promoting the circulation of blood to remove blood stasis.

Effect: Clearing up the *Ying* system to remove pathogenic heat, nourishing *Yin* and promoting the circulation of blood.

Indications: Syndrome appeared in the beginning of the invasion of pathogenic heat into the *Ying* system, marked by fever which is severe at night, fidget, insomnia, delirium, tending to open or close the eyes, thirst or no thirst, or mild skin eruption, crimson dry tongue, and repid pulse; including such diseases with the above symptoms as epidemic cerebrospinal meningitis, encephalitis B, typhus and scarlet fever.

Administration: Decocted in water for oral dose to be taken 3 times

Case Study: Modified *Qingying Tang* was clinically used to treat 5 cases of mucocutaneous lymph node syndrome. In the acute stage, such a prescription was prescribed:

Shui Niu Jiao (Cornu Bubali) 10 g, *Sheng Di* (Radix Rehmanniae) 10 g, *Chi Shao* (Radix Paeoniae Rubra) 10 g, *Dan Shen* (Radix salviae Miltiorrhizae) 10 g, *Yin Hua* (Flos Lonicerae) 10 g, *Lian Qiao* (Fructus Forsythiae) 10 g, *Yuan Shen* (Radix Scrophulariae) 10 g, *Lu Gen* (Rhizoma Phragmitis) 10 g, *Mai Dong* (Radix Ophiopogonis) 10 g, *Gan Cao* (Radix Glycyrrhizae) 10 g.

In the convalescence, 10 g of *Hong Hua* (Flos Carthami) and 10 g of *Chuan Xiong* (Rhizoma Chuanxiong) were added to the above prescription. It took 11—16 days for the fever to subside, averaging 13.5 days, 5—7 days for the skin eruption to vanish, averaging 6 days. Short—term treatment cured 4 cases and improved 1 case. Follow—up was given to 4 cases, none was found to be complicated by angiocardiopathy.

Modified *Qingying Tang* was used to treat 1 case of obstinate night sweating, which had persisted for 12 years and failed to respond to the prolonged treatment of both Western medicine and TCM. This disorder was included in the syndrome due to *Yin* deficiency of the *Ying* system and retention of pathogenic heat in the interior, marked by night sweating starting in early winter, baked sensation before sweating followed by cool body and aversion to cold, dry mouth and tongue, lassitude, edema of the face and feet, and thready rapid pulse, The therapeutic method used was "clearing away heat in the *Ying* system and nourishing *Yin*". The drugs administered were:

Xi Jiao (Cornu Rhinoceri), *Sheng Di* (Radix Rehmanniae), *Yuan Shen* (Radix Scrophulariae), *Dan Pi* (Cortex Moutan), *Mai Dong* (Radix Ophiopogonis), *Bai Wei* (Radix Cynanchi Atrati). The disorder was gradually cured, one year of follow—up didn't see its relapse.

4.8   The Prescription of *Xijiao Dihuang Tang*

Name: Decoction of Rhinoceros Horn and Rehmannia
Source: The book *Bei Ji Qian Jin Yao Fang*
Ingredients:

Xi Jiao (Cornu Rhinoceri) 1.5—3 g *Sheng Di* (Radix Rehmanniae) 30 g, *Chi Shao* (Radix Paeoniae Rubra) 12 g, *Mu Dan Pi* (Cortex Moutan) 9 g.

Explanation:

Xi Jiao: The principal drug, being salty in flavor and cold in nature, clearing away beart—fire, dispelling heat from the blood, removing toxic material.

Sheng Di: Removing heat from the blood, arresting bleeding, nourishing *Yin,* reducing fever.

Chi Shao and *Dan Pi:* Removing heat from the blood, dissipating blood stasis.

Effect; Removing pathogenic heat and toxic material, eliminating heat from the blood and dissipating blood stasis.

Indications: Syndrome due to the invasion of pathogenic heat into the blood system, marked by hemoptysis, nasal bleeding, hematochezia, forgetfulness as if something has gone wrong with the mind, no desire for drinking, restlessness, pain in the thorax, fullness in the abdomen, loose black stools, coma, mania, delirium, purplish skin eruption, and deep red tongue with pricks; including such diseases with the above symptoms as acute leukemia, acute yellow atrophy of liver, thrombocytopenic purpura, epidemic cerebrospinal meningitis, encephalitis B, typhus, hepatic coma, urin aemia, etc.

Administration: Decocted in water for oral dose to be taken 3 times

Case Study: *Xijiao Dihuang Tang* was mainly used clinically to treat 11 cases of primary thrombocytopenic purpura. All the cases suffered from hemorrhage. subcutaneous hemorrhage was found in 11 cases; oral mucosal hemorrhage in 9; nasal hemorrhage in 7; hematochezia in 6; hematuria in 2; hematemesis in 2; conjunctival hemorrhage in 2; coma due to hematorrhea in 2. Platelet count was below $60,000mm^3$ in 5 cases, between $60,000-80,000mm^3$ in the rest. All the 11 cases had the following symptoms: fever, dry mouth but no desire for drinking, dysphoria, flushed face, dark urine, hemorrhage, red dry tongue with thin coating, and slipper rapid pulse, all of which are the signs due to intense heat in the interior. The treatment result was that 6 cases were cured, 4 showed effectiveness, 1 died of the disease.

1 case of acute aplastic anemia was treated with *Xijiao Dihuang Tang* plus:

Da Huang (Radix et Rhizoma Rhei), *Huang Qin* (Radix

Scutellariae), *Ban Lan Gen* (Radix Isatidis), *Lian Qiao* (Fructus Forsythiae), *Shi Gao* (Gypsum Fibrosum), *Zhi Mu* (Rhizoma Anemarrhenae), *Ge Gen* (Radix Puerariae), *Jin Yin Hua* (Flos Lonicerae), *Gan Cao* (Radix Glycyrrhizae).

2 doses taken, the fever subsided from 40.7℃ to 36.5℃, the constipation was relieved, the skin eruption disappeared, the soreness of the throat was alleviated, the low spirits became higher, the amount of hemoglobin reached 9.4 g, the red blood cells increased from 2,800,000 / mm^3 to 3,480,000 / mm^3, the white blood cells rose from 1,600 / mm^3 to 2,800 / mm^3, the lymphocytes reduced from 94% to 44%. Then, instead of the above prescription, prescriptions for clearing away the heat in the *Qi* system, replenishing *Qi* and nourishing *Yin* were used to continue the treatment. At last, the case was cured.

4.9   Prescriptions for Removing Pathogenic Heat and Toxic Material

This kind of prescriptions are mainly composed of drugs with the action of clearing away heat and eliminating toxic material. They are indicated for the syndromes due to serious noxious heat such as epidemic febrile disease, virulent heat pathogen or skin and external diseases; marked by dysphoria, mania, spitting blood or nasal bleeding, or reddish and swelling face, aphthous stomatitis, and sore thoat. The representative prescriptions are *Huanglian Jiedu Tang, Puji Xiaodu Yin, Xianfang Huoming Yin,* ect., in which the commonly used drugs are:

Huang Lian (Rhizoma Coptidis), *Huang Qin* (Radix Scutellariae), *Huang Bai* (Cortex Phellodendri), *Zhi Zi* (Fructus Gardeniae), *Shi Gao* (Gypsum Fibrosum), *Lian Qiao* (Fructus

Forsythiae), *Ban Lan Gen* (Radix Isatidis), *Sheng Ma* (Rhizoma Cimicifugae), *Xuan Shen* (Radix Scrophulariae), *Pu Gong Ying* (Herba Taraxaci), *Zi hua Di Ding* (Herba Violae).

4.10 The Prescription of *Huanglian Jiedu Tang*

Name: Antidotal Decoction of Coptis

Source: The book *Wai Tai Mi Yao*

Ingredients:

Huang Lian (Rhizoma Coptidis) 9 g, *Huang Qin* (Radix Scutellariae) 6 g, *Huang Bai* (Cortex Phellodendri) 6 g, *Zhi Zi* (Fructus Gardeniae) 9 g.

Explanation:

Huang Lian: The principal drug, being bitter in flavor and cold in nature, dispelling pathogenic fire from the heart and the middle—*Jiao.*

Huang Qin: Purging fire in the upper—*Jiao.*

Huang Bai: Removing fire in the lower—*Jiao.*

Zhi Zi: Clearing away fire in the tri—*Jiao,* leading fire to go downward.

Effect: Purging pathogenic fire to detoxicate.

Indications:

Syndrome due to intense heat in the tri—*Jiao* which hasn't impaired body fluids, marked by high fever, dysphoria, dry mouth and thoat, delirium, insomnia, or spitting blood, skin eruption, skin and external diseases of surgery, reddish tongue with yellowish coating, and rapid forceful pulse; including such diseases with the above symptoms as acute purulent infections such as phlegmon, hematosepsis, pyemia, dysentery, pneumonia and hematopathy.

Administration: Decocted in water for oral dose to be taken twice

Case Study: 56 cases of encephalitis B, among which 31 were of severe or fulminat form, 25 were of mild or neutral form, were clinically treated with modified *Huanglian Jiedu Tang,* whose main ingredients were:

Huang Lian (Rhizoma Coptidis) 9 g, *Huang Qin* (Radix Scutellariae) 15 g, *Huang Bai* (Cortex Phellodendri) 15 g, *Zhi Zi* (Fructus Gardeniae) 9 g, *Ban Lan Gen* (Radix Isatidis) 15 g, *Jin Yin Hua* (Flos Lonicerae) 15 g.

In case of persistent fever, *Zhi Mu* (Rhizoma Anemarrhenae) was added. In case of vomting, *Zhu Ru* (Caulis Bambusae in Taeniam) and *Dai Zhe Shi* (Haematitum) were added. In case of clonic convulsions, *Zhijing San* (spasmolytic powder) was added. In case of delirium and coma, *Niuhuang Wan* (cow—bezoare pill) and *Zixue Dan* were added. The result was that 51 cases were cured, 1 case was improved, 4 cases died of the disease.

12 cases of epidemic cerebrospinal meningitis were treated with *Huanglian Jiedu Tang,* which was composed of the same dose of *Huang Lian* (Rhizoma Coptidis), *Huang Bai* (Cortex Phellodendri) and *Zhi Zi* (Fructus Gardeniae). In case of new affection of exterior syndrome, *Yin Hua* (Flos Lonicerae) and *Lian Qiao* (Fructus forsythiae) were added; in case of headache, *Sheng Shi Jue* (Choncha Haliotidis), *Hang Bai Shao* (Radix Paeoniae Alba), *Ci Ji Li* (Fructus Tribuli) and *Tian Ma* (Rhizoma Gastrodiae); in case of constipation, the decoction of *Chengqi Tang;* in case of high fever and restlessness and thirst, *Shi Gao* (Gypsum Fibrosum), *Zhu Ye* (Herba Lophatheri) and *Mai Dong* (Radix Ophiopogonis); in case of profuse expectorations, the

decoction of *Ditan Tang;* in case of delirium. pill of *Zi Xue Dan* and pill of *Niuhuang* Wan; in case of coma, *Shi Chang Pu* (Rhizoma Acori Tatarinowii). *Yuan Zhi* (Radix Polygalae) and *Zhu Li* (Succus Bambosae); in case of nasal bleeding and skin eruption, *Dan Pi* (Cortex Moutan) and *Sheng Di* (Radix Rehamnniae). The treatment result was that all the 12 cases were cured, each of the 4 cases took 3 doses; either of the 2 took 4; each of the 5 took 5; 1 case took 6 doses; none with any sequel.

4.11　The Prescription of *Liangge San*

Name: Powder for Removing Heat from the Diaphram

Source: The book *Tai Ping Hui Min He Ji Ju Fang*

Ingredients:

Da Huang (Radix et Rhizoma Rhei) 600 g, *Po Xiao* (Natrii Sulfas) 600 g. *Zhi Gan Cao* (Radix Glycyrrhizae Preparata) 600 g, *Zhi Zi* (Fructus Gardeniae) 300 g, *Bo He* (Herba Menthae) 300 g, *Huang Qin* (Radix Scutellariae) 300 g, *Lian Qiao* (Fructus Forsythiae) 1,200 g, *Zhu Ye* (Herba Lophatheri) adequate amount, *Feng Mi* (Mel) adequate amount.

Explanation:

Lian Qiao: The principal drug, being bitter in flavor and slightly cold in nature, clearing away heat and toxic material.

Huang Qin: Removing stagnated heat pathogens from the heart and chest.

Zhi Zi: Purging intense heat in the tri—*Jiao* and directing it to go downward.

Bo He and *Zhu Ye:* Dispelling heat in the lung, stomach and heart.

Mang Xiao and *Da huang:* Getting rid of pathogenic heat in the diaphragm and leading heat to go downward.

Bai Mi and *Gan Cao:* Relieving the drastic purgation of *Mang Xiao* and *Da Huang* and assisting them in promoting downward flow of heat.

Effect: Purging intense heat to relieve constipation ,leading heat to go downward and getting rid of it by purgation.

Indications: Syndrome due to heat produced by the accumulated pathogens in the upper and middle *Jiao,* marked by fever, thirst, flushed face and dry lips, burning sensation in the chest, aphthae, or sore throat, spitting blood , nasal bleeding, constipation, reddish urine, reddened tongue with yellowish coating, and slippery rapid pulse; including such diseases with the above sypmtoms as measles, pneumonia, tumor in the mediastinum, pulmonary abscess, etc.

Administration: The ingredients except *Zhu Ye* and *Feng Mi* were ground into powder, 6 g of which was mixed with 3 g of *Zhu Ye* and small amount of *feng Mi* and decocted in water for the decoction, which was taken after meal, 3 times daily. (Or used as a decoction dose, whose dosage was reduced according to the proportions of the ingredients in the original prescription.)

Case Study: 32 cases of infantile acute tonsillitis, a syndrome due to stagnated pathogenic heat in the lung and stomach complicated by wind pathogens, were clinically treated with modified *Liangge San,* whose main ingredients were:

Jiao Shan Zhi (Fructus Gardeniae Scorched) 6–9 g, *Yin Hua* (Flos Lonicerae) 6–9 g, *Lian Qiao* (Fructus Forsythiae) 6–9 g, *Dan Zhu Ye* (Herba Lophatheri) 6–9 g, *Tu Niu Xi* (Radix Achyranthis Bidentatae) 6–9 g, *Xuan Shen* (Radix Scrophulariae) 6–9 g, *Shi Gao* (Gypsum Fibrosum) decocted first

20 – 30 g, *Chuan Jun* (Radix et Rhizoma Rhei) decocted last 3–5 g, *Sheng Gan Cao* (Radix Glycyrrhizae) 3–5 g, *Da Qing Ye* (Folium Isatidis) 9–15 g, *Huang Qin* (Radix Scutellariae) 4.5–6 g.

The youngest case was 16 months old, the oldest 12 years old, all of whom had been treated with antibiotics. After the treatment, they were all cured except two who were not treated continually because of their vomiting.

In addition, 1 case of lobar pneumonia, 1 case of bronchiectasis, 1 case of hypertensive cerebral hemorrhage, and 1 case of tumor in the mediastinum were treated with modified *Liangge San* and remarkable curative effects were achieved in all of them.

4.12   The Prescription of *Puji Xiaodu Yin*

Name: Universal Relief Decoction for Disinfection

Source: The book *Dong Yuan Shi Xiao Fang*

Ingredients:

Huang Qin (Radix Scutellariae) parched with liquor 9 g, *Huang Lian* (Rhizoma Coptidis) parched with liquor 9 g, *Chen Pi* (Pericarpium Citri Reticulatae) 6 g, *Gan Cao* (Radix Glycyrrhizae) 6 g, *Xuan Shen* (Radix Scrophulariae) 6 g, *Chai Hu* (Radix Bupleuri) 6 g, *Jie Geng* (Radix Platycodi) 6 g, *Lian Qiao* (Fructus Forsythiae) 3 g, *Ban Lan Gen* (Radix Isatidis) 3 g, *Ma Bo* (Lasios phaera seu Calvatia) 3 g, *Niu Bang Zi* (Fructus Arctii) 3 g, *Bo He* (Herba Menthae) 3 g, *Jiang Can* (Bombyx Batryticatus) 2 g, *Sheng Ma* (Rhizoma Cimicifugae) 2 g.

Explanation:

Huang Lian and *Huang Qin:* The principal drugs, being bitter in flavor and cold in nature and good at eliminating noxious heat in the head and face after being stir—fried with liquor.

Niu Bang Zi, Lian Qiao, Bo He and *Jiang Can:* Dispersing wind—heat pathogens in the upper —*Jiao*

Xuan Shen, Ma Bo, Ban Lan Gen, Jie Geng and *Gan Cao:* Clearing away noxious heat in the throat, head and face.

Chen Pi: Regulating the flow of *Qi* to remove stasis.

Sheng Ma and *Chai Hu:* Expelling wind—heat and assisting all the other drugs in exerting their actions on the head and face.

Effect: Expelling wind pathogen and clearing away noxious heat

Indications: Syndrome due to noxious heat in the head and face, marked by aversion to cold, fever, redness and swelling and pain of the head and face, difficulty in opening eyes, throat disorder, dry tongue, thirst, reddened tongue with yellowish coating, and rapid forceful pulse; including such diseases with the above symptoms as epidemic parotitis, acute submaxillary lymphnoditis, acute tonsillitis, etc.

Administration: Decocted in water for oral dose to be taken 3 times (Taken originally as a powder)

Case Study: *Puji Xiaodu Yin* was clinically used to treat 69 cases of acute tonsillitis, marked by fever, sore throat, sweating , dry stools or constipation, poor appetite, yellowish urine or oliguria, reddened tongue with thick whitish or yellowish tongue coating , and floating rapid pulse. Congestion of throat was seen in all the 69 cases, First degree of antiadoncus was seen in 9 cases. second degree in 60. pus specks were seen in 53 cases. The result was: 65 cases were cured, 3 improved, 1 unimproved, the general effective rate being 98.6%.

100 cases of epidemic parotitis were treated with modified *Puji Xiaodu Yin,* whose main ingredients were:

Yin Hua (Flos Lonicerae), *Lian Qiao* (Fructus Forsythiae), *Niu Bang Zi* (Fructus Arctii), *Zhi Zi* (Fructus Gardeniae), *Ban Lan Gen* (Radix Isatidis), *Ma Bo* (Lasiophaera seu Calvatia), *Pu Gong Ying* (Herba Taraxaci), *Jie Geng* (Radix Platycodi).

In case of severe fever and headache, such drugs were added: *sang Ye* (Folium Mori), *Ju Hua* (Flos Chrysanthemi) and *Bo He* (Herba Menthae). In case of constipation, drugs added were : *Yuan Ming Fen* (powder of Natrii sulfas) and *Yuan Shen* (Radix Scrophulariae). In case of high fever, pill of *Zixue Dan* was also prescribed or pill of *Liushen Wan* was sucked in the mouth, 3-5 pills each time, 2 or 3 times daily. It took 2 days for 31 cases to be cured, 4 days for 46 cases , 6 days for 18 cases, 8-10 days for 5 cases.

Puji Xiaodu Yin is known to have better bacteriostatic action on a-hemolytic or beta-hemolytic streptococcus, Diplococcus pneumoniae, Staphylococcus aureus and Staphylococcus albus. On bacteria of other kinds its bacteriostatic action is different in degree.

4.13 Prescriptions for Clearing away Heat from *Qi* and Blood Systems

This kind of prescriptions are mainly made up of drugs with the action of clearing up the *Qi* system and removing heat from the blood system. They are suitable for the syndromes due to epidemic febrile troubles or noxious heat which are in full swing both in the interior and in the exterior and disturbing both the *Qi* and blood systems, marked by high fever, fidgets, thirst, spitting blood, nasal bleeding, skin eruption, coma and delirium. Drugs with the action of clearing up the *Qi* system such as *Shi Gao* (Gypsum Fibrosum) and *Zhi Mu* (Rhizoma Anemarrhenae) are often compatible with drugs with the action of removing heat in the blood such as *Xi Jiao* (Cornu Rhinoceri) and *Di Huang* (Radix Rehmanniae) in this kind of prescriptions, whose representatives are *Qingwen Baidu Yin* and the like.

4.14 The Prescription of *Qingwen Baidu Yin*

Name: Antipyretic and Antitoxic Decoction
Source: The book *Yi Zhen Yi De*
Ingredients:

Shi Gao (Gypsum Fibrosum) 30 g, *Sheng Di* (Radix Rehmanniae) 12 g, *Xi Jiao* (Cornu Rhinocerotis) 6 g, *Huang Lian* (Rhizoma Coptidis) 6 g, *Huang Qin* (Radix Scutellariae) 6 g, *Zhi Zi* (Fructus Gardeniae) 10 g, *Mu Dan Pi* (Cortex Moutan) 6 g, *Xuan Shen* (Radix Scrophulariae) 10 g, *Lian Qiao* (Fructus Forsythiae) 15 g, *Chi Shao* (Radix Paeoniae Rubra) 6 g, *Zhi Mu* (Rhizoma Anemarrhenae) 6 g, *Jie Geng* (Radix Platycodi) 9 g, *Zhu Ye* (Herba Lophatheri) 6 g, *Gan Cao* (Radix Glycyrrhizae) 6 g.

Explanation:

Shi Gao: Being pungent in taste and cold in nature, removing heat and purging fire.

Xi Jiao: One of the principal drugs, being salty in flavor and cold in nature, clearing away heat in the blood and nourishing *Yin.*

Sheng Di: The other principal drug, being sweet and bitter in flavor and cold in nature, removing heat in the blood and nourishing *Yin*.

Zhi Mu: Nourishing *Yin* and purging fire.

Zhi Zi, Huang Lian, Huang Qin, Lian Qiao and *Xuan Shen:* Clearing away heat and toxic material.

Dan Pi and *Chi Shao:* Removing heat in the blood and promoting the circulation of blood.

Jie Geng and *Zhu Ye:* Making the potency of the drugs go upward.

Gan Cao: Clearing away heat and toxic material and tempering the actions of all the other ingredients.

Effect: Clearing away heat and toxic material, removing heat in the blood and purging fire.

Indications: Syndrome due to noxious heat at the full in both the *Qi* and blood systems, marked by high fever, thirst with strong desire for drinking, headache as if the head were being splitted, coma and delirium, blurred vision, or skin eruption, or spitting blood, epistaxis, convulsion of the limbs or cold limbs, crimson tongue, very dry lips, and deep rapid pulse or deep thready rapid pulse or floating large rapid pulse; including such diseases with the above symptoms as epidemic cerebrospinal meningitis, severe influenza, epidemic hemorrhagic fever and hematosepsis.

Administration: Decocted in water for oral dose to be taken 3 times. *Shi Gao* was decocted first for about 10 seconds after the content was boiling, and, then , the other ingredients except *Xi Jiao* were put into the boiling content and decocted for the decoction . *Xi Jiao* was ground into powder in a small amount of water and drunk with the decoction.

Case Study: 23 cases of measles with severe noxious heat, a

syndrome due to intense heat in both the *Qi* and blood systems, marked by high fever, sweat or difficulty in sweating, thirst with desire for drinking, maroon and reddened tongue with yellowish dry coating, were clinically treated with modified *Qingwen Baidu Yin,* whose main ingredients were:

Sheng Shi Gao (Gypsum Fibrosum) 24 g, *Sheng Di* (Radix Rehmanniae) 9 g, *Lian Qiao* (Fructus Forsythiae) 9 g, *Shan Zhi* (Fructus Gardeniae) 9 g, *Huang Qin* (Radix Scutellariae) 4.5 g, *Dan Pi* (Cortex Moutan) 9 g, *Huang Lian* (Rhizoma Coptidis) 1.5 g, *Chi Shao* (Radix Paeoniae Rubra) 9 g, *Xuan Shen* (Radix Scrophulariae) 6 g, *Jin Yin Hua* (Flos Lonicerae) 9 g, *Lu Gen* (Rhizoma Phragmitis) 30 g.

In case of asthma and cough with flaring of nares, pale complexion and dry lips, *Chi Shao* and *Xuan Shen* were omitted, but *Ma Huang* (Herba Ephedrae), *Xing Ren* (Semen Armeniacae Amarum) and *Hou Zao San* (Calculus Macacae powder) were added. In case of hoarse voice, red and swollen throat and choke in drinking, *Shan Dou Gen* (Radix Sophorae Tonkinensis) and *Gua Jin Deng* (Calyx seu Fructus Physalis) were added. In case of frequent yellow sticky hot stools with disagreeable odor, *Ge Gen* (Radix Puerariae) was added, *Huang Qin* was omitted, and *Huang Lian* was parched. In case of halitosis and ulcerative gingivitis, *Ban Lan Gen* (Radix Isatidis) was added. After the treatment, all the 23 cases, of which 15 were complicated by pneumonia, were cured.

1 case of cerebritis due to tetracoccus was treated with modified *Qingwen Baidu Yin.* The patient was a child at the age of 6. It had been one and a half months since he suddenly had the symptoms of vomiting and fever followed by abdominal pain,

headache with the head tilted to the left , bent upper extremities, prolapse of the left shoulder, weak fingers with difficulty in holding things, and falling down in walking due to weak legs. The patient had been admitted to hospital for treatment with the symptoms relieved. Soon after being discharged from hospital , he suffered from a relapse of the disease manifested as the head tilted to the left, low prolapse of the left shoulder, mild fever in the morning , high fever and sweating in the afternoon, tiredness with desire for sleep, pale and yellowish complexion, reddened tongue without coating, and rapid pulse. Being treated mainly with the above modified prescription, the patient was completely cured. Follow—up proved that he was as well as usual.

4.15   Prescriptions for Clearing away Heat in *Zang—Fu* Organs

This kind of prescriptions are mainly composed of drugs with the action of removing heat from *Zang* or *Fu* organs. They are suitable for the syndromes due to pathogenic fire resulting from too much pathogenic heat in a *Zang* or *Fu* organ. Heat—evil in excess may be located in different *Zang* or *Fu* organs. Therefore, drug therapy used to treat this kind of syndromes is different accordingly. For instance, syndrome due to excess pathogenic heat in the Heart Channel is treated with drugs having the action of clearing away the heart—fire, such as *Huang Lian* (Rhizoma Coptidis), *Zhi Zi* (Fructus Gardeniae), *Lian Zi Xin* (Plumula Nelumbinis) and *Mu Tong* (Caulis Aristolochiae Manshuriensis). Syndrome due to excess fire in the liver and gallbladder is treated with drugs having the action of purging pathogenic heat from the liver, such as *Long Dan Cao* (Radix Gentianae), *Xia Ku Cao*

(Spica Prunellae) and *Qing Dai* (Indigo Naturalis). Syndrome due to pathogenic heat in the lung is treated with drugs having the action of clearing away the lung—heat, such as *Huang Qin* (Radix Scutellariae), *Sang Bai Pi* (Cortex Mori) and *Shi Gao* (Gypsum Fibrosum). When excessive heat is in the spleen and stomach, *Fang Feng* (Radix Saposhinkoviae), *Shi Gao* and *Shan Zhi* (Fructus Gardeniae) are, on one hand, used to disperse accumulated heat in the spleen and stomach; on the other hand, *Huang Lian*, *Sheng Ma*(Rhizoma Cimicifugae) and *Sheng Di* (Radix Rehmanniae) are used to remove heat from the stomach and blood. In case of stomach—heat and *Yin* deficiency, *Shi Gao, Shu Di* (Radix Rehmanniae Praeparata) and *Mai Dong* (Radix Ophiopogonis) are used to clear away the stomach—heat and nourish *Yin*. If heat evil is in the intestines, *Bai Tou Weng* (Radix Pulsatillae), *Huang Lian* and *Huang Bai* (Cortex Phellodendri) are used to purge noxious heat in the intestines . The representative prescriptions are *Daochi San* for removing heat from the Heart Channel, *Longdan Xiegan Tang* for removing excess fire from the liver and gallbladder, *Xiebai San* for removing heat from the lung, *Xiehuang San* and *Qingwei San* for removing heat from the spleen and stomach, *Yunü Jian* for removing heat from the stomach and nourishing *Yin,* and *Baitouweng Tang* and *Shaoyao Tang* for removing damp—heat from the intestines.

4.16   The Prescription of *Daochi San*

Name: Powder for Treating Dark Urine
Source: The book *Xiao Er Yao Zheng Zhi Jue*
Ingredients:
Sheng Di (Radix Rehmanniae) 9 g, *Mu Tong* (Caulis

Aristolochiae Manshuriensis) 6 g, *Gan Cao* (Radix Glycyrrhizae) 6 g, *Zhu Ye* (Herba Lophatheri) 9 g.

Explanation:

Sheng Di: The principal drug, being sweet and bitter in flavor and cold in nature, removing pathogenic heat from the blood and nourishing *Yin.*

Mu Tong: Clearing away pathogenic heat both in the Heart Channel and in the small intestine to promote diuresis.

Gan Cao: Removing heat and toxic material, tempering the actions of all the other ingredients.

Zhu Ye: Dispelling pathogenic heat from the heart and relieving restelessness.

Effect: Removing pathogenic heat from the heart, nourishing *Yin,* promoting diuresis.

Indications: Syndrome due to pathogenic heat accumulated in the Heart Channel and the small intestine, marked by restlessness and hot feeling in the chest, thirst, flushed face, preference for cold drink, aphthae, or dark urine excreted with difficulty and stabbing pain, reddened tongue, and rapid pulse; including such diseases with the above symptoms as acute infection of the urinary tract, stomatitis and stone of the urinary system.

Administration: Decocted in water for oral dose to be taken twice (Taken originally as a powder)

Case Study: Modified *Daochi San* was clinically used to treat 15 cases of stranguria, among which 5 cases were from urolithiasis, 7 cases were caused by disorder of *Qi,* 3 cases were complicated by hematuria. The manifestations were: strangury with pain referring to the umbilical region, and even distention or pain of the loins, whitish greasy or thin yellowish tongue coating, and floating rapid or thready rapid pulse. In the treatment of stranguria from urolithiasis, *Hai Jin Sha* (Spora Lygodii), *Bian Xu* (Herba Polygoni Avicularis) and *Jin Qian Cao* (Herba Lysimachiae) were added to the prescription of *Daochi San;* in stranguria complicated by hematuria, *Bai Mao Gen* (Rhizoma Imperatae), *Sheng Ce Bai* (Cacumen Biotae) and *Xiao Ji* (Herba Cirri) were added; in stranguria caused by disorder of *Qi, Hou Po* (Cortex Magnoliae Officinalis) and *Xiang Fu* (Rhizoma Cyperi) were added . The result was that 9 cases were cured, 6 cases were improved.

Modified *Daochi San* was also used to treat 50 cases of infantile disorders in the hand, foot and mouth. The cases were in three types. 26 cases of damp—heat type were treated with the prescription of *Daochi San* plus:

Ban Lan Gen (Radix Isatidis), *Chong Lou* (Rhizoma Paridis), *Huang Qin* (Radix Scutellariae).

15 cases of heat—over—dampness type were treated with *Daochi San* plus:

Shi Gao (Gypsum Fibrosum), *Zhi Mu* (Rhizoma Anemarrhenae), *Zhi Zi* (Fructus Gardeniae), *Lian Qiao* (Fructus Forsythiae), *Ban Lan Gen* (Radix Isatidis), *Da Qing Ye* (Folium Isatidis), *Chong Lou* (Rhizoma Paridis), *Jiang Can* (Bombyx Batryticatus).

9 cases of dampness—over—heat type were treated with *Daochi San* plus:

Fu Ling (Poria), *Ze Xie* (Rhizoma Alismatis), *Cang Zhu* (Rhizoma Atractylodis), *Huang Bai* (Cortex Phellodendri), *Ban Lan Gen* (Radix Isatidis), *Chong Lou* (Rhizoma Paridis), *Hua Shi* (Talcum).

but minus *Sheng Di* (Radix Rehmanniae) . The result was: 34 cases were cured after 3 doses were taken by each of them, 12 cases were cured after 6 doses were taken by each of them, ineffectiveness and relapse after the treatment were seen in 4 cases, the total effective rate was 92%. .

4.17   The Prescription of *Longdan Xiegan Tang*

Name: Decoction of Gentiana for Purging Liver—fire
Source: The book *Yi Fang Ji Jie*
Ingredients:

Long Dan Cao (Radix Gentianae) stir—fried with liquor 6 g, *Huang Qin* (Radix Scutellariae) parched 6 g, *Zhi Zi* (Fructus Gardeniae) stir—fried with liquor 9 g, *Ze Xie* (Rhizoma Alismatis) 12 g, *Mu Tong* (Caulis Aristolochiae Manshuriensis) 9 g, *Che Qian Zi* (Semen Plantaginis) 9 g, *Dang Gui* (Radix Angelicae Sinensis) washed with liquor 3 g, *Sheng Di* (Radix Rehmanniae) stir—fried with liquor 9 g, *Chai Hu* (Radix Bupleuri) 6 g, *Gan Cao* (Radix Glycyrrhizae) 6 g.

Explanation:

Long Dan Cao: The principal drug, being bitter in taste and cold in nature , purging excess fire in the liver and gallbladder, removing damp—heat from the lower—*Jiao*.

Huang Qin and *Zhi Zi:* Being bitter in flavor and cold in nature, purging pathogenic fire.

Ze Xie, Mu Tong and *Che Qian Zi:* Removing heat and promoting diuresis, discharging damp—heat by way of the urinary tract.

Sheng Di and *Dang Gui:* Nourishing *Yin* and blood. Heat in the Liver Channel tends to impair *Yin*—blood. If drugs being bitter in flavor and cold in nature and capable of drying dampness are used , the *Yin* will be further exhausted. That's why *Sheng Di* and *Dang Gui* are used.

Chai Hu: Soothing the liver and gallbladder to promote the circulation of *Qi*.

Gan Cao: Regulating the middle—*Jiao* and tempering the actions of all the other ingredients.

Effect: Purging excessive pathogenic fire in the liver and gallbladder, clearing away damp—heat in the lower—*Jiao*.

Indications: Syndrome due to excessive pathogenic fire in the liver and gallbladder or downward flow of damp—heat in the liver Channel to the lower—*Jiao* , marked by headache, reddened eyes, pain in the hypochondriac region, bitter taste in the mouth, deafness, swelling of ears, or swelling of vulva, pruritus vulvae, turbid and dripping urine, and leukorrhea of damp—heat type; including such diseases with the above symptoms as acute conjunctivitis, otitis media acuta, hypertension, acute icterohepatitis, acute cholecystitis, herpes zoster, acute pyelonephritis, oystitis, urethritis, acute pelvitis of pelvic cavity, and acute prostatitis.

Administration: Decocted in water for oral dose to be taken twice

Contraindication: Patients whose spleen and stomach are in the deficient and cold state should not be treated with this prescription, for most of the drugs in the prescription are bitter in flavor and cold in nature.

Case Study:

172 cases of acute icterohepatitis included in the syndrome due to damp—heat pathogens in the liver and gallbladder, marked

by anorexia , yellow urine, moderately yellowish sclera and skin, hepatomegaly and impairment of liver function were clinically treated with the prescription of *Longdan Xiegan Tang* minus:

Ze Xie (Rhizoma Alismatis), *Che Qian Zi* (Semen Plantaginis), *Zhi Zi* (Fructus Gardeniae), but plus: *Yin Chen* (Herba Artemisiae Scopariae), *Hong Zao* (Fructus Jujubae). Each of the cases took 30—40 doses without any interval and they were cured with the course for the treatment averaging 28 days.

1 case of rapidly progressing hypertension manifested as dizziness, headache, dry and bitter sensation in the mouth, palpitation, dreamfulness, restlessness, irritability, yellowish and dark urine, reddened tongue with yellowish greasy coating , taut slippery pulse, blood pressure being 200 / 148 mmHg, urinary protein being +++, kidney function being NPN 60 mg, and papilledema, was treated with the prescription of *Longdan Xiegan Tang* minus *Dang Gui* and *Sheng Di* but plus:

Xia Ku Cao (Spica Prunellae), *Sheng Long Gu* (Os Draconis Fossilia), *Sheng Mu Li* (Concha Ostreae), *Jiang Can* (Bombyx Batryticatus), *Shi Chang Pu* (Rhizoma Acori Tatarinowii). All the symptoms vanished after 4 doses were taken with the blood pressure returned to 120 / 86 mmHg. 2 months later, the case was cured.

4.18 The Prescription of *Zuojin Wan*

Name: Pill for Treating the Lung
Source: The book *Dan Xi Xin Fa*
Ingredients:

Huang Lian (Rhizoma Coptidis) 9 g, *Wu Zhu Yu* (Fructus Euodiae) 1.5 g.

Explanation:

Huang Lian: The principal drug, being bitter in flavor and cold in nature, removing heat, purging fire.

Wu Zhu Yu: Being pungent in taste and hot in nature, restricting the cold nature of *Huang Lian,* exerting its potency to the liver to descend the adverse flow of Qi, promoting the coordination between the stomach and the liver.

Effect: Clearing away pathogenic heat and fire from the liver, descending the adverse flow of *Qi* to arrest vomiting.

Indications: Syndrome due to pathogenic fire in the liver produced by stagnation of the liver—Qi and due to attacking of the liver—fire on the stomach, marked by distending pain in the hypochondriac region, heart—burning, regurgitation of sour fluid, vomiting, bitter taste in the mouth, fullness sensation in the stomach, eructation, reddened tongue with yellowish coating, and taut rapid pulse; including such diseases with the above symptoms as acute gastritis, gastroduodenal ulcer and nonicteric infective hepatitis.

Administration: Decocted in water for oral dose to be taken twice (Taken originally in the form of pills)

Case Study: 24 cases of ulcerative disorders were clinically treated with the modification of *Zuojin Wan,* whose main ingredients were:

Huang Qin (Radix Scutellariae) instead of Huang Lian 12 g, *Wu Zhu Yu* (Fructus Evodiae) 1.5 g, If the syndrome was due to incoordination between the liver and the stomach, *Sini San* (a powder) was also prescribed together with the modification. If the syndrome was caused by damp—heat in the spleen and stomach, *Pingwei San* (a powder) was used in combination with the modifiaction. Provided that the syndrome was brought about by the accumulated dampness due to deficiency of the spleen, *Liujunzi Tang* and the modification were administered at the same time. After the treatment, the main symptoms such as pain in the stomach and anorexia were relieved to different extent.

4.19 The Prescription of *Xiebai San*

Name: Lung—heat Expelling Powder

Source: The book *Xiao Er Yao Zheng Zhi Jue*

Ingredients:

Di Gu Pi (Cortex Lycii) 12 g, *Sang Bai Pi*(Cortex Mori) 12 g, *Zhi Gan Cao* (Radix Glycyrrhizae Preparata) 3 g, *Jing Mi* (Semen Oryzae Sativae) 6 g.

Explanation:

Sang Bai Pi: The principal drug, being sweet in flavor and cold in nature, removing heat from the lung and clearing away accumulated heat.

Di Gu Pi: Purging fire pathogen hidden in the lung, relieving fever of deficiency type.

Zhi Gan Cao and *Jing Mi:* Nourishing and regulating the stomach to support the lung—*Qi*.

Effect: Removing heat from the lung, relieving cough and asthma.

Indications: Syndrome due to accumulated heat resulting from fire pathogen hidden in the lung, marked by cough even leading to asthma, hot and damp skin which is severe at 3—5 o'clock in the afternoon, reddened tongue with yellowish coating, and thready rapid pulse; including such diseases with the above symptoms as acute bronchitis, bronchial asthma, pulmonary emphysema complicated by infection, infantile pneumonia, etc.

Administration: Decocted in water for oral dose to be taken twice (Taken originally in the form of powder)

Case Study: 63 cases of chin cough in the stage of spasmodic cough, mainly marked by uninterrupted cough with sound produced when inhaling and which is relieved a little after thick sputum is expectorated, were treated clinically with the prescription of *Xiebai San*. Among the 63 cases , 23 were due to pathogenic fire hidden in the lung. They were treated with the prescription plus:

Bai Bu (Radix Stemonae), *Ma Dou Ling* (Fructus Aristolochiae), *Xing Ren* (Semen Armeniacae Amarum), *Bei Mu* (Bulbus Fritillariae Cirrhosae), *Huang Qin* (Radix Scutellariae), *Gua Lou Pi* (Pericarpium Trichosanthis), *Pi Pa Ye* (Folium Eriobotryae).

in order to purge the pathogenic fire in the lung. If the syndrome was complicated by hemoptysis and nasal bleeding , drugs added to the prescription were:

Ce Bai Ye (Cacumen platyclad) *Dan Pi* (Cortex Moutan) *Ou Jie* (Nodus Nelumbinis Rhizomatis)

in order to remove heat from the blood and stop bleeding. 28 cases were due to wind—heat in the exterior. They were treated with the prescription plus:

Bo He (Herba Menthae), *Niu Bang Zi* (Fructus Arctii), *Zhu Ye* (Herba Lophatheri), *Xing Ren* (Semen Armeniacae Amarum), *Lian Qiao* (Fructus Forsythiae), *Bai Bu* (Radix Stemonae).

12 cases were due to attack of wind—cold on the exterior. They were treated with the prescription plus:

Ma Huang (Herba Ephedrae), *Xing Ren* (Semen Armeniacae

Amarum), *Qian Hu* (Radix Peucedani), *Pi Pa Ye* (Folium Eriobotryae), *Zhu Ru* (Caulis Bambusae in Taeniam), *Fang Feng* (Radix Saposhinkoviae).

All the 63 cases were cured, each of them taking 4—8 doses.

4.20   The Prescription of *Qingwei San*

Name: Powder for Clearing the Stomach—heat

Source: The book *Lan Shi Mi Cang*

Ingredients:

Sheng Di Huang (Radix Rehmanniae) 12 g, *Dang Gui* (Radix Angelicae Sinensis) 6 g, *Mu Dan Pi* (Cortex Moutan) 9 g, *Huang Lian* (Rhizoma Coptidis) 4.5 g, *Sheng Ma* (Rhizoma Cimicifugae) 6 g.

Explanation:

Huang Lian: The principal drug, being bitter in flavor and cold in nature, removing accumulated heat in the stomach.

Sheng Di: Removing heat from the blood, nourishing *Yin*.

Dan Pi: Removing heat from the blood to clear away heat pathogens.

Dang Gui: Nourishing and regulating the blood.

Sheng Ma: Dispersing fire pathogen to detoxicate.

Effect: Removing heat from the stomach and blood

Indications: Syndrome due to accumulated heat in the stomach and flaring—up of the stomach—fire, marked by headache induced by toothache, hotness in the cheeks, teeth averse to heat but preferable for cold, or ulceration of gums, or gingival atrophy with bleeding, or swelling and pain in the lips, tongue and cheeks, or hot foul breath, dry mouth and tongue, reddened tongue with yellowish coating, and slippery full rapid pulse; including such diseases with the above symptoms as prosopalgia, stomatitis, periodontitis, chronic gastritis, etc.

Administration: Decocted in water for oral dose to be taken twice (Taken originally in the form of powder)

Case Study: Toothache and 60 cases of pulpitis or periodontitis due to pathogenic fire in the stomach were clinically treated with modified *Qingwei San*, whose ingredients were :

those in the prescription of *Qingwei San*

Shi Gao (Gypsum Fibrosum), *Zhi Mu* (Rhizoma Anemarrhenae), *Yin Hua* (Flos Lonicerae), *Lian Qiao* (Fructus Forsythiae).

Satisfactory curative effects were achieved.

56 cases of recurrent aphtha were treated with modified *Qingwei San*, whose ingredients were :

Huang Lian (Rhizoma Coptidis) 9 g, *Sheng Di* (Radix Rehmanniae) 45 g, *Dang Gui* (Radix Angelicae Sinensis) 12 g, *Dan Pi* (Cortex Moutan) 16 g, *Sheng Ma* (Rhizoma Cimicifugae) 12 g, *Shuang Hua* (Flos Lonicerae) 12 g, *Gong Ying* (Herba Taraxaci) 16 g, *Lian Qiao* (Fructus Forsythiae) 16 g, *Dan Zhu Ye* (Herba Lophatheri) 12 g, *Gan Cao* (Radix Glycyrrhizae) 6 g. The treatment result was: effectiveness was seen in 31 cases, improvement in 18, failure in 7, the total effective rate being 87.5%.

4.21　The Prescription of *Xiehuang San*

Name: Powder for Expelling Pathogenic Fire in the Spleen and Stomach

Source: The book *Xiao Er Yao Zheng Zhi Jue*

Ingredients:

Huo Xiang (Herba Agastachis) 12 g, *Shan Zhi Ren* (Semen

Gardeniae) 6 g, *Shi Gao* (Gypsum Fibrosum) 15 g, *Gan Cao* (Radix Glycyrrhizae) 6 g, *Fang Feng* (Radix Saposhinkoviae) 9 g.

Explanation:

Shi Gao: One of the principal drugs, being pungent and sweet in flavor and very cold in nature, clearing away accumulated heat in the spleen and stomach.

Zhi Zi: The other principal drug, being bitter in taste and cold in nature, removing heat retained in the spleen and stomach.

Fang Feng: Dispersing pathogenic fire hidden in the spleen.

Huo Xiang: Being aromatic and promoting functioning of the spleen, assisting *Fang Feng* in dispersing heat in the spleen and stomach.

Gan Cao: Purging pathogenic fire, regulating the stomach, tempering the actions of all the other ingredients.

Effect: Purging latent pathogenic fire in the spleen and stomach

Indications: Syndrome due to latent pathogenic fire in the spleen and stomach, marked by aphthae, halitosis, restlessness, thirst, hungriness, dry mouth and lips, reddened tongue, and rapid pulse; including such diseases with the above symptoms as stomatitis and periodontitis.

Administration: Decocted in water for oral dose to be taken twice (Taken originally in the form of powder).

4.22   The Prescription of *Yunü Jian*

Name: Gypsum Decoction
Source: The book *Jing Yue Quan Shu*
Ingredients:

Shi Gao (Gypsum Fibrosum) 18 g, *Shu Di* (Radix Rehmanniae Preparata) 15 g, *Mai Dong* (Radix Ophiopogonis) 6 g, *Zhi Mu* (Rhizoma Anemarrhenae) 4.5 g, *Niu Xi* (Radix Achyranthis Bidentatae) 4.5 g.

Explanation:

Shi Gao: The principal drug, being pungent and sweet in flavor and very cold in nature, removing lingering heat in the stomach.

Shu Di: Nourishing *Yin*.

Zhi Mu: Being moisture in nature, assisting *Shi Gao* in expelling heat from the stomach.

Mai Dong: Nourishing *Yin*, helping *Shu Di* with the nourishment of the stomach—*Yin*.

Niu Xi: Inducing heat and blood to go downward to descend fire flaring up and arrest the adverse flow of blood.

Effect: Clearing away heat in the stomach and nourishing *Yin*.

Indications: Syndrome due to heat in the stomach and *Yin* deficiency, marked by headache, toothache, odontoseisis, gingival bleeding, restlessness, thirst, dry and reddened tongue with yellowish and dry coating; including such diseases with the above symptoms as acute stomatitis, glossitis, diabetes and neurotic toothache.

Administration: Decocted in water for oral dose to be taken twice

Case Study: 15 cases of toothache which was caused mainly by dental caries, a syndrome due to pathogenic fire in the stomach, marked by toothache which even induced headache when severe, or reddish and swelling of gums, or reddish and swelling and hot cheeks, all of the above were accompanied by disturbed sleep, incapability of chewing, thirst with desire for drinking, constipation, reddened tongue with thin yellowish coating, and floating taut slippery or rapid pulse, were treated clinically with modified *Yunü Jian,* whose ingredients were:

those of the prescription of *Yunü Jian* plus:

Fang Feng (Radix Saposhinkoviae), *Zhu Ye* (Herba Lophatheri) *Huai Shan Yao* (Rhizoma Dioscoreae).

In general, 2—7 doses cured a case with the ache relieved.

1 case of Wright's disease whose manifestations were fever after bacillary dysentery, swelling and pain of the joints, limited motivity, all of which were accompanied by urethritis, conjunctival congestion, stomatocace and genital erosion, was treated with the modification of *Yunü Jian* after the treatment with antibiotics, antirheumatics and hormon es had not achieved any remarkable curative effects. The ingredients of the modification were:

Sheng Di (Radix Rehmanniae) 30 g, *Zhi Mu* (Rhizoma Anemarrhenae) 9 g, *Shi Gao* (Gypsum Fibrosum) 30 g, *Niu Xi* (Radix Achyranthis Bidentatae) 9 g, *Qin Jiao* (Radix Gentianae Macrophyllae) 15 g, *Ren Dong Teng*(Caulis Lonicerae) 15 g, *Yin Hua* (Flos Lonicerae) 15 g, *Chi Shao* (Radix Paeoniae Rubra) 12 g, *Dan Pi* (Cortex Moutan) 12 g, *Fang Feng* (Radix Saposhinkoviae) 12 g, *Mu Gua* (Fructus Chaenomelis) 12 g, *Fu Ling* (Poria) 9 g, *Chen Pi* (Pericarpium Citri Reticulatae) 9 g, *Sang Ye* (Folium Mori) 30 g, *Xun Gu Feng* (Herba Aristologchiae Mollissimae) 30 g.

After one month of treatment, the case returned to normal. Follow—up half a year later after the case was discharged from hospital found out that the condition was still better.

4.23 The Prescription of *Shaoyao Tang*

Name: Peony Decoction

Source: The book *Yi Xue Liu Shu*

Ingredients:

Shao Yao (Radix Paeoniae) 15 g, *Dang Gui* (Radix Angelicae Sinensis) 9 g, *Huang Lian* (Rhizoma Coptidis) 9 g, *Bing Lang* (Semen Arecae) 5 g, *Mu Xiang* (Radix Aucklandiae) 5 g, *Gan Cao* (Radix Glycyrrhizae) 5 g, *Da Huang* (Radix et Rhizoma Rhei) 9 g, *Huang Qin* (Radix Scutellariae) 9 g, *Rou Gui* (Cortex Cinnamomi) 3 g.

Explanation:

Bai Shao: The principal drug, being bitter and sour in flavor and slightly cold in nature, regulating *Ying* and blood, treating dysentery and relieving pain.

Huang Lian, Huang Qin and *Da Huang:* Removing heat and toxic material.

Dang Gui and *Rou Gui:* Regulating *Ying* and promoting the circulation of blood.

Mu Xiang and *Bing Lang:* Resolving stasis and regulating *Qi*.

Gan Cao: Removing heat and toxic material, coordinating the actions of all the other ingredients, getting together with *Bai Shao* to relieve spasm and pain.

Effect: Regulating *Qi* and blood, removing heat and toxic material.

Indications: Syndrome due to damp−heat accumulated in the intestines and leading to stagnation of *Qi*, marked by abdominal pain, pus and blood stools, rectal tenesmus, calor of anus, scanty dark urine, yellowish greasy tongue coating, and slippery rapid pulse; including such diseases with the above symptoms as bacillary dysentery, amebic dysentery, allergic enteritis and acute enteritis.

Administration: Decocted in water for oral dose to be taken twice (Taken originally in the form of powder)

Case Study: *Shaoyao Heji (Shaoyao Tang* minus *Da Huang)* was clinically used to treat 46 cases of Escherihia coli dysentery manifested as sudden onset, fever, abdominal pain, mucous stools with pus and blood, rectal tenesmus, anorexia, pus cells and red blood cells in feces found through microscopy. It took less than 1 day for the fever to subside in 18 cases, less than 2 days in 1 case, the other 27 cases having normal body temperature when admitted to hospital. It took less than 3 days for the bowel movement to be returned to normal in 19 cases, less than 4 days in 6 cases, less than 7 days in 11 cases, and more than 7 days in 10 cases. And it took less than 5 days for the abdominal pain and rectal tenesmus to vanish basically. At last all the cases were cured.

Modified *Shaoyao Tang* was also used to treat 18 cases of infantile Escherihia coli dysentery, manifested as fever of 37℃ −39℃ before admitted to hospital, vomiting, diarrhea, abdominal pain, rectal tenesmus, clonic convulsion, coma, red blood cells and mucus in feces found through microscopy and leukocytosis. The ingredients of the modification were:

Bai Shao (Radix Paeoniae Alba) 9 g, *Huang Qin* (Radix Scutellariae) 4.5 g, *Huang Lian* (Rhizoma Coptidis) 4.5 g, *Bing Lang* (Semen Arecae) 4.5 g, *Mu Xiang* (Radix Aucklandiae) 3 g, *Dang Gui* (Radix Angelicae Sinensis) 3 g, *Zhi Qiao* (Fructus Aurantii) 4.5 g, *Chen Pi* (Pericarpium Citri Reticulatae) 4.5 g,

Yin Hua (Flos Lonicerae) 6 g, *Jiao Zha* (Fructus Crataegi) 3 g. The ingredients were decocted in water for oral dose to be taken 6 times, 3 times daily. All the 18 cases were cured, the duration for them to stay in hospital averaging 4.44 days. Comparision between the cases treated with this modification and the 20 cases with sintomycin showed that this modification was more effective than sintomycin in treating this disorder.

4.24   The Prescription of *Baitouweng Tang*

Name: Pulsatilla Decoction
Source: The book *Shang Han Lun*
Ingredients:

Bai Tou Weng (Radix Pulsatillae) 15 g, *Huang Bai* (Cortex Phellodendri) 12 g, *Huang Lian* (Rhizoma Coptidis) 6 g, *Qin Pi* (Cortex Fraxini) 12 g.

Explanation:

Bai Tou Weng: The principal drug, being bitter in flavor and cold in nature, clearing away noxious heat in the blood system.

Huang Lian, Huang Bai and *Qin Pi:* Removing heat and toxic material, drying dampness and relieving dysentery.

Effect: Removing heat and toxic material, clearing away pathogenic heat in blood, relieving dysentery.

Indications: Dysentery with bloody stool due to noxious heat, marked by abdominal pain, rectal tenesmus, burning sensation in the anus, discharge of pus and blood with the latter more than the former, thirst with desire for drink, reddened tongue with yellowish coating, and taut rapid pulse; including such diseases with the above symptoms as acute bacillary dysentery, amebic dysentery, ulcerative colitis, trichomonal enteritis, lobar pneumonia and bronchial pneumonia.

Administration: Decocted in water for oral dose to be taken twice

Case Study: 48 cases of acute bacillary dysentery were clinically treated with the combination of *Baitouweng Tang* and *Dahuang Tang*, whose ingredients were:

Bai Tou Weng (Radix Pulsatillae) 8 g, *Huang Lian* (Rhizoma Coptidis) 6 g, *Huang Bai* (Cortex Phellodendri) 10 g, *Qin Pi* (Cortex Fraxini) 12 g, *Chao Da Huang* (parched Radix et Rhizoma Rhei) 10 g.

When there were exterior symptoms in the beginning of the disorder, the drugs added were:

Jing Jie (Herba Schizonepetae), *Fang Feng* (Radix Saposhinkoviae), Ge Gen (Radix Puerariae).

When heat—evil was more severe than damp—evil, the drugs added were:

Ma Chi Xian (Herba Portulacae), *Ku Shen* (Radix Sophorae Flavescentis), Di Yu Tan (Radix Sanguisorbae).

When damp—evil was more severe than heat—evil, the drugs added were:

Cang Zhu (Rhizoma Atractylodis), *Huo Xiang* (Herba Agastachis), Hou Po (Cortex Magnoliae Officinalis).

When there were severe abdominal pain and rectal tenesmus, the drugs added were:

Bing Lang (Semen Arecae), *Mu Xiang* (Radix Aucklandiae), Jiao Zha (Fructus Crataegi).

The treatment cured all the 48 cases, among whom 29 were cured in 3 days, 11 in 5, and 8 in 7.

Baitouweng Tang was used to treat 67 cases of pneumonia, a syndrome due to pathogenic heat accumulated in the lung and caused by the heat in the large intestine. Among the cases, 48 were male, 19 were female; the oldest was 56 years old, the youngest was 3; the highest body temperature was 41.4 C. the lowest was 38.2 C; 41 cases were lobar pneumonia, 26 were bronchial pneumonia. The ingredients of the basic prescription were:

Bai Tou Weng (Radix Pulsatillae) 16 g, *Huang Lian* (Rhizoma Coptidis) 6 g, *Huang Bai* (Cortex Phellodendri) 6 g, *Qin Pi* (Cortex Fraxini) 9 g.

For patients at the age of below 16, the dosage was reduced. When there was wind–heat in the lung, the drugs added were:

Xing Ren (Semen Armeniacae Amarum), *Ma Huang* (Herba Ephedrae), *Yu Xing Cao* (Herba Houttuyniae), *Jiang Can* (Bombyx Batryticatus), *Da Qing Ye* (Folium Isatidis), *Shi Gao* (Gypsum Fibrosum), *Ting Li Zi* (Semen Lepidii seu Descurainiae).

In case of edema due to phlegm–heat, the drugs added were:

Huang Qin (Radix Scutellariae), *Sheng Shi Gao* (Gypsum Fibrosum), *Sheng Gan Cao* (Radix Glycyrrhizae), *Ting Li Zi* (Semen Lepidii seu Descurainiae), *Dan Shen* (Radix Salviae Miltiorrhizae), *Bai Hua She Cao* (Herba Hedyotis Diffusae).

In case of excessive heat in the *Ying* system which had been attacking *Yin*, the drugs added were:

Sheng Di (Radix Rehmanniae), *Xuan Shen* (Radix Scrophulariae), *Bei Tiao Shen* (Radix Glehniae), *Dan Shen* (Radix Salviae Miltiorrhizae), *Mai Dong* (Radix Ophiopogonis), *Hua Fen* (Radix Trichosanthis).

For the treatment of intense heat in both the *Qi* and blood systems, the drugs added were:

Sheng Di (Radix Rehmanniae), *Xuan Shen* (Radix Scrophulariae), *Mai Dong* (Radix Ophiopogonis), *Nan Sha Shen* (Radix Adenophorae).

If there was coma and delirium, pill of *Zixue Dan* was also prescribed. After the treatment, cure resulted in 56 cases, ineffectiveness in 11 cases, Among the 56 cases cured, 8 had their body temperature normalized in 3 days, 37 in 5–6 days, and 11 in 8–14 days.

4.25 Prescriptions for Clearing away Pathogenic Heat of Deficiency Type

This kind of prescriptions are mainly made up of drugs with the action of dispersing excessive heat of deficiency type. They are indicated for the syndrome in the later stage of febrile diseases due to lingering heat in the *Yin* system which has impaired *Yin*–fluid, or deficiency and impairment of the liver and kidney, or standing fever of deficiency type, marked by fever high in the evening and low in the morning, bone heat, tidal fever, reddened tongue with little coating, and rapid or thready rapid pulse. Drugs such as

Qing Hao (Herba Artemisiae Annuae), *Bie Jia* (Carapax Trionycis), *Di Gu Pi* (Cortex Lycii), *Zhi Mu* (Rhizoma Anemarrhenae).

are commonly used in these prescriptions, whose representatives are *Qinghao Biejia Tang*, *Qinjiao Biejia San*, *Qinggu San*, etc.

4.26 The Prescription of *Qinghao Biejia Tang*

Name: Sweet Wormwood and Turtle Shell Decoction

Source: The book *Wen Bing Tiao Bian*

Ingredients:

Qing Hao (Herba Artemisiae Annuae) 6 g, *Bie Jia* (Carapax Trionycis) 15 g, *Sheng Di* (Radix Rehmanniae) 12 g, *Zhi Mu* (Rhizoma Anemarrhenae) 6 g, *Dan Pi* (Cortex Moutan) 9 g.

Explanation:

Bie Jia: One of the principal drugs, being salty in flavor and cold in nature, nourishing *Yin* and relieving fever of deficiency type.

Qing Hao: The other principal drug, being bitter and pungent in flavor and cold in nature, removing heat from the collaterals and inducing pathogens to go outside of the body to nourish *Yin* and subdue fever.

Sheng Di and *Zhi Mu:* Replenishing *Yin,* dispelling heat, assisting *Bie Jia* in erasing fever of deficiency type.

Dan Pi: Clearing away heat from blood, helping *Qing Hao* with the erasion of the heat hidden in the collaterals.

Effect: Nourishing *Yin* and expelling heat

Indications: Syndrome due to deficient *Yin* and retained pathogens in the later stage of febrile diseases, marked by fever high in the night and low in the morning, subsiding of fever without sweating, reddened tongue with little coating, and thready rapid pulse; including such diseases with the above symptoms as chronic pyelonephritis, renal tuberculosis and summer fever of children.

Administration: Decocted in water for oral dose to be taken twice

Case Study: Modified *Qinghao Biejia Tang* was clinically used to treat 100 cases of low fever after gynecologic operations. Among them, 82 cases were subjected to total hysterectomy and 7 cases to subtotal hysterectomy because of hysteromyoma, endometriosis, carcinoma of uterine body and dysfunctional uterine bleeding, and 11 cases to adnexectomy because of oophoritic cyst, ectopic pregnancy and tubo-ovarian dropsy. 11 cases still had a standing fever, 37.3℃-38℃ or so after being treated with antibiotics, Examination didn't show any positive sign of infection. The ingredients of the modification were:

Sheng Di (Radix Rehmanniae) 15 g, *Bie Jia* (Carapax Trionycis) roasted 12 g, *Qing Hao* (Herba Artemisiae Annuae) 10 g, *Zhi Mu* (Rhizoma Anemarrhenae) 10 g, *Dan Pi* (Cortex Moutan) 10 g, *Bai Wei* (Radix Cynanchi Atrati) 10 g, *Yin Chai Hu* (Radix Stellariae) 10 g, *Bai Shao* (Radix Paeoniae Alba) 10 g, *Sheng Gan Cao* (Radix Glycyrrhizae) 5 g.

81 cases began to take the decoction of this prescription from 5-10 days after the operation; 19 cases from 11-15 days. 82 cases were treated only with this prescription; 18 cases were treated with a combination of this prescription and antibiotics, most of which were prescribed in the first period of taking the decoction of this prescription. Remarkable effectiveness was seen in 70 cases, whose body temperature returned to normal after 1-3 doses were taken by each of them. Effectiveness was seen in 28 cases, whose body temperature returned to normal after 4-5 doses were taken by each of them. Ineffectiveness was seen in the rest cases.

19 cases of phlyctenular conjunctivitis, a syndrome due to dryness-heat in the Lung Channel, were treated with the modification of *Qinghao Biejia Tang*, whose basic ingredients were: those of the prescription of *Qinghao Biejia Tang* minus:

Dan Pi (Cortex Moutan), *Sheng Di* (Radix Rehmanniae) but plus: *Chai Hu* (Radix Bupleuri), *Gou Teng* (Ramulus Uncariae cum Uncis), *Chen Pi* (Pericarpium Citri Reticulatae), *Bai Zhu* (Rhizoma Atractylodis Macrocephalae).

All the cases were cured, each of them taking several or more than ten doses, and the curative rate being 100%.

4.27 The Prescription of *Qinjiao Biejia San*

Name: Decoction of Large—leaf Gentian Root and Turtle Shell

Source: The book *Wei Sheng Bao Jian*

Ingredients:

Di Gu Pi (Cortex Lycii) 12 g, *Chai Hu* (Radix Bupleuri) 9 g, *Bie Jia* (Carapax Trionycis) 15 g, *Qin Jiao* (Radix Gentianae Macrophyllae) 12 g, *Zhi Mu* (Rhizoma Anemarrhenae) 9 g, *Dang Gui* (Radix Angelicae Sinensis) 9 g, *Qing Hao* (Herba Artemisiae Annuae) 6 g, *Wu Mei* (Fructus Mume) 3 g.

Explanation:

Bie Jia: One of the principal drugs, being salty in taste and cold in nature, nourishing *Yin* and removing heat.

Qin Jiao: The other principal drug, being bitter and pungent in flavor and slightly cold in nature, clearing away bone—heat.

Zhi Mu, Qing Hao and *Di Gu Pi:* Dispersing heat in the interior to eliminate bone—heat.

Dang Gui: Tonifying and coordinating blood.

Chai Hu: Dispelling wind pathogens from the superficies of the body.

Wu Mei: Astringing *Yin* to stop sweating.

Effect: Nourishing *Yin* and blood, removing bone—heat.

Indications: Consumptive syndrome due to pathogenic wind, marked by bone-heat sensation, night sweating, emaciation, reddish lips and cheeks, tidal fever after noon, cough, lassitude, reddened tongue with little coating, and feeble rapid pulse; including such diseases with the above symptoms as lung tuberculosis and bone tuberculosis.

Administration: Decocted in water for oral dose to be taken twice (Taken originally in the form of powder)

4.28   The Prescription of *Qinggu San*

Name: Powder of Relieving Bone-heat
Source: The book *Zheng Zhi Zhun Sheng*
Ingredients:

Yin Chai Hu (Radix Stellariae) 10 g, *Hu Huang Lian* (Rhizoma Picrorhizae) 6 g, *Qin Jiao* (Radix Gentianae Macrophyllae) 6 g, *Bie Jia* (Carapax Trionycis prepared with vinegar) 6 g, *Di Gu Pi* (Cortex Lycii) 6 g, *Qing Hao* (Herba Artemisiae Annuae) 6 g, *Zhi Mu* (Rhizoma Anemarrhenae) 6 g, *Gan Cao* (Radix Glycyrrhizae) 4 g.

Explanation:

Yin Chai Hu: The principal drug, being sweet in flavor and slightly cold in nature and good at clearing away bone-heat due to consumption.

Zhi Mu, Hu Huang Lian and *Di Gu Pi:* Being good at reducing asthenia-type fever and removing bone-heat with sweat.

Bie Jia: Nourishing *Yin* and suppressing hyperactive *Yang* to reduce asthenia-type fever.

Qing Hao and *Qin Jiao:* Dispelling bone-heat without sweat.

Gan Cao: Tempering the actions of all the other ingredients

Effect: Alleviating asthenic fever and removing bone—heat

Indications:

Syndrome due to bone—heat resulting from consumption or prolonged low fever; including tuberculosis and hematopathy

Administration: Decocted in water for oral dose to be taken twice (Taken originally in the form of powder)

Case Study: 21 cases of fever due to trauma were clinically treated with modified *Qinggu San,* whose ingredients were as follows:

Yin Chai Hu(Radix Stellariae) 18 g, *Di Gu Pi* (Cortex Lycii) 18 g, *Huang Lian* (Rhizoma Coptidis) 9 g, *Zhi Mu* (Rhizoma Anemarrhenae) 9 g, *Qin Jiao* (Radix Gentianae Macrophyllae) 15 g, *Qing Hao* (Herba Artemisiae Annuae) added later 6 g, *Gan Cao* (Radix Glycyrrhizae) 6 g, *Bai Wei* (Radix Cynanchi Atrati) 30 g.

All the cases had a history of trauma, local hematoma, ecchymosis, rising of body temperature from noon to dusk and subsiding of it in the following morning, feverish sensation, absence of exterior syndrome, undisturbed mental state, elevating of leukocytic reaction at the early stage with it becoming normal several days later, reddened tongue with thin whitish or thin yellowish coating, and thready rapid pulse. Among the 21 cases, 20 were cured after 1—2 doses were taken by each of them, 1 showed no effectiveness.

4.29 The Prescription of *Danggui Liuhuang Tang*

Name: Decoction of Chinese Angelica and Six Yellow Ingredients

Source: The book *Lan Shi Mi Cang*

Ingredients:

Dang Gui (Radix Angelicae Sinensis) 9 g, *Sheng Di* (Radix Rehmanniae) 9 g, *Shu Di* (Radix Rehmanniae Preparata)9 g, *Huang Qin* (Radix Scutellariae) 9 g, *Huang Bai* (Cortex Phellodendri) 9 g, *Huang Lian* (Rhizoma Coptidis) 6 g, *Huang Qi* (Radix Astragali) 18 g.

Explanation:

Dang Gui, Sheng Di and *Shu Di:* The principal drugs, nourishing *Yin* and blood to clear away heat in the interior.

Huang Lian, Huang Qin and *Huang Bai:* Purging fire to arrest restlessness, clearing away heat to consolidate *Yin*.

Huang Qi: Invigorating *Qi* and strengthening superficial resistance to stop sweating.

Effect: Nourishing *Yin* and purging fire, consolidating the superficial resistance to arrest sweating.

Indications: Syndrome of fever and night sweating due to deficiency of *Yin* and flaring—up of fire, marked by flushed face, vexation dry mouth and lips, dry stools and deep—colored urine, reddened tongue, and rapid pulse; including such diseases with the above symptoms as tuberculosis, rheumatism and hematopathy.

Administration: Decocted in water for oral dose to be taken twice (Taken originally in the form of powder).

Case Study: *Danggui Liuhuang Tang* was clinically used to treat 1 case of night sweating, 1 case of menorrhagia, 1 case of recurrent aphtha and 1 case of chronic urinary tract infection, all of which were included in the syndrome due to incoordination between *Qi* and fire. After the treatment, all the cases were cured.

Danggui Liuhuang Tang plus:

Lian Zi Xin (Plumula Nelumbinis) *Mai Men Dong* (Radix Ophiopogonis) *Ma Huang Gen* (Radix Ephedrae) was used to treat 1 case of persistent high fever, marked by fever for 10 days with the body temperature reaching 39—40℃ in the night, night sweating all over before daybreak after which the body temperature returned to 38.5℃ or so , dry mouth, glossitis, vexation, reddened tongue with dry lusterless thin yellowish coating and with bright red tip, and slippery rapid pulse. The night sweating completely vanished and the night fever lowered after 5 doses were taken.

5 Prescriptions for Removing Summer-heat

5.1 Prescriptions for Removing Summer-heat

Prescriptions mainly composed of drugs with the action of expelling pathogenic summer heat and used to treat summer heat diseases are all known as "prescriptions for removing summer heat". Prevailing in summer, summer heat is included in the range of warm-heat or fire. Because summer heat tends to impair Qi, summer heat disease is usually manifested as the syndrome of "impairment of both fluids and Qi", marked by higher fever, thirst, vexation, and profuse sweat; because it is rainy in summer, summer heat disease is often complicated by pathogenic dampness; because it is hot in summer, and people are preferable for cold food and drink and exposure to wind and dew, summer heat disease is apt to be associated with exterior cold. According to these features of summer heat disease, prescriptions for removing summer heat may be classified as the following four kinds: those for removing summer-heat from the superficies of the body by diaphoresis, those for clearing away summer-heat by expelling pathogenic heat, those for removing summer-heat by inducing diuresis and those for eliminating summer-heat by invigorating Qi.

When prescriptions for removing summer-heat are prescribed, drugs with the action of removing dampness are often administered, for summer heat diseases are often complicated by pathogenic dampness. But attention must be paid to which is more severe, dampness or summer–heat. When summer–heat is more severe than dampness, dampness tends to transform into summer–heat, and drugs for removing dampness should not be too warm or dry in nature in order to prevent body fluids from being consumed by dryness. When dampness is more severe than summer–heat, summer–heat is liable to be obstructed by dampness, and drugs for removing summer–heat should not be too sweet in flavor and cold in nature lest the elimination of dampness be impeded by the drugs *Yin*–soft in nature.

5.2 Prescriptions for Clearing away Summer–heat by Expelling Pathogenic Heat

This kind of prescriptions are mainly made up of drugs with the action of removing pathogenic heat in summer. They are suitable for the syndrome due to the attack of summer–heat, marked by fever, restlessness, profuse sweat and thirst. Drugs such as

Xi Gua Cui Yi (Exocarpium Citrulli) *Yin Hua* (Flos Lonicerae) *Bian Dou Hua* (Flos Lablab) *He Ye* (Folium Nelumbinis)

are commonly used in these prescriptions, whose representatives are *Qingluo Yin,* etc.

5.3 The Prescription of *Qingluo Yin*

Name: Decoction for Removing Heat from the Lung Channel

Source: The book *Wen Bing Tiao Bian*

Ingredients:

Xian He Ye (Folium Nelumbinis) 6 g, *Xian Yin Hua* (Flos Lonicerae) 9 g, *Si Gua Luo* (Fasciculus Vascularia Luffae) 6 g, *Xi Gua Cui Yi* (Exocarpium Citrulli) 6 g, *Xian Bian Dou Hua* (Flos Lablab) 6 g, *Xian Zhu Ye* (Herba Lophatheri) 6 g.

Explanation:

Xian Yin Hua: One of the principal drugs, being sweet in flavor and cold in nature, getting together with the other principal drug *Xian Bian Dou Hua* aromatic in flavor to remove summer—heat.

Xi Gua Cui Yi: Removing summer—heat.

Si Gua Luo: Dispelling heat from the lung collaterals.

Xian He Ye: Dispersing and purging summer—heat.

Xian Zhu Ye: Purging heart—fire by inducing diuresis.

Effect: Expelling pathogenic summer—heat.

Indications: Syndrome due to attack of summer—heat on the lung and pathogens lodging in the *Qi* system, marked by mild fever and thirst, vague mind, dizziness, mild distention of the head, pale red tongue with thin whitish coating; including sun—stroke with the above symptoms.

Administration: Decocted in water for oral dose to be taken twice

5.4 Prescriptions for Removing Summer—heat from the Superficies of the Body by Diaphoresis

This kind of prescriptions are mainly composed of drugs with the action of removing summer—heat to relieve exterior syndrome. They are indicated for the syndrome due to summer heat hidden in the interior and complicated by exogenous wind—cold, marked by aversion to cold, fever, no sweat, headache, vexation and thirst. Drugs such as

Xiang Ru (Herba Elsholtziae), Yin Hua (Flos Lonicerae).
are commonly used in these prescriptions, whose representatives are *Xinjia Xiangru Yin,* etc.

5.5 The Prescription of *Xinjia Xiangru Yin*

Name: Decoction of Elsholtzia with Supplements
Source: The book *Wen Bing Tiao Bian*
Ingredients:
Xiang Ru (Herba Elsholtziae) 6 g, *Yin Hua* (Flos Lonicerae) 9 g, *Xian Bian Dou Hua* (Flos Dolichoris) 9 g, *Hou Po* (Cortex Magnoliae Officinalis) 6 g, *Lian Qiao* (Fructus Forsythiae) 9 g.
Explanation:
Xiang Ru: The principal drug, being pungent in flavor and slightly warm in nature, relieving exterior syndrome by inducing diaphoresis, removing summer—heat and eliminating dampness.
Xian Bian Dou Hua, Yin Hua and *Lian Qiao:* Clearing away summer—heat in the upper—*Jiao* to quench thirst.
Hou Po: Removing dampness and relieving distension.
Effect: Removing summer—heat by inducing diaphoresis, clearing away heat and eliminating dampness.
Indications: Syndrome of early summer fever complicated by exogenous cold, marked by fever, headache, aversion to cold, absence of sweat, thirst, flushed face, oppressed sensation in the chest, whitish greasy tongue coating, and floating rapid pulse; including common cold due to summer—heat and dampness with the above symptoms. "Absence of sweat" is the essential point for the application of this prescription when it is adopted to treat the

syndrome due to summer—heat complicated by exogenous cold. If the syndrome is caused by mere summer—heat and manifested as fever and sweating, this prescription can not be used dispite of the existence of the symptom aversion to cold.

Administration: Decocted in water for oral dose to be taken twice

5.6 Prescriptions for Removing Summer—heat by Inducing Diuresis

This kind of prescriptions are mainly made up of drugs with the action of removing summer—heat and inducing diuresis. They are suitable for common cold complicated by damp pathogens, marked by fever, restlessness, thirst, fullness in the chest and stomach, difficulty in urinating, etc. Drugs such as

Hua Shi (Talcum), *Fu Ling* (Poria), *Ze Xie* (Rhizoma Alismatis). are commonly used in these prescriptions, whose representatives are *Liu Yi San, Guiling Ganlu San*,etc.

5.7 The Prescription of *Liu Yi San*

Name: Six to One Powder

Source: The book *Shang Han Zhi Ge*

Ingredients:

Hua Shi (Talcum) 180 g, *Gan Cao* (Radix Glycyrrhizae) 30 g.

Explanation:

Hua Shi: The principal drug, being sweet and tasteless in flavor and cold in nature, having the particular action of clearing away heat and inducing diuresis.

Gan Cao: Being sweet in flavor and cold in nature, dispelling heat, regulating the stomach, combining *Hua Shi* to promote the production of body fluid and inducing diuresis to make body fluid not be damaged.

Effect: Removing summer—heat and inducing diuresis.

Indications: Syndrome due to affection of summer—heat and dampness, marked by fever, intense thirst, dysuria, or diarrhea; including such diseases with the above symptoms as mild sun—stroke, cystitis and stone of the urinary tract.

Administration: Ground into powder and 9—18 g of the powder is taken each time, or wrapped in cloth and decocted in water for oral dose to be taken twice.

Case Study: 1 case of stranguria due to urinary stone, marked by soreness of the loins, intermittent difficult urination, turbid and deep—colored urine, dripping urination with stabbing pain, whitish greasy tongue coating, and taut pulse, was clinically treated with modified *Liu Yi San,* whose ingredients were:

Fei Hua Shi (Talcum) refined with water 30 g, *Gan Cao* (Radix Glycyrrhizae) 6 g, *Ji Nei Jin* (Endothelium Corneum Gigeriae Galli) 18 g, *Hu Po* (Succinum) 12 g.

The above ingredients were ground into fine powder, which was wrapped in 9 packets, each of which was taken each time with the decoction of :

Jin Qian Cao (Herba Lysimachiae) 60 g, *Che Qian Cao* (Herba Plantaginis) 60 g.

Free urination occurred 2 days later.   At noon of the 3rd day, 2 pieces of stone were discharged out. 5 days later, 11 pieces of stone were discharged out one after another. After that, the pain in the loins and the abdominal distention disappeared,   and normal urination occurred. The treatment was continued by taking the decoction of *Jin Qian Cao* and *Che Qian Cao* for another week, and finally the case was cured.

5.8   The Prescription of *Guiling Ganlu Yin*

Name: Decoction of Cinnamom Twig and Poria

Source: The book *Xuan Ming Lun Fang*

Ingredients:

Fu Ling (Poria) 30 g, *Gan Cao* (Radix Glycyrrhizae) 6 g, *Bai Zhu* (Rhizoma Atractylodis Macrocephalae) 12 g, *Ze Xie* (Rhizoma Alismatis) 15 g, *Guan Gui* (Ramulus Cinnamomi) 3 g, *Shi Gao* (Gypsum Fibrosum) 30 g, *Han Shui Shi* (Calcitum) 30 g, *Hua Shi* (Talcum) 30 g, *Zhu Ling* (Polyporus) 15 g.

Explanation:

Hua Shi: The principal drug, being sweet and tasteless in flavor and cold in nature, clearing away heat, eliminating dampness by inducing diuresis.

Shi Gao and *Han Shui Shi:* Expelling summer—heat.

Guan Gui: Promoting functional activity of the *Qi* of the lower—*Jiao*.

Zhu Ling, Fu Ling and *Ze Xie:* Inducing diuresis.

Bai Zhu: Strengthening the spleen.

Gan Cao: Tempering the actions of all the other ingredients, working together with *Hua Shi* to enhance the elimination of heat and promotion of diuresis.

Effect: Clearing away summer—heat, promoting functional activity of *Qi,* inducing diuresis.

Indications: Syndrome due to affection of summer—heat and dampness, marked by fever, headache, restlessness, thirst with desire for drinking, dysuria, and severe vomiting and diarrhea ; including such diseases with the above symptoms as sunstroke and common cold of gastrointestinal type in summer.

Administration: Ground into powder, 9 g of which is taken after being mixed with warm liquid each time, 2 times daily. Liquid of *sheng Jiang* (Rhizoma Zingiberis Recens) is preferable.

5.9 Prescriptions for Removing Summer—heat by Invigorating *Qi*

This kind of prescriptions are mainly composed of drugs with the action of clearing away summer—heat and replenishing *Qi*. They are indicated for the syndrome due to impairment of *Qi* and body fluids by summer—heat, marked by fever, intense thirst, lassitude, shortness of breath, profuse sweat, and weak pulse. Drugs such as

Xi Yang Shen (Radix Panacis Quinquefolii)

Xi Gua Cui Yi (Exocarpium Citrulli)

Shi Hu (Herba Dendrobii)

Zhi Mu (Rhizoma Anemarrhenae)

are commonly used in these prescriptions, whose representatives are *Wangshi Qingshu Tang*, etc.

5.10 The Prescription of *Qingshu Yiqi Tang*

Name: Decoction for Clearing away Summer—heat and Reinforcing *Qi*

Source: The book Wen Re Jing Wei

Ingredients: .

Xi Yang Shen (Radix Panacis Quinquefolii) 5 g, *Shi Hu* (Herba Dendrobii) 15 g, *Mai Dong* (Radix Ophiopogonis) 9 g, *Huang Lian* (Rhizoma Coptidis) 3 g, *Zhu Ye* (Herba Lophatheri)

6 g, *He Geng* (Petiolus Nelumbinis) 15 g, *Zhi Mu* (Rhizoma Anemarrhenae) 6 g, *Gan Cao* (Radix Glycyrrhizae) 3 g, *Jing Mi* (Semen Oryzae Sativae) 15 g, *Xi Gua Cui Yi* (Exocarpium Citrulli) 30 g.

Explanation:

Xi Yang Shen: One of the principal drugs, being sweet and slightly bitter in flavor and cool in nature, reinforcing *Qi* to promote the production of body fluids, nourishing *Yin* and removing heat.

Xi Gua Cui Yi: The other principal drug, being sweet in flavor and cold in nature, eliminating summer—heat.

He Geng: Assisting *Xi Gua Cui Yi* in driving away summer—heat.

Shi Hu and *Mai Dong:* Aiding *Xi Yang Shen* in nourishing *Yin* and removing heat.

Zhi Mu and *Zhu Ye:* Dispelling heat to arrest restlessness.

Gan Cao and *Jing Mi:* Reinforcing *Qi* and invigorating the stomach.

Effect: Removing summer—heat, reinforcing *Qi,* nourishing *Yin,* promoting the production of body fluids.

Indications: Syndrome due to attack of summer—heat and impairment of both *Qi* and body fluids, marked by fever, profuse sweat, vexation, thirst, scanty and deep—colored urine, lassitude, shortness of breath, poor mental state, and weak rapid pulse; including sunstroke and the like with the above symptoms.

6 Prescriptions for Warming the Interior

6.1 Prescriptions for Warming the Interior

Prescriptions which consist of drugs warm or heat in nature, have the function of warming the interior to support *Yang* and removing pathogenic cold from the channels, and are used to treat the syndromes due to *Yin*—cold in the interior are all known as "prescriptions for warming the interior". Diseases due to cold pathogens may be in the exterior or in the interior. Those in the exterior should be treated with prescriptions consisting of drugs pungent in flavor and warm in nature and having the function of relieving the exterior syndromes, while those in the interior, with prescriptions having the function of warming the interior. Syndromes due to cold pathogens in the interior are caused by cold originating from the interior due to *Yang*—deficiency of the constitution, by exogenous pathogenic cold attacking directly *Zang*—*Fu* organs, by cold pathogens entering the interior due to improper treatment of an exterior cold syndrome, or by impairment of *Yang*—*Qi* due to over—intake of drugs cold in nature. According to the difference in severity and location of syndromes due to cold in the interior, prescriptions for warming the interior are classified as the following three types: warming the middle—*Jiao* to dispel pathogenic cold, recuperating depleted *Yang* to rescue the patient from collapse, and warming the channels to expel pathogenic cold.

Because the prescriptions of this kind are mainly composed of drugs pungent in flavor and warm,　dry and heat in nature, they are contraindicated for heat syndromes with pseudo—cold symptoms. Therefore, before they are prescribed, the true or false of a cold syndrome must be first made clear. Besides, they should not be over—administered for a patient with the syndrome of *Yin*—deficiency of the symptom of loss of blood lest his *Yin* be reimpaired, heat pathogen be produced with the cold one removed, and the drugs pungent in flavor and heat in nature consume his *Yin* to cause bleeding. Meanwhile, their dosage should be appropriately adjusted according to the variation of cold and hotness of the climate of the four seasons, Other prescriptions for warming and restoring should be chosen instead when prescriptions for warming the interior has been used to treat a patient with *Yang*—deficient constitution and the cold in his interior has been removed but his *Yang* still remains deficient, Once a syndrome due to cold in the interior is cured, prescriptions for warming the interior should not be used any longer.

6.2　Prescriptions for Warming the Middle—*Jiao* to Dispel Pathogenic Cold

This kind of prescriptions are mainly made up of drugs with the action of warming the middle—*Jiao* and dispelling pathogenic cold. They are suitable for the syndrome due to cold of deficiency type in the middle—*Jiao,* marked by distending pain in the stomach, lassitude,cold extremities, or regurgitation of sour fluid, salivation, nausea, vomiting, or abdominal pain, loose stools, anorexia, tastelessness in the mouth , no thirst, whitish slippery tongue coating, and deep thready or deep slow pulse. Drugs such as.

Gan Jiang (Rhizoma Zingiberis), *Wu Zhu Yu* (Fructus Euodiae), *Shu Jiao* (Pericarpium Zanthoxyli), *Sheng Jiang* (Rhizoma Zingiberis Recens).
are usually used in these prescriptions, whose representatives are *Lizhong Wan* , *Wuzhuyu Tang, Xiao Jianzhong Tang* and *Da Jianzhong Tang.*

6.3 The Prescription of *Lizhong Wan*

Name: Pill for Regulating the Function of the Middle—*Jiao*
Source: The book *Shang Han Lun*
Ingredients:
Ren Shen (Radix Ginseng) 6 g, *Gan Jiang* (Rhizoma Zingiberis) 5 g, *Gan Cao* (Radix Glycyrrhizae Preparata) 6 g, *Bai Zhu* (Rhizoma Atractylodis Macrocephalae) 9 g.
Explanation:
Gan Jiang: The principal drug, being pungent in flavor and heat in nature, warming the spleen and stomach to remove cold in the interior.
Ren Shen: Invigorating primodial *Qi,* aiding in transporting and transforming nutrients and regulating the ascending and descending movement of *Qi.*
Bai Zhu: Strengthening the spleen and drying dampness.
Zhi Gan Cao: Replenishing *Qi* and regulating the stomach.
Effect: Warming the stomach to remove cold, invigorating the spleen to replenish *Qi.*
Indications: Syndrome due to deficiency and cold in the middle—*Jiao,* marked by loose stools, no thirst, vomiting, abdom-

inal pain, anorexia, pale tongue with whitish coating, and deep slow pulse; including such diseases with the above symptoms as gastroduodenal ulcer, chronic gastritis , chronic colitis,regional enteritis and bacillary dysentery.

Administration: Ground into fine powder and made with honey into boluses, each of which is as big as an egg yolk and ground into particles to be taken warm each time, 3 times daily. (Used also as a decoction, the dosage of the drugs is decided on according to the proportions of the ingredients in the original prescription.)

Case Study: *Lizhong Tang* was clinically used to treat 1 case of severe abdominal distention. The patient had been admitted to hospital with the complaints of fever, severe abdominal distention, vomiting and paroxysmal abdominal pain.When treated with this prescription, he or she was found to have the following symptoms: no intake of food and water for 10 days, body temperature lowered to 35℃ frequent vomiting, severe abdominal distention, 3-day-absence of laxation.The ingredients administered were:

those in *Lizhong Tang* plus:

Gui Zhi (Ramulus Cinnamomi), *Da Huang* (Radix et Rhizoma Rhei), *Mang Xiao* (Natrii Sulfas), *Shi Gao* (Gypsum Fibrosum), *Zhi Mu* (Rhizoma Anemarrhenae).

with rice and *He Ye* (Folium Nelumbinis) as the guiding drugs. 1 dose taken, the symptoms were relieved; another 3 doses of the modification of the above prescription taken, they were remarkable alleviated.

Modified *Lizhong Tang* was employed to treat 1 case of chronic aphthae which had been lasting for 3 years, marked by recurrent ulcer with burning sensation,foul odor sometimes in the mouth , gingival bleeding, feverish sensation in the palms and soles, all of which were gradually worsened in the last 2 months.When received , the patient was found to have such symptoms as aphthae with burning sensation, moderate appetite, lassitude, dry mouth without desire for drinking, diluted urine, pale tongue with thin whitish coating, and thready slow pulse. The drugs administered were as follows:

Fu Zi (Radix Aconiti Lateralis Preparata) 9 g, *Dang Shen* (Radix Codonopsis) 15 g,*Pao Jiang* (Rhizoma Zingiberis) 6 g, *Bai Zhu* (Rhizoma Atractylodis Macrocephalae) 9 g,*Shu Di* (Radix Rehmanniae Preparata) 15 g, *Gan Cao* (Radix Glycyrrhizae) 4.5 g.

4 doses remarkably relieved the ulcer. Another 3 doses cured the aphthae.

6.4   The Prescription of *Wuzhuyu Tang*

Name: Decoction of Root of Medicinal Evodia

Source: The book *Shang Huan Lun*

Ingredients:

Wu Zhu Yu (Fructus Euodiae) 3 g, *Ren Shen* (Radix Ginseng) 6 g,*Da Zao* (Fructus Jujubae) 4 dates, *Sheng Jiang* (Rhizoma Zingiberis Recens) 18 g.

Explanation:

*Wu Zhu Yu:*The principal drug, being pungent and bitter in flavor and heat in nature, warming the stomach to disperse cold , removing stagnated food , descending *Qi* to lower the turbid.

Ren Shen: Invigorating primodial *Qi* and benifiting *Yin*.

Sheng Jiang: Warming the stomach to purge cold.

Da Zao: Replenishing *Qi* and nourishing the spleen , working together with *Sheng Jiang* to regulate *Ying* and *Wei.*

Effect: Warming the middle—*Jiao* to tonify the spleen and stomach, keeping the adverse flow of the stomach—*Qi* going down to stop vomiting.

Indications:

Syndrome due to deficiency—cold in the stomach, marked by nausea after meal,fullness in the chest and gastric region, gastric pain, gastric discomfort with acid regurgitation ,or due to *Jueyin* disease marked by headache and vomiting with foams, or due to *Shaoyin* disease marked by vomiting and diarrhea; including such diseases with the above symptoms as chronic gastritis, nervous headache,vomiting in pregnancy, gastrointestinal neurosis, Meniere's disease, drug anaphylactic vomiting, etc.

Administration: Decocted in water for oral dose to be taken 3 times

Case Study:

Modified *Wuzhuyu Tang* was clinically used to treat 34 cases of peptic ulcer, a syndrome due to deficiency—cold in the stomach marked by recurrent and protracted gastric pain which was preferable for palpation and warmth but averse to cold and worsened by hunger but relieved by food intake, poor appetite,nausea or vomiting of watery fluid, no thirst, pale tongue with whitish slippery coating, and slow pulse. After the treatment, remarkable effectiveness was seen in 25 cases, improvement in 8 cases, ineffectiveness in 1 case. The paindisappeared winthin 3—25 days.

Modified *Wuzhuyu Tang* was used to treat 3 cases of chronic cholecystitis, whose *Yang—Qi* of the middle—*Jiao* had been injured due to over—taking of drugs bitter in flavor and cold in nature, which resulted in the attack of cold pathogens on the stomach, adverse flow of the stomach—*Qi* and vomiting of foamy fluid. The treatment ensured remarkable effectiveness.

6.5 The Prescription of *Xiao Jianzhong Tang*

Name: Minor Decoction of Strengthening the Middle—*Jiao*
Source: The book *Shang Han Lun*
Ingredients:

Shao Yao (Radix Paeoniae parched with liquor) 18 g. *Gui Zhi* (Ramulus Cinnamomi) 9 g,*Zhi Gan Cao* (Radix Glycyrrhizae Preparata) 6 g, *Sheng Jiang* (Rhizoma Zingiberis Recens) 10 g, *Da Zao* (Fructus Jujubae) 4 dates, *Yi Tang* (Saccharum Granorum) 30 g.

Explanation:

Yi Tang: The principal drug, being sweet in flavor and warm in nature, replenishing the spleen—*Qi* to nourish the spleen—*Yin*, warming and tonifying the middle—*Jiao*, nourishing the liver to relieve pain, moisturizing the dryness of the lung.

*Gui Zhi :*Warming *Yang—Qi*.

Shan Yao: Replenishing *Yin*—blood.

Zhi Gan Cao: Being sweet in flavor and warming nature benefiting *Qi* , not only assisting *Yi Tang* and *Gui Zhi* in replenishing *Qi* and warming the middle—*Jiao* but also getting together with *Shao Yao* which is sour and sweet in taste to promote the production of *Yin*—fluid, thus invigorating the liver and nourishing the spleen.

Sheng Jiang: Warming the stomach.

Da Zao: Tonifying the spleen , working together with *Sheng Jiang* to regulate *Ying* and *Wei*.

Effect: Warming the middle—*Jiao* to nourish the spleen and stomach, regulating the function of the middle—*Jiao* to relieve pain.

Indications: Syndrome of abdominal pain due to consumption, marked by paroxysmal abdominal pain relieved by warmth and palpation, pale tongue with whitish coating, and taut thready but slow pulse, or palpatation, vexation, lustreless complexion, of aching of the limbs, feverish sensation of the hands and feet, dry mouth and throat; including such diseases with the above symptoms as gastroduodenal ulcer, neurosism, aplastic anemia and thrombocytopenic penic purpura.

Administration: The first 5 ingredients in the prescription were decocted twice for the decoction , into which *Yi Tang* was put, taken warm twice.

Case Study: 1 case of emission of more than 2 years, marked by occurance of emission every 1—2 days, dim complexion, poor appetite, lassitude,dizziness, palpatation, tinnitus, soreness of the loins, dreaminess, bright tongue without coating, and thready weak pulse, was clinically treated with modified *Xiao Jianzhong Tang,* whose ingredients were:

Gui Zhi (Ramulus Cinnamomi) 15 g, *Yi Tang* (Saccharum Granorum) 60 g,*Shao Yao* (Radix Paeoniae) 30 g, *Zhi Gan Cao* (Radix Glycyrrhizae Preparata) 9 g,*Sheng Jiang* (Rhizoma Zingiberis Recens) 3 pieces, *Da Zao* (Fructus Jujubae) 3 dates,*Mu Li* (Concha Ostreae) 24 g, *Long Gu* (Os Draconis Fossilia) 24 g. After 3 doses were taken , the emission was ceased, dreaminess and the other symptoms were relieved and the patient could have a sound sleep.

3 cases of ascaris abdominal pain were treated with modified

Xiao Jianzhong Tang, whose ingredients were:

Gui Zhi (Ramulus Cinnamomi) 6 g, *Bai Shao* (Radix Paeoniae Alba) 6 g,*Zhi Gan Cao* (Radix Glycyrrhizae Preparata) 6 g, *Da Zao* (Fructus Jujubae) 4 dates, *Sheng Jiang* (Rhizoma Zingiberis Recens) 3 pieces, *Wu Mei* (Fructus Mume) 6 g, *Yi Tang* (Saccharum Granorum) 30 g.

Each of the 3 cases was cured by taking 2—3 doses.

6.6 The Prescription of *Da Jianzhong Tang*

Name: Major Decoction for Rehabilitating the Middle—*Jiao*

Source: The book *Jin Gui Yao Lue*

Ingredients:

Shu Jiao (Pericarpium Zanthoxyli) 3 g, *Gan Jiang* (Rhizoma Zingiberis) 4.5 g,*Ren Shen* (Radix Ginseng) 6 g, *Yi Tang* (Saccharum Granorum) 30 g.

Explanation:

Shu Jiao: The principal drug, being pungent in flavor and hot in nature, warming the spleen and stomach , aiding the fire of *Ming Men* , thus expelling cold and removing dampness , descending *Qi* to relieve stagnation.

Gan Jiang: Warming the middle—*Jiao* to dispel cold, assisting *Shu Jiao* in rehabilitating the Yang—*Qi* of the middle—*Jiao* and dispersing the *Qi* adversely flowing, relieving pain and stopping vomiting.

Ren Shen and *Yi Tang:* Being sweet in flavor and warm in nature, warming and invigorating the middle—*Jiao* to replenish the spleen and stomach.

Effect: Warming the middle—*Jiao* to nourish the spleen and stomach, discending the adverse flow of *Qi* to relieve pain.

Indications: Syndrome due to weakened *Yang—Qi* of the middle—*Jiao* and excessive *Yin*—cold in the interior, marked by colic pain in the chest and epigastric region, inability to take food due to vomiting, clear—cut and mobile and painful abdominal masses averse to palpation due to cold within the abdomen , whitish slippery tongue coating, thready tense pulse, even cold limbs and hidden pulse, or borborygmus; including such diseases with the above symptoms as chronic gastritis, peptic ulcer, chronic pancreatitis, chronic cholecystitis, biliary ascariasis and intestinal tuberculosis.

Administration: The first 3 ingredients in the prescription were first decocted twice for the decoction , into which 30 g of *Yi Tang* was put , taken warm twice.

Case Study: 45 cases of biliary ascariasis were clinically treated with modified *Da Jianzhong Tang,* whose ingredients were:

Gan Jiang (Rhizoma Zingiberis) 9 g, *Chuan Jiao* (Pericarpium Zanthoxyli) 9 g, *Wu Mei* (Fructus Mume) 9 g, *Ku Lian Pi* (Cortex Meliae) 9 g, *Bing Lang* (Semen Arecae) 9 g, *Dang Shen* (Radix Codonopsis) 9 g, *Yi Tang* (Saccharum Granorum) 60 g, *Huang Lian* (Rhizoma Coptidis) 4.5 g, *Zhi Gan Cao* (Radix Glycyrrhizae Preparata) 4.5 g.

(half amount of the ingredients for children).

After the treatment , 39 cases were cured, and 4 improved.

Da Jianzhong Tang was used to treat 6 cases of severe pain due to cold in the chest and epigastric region complicated by vomiting and inability to take food, a syndrome due to weakened *Yang—Qi* of the middle—*Jiao* and up—attacking of *Yin*—cold. The disease duration ranged from 2 days to 3 years.

In case of distention and fullness in the abdomen, the drugs added were.

Hou Po (Cortex Magnoliae Officinalis), *Sha Ren* (Fructus Amomi).

In case of intense cold or dizziness, the drug added was:

Wu Zhu Yu (Fructus Euodiae).

In case of severe chills, the drug added was:

Pao Fu Zi (Radix Aconiti Lateralis Preparata).

In case of vomiting the drugs added were:

Ban Xia (Rhizoma Pinelliae), *Sheng Jiang* (Rhizoma Zingiberis Recens).

In case of deficiency of the spleen, the drug added was:

Bai Zhu (Rhizoma Atractylodis Macrocephalae).

In case of blood—deficiency, the drug added was:

Dang Gui (Radix Angelicae Sinensis).

In case of dry mouth , the drug added was:

Bai Shao (Radix Paeoniae Alba).

In case of weakness or paralysis of the extremities, the drug added was:

Gui Zhi Jian (Ramulus Cinnamomi).

The treatment resulted in satisfactory curative effects in all the cases.

6.7 Prescriptions for Recuperating Depleted *Yang* and Rescuing Patients from Collapse

This kind of prescriptions are mainly composed of drugs with the action of restoring *Yang* and saving patients in danger. They are suitable for the syndromes due to weakened and feeble *Yang—Qi,* cold in both the interior and exterior, *Yang* kept in the exterior by excessive *Yin* or floating *Yang,* marked by cold limbs, aversion to cold, lying with the limbs drawn up, vomiting, abdominal pain, diarrhea with undigested food, listlessness, deep thready of deep feeble pulse.

Drugs such as

Fu Zi (Radix Aconiti Lateralis Preparata), *Gan Jiang* (Rhizoma Zingiberis), *Rou Gui* (Cortex Cinnamomi)

are usually used in these prescriptions, whose representatives are *Sini Tang*, *Huiyang Jiuji Tang*, etc.

6.8   The Prescription of *Sini Tang*

Name: Decoction for Resuscitation

Source: The book *Shang Han Lun*

Ingredients:

Fu Zi (Radix Aconiti Lateralis Preparata) 5—10 g, *Gan Jiang* (Rhizoma Zingiberis) 6—9 g, *Zhi Gan Cao* (Radix Glycyrrhizae Preparata) 6 g.

Explanation:

Fu Zi: The principal drug, being pungent and sweet in flavor and very hot and toxic in nature, being good at supporting the congenital true fire of *Mingmen,* promoting the circulation of *Qi* and blood throughout the twelve regular channels, used raw to act on the whole body rapidly to warm up *Yang—Qi* and dispel cold.

Gan Jiang: warming the *Yang—Qi* of the middle—*Jiao* to remove cold in the interior, assisting *Fu Zi* in promoting the generation of *Yang—Qi.*

Zhi Gan Cao: Detoxicating and relieving the drastic and pungent nature of *Gan Jiang* and *Fu Zi.*

Effect: Recuperating depleted *Yang* and rescuing patients

from collapse

Indications: *Shaoyin* disease manifested as cold limbs, aversion to cold, lying with the extremities drawn up, vomiting, no thirst , abdominal pain, diarrhea,listlessness, inclination to sleep , whitish slippery tongue coating and feeble thready pulse, or syndrome due to *Yang* depletion from misuse of diaphoresis; including such diseases with the above symptoms as chronic colitis, cor pulmonale, pneumonia , dehydration, etc.

Administration: *Fu Zi* is decocted in water for 1 hour and then all the other drugs are added and decocted together for the decoction. The decoction is taken warm twice. The drugs of this prescription are most warm and dry . When used to treat a patient with flushed face and restlessness, a sign of the syndrome of "true cold in nature with pseudo−heat symptoms", the decoction should be taken cold . Or else , dryness in the upper−*Jiao* will be made severe, resulting in nasal bleeding.

Case Study: Acupuncture, modified *Sini Tang* and therapies of Western medicine were clinically co−used to rescue 1 case of cardiac arrest due to lightening stroke. The patient was a male at the age of 38 and had the following symptoms and signs: coma , pale complexion, cyanotic lips, cold limbs, feeble breathing and disappearance of heart sounds. Closed cardiac massage, needling of the acupoints *Ren Zhong, He Gu* and *Yong Quan,* intramuscular injection of 0.375 mg of nikethamide intravenous injection 50 ml of 50% glucose were performed. Half an hour after that, the condition was: intermittent feeble heart sounds, arrhythmia, and 28 times per minute of the heart rate. Whereupon, 1 dose of *Sini Tang* (in which the dosage of *Fu Zi* was changed from 5−10 g to 25g.) plus:

Dang Shen (Radix Codonopsis), *Huang Qi* (Radix Astragali), was used. 1 hour later after the drcoction was taken, the cold limbs became warm, the heart rate reached 50 times per minute, the patient complained of precardial pain. Then, 1 dose of the above prescription plus:

Hong Hua (Flos Carthami), *Dang Gui* (Radix Angelicae Sinensis), was used and the disease condition was further improved. Finally, the above prescription, in which the dosage of *Fu Zi* was reduced to 12.5 g, was again used and 2 doses cured the case.

70 cases of infantile diarrhea marked by loose stools, mild fever, cold limbs, feeble pulse and whitish thin tongue coating were treated with *Sini Tang,* whose ingredients were:

Fu Zi (Radix Aconiti Lateralis Preparata) 15 g, *Gan Jiang* (Rhizoma Zingiberis) 9 g,*Gan Cao* (Radix Glycyrrhizae) 9 g, *Huang Lian* (Rhizoma Coptidis) 9 g.

The first three ingredients were decocted in 350 ml of water until the time when 150 ml was left and , then, *Huang Lian* was added. The mixture was decocted on gentle fire until 80 ml of the decoction was got through filtrating. Finally,appropriate amount of sugar was added to the decoction, which was boiled for use. 3−5 ml of the decoction was taken each time, 1 time every 4 hours by the infants below 5 months, 5−8 ml by the infants between 6−10 months, 8−10 ml by the infants at the age of 1−1.5 years old. The result showed that 58 cases were cured,effectiveness resulted in 8 cases, ineffectiveness in 4, the treatment duration averaging 4 days.

6.9　The Prescription of *Huiyang Jiuji Tang*

Name: Decoction for Restoring *Yang* from Collapse
Source: The book *Shang Han Liu Shu*
Ingredients:

Shu Fu Zi (Radix Aconiti Lateralis Preparata) 9 g, *Gan Jiang* (Rhizoma Zingiberis) 5 g, *Rou Gui* (Cortex Cinnamomi) 3 g, *Ren Shen* (Radix Ginseng) 6 g,*Bai Zhu* (parched Rhizoma Atractylodis Macrocephalae) 9 g, *Fu Ling* (Poria) 9 g,*Chen Pi* (Pericarpium Citri Reticulatae) 6 g, *Gan Cao* (Radix Glycyrrhizae Preparata) 5 g,*Wu Wei Zi* (Fructus Schisandrae) 3 g, *Zhi Ban Xia* (Rhizoma Pinelliae Preparata) 9 g,*Sheng Jiang* (Rhizoma Zingiberis Recens) 3 pieces, *She Xiang* (Moschus) 0.1 g.

Explanation:

Fu Zi: The principal drug, being pungent and sweet in flavor and very hot in nature, warming the interior, restoring *Yang,* removing cold accumulation through expelling cold pathogen.

Gan Jiang: Warming the middle—*Jiao* and purging cold .

Rou Gui: Warming and strengthening the kidney—*Yang*.

Ren Shen, Bai Zhu, Fu Ling, Gan Cao, Chen Pi and *Ban Xia:*Invigorating the spleen and stomach, drying dampness and resolving phlegm.

*She Xiang:*Activating the flow of *Qi* and blood throughout the twelve channels.

Wu Wei Zi: Being sour in flavor, functioning in astringing while dispersing, working together with *Ren Shen* to replenish *Qi* and promote the production of blood.

Effect: Recuperating depleted *Yang* and rescuing the patient from collapse, replenishing *Qi* and promoting the circulation of blood.

Indications: Syndrome of weakness of the kidney—*Yang* due to direct attack of cold pathogen on the three *Yin* channels, marked by aversion to cold , lying with the extremities drawn up, cold limbs, vomiting, diarrhea, abdominal pain , no thirst, listlessness with desire for sleep, or shiver with cold , or dark purplish nails and lips, or vomiting of foamy fluid, pale tongue with whitish coating, and deep feeble or even unfelt pulse; including such diseases with the above symptoms as chronic colitis, chronic diarrhea, salmonellal infection and toxic dysentery.

Administration: Decocted in water for oral dose to be taken twice. *She Xiang* is added when the decoction is about to be taken.

This prescription is mainly composed of drugs warm and dry in nature, so it should not be administered any longer once the cold limbs of a patient become warm.

6.10 The Prescription of *Heixi Dan*

Name: Black Tin Pill
Source: The book *Tai Ping Hui Min He Ji Ju Fang*
Ingredients:

Chuan Lian Zi (steamed Fructus Meliae Toosendan) 30 g, *Hu Lu Ba* (Semen Trigonellae steeped in liquor and then parched) 30 g, *Mu Xiang* (Radix Aucklandiae) 30 g, *Fu Zi* (Radix Aconiti Lateralis Preparata) 30 g, *Rou Dou Kou* (Semen Myristicae enclosed in flour paste and then baked) 30 g, *Po Gu Zhi* (Fructus Psoraleae steeped in Liquor and then parched) 30 g, *Chen Xiang* (Lignum Aquilariae Resinatum) 30 g, *Hui Xiang* (parched

Fructus Foeniculi) 30 g, *Yang Qi Shi* (Actinolitum boiled in liquor and baked and ground) 30 g, *Rou Gui* (Cortex Cinnamomi) 15 g, *Hei Xi* (cleaned Stannum Nigrum) 60 g, *Liu Huang* (Sulfur) 60 g.

Explanation:

Hei Xi: One of the principal drugs, being sweet in flavor and cold in nature, suppressing floating *Yang*, keeping the up-ward adverse flow of *Qi* downward to relieve asthma.

Liu Huang: The other principal drug, being sour in flavor and hot in nature, warming and tonifying the fire of *Mingmen*, warming the kidney to expel pathogenic cold.

Fu Zi and *Rou Gui:* Warming the kidney and supporting *Yang*, conducting the fire back to its origin.

Yang Qi Shi, Po Gu Zhi and *Hu Lu Ba:* Warming *Mingmen* to remove pathogenic cold.

Hui Xiang, Chen Xiang and *Rou Dou Kou:* Warming the middle—*Jiao* and regulating the flow of *Qi*, keeping the adverse flow of *Qi* downward to remove phlegm, and warming the kidney.

Chuan Lian Zi: Being bitter in flavor and cold in nature, restricting the warm and dry nature of the other ingredients, regulating the flow of *Qi* and relieving liver depression.

Effect: Warming and strengthening the primordial *Qi* in the lower—*Jiao*, suppressing floating *Yang*.

Indications: Syndrome due to insufficiency of the kidney—*Yang* and inability of the kidney to govern reception of *Qi*, marked by accumulation of phlegm in the chest, dyspnea, cold limbs, profuse cold sweating, pale tongue with whitish coating, and deep weak pulse, or due to up—rushing of *Qi* to the chest, marked by a sensation of *Qi* rushing like a running piggy and distention in the chest and hypochondrium, or due to periumbilical colic from invasion of cold complicated by borborygmus and lingering diarrhea or impotence and cold sperm in males or cold and deficiency of the uterus marked by thin and diluted leukorrhea in females; including such diseases with the above symptoms as asthma and impotence.

Administration: Ground into fine powder, which is made into pills with flour paste and liquor and taken with salt water. 5 g of the pills each time for adults,2—3 g each time for young children, 9 g each time for first aid.

This prescription is composed of drugs with the action of warming the kidney , descending *Qi* and suppressing floating *Yang,* so it is suitable for first aid but it should not be used often or for a long time lest lead poisoning result.

Caes Study: *Heixi Dan* was clinically used to treat 1 case of asthma. The patient had suffered from the disorder for several years. Asthma recurred 1—10 or so times daily with the following symptoms and signs: shortness of breath as if air in the chest could not be exhaled and air outside could not be inhaled, profuse sweat, spitting sputum with foam, thirst with desire for hot food, whitish thin tongue coating, 5—6 times of recurrence round the clock, sitting with the body twisted and inability to lie flat in the course of recurrence. *Heixi Dan* was taken 1—3 times daily, 30 pills each time. 3 days later, the disorder recurred 1 time daily or every two days. 10 days later, the asthma vanished. Another 10 days' taking of the medicine swept away all the symptoms and signs.

6.11 Prescriptions for Warming the Channels and Removing Cold

This kind of prescriptions are mainly made up of drugs with the action of warming the channels to eliminate pathogenic cold and nourishing blood to promote its circulation through the channels. They are suitable for the syndromes due to deficiency of *Yang—Qi* and *Yin*—blood complicated by invasion of exogeous pathogenic cold into the channels and sluggish flow of blood in the vessels. Drugs with the action of warming the channels to eliminate cold such as

Gui Zhi (Ramulus Cinnamomi), *Xi Xin* (Herba Asari), are usually compatible with drugs with the action of nourishing blood to promote its circulation through the channels such as

Dang Gui (Radix Angelicae Sinensis), *Shao Yao* (Radix Paeoniae),

in these prescriptions, whose representatives are *Danggui Sini Tang*, etc.

6.12 The Prescription of *Danggui Sini Tang*

Name: Chinese Angelica Decoction for Restoring *Yang*

Source: The book *Shang Han Lun*

Ingredients:

Dang Gui (Radix Angelicae Sinensis) 12 g, *Gui Zhi* (Ramulus Cinnamomi) 9 g, *Shao Yao* (Radix Paeoniae) 9 g, *Xi Xin* (Herba Asari) 1.5 g, *Zhi Gan Cao* (Radix Glycyrrhizae Preparata) 5 g, *Tong Cao* (Medulla Tetrapanacis) 3 g, *Da Zao* (Fructus Jujubae) 8 dates.

Explanation:

Dang Gui: The principal drug, being pungent and sweet in flavor and warm in nature, nourishing blood and activating the flow of it.

Gui Zhi: Warming the channels to promote the circulation of blood.

Bai Shao: Enriching blood and regulating *Ying*.

Xi Xin: Promoting the circulation of blood through the channels to disperse pathogenic cold.

Da Zao and *Zhi Gan Cao:* Replenishing the spleen—*Qi* and tempering the actions of all the other ingredients.

Tong Cao: Removing obstructions from the channels.

Effect: Warming the channels to expel pathogenic cold, nourishing blood and promoting the flow of it.

Indications: Syndrome due to blood deficiency and exposure to cold, marked by cold limbs, pale tongue with whitish coating, deep thready or indistinct pulse; including such diseases with the above symptoms as thromboangiitis obliterans, peripheral phlebitis polyneuritis and frostbite.

Administration: Decocted in water for oral dose to be taken 3 times

Case Study: 10 cases of thromboangiitis obliterans were clinically treated with modified *Danggui Sini Tang,* whose ingredients were:

Dang Gui (Radix Angelicae Sinensis), *Gui Zhi* (Ramulus Cinnamomi), *Chi Shao* (Radix Paeoniae Rubra), *Tong Cao* (Medulla Tetrapanacis),*Chuan Jiao* (Pericarpium Zanthoxyli), *Da Zao* (Fructus Jujubae),*Dan Shen* (Radix Salviae Miltiorrhizae), *Yi Mu Cao* (Herba Leonuri),*Wang Bu Liu Xing* (Semen Vaccariae), *Yu Jin* (Radix Curcumae),*Pu Gong Ying* (Herba

Taraxaci), *Yin Hua* (Flos Lonicerae),*Xuan Shen* (Radix Scrophulariae), *Fu Zi* (Radix Aconiti Lateralis Preparata),*Lu Jiao Jiao* (Colla Cornus Cervi), *Ji Xue Teng* (Caulis Spatholobi),*Dang Shen* (Radix Codonopsis), *Huang Qi* (Radix Astragali),*Chuan Niu Xi* (Radix Achyranthes bidentata).

The disease's duration varied from 2 months to 3 years. After the treatment, 9 cases were cured.

2 cases of early Reynaud's disease, a syndrome due to inability of deficient *Yang* to warm and nourish the extremities complicated by invasion of exogenous pathogenic cold resulting in stagnation and sluggish flow of blood in the vessels, were treated with modified *Danggui Sini Tang*. 1 case was cured by taking over 30 doses of the prescription plus:

Ai Ye (Folium Artemisiae Argyi), *Hong Hua* (Flos Carthami),

and the other by taking 18 doses. Follow–up found no recurrence at all.

7 Prescriptions for Expelling Pathogenic Factors from Both the Exterior and Interior

7.1 Prescriptions for Expelling Pathogenic Factors from Both the Exterior and Interior

This kind of prescriptions are mainly composed of exterior—syndrome—relieving drugs which are compatible with drugs of reducing bowel movements or drugs of removing heat and warming the interior. Being capable of expelling pathogenic factors from both the exterior and interior, they are used to treat diseases involving the exterior as well as the interior. When the exterior syndrome has not been cured but the interior one is in full swing, if mere prescriptions for relieving exterior syndrome are prescribed, pathogens in the interior can't be expelled; if attention is only paid to expel pathogenic factors in the interior, pathogens in the exterior won't be swept away. Under this conditon, therefore, prescriptions for expelling pathogenic factors in both the exterior and interior should be used to dispel the pathogenic factors separately. According to the different nature of diseases involving both the exterior and interior, prescriptions of this kind are subdivided into the following three: those for relieving exterior syndrome to expel interior pathogens with purgatives, those for relieving exterior syndrome to remove pathogenic heat in the interior, and those for relieving exterior syndrome to warm the interior. As to the prescriptions for relieving exterior syndrome and tonifying the interior, which are suitable for the syndromes due to unrelieved exterior disorders complicated by deficiency of vital—Qi, they have been introduced in the above and won't be rementioned here.

Prescriptions for expelling pathogenic factors from both the exterior and interior should be only prescribed to treat syndromes with both the exterior and interior symptoms. Most effective ones will be selected exactly through differentiating the disease condition such as the cold / heat nature, and the deficiency / excess of the exterior, and interior syndromes. The proportions of the drugs for relieving exterior syndrome and the drugs for expelling pathogenic factors from the interior will be right determined and no too potent or too mild prescriptions will be prescribed if only which is more severe and which is the dominative one, the exterior syndrome or the interior one, have been made clear.

7.2 Prescriptions for Relieving Exterior Syndrome to Expel Interior Pathogens with Purgatives

This kind of prescriptions are mainly composed of diaphoretics and purgatives. They are suitable for the syndrome due to cold or heat pathogens in the exterior and excessive pathogenic factors in the interior. Drugs such as

Ma Huang (Herba Ephedrae), *Gui Zhi* (Ramulus Cinnamomi), *Jing Jie* (Herba Schizonepetae), *Fang Feng* (Radix Saposhinkoviae),*Chai Hu* (Radix Bupleuri), *Bo He* (Herba Menthae),*Da Huang* (Radix et Rhizoma Rhei), *Mang Xiao* (Natrii Sulfas).

are usually used in these prescriptions, whose representatives are *Da Chaihu Tang, Fangfeng Tongsheng San*, etc.

7.3 The Prescription of *Da Chaihu Tang*

Name: Major Bupleurum Decoction

Source: The book *Jin Gui Yao Lue*

Ingredients:

Chai Hu (Radix Bupleuri) 15 g, *Huang Qin* (Radix Scutellariae),9 g, *Shao Yao* (Radix Paeoniae) 9 g, *Ban Xia* (Rhizoma Pinelliae), 9 g, *Zhi Zhi Shi* (Fructus Aurantii Immaturus Preparata) 9 g,*Da Huang* (Radix et Rhizoma Rhei) 6 g, *Sheng Jiang* (Rhizoma Zingiberis Recens) 15 g, *Da Zao* (Fructus Jujubae) 5 dates.

Explanation:

Chai Hu: The principal drug, being bitter and pungent in flavor and slightly cold in nature, clearing away heat through the superficies of the body to relieve exterior syndrome.

Huang Qin: Working together with *Chai Hu* to clear away heat and mediate *Shaoyang* and expel pathogens in it.

Da Huang and *Zhi Shi:* Purging accumulated pathogenic heat in *Yangming*.

Shao Yao: Relieving spasm and pain, getting together with *Da Huang* to treat abdominal pain of excess type, combining *Zhi Shi* to treat incoordination between *Qi* and blood.

Ban Xia: Keeping the adverse flow of *Qi* downward to arrest vomiting, treating obstinate vomiting and hiccup in large dose and compatible with *Sheng Jiang*.

Da Zao and *Sheng Jiang:* Working together to regulate *Ying* and *Wei* and temper the actions of all the other ingredients.

Effect: Mediating *Shaoyang* and purging accumulated heat in the interior

Indications: Combined syndrome of *Shaoyang* and *Yangming,* marked by alternative attack of fever and chills, fullness in the chest and hypochondrium, intractable vomiting, mental depression and mild restlessness, distending pain in the epigastrium or epigastric fullness and rigidity, constipation or diarrhea with heat, yellow tongue coating and wiry forceful pulse; including such diseases with the above symptoms as acute simple intestinal obstruction, acute pancreatitis, acute cholecystitis and biliary calculi.

Administration: Decocted in water for oral dose to be taken twice

Case Study: *Da Chaihu Tang* plus:

Chuan Lian Zi (Fructus Toosendan), *Yan Hu Su* (Rhizoma Corydalis),

was clinically prescribed to treat 40 cases of acute cholecystitis manifested as pain in the chest and hypochondriac region, tenderness in the liver which is, in most cases, radiates to the right back and shoulder, aversion to cold, fever, nausea, vomiting, tension of the abdominal muscles and icteric sclera, and as well as dry throat , bitter taste in the mouth, palpable enlarged bile—cyst or inflammatory adhesive mass in the right hypochondriac region in about half of the cases,   As a result of this treatment, 35 cases were cured, 5 improved and 3 relapsed.

Da Chaihu Tang plus:

Yan Hu Su (Rhizoma Corydalis), *Mu Xiang* (Radix Aucklandiae),

was used to treat 22 cases of acute pancreatitis marked by severe epigastric pain with local tenderness, nausea , vomiting, elevated body temperature at different level in most of the cases, yellow thick or yellow dry tongue coating, and taut slippery pulse. Of the cases, increased leukocyte count was found in 18 cases, amylase in urine reached 128 in 2 cases and over 256 in all the others. Among the 19 cases whose serum amylase were tested, the serum level of amylase was above 128 in 8 cases. Treated with this decoction combined with transfusion, atropine and dolantin, all the cases were cured.

7.4   The Prescription of *Fangfeng Tongsheng San*

Name: Miraculous Powder of Ledebouriella

Source: The book *Xuan Ming Lun Fang*

Ingredients:

Fang Feng (Radix Saposhinkoviae) 15 g, *Jing Jie* (Herba Schizonepetae) 15 g, *Lian Qiao* (Fructus forsythiae) 15 g, *Ma Huang* (Herba Ephedrae) 15 g, *Bo He* (Herba Menthae) 15 g, *Chuan Xiong* (Rhizoma Chuanxiong) 15 g, *Dang Gui* (Radix Angelicae Sinensis) 15 g, *Bai Shao* (parched Radix Paeoniae Alba) 15 g, *Bai Zhu* (Rhizoma Atractylodis Macrocephalae) 15 g,*Shan Zhi* (Fructus Gardeniae) 15 g, *Da Huang* (Radix et Rhizoma Rhei steamed with liquor) 15 g,*Mang Xiao* (Natrii Sulfas added later) 15 g, *Shi Gao* (Gypsum Fibrosum) 30 g,*Huang Qin* (Radix Scutellariae) 30 g, *Jie Geng* (Radix Platycodi) 30 g,*Gan Cao* (Radix Glycyrrhizae) 60 g, *Hua Shi* (Talcum) 90 g, *Sheng Jiang* (*Rhizoma Zingiberis Recens*) 3 pieces.

Explanation:

Fang Feng: The pricipal drug, being pungent and sweet in flavor and slightly warm in nature, dispersing wind pathogen to relieve exterior syndrome, working together with *Jing Jie, Ma Huang* and *Bo He* to strongly dispel wind pathogen by diaphoresis.

Da Huang and *Mang Xiao:* Removing heat pathogen to relieve constipation, working together with *Shi Gao, Huang Qin, Lian Qiao* and *Jie Geng* to expel heat in the lung and stomach.

Shan Zhi and *Hua Shi:* Clearing away pathogenic demp—heat through promoting the discharge of feces and urine.

Dang Gui, Chuan Xiong and *Bai Shao:* Nourishing blood and promoting the flow of it.

Bai Zhu: Strengthenig the spleen and drying dampness.

Gan Cao: Regulating the middle—*Jiao* and relieving pain.

Sheng Jiang: Regulating the stomach and descending the adverse flow of *Qi.*

Effect: Dispelling wind pathogen to relieve exterior syndrome, clearing away heat pathogen to relieve constipation.

Indications:

Syndrome due to excessive wind and heat pathogens in both the exterior and interior, marked by great aversion to cold, high fever, dizziness, reddened and painful eyes, bitter and dry sensation in the mouth, sore throat, fullness in the chest, cough, vomiting, asthma, thick nasal discharges and saliva, constipation, scanty and deep—clored urine; including such diseases with the above symptoms as urticaria, neurogenic headache, psoriasis and allergic purpura.

Administration: The ingredients except *Sheng Jiang* are gound into powder, 9 g of which is mixed with 3 pieces of *Sheng*

Jiang. The mixture is decocted in water for the decoction to be taken twice. (Taken also in the form of pills)

Case Study:

Fangfeng Tongsheng San plus:

Chen Pi (Pericarpium Citri Reticulatae), *Ban Xia* (Rhizoma Pinelliae),

was clinically used to treat 1 case of intractable headache, marked by headache more severe in the right side of the head and in the left cheek, high blood pressure, mild neuroparalysis of the left face and mild dysphasia occurred one month ago, one bowel movement every week ,taut forceful pulse, little tongue coating , mild inflation of the abdomen , mild guarding in the epigastric region, 170 / 90 mmHg of blood pressure. 3 doses cured the patient of his / her headache with the dysphasia remarkably improved.

7.5　Prescriptions for Relieving Exterior Syndrome to Remove Pathogenic Heat in the Interior

This kind of prescriptions are mainly composed of drugs with the action of alleviating exterior syndrome and expelling heat pathogen. They are indicated for the syndrome due to pathogenic cold or heat in the exterior complicated by pathogenic heat in the interior.

Drugs such as

Ma Huang (Herba Ephedrae), *Dan Dou Chi* (Semen Sojae Preparatum), *Ge Gen* (Radix Puerariae), *Huang Qin* (Radix Scutellariae), *Huang Lian* (Rhizoma Coptidis), *Huang Bai* (Cortex Phellodendri), are usually used in these prescriptions, whose representatives are *Gegen Huangqin Huanglian Tang* and *Shigao Tang*.

7.6 The Prescriptions of *Gegen Huangqin Huanglian Tang*

Name: Decoction of Pueraria, Scutellaria and Coptis

Source: The book *Shang Han Lun*

Ingredients:

Ge Gen (Radix Puerariae) 15 g, *Zhi Gan Cao* (Radix Glycyrrhizae Preparata) 6 g, *Huang Qin* (Radix Scutellariae) 9 g, *Huang Lian* (Rhizoma Coptidis) 9 g.

Explanation:

Ge Gen: The principal drug, being sweet and pungent in flavor and cold in nature, removing pathogenic heat from the exterior, ascending the *Qi* of the spleen and stomach to treat diarrhea.

Huang Qin and *Huang Lian:* Clearing away heat pathogen from the stomach and intestines and dry dampness in them.

Gan Cao: Regulating the *Qi* of the middle—*Jiao* and tempering the actions of all the other ingredients.

Effect: Relieving exterior syndrome and removing heat

Indications: Unrelieved exterior syndrome complicated by pathogenic heat in the interior, marked by fever, loose stools with disagreeable odour, buring sensation in the anus, restless and heat sensation in the chest and epigastric region, dry mouth, thirst, asthma, sweating, yellowish tongue coating , and rapid pulse; including such diseases with the above symptoms as bacillary dysentery, ileotyphus, acute enteritis and infantile diarrhea.

Administration: Decocted in water for oral dose to be taken

twice

Case Study: 40 cases of acute bacillary dysentery were clinically treated with *Gegen Huangqin Huanglian Tang*. The result was that all the cases were cured, each case taking 2—12 doses. The shortest duration for the fever to subside was 4 hours. The duration for the abdominal pain to disappear averaged 4.51 days, for the rectal tenesmus to vanish 3.47 days, for the poor appetite to return to normal 2.5 days for the number of bowel movements to return to normal and for the feces microscopy to show negative findings 4 days, for the acute symptoms and signs to vanish 3.44 days Clinical symptoms and signs disappeared completely in 39 cases.

129 cases of poliomyelitis were treated with modified *Gegen Huangqin Huanglian Tang*, whose ingredients were:

Ge Gen (Radix Puerariae), *Huang Qin* (Radix Scutellariae), *Huang Lian* (Rhizoma Coptidis), *Gan Cao* (Radix Glycyrrhizae), *Sheng Shi Gao* (Gypsum Fibrosum), *Yin Hua* (Flos Lonicerae), *Bai Shao* (Radix Paeoniae Alba), *Quan Xie* (Scorpio), *Wu Gong* (Scolopendra).

After the treatment, among the 52 severe cases whose affected legs were in the state of deep complete paralysis and lost paleocinetic function, 17 were cured, 35 improved; among the 67 moderately severe cases who had paleocinetic legs but could not walk and stand, 33 were cured, 34 improved; the 10 mild cases who could stand and walk with paleocinetic but weak legs were all cured. Most of the mild and moderately severe cases were cured within one month or so with one case cured in one week.

7.7   The Prescription of *Shigao Tang*

Name: Gypsum Decoction

Source: The book *Wai Tai Mi Yao*

Ingredients:

Shi Gao (Gypsum Fibrosum) 30 g, *Huang Lian* (Rhizoma Coptidis) 6 g, *Huang Bai* (Cortex Phellodendri) 6 g, *Huang Qin* (Radix Scutellariae) 6 g, *Dan Dou Chi* (Semen Sojae Preparatum) 9 g, *Zhi Zi* (Fructus Gardeniae) 9 g, *Ma Huang* (Herba Ephedrae) 9 g.

Explanation:

Shi Gao: The principal drug, being pungent and sweet in flavor and very cold in nature, removing heat and restlessness.

Ma Huang and *Dou Chi:* Removing the pathogenic factors in the exterior through the superficies of the body.

Huang Lian, Huang Qin, Huang Bai and *Zhi Zi:* Purging fire and removing toxic materials, expelling fire in the tri–*Jiao* from the interior.

Effect: Removing heat and toxic materials, relieving exterior syndrome through diaphoresis.

Indications: Syndrome of intense heat due to febrile disease in the interior complicated by unrelieved exterior syndrome , marked by high fever, no sweat, heavy and strain sensation of the body , dry nose, thirst, restlessness, insomnia, coma, delirium ,or skin eruption, and slippery rapid pulse; including such diseases with the above symptoms as hematosepsis, cholecystitis, pelvic inflammation, pancreatitis and appendicitis.

Administration: Decocted in water for oral dose to be taken 3 times

7.8　Prescriptions for Relieving Exterior Syndrome to Warm the Interior

This kind of prescriptions are mainly made up of drugs with the action of expelling pathogenic factors from the exterior and eliminating pathogenic cold from the interior. They are suitable for the syndrome due to unrelieved exterior syndrome complicated by cold pathogens in the interior. Drugs with the action of relieving exterior syndromes such as

Ma Huang (Herba Ephedrae), *Bai Zhi* (Radix Angelicae Dahuricae),

are usually used compatibly with drugs with the action of warming the interior to dispel pathogenic cold such as

Gan Jiang (Rhizoma Zingiberis), *Rou Gui* (Cortex Cinnamomi),

in these prescriptions, whose representatives are *Wuji San,* etc.

7.9　The prescription of *Wuji San*

Name: Powder for Relieving Five Kinds of Accumulation in the Abdomen

Source: The book *Tai Ping Hui Min He Ji Ju Fang*

Ingredients:

Bai Zhi (Radix Angelicae Dahuricae) 90 g, *Chuan Xiong* (Rhizoma Chuanxiong) 90 g, *Zhi Gan Cao* (Radix Glycyrrhizae Preparata) 90 g, *Fu Ling* (Poria) 90 g, *Dang Gui* (Radix Angelicae Sinensis) 90 g, *Rou Gui* (Cortex Cinnamomi) 90 g, *Shao Yao* (Radix Paeoniae) 90 g, *Ban Xia* (Rhizoma Pinelliae) 90 g, *Chen Pi* (Pericarpium Citri Reticulatae) 180 g, *Zhi Qiao* (parched Fructus Aurantii) 180 g, *Ma Huang* (Herba Ephedrae)

180 g, *Cang Zhu* (Rhizoma Atractylodis) 720 g, *Gan Jiang* (baked Rhizoma Zingiberis) 120 g, *Jie Geng* (Radix Platycodi) 360 g, *Hou Po* (Cortex Magnoliae Officinalis) 120 g, *Sheng Jiang* (Rhizoma Zingiberis Recens) 3 pieces.

Explanation:

Ma Huang and *Bai Zhi:* The principal drugs, relieving exterior syndrome through diaphoresis.

Gan Jiang and *Rou Gui:* The principal drugs, warming the interior to remove cold pathogen.

Gang Zhu and *Hou Po:* Drying dampness and strengthening the spleen.

Chen Pi, Ban Xia and *Fu Ling:* Regulating the flow of *Qi* to resolve phlegm.

Dang Gui, Chuan Xiong and *Shao Yao:* Promoting the circulation of blood to relieve pain.

Jie Geng and *Zhi Qiao:* Activating the flow of *Qi* to remove stagnations.

Gan Cao: Regulating the *Qi* of the middle—*Jiao* to strengthen the spleen , tempering the actions of all the other ingredients.

Effect: Relieving exterior syndrome through diaphoresis, warming the interior to dispel pathogenic cold, activating the flow of *Qi* to remove phlegm, promoting the circulation of blood and digestion.

Indications: Syndrome due to affection of exogenous wind—cold and impairment done by raw and cold pathogens in the interior, marked by fever without sweat, headache and general aching, muscular rigidity in the back and neck, fullness in the chest, anorexia, vomiting, abdominal pain, pain in the abdomen and irregular menstruation in women due to derangement of *Qi* and blood ; including such diseases with the above symptoms as habitual common cold, gastrointestinal neurosis, irregular menstruation, chronic gastroenteritis and chronic hepatitis.

Administration:

All the ingredients except *Sheng Jiang, Rou Gui* and *Zhi Qiao* are ground into coarse powder, The powder is parched until it's color has been changed. The parched powder is spread to be cooled and then mixed with the powder of *Rou Gui* and *Zhi Qiao*. 9 g of the mixed powder and *Sheng Jiang* are decocted in water for the decoction, which is taken warm 2 times in one day. (The ingredients of this prescription may be decocted in water for oral dose. In so doing , the dosage of the drugs should be deterimined according to the proportions of the drugs in the original prescription.)

8 Prescriptions for Tonification

8.1 Prescriptions for Tonification

This kind of prescriptions are mainly composed of drugs with the action of tonifying, Being capable of nourishing and invigorating the *Qi,* blood, *Yin* and *Yang* of the body, they are used to treat various syndromes of deficiency type. As syndromes of deficiency type can be summarized as *Qi* deficiency, blood deficiency, *Yin* deficiency, *Yang* deficiency and deficiency of both *Qi* and blood, prescriptions of this kind are classified, accordingly, as the following five: those for invigorating *Qi,* those for enriching blood, those for replenishing *Yin,* those for tonifying *Yang,* and those for reinforcing both *Qi* and blood.

Qi, blood, *Yin* and *Yang* are inseparably related to each other. Just as the theories indicate: *Qi* and blood generate mutually; *Qi* were the commander of blood; blood were the mother of *Qi,* Therefore, drugs for invigorating *Qi* are used in prescriptions for enriching blood, and drugs for enriching blood are used to treat syndromes due to *Qi* deficiency complicated by blood deficiency. Similarly, drugs for tonifying *Yang* are used in prescriptions for replenishing *Yin,* and drugs for replenishing *Yin* are used in prescriptions for tonifying *Yang,* for the purpose of "tonifying *Yang* by replenishing *Yin*" and "replenishing *Yin* by tonifying *Yang*". This is based on the theory that *Yin* and *Yang* depend on and assist each other, they are physiologically related to and pathologically influenced each other. As for the hypoactivities of the spleen and stomach, drugs which should be prescribed are those with the action of strengthening the spleen and benefiting the stomach.

Drugs in prescriptions for tonification should be decocted with gentle heat for a longer time, and it is better to take their decoction on an empty stomach or before meal. Before prescriptions for tonification are prescribed, the true or false of a deficiency syndrome must be identified. When exogenous pathogens still linger, the first thing is to expel them instead of tonifying. If tonification is really needed, drugs for tonification must be used together with drugs for removing pathogens

8.2   Prescriptions for Invigorating *Qi*

This kind of prescriptions are mainly made up of drugs with the action of invigorating *Qi*. They are suitable for the syndrome due to *Qi* deficiency of the spleen and lung, marked by lassitude, shortness of breath, lower voice, languor, pale complexion loss of appetite, pale tongue with whitish coating, floating or feeble large pulse, or fever of deficiency type, spontaneous sweating, or proctoptosis prolapse of the uterus, etc. Drugs such as

Ren Shen (Radix Ginseng), *Huang Qi* (Radix Astragali), *Bai Zhu* (Rhizoma Atractylodis Macrocephalae), *Zhi Gan Cao* (Radix Glycyrrhizae Preparata),

are usually used in these prescriptions, whose representatives are *Si Jun Zi Tang*, *Shenling Baizhu San* and *Buzhong Yiqi Tang*.

8.3   The Prescription of *Si Jun Zi Tang*

Name: Decoction of Four Noble Drugs

Source: The book *Tai Ping Hui Min He Ji Ju Fang*

Ingredients:

Ren Shen (Radix Ginseng) 10 g, *Bai Zhu* (Rhizoma Atractylodis Macrocephalae) 9 g, *Fu Ling* (Poria) 9 g, *Zhi Gan Cao* (Radix Glycyrrhizae Preparata) 6 g.

Explanation:

Ren Shen: The principal drug, being sweet in flavor and warm in nature, invigorating primordial *Qi,* strengthening the spleen and stomach.

Bai Zhu: Strengthening the spleen and drying dampness.

Fu Ling: Inducing diuresis and strengthening the spleen,assisting *Bai Zhu* in promoting the transforming and transporting function of the spleen.

Zhi Gan Cao: Invigorating *Qi,* regulating the stomach, tempering the actions of all the other ingredients.

Effect: Invigorating *Qi* and strengthening the spleen

Indications:

Syndrome due to *Qi* deficiency of the spleen and stomach, marked by pale complexion, lower voice, weakness of the limbs, poor appetite or loose stools, pale tongue, thready and slow pulse; including such diseases with the above symptoms as chronic gastritis and gastroduodenal ulcer.

Administration: Decocted in water for oral dose to be taken twice.

Case Study: The way to take decoction of *Si Jun Zi Tang* was clinically used to replace or reduce postgastric operation fluid transfusion in 154 cases with satisfactory effects.The prescription prescribed consisted of :

Dang Shen (Radix Codonopsis) 9 g, *Bai Zhu* (Rhizoma

Atractylodis Macrocephalae) 6 g, *Fu Ling* (Poria) 6 g, *Gan Cao* (Radix Glycyrrhizae) 3 g, *Shou Wu* (Radix Polygoni Multiflori) 6 g, *Bai Shao* (Radix Paeoniae Alba) 6 g.

The above ingredients were decocted in water for oral dose and 3 doses were taken in the whole course of treatment. The first dose was taken at 16th – 24th hours after the operation, the second at 48th hour, and the third at 72th hour.

Pharmacology:

The decoction of *Si Jun Zi Tang* acts on the hepatic glycogen and RNA of a mouse. An experiment showed that in the group of administration (40%), the hepatic glycogen was remarkably increased and the glycogen particles were accumulated into masses, especially in the centre.

A certain amount of the decoction of *Si Jun Zi Tang* exerted inhibitory influence on the movements of isolated small intestine of a rabbit. This was mainly related to the decoction's anti–acetylcholine action, which was marked by relaxing the tension of the movements of the intestinal canals rather than inhibiting their contraction.

The decoction also had evident anti–histamine action. This may be the reason that the patients with gastrointestinal disorders will get well after they take the decoction of *Si Jun Zi Tang*, suggesting that the decoction has the anti–adrenalin action as well as the anti–acetylcholine and anti–histamine actions.

8.4 The Prescription of *Liu Jun Zi Tang*

Name : Decoction of Six Ingredients
Source: The book *Fu Ren Liang Fang*
Ingredients:

Ren Shen (Radix Ginseng) 10 g, *Bai Zhu* (Rhizoma Atractylodis Macrocephalae) 9 g, *Fu Ling* (Poria) 9 g, *Zhi Gan Cao* (Radix Glycyrrhizae Preparata) 6 g, *Chen Pi* (Pericarpium Citri Reticulatae) 9 g, *Ban Xia* (Rhizoma Pinelliae) 9 g.

Explanation:

Ren Shen, Bai Zhu, Fu Ling and *Zhi Gan Cao:* Working together to invigorate *Qi* and reinforce the spleen.

Chen Pi: Regulating the flow of *Qi* and stomach, removing dampness and dissolving phlegm.

Ban Xia: Removing dampness and resolving phlegm, descending the upward adverse flow of *Qi* to arrest vomiting.

Effect: Strengthening the spleen to arrest vomiting.

Indications: Syndrome due to *Qi* deficiency of the spleen and stomach complicated by damp—phlegm, marked by loss of appetite, nausea, vomiting, full and depressing sensation in the chest and epigastric region, loose stools, or productive cough with whitish watery sputum; including such diseases with the above symptoms as vomiting in pregnancy, chronic gastritis and gastroduodenal ulcer.

Administration: Decocted in water for oral dose to be taken twice.

Case Study: 52 cases of pernicious vomiting were clinically treated with modified *Liu Jun Zi Tang*. The vomiting in all the cases was stopped 24—96 hours later after the decoction was taken (It reoccurred in 4 cases), and the appetite was rapidly improved. Each of 42 cases (80.77%) took 1—5 doses and they were all cured, 9 cases (17.3%) were improved, and 1 case (1.93%) was unimproved.

8.5 The Prescription of *Xiangsha Liujunzi Tang*

Name: Decoction of Cyperus and Amomum with Six Noble Ingredients

Source: The book *Yi Fang Ji Jie*

Ingredients:

Ren Shen (Radix Ginseng) 10 g, *Bai Zhu* (Rhizoma Atractylodis Macrocephalae) 9 g, *Fu Ling* (Poria) 9 g, *Zhi Gan Cao* (Radix Glycyrrhizae Preparata) 6 g, *Chen Pi* (Pericarpium Citri Reticulatae) 9 g, *Ban Xia* (Rhizoma Pinelliae) 9 g, *Mu Xiang* (Radix Aucklandiae) 6 g, *Sha Ren* (Fructus Amomi) 6 g.

Explanation:

Ren Shen, Bai Zhu, Fu Ling and *Zhi Gan Cao:* Invigorating *Qi* and strengthening the spleen.

Ban Xia: Removing dampness and resolving phlegm, keeping the adverse flow of *Qi* downward to arrest vomiting.

Chen Pi, Mu Xiang and *Sha Ren:* Promoting the flow of *Qi* to regulate the stomach and relieve pain.

Effect: Strengthening the spleen, regulating the stomach, promoting the flow of *Qi*, relieving pain.

Indications:

Syndrome due to hypofunction of the spleen and stomach and cold—dampness retained in the interior, marked by full and depressing sensation in the chest and epigastric region, vomiting, nausea, poor appetite, diarrhea, or stomachache of cold—type; including such diseases with the above symptoms as chronic gastritis, peptic ulcer and vomiting in pregnancy.

Administration: Decocted in water for oral dose to be taken twice

8.6 The Prescription of *Shenling Baizhu San*

Name: Powder of Ginseng, Poria and Bighead Atractylodes

Source: The book *Tai Ping Hui Min He Ji Ju Fang*

Ingredients:

Lian Zi Rou (Semen Nelumbinis) 500 g, *Yi Yi Ren* (Semen Coicis) 500 g, *Sha Ren* (Fructus Amomi) 500 g, *Jie Geng* (Radix Platycodi) 500 g, *Bai Bian Dou* (Semen Lablab Album) 750 g, *Fu Ling* (Poria) 1,000 g, *Bai Zhu* (Rhizoma Atractylodis Macrocephalae) 1,000 g, *Ren Shen* (Radix Ginseng) 1,000 g, *Shan Yao* (Rhizoma Dioscoreae) 1,000 g, *Zhi Gan Cao* (Radix Glycyrrhizae Preparata) 1,000 g.

Explanation:

Ren Shen, Shan Yao and *Lian Zi Rou:* The principal drugs, invigorating *Qi* and strengthening the spleen, regulating the stomach to treat diarrhea.

Bai Zhu, Fu Ling, Yi Yi Ren and *Bian Dou:* Promoting water metabolism and strengthening the spleen.

Sha Ren: Regulating the stomach and enlivening the spleen, promoting the flow of *Qi* to relieve chest depression.

Jie Geng: Facilitating the flow of the lung–*Qi* and guiding the action of other drugs to the upper–*Jiao*.

Zhi Gan Cao: Replenishing *Qi* and regulating the function of the middle–*Jiao*, tempering the actions of all other ingredients.

Effect: Strengthening the spleen, invigorating *Qi*, regulating the stomach, removing dampness.

Indications: Syndrome due to *Qi* deficiency of the spleen and stomach complicated by dampness pathogen, marked by poor appetite, loose stools, or vomiting and diarrhea, weakness of the limbs, emaciation, depressing and distending sensation in the chest and epigastric region, sallow complexion, whitish greasy tongue coating, and weak slow pulse; including such diseases with the above symptoms as chronic gastroenteritis, anemia, tuberculosis of lung chronic nephritis, and other chronic consumptive diseases.

Administration: All the ingredients are ground into fine powder, 6 g of which is taken with the decoction of *Da Zao* (Fructus Jujubae). (Taken also in the form of decoction with the dosages of the drugs properly reduced according to the original proportions of the ingredients in the prescription).

Case Study: 18 cases of diarrhea due to spleen deficiency, marked by emaciation, listlessness, pale or sallow complexion, distention and fullness in the abdomen, abdominal pain with preference for palpation, protracted diarrhea or loose stools with undigested food, poor appetite, pale tongue with thin whitish coating, thready slow pulse, and light indistinct supericial venule of the index finger, were clinically treated with *Shenling Baizhu San* modified according to the symptoms. The result was: 13 cases were cured, 4 cases improved, and 1 case unimproved.

8.7 The Prescription of *Buzhong Yiqi Tang*

Name: Decoction for Reinforcing the Middle—*Jiao* and Replenishing *Qi*

Source: The book *Pi Wei Lun*

Ingredients:

Huang Qi (Radix Astragali) 15 g, *Zhi Gan Cao:* (Radix Glycyrrhizae Praeparata) 6 g, *Ren Shen* (Radix Ginseng) 6 g,

Dang Gui (Radix Angelicae Sinensis) 9 g, *Ju Pi* (Pericarpium Citri Reticulatae) 6 g, *Chai Hu* (Radix Bupleuri) 3 g, *Sheng Ma* (Rhizoma Cimicifugae) 3 g, *Bai Zhu* (Rhizoma Atractylodis Macrocephalae) 10 g.

Explanation:

Huang Qi: The principal drug, invigorating *Qi* to consolidate the superficial resistance, elevating *Yang—Qi* to treat prolapse.

Dang Gui: Working with *Huang Qi* to replenish *Qi* and promote the generation of blood.

Chen Pi: Regulating the flow of *Qi* and the stomach, making this tonifying prescription not cause any stagnation.

Sheng Ma and *Chai Hu:* Aiding *Huang Qi* in elevating *Yang—Qi* and regulating the stomach.

Effect: Reinforcing the middle—*Jiao* and invigorating *Qi,* elevating *Yang—Qi* to treat prolapse.

Indications: Syndrome due to *Qi* deficiency of the spleen and stomach, marked by fever, sweating, headache, aversion to cold, thirst with prefernce for hot drink, shortness of breath, languor, or tastelessness in the mouth, weakness of the limbs, pale tongue with whitish coating, weak feeble pulse, including such disorders due to weak *Qi* of the middle—*Jiao* as proctoptosis, hysteroptosis, gastroptosis, prolonged diarrhea or dysentery as well as easy affection of common cold.

Administration: Decocted in water for oral dose to be taken twice (Taken also in the form of bolus, in which the proportions of the drugs are according to those in the original prescription. 10--15 g of the bolus is taken each time, 2--3 times daily.).

Contraindication: This prescription is contraindicated for the patients with heat pathogen in the interior due to *Yin* deficiency, for the drugs in it are sweet in flavor and damp in nature.

Case Study: *Buzhong Yiqi Tang* was clinically used to treat 23 cases of prolapse of the uterus, 1 dose being taken daily and 1 course of treatment involving 2 weeks. During the treatment, the patients were asked to take the chest—knee position and do the exercise of lifting anus and contracting the anal sphincter for 10—20 minutes both in the morning and evening, and avoid heavy physical labor and sudden rage. The result was: the treatment was stopped within 1 course in 2 cases but continued in all the other 21 cases, 76.2% of whom were cured, 6.5% improved, and 14.2% unimproved.

Buzhong Yiqi Tang was also used to treat 3 cases of blepharoptosis manifested as nearly—closed eyes due to inability of the upper eyelid to be lifted, dryness and soreness of the eyes and intermittent pain in the eyes. Half a month later, effectiveness was seen in all the 3 cases.

8.8 The Prescription of *Shengmai San*

Name: Pulse—activating Powder

Source: The book *Nei Wai Shang Bian Huo Lun*

Ingredients:

Ren Shen (Radix Ginseng) 10 g, *Mai Dong* (Radix Ophiopogonis) 15 g, *Wu Wei Zi* (Fructus Schisandrae) 6 g.

Explanation:

Ren Shen: The principal drug, replenishing the lung—*Qi*, promoting the production of body fluids.

Mai Dong: Nourishing *Yin*, clearing away heat, promoting the production of body fluids.

Wu Wei Zi: Astringing the lung to stop thirst, promoting the production of body fluids.

Effect: Working together to exert the action of tonifying, clearing away heat and astringing, and produce the effect of replenishing *Qi*, promoting the secretion of body fluids, astringing *Yin* and arresting sweating.

Indications: Syndrome due to impairment of both *Qi* and body fluid by pathogenic heat or lung—deficiency from prolonged cough, marked by profuse sweating, lassitude , shortness of breath, thirst, weak rapid pulse, or by cough with little sputum, shortness of breath, spontaneous sweating, dry tongue and mouth, and weak rapid pulse; including such diseases with the above symptoms as febrile disease at its later stage, tuberculosis of lung, chronic bronchitis, heart failure and acute infectious diseases in the convalescence.

Administration: Decocted in water for oral dose to be taken twice

Case Study: Compound injection of *Shengmai San* and *Sini San* was clinically adopted to treat 17 cases of acute myocardiac infarction complicated by cardiogenic shock with satisfactory curative effects. Of all the cases, failure of the left heart in the acute state was seen in 4 ones, ventricular tachycardia in one, supraventricular tachycardia in one, and second degree atrioventricular block in one. The result was: the blood pressure was retured to normal in all the cases except the one who had died in the course of treatment.

8.9 The Prescription of *Renshen Gejie San*

Name: Powder of Ginseng and Gecko
Source: The book *Wei Sheng Bao Jian*

Ingredients:

Ge Jie (Gecko) 1 pair, *Xing Ren* (Semen Armeniacae Amarum) 150 g, *Zhi Gan Cao* (Radix Glycyrrhizae Preparata)150 g, *Ren Shen* (Radix Ginseng) 60 g, *Fu Ling* (Poria) 60 g, *Bei Mu* (Bulbus Fritillariae Cirrhosae) 60 g, *Sang Bai Pi* (Cortex Mori) 60 g, *Zhi Mu* (Rhizoma Anemarrhenae) 60 g.

Explanation:

Ge Jie: The principal drug, improving inspiration to relieve asthma by invigorating the kidney−*Qi*.

Ren Shen: Reinforcing the primordial *Qi*, benefiting the spleen and lung.

Fu Ling: Strengthening the spleen to remove dampness.

Sang Pi and *Xing Ren:* Descending the adverse flow of *Qi* downward to relieve asthma.

Bei Mu: Clearing away heat, moisturizing the lung, resolving phlegm.

Zhi Mu: Clearing away lung−heat, nourishing the kidney, improving inspiration.

Zhi Gan Cao: Invigorating *Qi*, regulating the stomach, tempering the actions of all the other ingredients.

Effect: Replenishing *Qi*, clearing away lung−heat, relieving cough and asthma.

Indications: Syndrome due to lung−deficiency and prolonged cough, marked by cough, asthma, thick yellowish sputum, or cough, vomiting of pus and blood, restless and feverish sensation in the chest, emaciation, and floating weak pulse; including such diseases with the above symptoms as tuberculosis and chronic bronchitis.

Administration: The ingrediants are ground into powder.6 g of it is taken on an empty stomach with boiled water each time, twice daily, in the morning and evening.

8.10 Prescriptions for Enriching Blood

This kind of prescriptions are mainly made up of drugs with the action of tonifying blood. They are suitable for the syndrome of blood–deficiency manifested as dizziness, sallow complexion, pallor fingernails or toenails, palpitation, insomnia, scanty and light–colored menstruation, and thready rapid weak pulse.Drugs such as

Dang Gui (Radix Angelicae Sinensis), *Shu Di* (Radix Rehmanniae Preparata), *E Jiao* (Colla Corii Asini), *He Shou Wu* (Radix Polygoni Multiflori), are usually used in these prescriptions, whose representatives are *Siwu Tang* and *Guipi Tang*.

8.11 The Prescription of *Siwu Tang*

Name: Decoction of Four Ingredients
Source: The book *Tai Ping Hui Min He Ji Ju Fang*
Ingredients:

Dang Gui (Radix Angelicae Sinensis) 10 g, *Shu Di* (Radix Rehmanniae Preparata) 15 g, *Bai Shao* (Radix Paeoniae Alba) 10 g, *Chuan Xiong* (Rhizoma Chuanxiong) 6 g.

Explanation:

Shu Di: The principal drug, nourishing *Yin,* enriching blood, supplementing essence of the kidney.

Dang Gui: Tonifying and coordinating blood, regulating menstruation.

Bai Shao: Nourishing blood and astringing *Yin.*

Chuan Xiong: Promoting the circulation of blood and removing the stagnation of *Qi,* thus preventing other sticky—natured tonics in this prescription from bringing about the stagnation of *Qi* and blood.

Effect: Enriching blood and regulating menstruation.

Indications: Syndrome due to blood deficiency and blood stasis, marked by palpitation, dizziness, blurred eyes, tinnitus, pallor lips and finger / toe nails, scanty menstruation, or amenorrhea, pain around the umbilicus, pale tongue, and taut thready or thready uneven pulse; including such diseases with the above symptoms as anemia and irregular menstruation.

Contraindication: Because *Shu Di* and *Shao Yao* are liable to cause stagnation of *Qi* and impairment of *Yang—Qi* due to their *Yin*—soft nature, this prescription should not be used to treat cases with *Yang* deficiency of the spleen and stomach, marked by poor appetite and loose stools.

Administration: Decocted in water for oral dose to be taken twice

Case Study: Modified *Siwu Tang* was clinically employed to treat 44 cases of neurogenic headache, marked by oppressed, distending or pricking pain in the head complicated by dizziness, insomnia, palpitation, soreness of the loins, and thready weak pulse. Short—term control was obtained in 23 cases(no recurrence in 6 months),remarkable improvement in 13, improvement in 7,and unimprovement in 1.

100 cases of abnormal fetal position were corrected with modified Siwu Tang,whose ingredients were:

Dang Gui (Radix Angelicae Sinensis) 6 g, *Bai Shao* (Radix Paeoniae Alba) 9 g, *Chuan Xiong* (Rhizoma Chuanxiong) 1.5 g,

Bai Zhu (Rhizoma Atractylodis Macrocephalae) 9 g, *Fu Ling* (Poria) 9 g.

3 doses were taken by each of them, 1 dose daily. The treatment result was: In the 87 cases reexamined, correction of the abnormal fetal position was seen in 73, and in effectiveness in 9. This modified *Siwu Tang* is contraindicated for those with hemorrhage.

8.12 The Prescription of *Danggui Buxue Tang*

Name: Chinese Angelica Decoction for Enriching Blood
Source:The book *Nei Wai Shang Bian Huo Lun*
Ingredients:

Huang Qi (Radix Astragali) 30 g, *Dang Gui* (Radix Angelicae Sinensis) 6 g.

Explanation:

Huang Qi: Used in large dose to invigorate strongly the *Qi* of the spleen and lung so as to promote the production of blood.

Dang Gui: Enriching blood and regulating *Ying*, working together with *Huang Qi* to result in the growth of both *Yang* and *Yin* and the generation of both *Qi* and blood.

Effect: Supplementing *Qi* to promote the production of blood.

Indications: Syndrome of fever due to blood deficiency, marked by muscle—heat and flushed face, excessive thirst with desire for drinking, full large but weak pulse, or headache during menstruation or after giving birth, or unhealing opening of a carbuncle or furuncle; including such diseases with the above manifestations as various anemia, allergic purpura, dysfunctional uterine bleeding, leukopenia and neurosism.

Administration: Decocted in water for oral dose to be taken

twice.

8.13 The Prescription of *Guipi Tang*

Name: Decoction for Invigorating the Spleen and Nourishing the Heart

Source: The book *Ji Sheng Fang*

Ingredients:

Bai Zhu (Rhizoma Atractylodis Macrocephalae) 9 g, *Fu Shen* (Poria cum Ligno Hospite) 10 g, *Huang Qi* (Radix Astragali) 12 g, *Long Yan Rou* (Arillus Longan) 10 g, *Suan Zao Ren* (Semen Ziziphi Spinosae) 10 g, *Ren Shen* (Radix Ginseng) 12 g, *Mu Xiang* (Radix Aucklandiae) 5 g, *Gan Cao* (Radix Glycyrrhizae) 5 g, *Dang Gui* (Radix Angelicae Sinensis) 10 g, *Yuan Zhi* (Radix Polygalae) 10 g, *Sheng Jiang* (Rhizoma Zingiberis Recens) 6 g, *Da Zao* (Fructus Jujubae) 3 dates.

Explanation:

Huang Qi and *Ren Shen:* The principal drugs, invigorating *Qi* and strengthening the spleen.

Dang Gui and *Long Yan Rou:* Nourishing blood and coordinating *Ying,* assisting the principal drugs in invigorating *Qi* and enriching blood.

Bai Zhu and *Mu Xiang:* Strengthening the spleen and regulating the flow of *Qi* to cause the stagnation to be avoided which is prone to be brought about by the tonics in the prescription.

Fu Shen, Yuan Zhi and *Suan Zao Ren:* Nourishing the heart to calm the mind.

Gan Cao, Sheng Jiang and *Da Zao:* Regulating the stomach and strengthening the spleen.

Effect: Invigorating *Qi* and nourishing blood, strengthening the spleen and tonifying the heart.

Indications: Syndrome due to deficiency of both the heart and spleen or inability of the spleen to control the flow of blood, marked by palpatation, amnesia, insomnia, dreamful sleep, tending to be frightened, fever of deficiency type, lassitude, poor appetite, sallow complexion, pale tongue with thin whitish coating, and thready weak pulse, or hematochezia, metrorrhagia and metrostaxis, preceded menstrual cycle with profuse and light–colored menses; including such diseases with the above symptoms as neurosism, heart disease, dysfunctional uterine bleeding, thrombocytopenic purpura, aplastic anemia and bleeding due to gastroduodenal ulcer.

Administration: Decocted in water for oral dose to be taken twice

Case Study: 720 cases of neurosism were treated with *Guipi Tang* clinically.2.2% of them were cured, 46.4% almost cured, 28% improved.

Modified *Guipi Tang* was selected to treat 88 cases of post–traumatic brain syndrome which had been diagnosed as closed injury of the brain such as concussion of brain or brain contusion. The result was: 41 cases (45.5%) were cured, 30 (34%) remarkable improved, and 17 (20.5%) improved.

8.14   The Prescription of *Zhi Gancao Tang*

Name: Decoction of Prepared Licorice
Source: The book *Shang Han Lun*
Ingredients:
Zhi Gan Cao (Radix Glycyrrhizae Preparata) 12 g, *Ren Shen* (Radix Ginseng) 6 g, *Sheng Di Huang* (Radix Rehmanniae) 30 g,

Gui Zhi (Ramulus Cinnamomi) 9 g, E Jiao (Colla Corii Asini) 6 g, Mai Dong (Radix Ophiopogonis) 10 g, Ma Ren (Frutus Cannabis) 10 g, Sheng Jiang (Rhizoma Zingiberis Recens) 10 g, Da Zao (Fructus Jujubae) 5 dates.

Explanation:

Zhi Gan Cao: The principal drug, being sweet in flavor and warm in nature, used in large dosage to replenish Qi, relieve spasm and nourish the heart.

Ren Shen and Da Zao: Invigorating Qi, strengthening the spleen, nourishing the heart.

Sheng Di, Mai Dong, Ma Ren and E Jiao: Enriching Yin-blood.

Gui Zhi and Sheng Jiang: Warming up Yang-Qi to promote the circulation of Qi and blood in the channels.

Effect: Replenishing Qi, nourishing blood, enriching Yin, restoring the circulation of blood.

Indications:Syndrome due to deficiency of both Qi and blood, marked by intermittent and knotted pulse, palpitation, or dry stools, light red tongue with little coating, dry cough without sputum or with blood-tinged sputum; including such diseases with the above symptoms as coronary heart disease, viral myocarditis, rheumatic heart disease and neurosism.

Contraindication: Because Zhi Gancao Tang is wet in nature, it can not be used to treat patients with interior heat due to Yin-deficiency.

Case Study: 28 cases, who had been suffering from arrhythmia for 3 months to 2 years and of whom 12 were male, 16 were female, the oldest was 56 years old, the youngest was 4, were treated clinically with modified Zhi Gancao Tang, whose ingredients were:

Dang Shen (Radix Codonopsis) 9 g, Gui Zhi (Ramulus Cinnamomi) 9 g, E Jiao (Colla Corii Asini) 9 g, Sheng Jiang (Rhizoma Zingiberis Recens) 9 g, Sheng Di (Radix Rehmanniae) 15 g, Mai Dong (Radix Ophiopogonis) 9 g, Ma Ren (Fructus Cannabis) 12 g, Da Zao (Fructus Jujubae) 10 dates.

all of which were decocted in water for oral dose, 1 dose daily. In case of restlessness, insomnia and night sweat, the drug added was:

Suan Zao Ren (Semen Ziziphi Spinosae).

In case of palpitation, the drugs added were:

Zhu Sha (Cinnabaris)

Long Gu (Os Draconis Fossilia)

Mu Li (Concha Ostreae).

The result was that remarkable improvement was obtained in 23 cases, improvement in 4, and ineffectiveness in 1.

150 cases of angina pectoris were treated with Zhi Gancao Tang minus:

Ma Ren (Fructus Cannabis), Sheng Jiang (Rhizoma Zingiberis Recens) but plus:

Wu Wei Zi (Fructus Schisandrae), Ji Xue Teng (Caulis Spatholobi), Gui Ban (Carapax et Plastrum Testudinis), Bing Tang (crystal sugar).

Clinical observation showed that remarkable improvement was seen in 48 cases, improvement in 90, and no improvement in 12.

8.15 Prescriptions for Reinforcing Both Qi and Blood

Prescriptions of this kind are mainly composed of drugs with the action of invigorating *Qi* and drugs of nourishing blood. They are applicable to the syndrome due to deficiency of both *Qi* and blood, marked by lustreless complexion, dizziness, blurred eyes, palpitation, shortness of breath, pale tongue, and weak thready pulse. Drugs with the action of invigorating *Qi* such as

Ren Shen (Radix Ginseng), *Huang Qi* (Radix Astragali), *Gan Cao* (Radix Glycyrrhizae),

are usually compatible with drugs with the action of enriching blood such as

Dang Gui (Radix Angelicae Sinensis), *Bai Shao* (Radix Paeoniae Alba), *Shu Wu* (Radix Polygoni Multiflori), *E Jiao* (Colla Corii Asini), *Long Yan Rou* (Arillus Longan),

in these prescriptions, whose representatives are *Bazhen Tang* and *Taishan Panshi San*.

8.16   The Prescription of *Bazhen Tang*

Name: Eight Precious Ingredients'. Decoction

Source: The book *Zheng Ti Lei Yao*

Ingredients: *Dang Gui* (Radix Angelicae Sinensis) 10 g, *Chuan Xiong* (Rhizoma Chuanxiong) 6 g, *Bai Shao* (Radix Paeoniae Alba) 10 g, *Shu Di* (Radix Rehmanniae Preparata) 15 g, *Ren Shen* (Radix Ginseng) 6 g, *Bai Zhu* (Rhizoma Atractylodis Macrocephalae) 10 g, *Fu Ling* (Poria) 10 g, *Zhi Gan Cao* (Radix Glycyrrhizae Preparata) 6 g, *Sheng Jiang* (Rhizoma Zingiberis Recens) 6 g, *Da Zao* (Fructus Jujubae) 3 dates.

Explanation:

Shu Di and *Ren Shen*: The principal drugs, invigorating *Qi* and nourishing blood.

Bai Zhu and *Fu Ling*: Strengthening the spleen to remove

dampness.

Dang Gui and *Bai Shao*:Nourishing blood and regulating Ying.

Chuan Xiong: Regulating blood and promoting the flow of *Qi*.

Zhi Gan Cao: Replenishing *Qi* and regulating the function of the middle—*Jiao*.

Sheng Jiang and *Da Zao:* Coordinating the spleen and stomach.

Effect: Reinforcing *Qi* and blood.

Indications: Syndrome due to deficiency of both *Qi* and blood, marked by pale or sallow complexion, dizziness, blurred eyes, lassitude, shortness of breath, languor, palpitation, poor appetite, pale tongue with thin whitish coating, and thready weak or weak large pulse; including such diseases with the above symptoms as weakness in the convalescence, various chronic diseases, irregular menstruation, postpartum blood deficiency, and carbuncle or furuncle with opening difficult to heal.

Administration: Decocted in water for oral dose to be taken twice.

Case Study: 38 cases who had been troubled by habitual abortion for 2—5 times were treated clinically with modified *Bazhen Tang*, whose ingredients were: *Dang Gui* (Radix Angelicae Sinensis), *Shu Di* (Radix Rehmanniae Preparata), *Bai Shao* (Radix Paeoniae Alba), *Chuan Xiong* (Rhizoma Chuanxiong), *Dang Shen* (Radix Codonopsis), *Fu Ling* (Poria), *Bai Zhu* (Rhizoma Atractylodis Macrocephalae), *Gan Cao* (Radix Glycyrrhizae), *Sha Ren* (Fructus Amomi), *Zi Su* (Caulis Perillae), *Sheng Jiang* (Rhizoma Zingiberis Recens), *Da Zao* (Fructus

Jujubae).

In case of *Qi* deficiency, the drug added was:

Huang Qi (Radix Astragali);

in case of blood deficiency, the drug added was:

E Jiao (Colla Corii Asini);

in case of vomiting due to exuberance of fire of deficiency type, drugs added were:

Huang Qin (Radix Scutellariae), *Zhu Ru* (Caulis Bambusae in Taeniam);

in case of dry mouth and throat due to fire of deficiency type, the drug omitted was:

Shu Di (Radix Rehmanniae Preparata) and the drugs added were:

Sheng Di (Radix Rehmanniae), *Yu Zhu* (Rhizoma Polygonati Odarati)

Effectiveness was seen in all the cases treated.

8.17   The Prescription of *Taishan Panshi San*

Name: Miscarriage Preventing Powder

Source: The book *Jing Yue Quan Shu*

Ingredients:

Ren Shen (Radix Ginseng) 5 g, *Huang Qi* (Radix Astragali) 10 g, *Dang Gui* (Radix Angelicae Sinensis) 10 g, *Chuan Duan* (Radix Dipsaci) 10 g, *Huang Qin* (Radix Scutellariae) 6 g, *Bai Zhu* (Rhizoma Atractylodis Macrocephalae) 10 g, *Chuan Xiong* (Rhizoma Chuanxiong) 3 g, *Shao Yao* (Radix Paeoniae Alba) 6 g, *Shu Di* (Radix Rehmanniae Preparata) 10 g, *Sha Ren* (Fructus Amomi) 3 g, *Zhi Gan Cao* (Radix Glycyrrhizae Preparata) 6 g, *Nuo Mi* (Semen Oryzae Glutinosae) 5 g.

Explanation:

Ren Shen, Huang Qi, Bai Zhu and Zhi Gan Cao: Strengthening the spleen to invigorate *Qi*.

Dang Gui, Shu Di, Shao Yao and *Xu Duan:* Tonifying the liver and kidney, nourishing blood and regulating its flow.

Huang Qin: Clearing away heat, working together with *Bai Zhu* to strengthen the spleen and remove pathogenic heat so as to prevent miscarriage.

Sha Ren: Regulating *Qi* and the middle—*Jiao* so as to ensure a successful gestation.

Chuan Xiong: Promoting the flow of *Qi* and coordinating blood.

Nuo Mi: Nourishing the spleen and stomach to prevent abortion.

Effect: Invigorating *Qi*, strengthening the spleen,nourishing blood, preventing abortion.

Indications: Syndrome of miscarriage due to deficiency of both *Qi* and blood, marked by threatened abortion or habitual abortion, pale complexion, lassitude, anorexia, pale tongue with thin whitish coating, and weak slippery pulse; including disorders with the above symptoms such as threatened abortion and habitual abortion.

Administration: Decocted in water for oral dose to be taken 3 times on an empty stomach.

8.18 Prescriptions for Replenishing *Yin*

This kind of prescriptions are mainly made up of drugs with the action of nourishing *Yin*. They are indicated for the syndrome due to *Yin* deficiency, marked by emaciation, wan and sallow complexion, dry mouth and throat, soreness and weakness of the loins and legs, dizziness, blurred eyes, dry stools, or hectic fever due to bone—heat, night sweat, dry cough without sputum, flushing of zygomatic region, reddened tongue with little coating, and thready rapid pulse. The commonly used drugs in these prescriptions are:

Di Huang (Radix Rehmanniae), Mai Dong (Radix Ophiopogonis), Tian Dong (Radix Asparagi), Gui Ban (Carapax et Plastrum Testudinis), Zhi Mu (Rhizoma Anemarrhenae),which may be prescribed together with drugs with the action of supporting Yang such as

Lu Jiao (cornus Corii Cervi), Tu Si Zi (Semen Cuscutae),

in order that Yin can be generated by means of reinforcing Yang. Liuwei Dihuang Wan and Zuogui Wan are the representative prescriptions.

8.19   The Prescription of Liuwei Dihuang Wan

Name: Chinese Foxglove Root Pills of Six Ingredients
Source: The book Xiao Er Yao Zheng Zhi Jue
Ingredients:

Shu Di Huang (Radix Rehmanniae Preparata) 24 g, Shan Zhu Yu (Fructus Corni) 12 g, Shan Yao (Rhizoma Dioscoreae) 12 g, Ze Xie (Rhizoma Alismatis) 9 g, Fu Ling (Poria) 9 g, Mu Dan Pi (Cortex Moutan) 9 g.

Explanation:

Shu Di: The principal drug, nourishing the kidney and replenishing essence.

Shan Zhu Yu: Warming up and tonifying the kidney and liver, arresting seminal emission.

Shan Yao: Reinforcing the kidney and benefiting the spleen, combining *Shu Di* and *Shan Zhu Yu* to enriching all the three *Yin*.

Ze Xie: Purging fire of the kidney and preventing *Shu Di* from resulting in stagnation of *Qi* due to its tonic and sticky nature.

Dan Pi: Clearing away pathogenic fire in the liver and restricting the warm nature of *Shan Zhu Yu*.

Fu Ling: Inducing diuresis to benefit the spleen, aiding *Shan Yao* in strengthening the spleen.

Effect: Nourishing and tonifying the liver and the kidney.

Indications: Syndrome of *Yin*—deficiency marked by weakness and soreness of the loins and knees, dizziness and vertigo, tinnitus and deafness, night sweat and emission, or hectic fever due to bone—heat, feverish sensation in the palms and soles, reddened tongue with little coating, and thready rapid pulse; including such diseases with the above symptoms as lung tuberculosis, renal tuberculosis, chronic pyelonephritis, hypertension and menopausal syndrome.

Administration: All the ingredients are ground into fine powder and made into boluses with honey, each of which weighs 15 g. 1bolus is taken by an adult, 3 times daily. This prescription may also be used in the form of decoction with the dosage of the ingredients reduced according to the primary proportions.

Case Study: *Liuwei Dihuang Wan* modified according to different symptoms and signs was clinically prescribed to treat 5 cases of central retina and central choroid disorder with 4 cases cured and 1 improved.

8.20   The Prescription of *Zuogui Wan*

Name: Bolus for Reinforcing the Kidney—*Yin*

Source: The book *Jing Yue Quan Shu*

Ingredients:

Shu Di (Radix Rehmanniae Preparata) 240 g, *Shan Yao* (Rhizoma Dioscoreae) 120 g, *Gou Qi* (Fructus Lycii) 120 g, *Shan Zhu Yu* (Fructus Corni) 120 g, *Chuan Niu Xi* (Radix Cyathulae) 90 g, *Tu Si Zi* (Semen Cuscutae) 120 g, *Lu Jiao* (Colla Cornus Cervi) 120 g, *Gui Jiao* (Colla Carapacis et Plastri Testudinis) 120 g.

Explanation:

Shu Di: The principal drug, nourishing the kidney and supplementing essence.

Shan Zhu Yu, Gou Qi Zi and *Tu Si Zi:* Tonifying the liver and kidney.

Shan Yao: Benefiting both the spleen and the kidney.

Gui Ban Jiao and *Lu Jiao Jiao:* Drastically tonifying blood and kidney—essence with Lu Jiao Jiao's another action of warming *Yang* to generate *Yin.*

Niu Xi: Strengthening the muscles and bones.

Effect: Nourishing and tonifying the kidney—*Yin*.

Indications: Syndrome due to deficiency of the kidney—*Yin*, marked by dizziness, vertigo, soreness and weakness of the loins and knees, spontaneous sweat and night sweat, dry mouth and throat, reddened tongue with little coating, and thready or rapid pulse; including such diseases with the above symptoms as chronic nephritis, renal tuberculosis and menopausal syndrome.

Administration: All the ingredients are ground into powder

and made with honey into boluses, each of which weighing 15 g. 1 bolus is taken each time on an empty stomach, twice daily in the morning and evening.

Prolonged taking of this bolus tends to cause the *Qi* of the spleen and stomach to be stagnated, for the prescription is mainly composed of *Yin*—soft natured drugs with the action of nourishing *Yin*. As a result, drugs with the action of promoting the flow of *Qi* and enlivening the spleen such as *Chen Pi* (Pericarpium Citri Reticulatae) and *Sha Ren* (Fructus Amomi) should be added when long—term use of it is needed.

8.21   The Prescription of *Yiguan Jian*

Name: An Ever Effective Decoction for Nourishing the. Liver and Kidney

Source: The book *Liu Zhou Yi Hua*

Ingredients:

Bei Sha Shen (Radix Glehniae) 10 g, *Mai Dong* (Radix Ophiopogonis) 10 g, *Dang Gui* (Radix Angelicae Sinensis) 10 g, *Sheng Di Huang* (Radix Rehmanniae) 30 g, *Gou Qi Zi* (Fructus Lycii) 12 g, *Chuan Lian Zi* (Fructus Toosendan) 5 g.

Explanation:

Sheng Di: The principal drug, used in large dose to nourish *Yin* and enrich blood so as to tonify the liver and kidney.

Sha Ren ,Mai Dong, Dang Gui and *Gou Qi Zi:* Replenishing *Yin* and nourishing the liver.

Chuan Lian Zi: Used in small dose to disperse the depressed liver—*Qi*. Although it is bitter in flavor and cold in nature, it will not bring about any damage to *Yin*, because it is used together with quite a number of drugs with the action of nourishing *Yin*

and blood.

Effect: Nourishing the liver and kidney, soothing the liver and regulating the circulation of *Qi*.

Indications: Syndrome due to *Yin* deficiency of the liver and kidney and depressed liver—*Qi,* marked by pain in the chest, epigastric and hypochondriac region, regurgitation of sour fluid, bitter taste in the mouth, dry throat and mouth, reddened tongue with dry coating, and thready weak or deficient taut pulse; including such diseases with the above symptoms as chronic hepatitis, peptic ulcer, neurosis, hypertension, pleurisy, intercostal neuralgia, and chronic testitis.

Administration: Decocted in water for oral dose to be taken twice.

Contraindication: Because this prescription is mainly made up of sticky—natured drugs with nourishing effects, it should not be prescribed to treat syndromes complicated by phlegm—accumulation and water—retention.

8.22   The Prescription of *Da Buyin Wan*

Name: Bolus for Replenishing Vitəl Essence

Source: The book *Dan Xi Xin Fa*

Ingredients:

Huang Bai (Cortex Phellodendri) 120 g, *Zhi Mu* (Rhizoma Anemarrhenae) 120 g, *Shu Di* (Radix Rehmanniae Preparata) 180 g, *Gui Ban* (Carapax et Plastrum Testudinis) 80 g, *Zhu Ji Sui* (spinal marrow of a pig) appropiate amount, *Feng Mi* (Mel) appropiate amount.

Explanation:

Shu Di and *Gui Ban:* Nourishing the kidney—*Yin* and suppressing floating *Yang* and fire.

Zhu Ji Sui and *Feng Mi:* As drugs from animal and with sweet taste and moistening nature, they are used to reinforce the kidney—*Yin* and essence so as to promote the production of body fluids.

Huang Bai: Being bitter in flavor and cold in nature, purging ministerial fire to consolidate the kidney—*Yin*.

Zhi Mu: Being bitter in taste and cold in nature, moisturizing the lung to clear away the lung—heat upward, replenishing the kidney—*Yin* downward.

Effect: Nourishing *Yin* to reduce pathogenic fire.

Indications: Syndrome of up—flaring of pathogenic fire of deficiency type due to *Yin*—deficiency of both the liver and kidney, marked by tidal fever due to bone—heat, night sweat, nocturnal emission, cough and hemoptysis, irritability, pain and hotness or flaccidity in the knees and feet, reddened tongue with little coating, and rapid forceful cubit pulse; including such diseases with the above symptoms as hyperthyroidism, renal tuberculosis and diabetes.

Administration: *Zhu Ji Sui* is steamed until it is done and pounded into paste, which is then mixed with melted *Feng Mi* evenly. The mixture is made into boluses with the powder of all the other ingredients, each bolus weighing 15 g. 1 bolus is taken with slightly salty boiled water each time, twice daily, in the morning and evening. Or its decoction is taken orally.

Contraindication: This prescription contains *Huang Bai* and *Zhi Mu* which are bitter in taste and cold in nature. As a result, it should be cautiously used for the syndromes complicated by poor appetite and loose stools due to hypofunction of the spleen and stomach.

Case Study: 10 cases of hemoptysis caused by tuberculosis, a syndrome diagnosed, in TCM, as "impairment of the lung vessels done by up—flaring of asthenic—fire due to *Yin*—deficiency of the lung and kidney", were clinically treated with modified *Da Buyin Wan* after they failed to respond to the combined remedies of Chinese and Western medicines. The drugs prescribed were:

Sheng Di (Radix Rehmanniae) 12 g, *Shu Di* (Radix Rehmanniae Preparata) 12 g, *Shan Zhi* (Fructus Gardeniae) 6 g, *Zhi Mu* (Rhizoma Anemarrhenae) 9 g, *Gui Ban* (Carapax et Plastrum Testudinis) 30 g, *Mai Dong* (Radix Ophiopogonis) 15 g, *Niu Xi* (Radix Achyranthis Bidentatae) 9 g, *Pi Pa Ye* (Folium Eriobotryae) 9 g, *Ce Bai Ye* (Cacumen Platycladi) 30 g, *Han Lian Cao* (Herba Ecliptae) 30 g.

Of the 10 cases, 9 were cured, 1 unimproved, Generally, 1 − 2 doses brought about remarkable effectiveness, another dose led to cure.

8.23　The Prescription of *Shihu Yeguang Wan*

Name : Bolus for Treating Eye Disorders
Source:The book *Yuan Ji Qi Wei*
Ingredients:

Tian Men Dong (Radix Asparagi) 60 g, *Ren Shen* (Radix Ginseng)60 g, *Fu Ling* (Poria) 60 g, *Shu Di Huang* (Radix Rehmanniae Preparata) 30 g, *Sheng Di Huang* (Radix Rehmanniae) 30 g, *Mai Men Dong* (Radix Ophiopogonis) 30 g, *Tu Si Zi* (Semen Cuscutae) 23 g, *Gan Ju Hua* (Flos Chrysanthemi) 23 g, *Cao Jue Ming* (Semen Cassiae) 23 g, *Xing Ren* (Semen Armeniacae Amarum) 23 g, *Gan Shan Yao*

(Rhizoma Dioscoreae) 23 g, *Gou Qi* (Fructus Lycii) 23 g, *Niu Xi* (Radix Achyranthis Bidentatae) 23 g, *Wu Wei Zi* (Fructus Schisandrae) 23 g, *Ji Li* (Fructus Tribuli) 15 g, *Shi Hu* (Herba Dendrobii) 15 g, *Rou Cong Rong* (Herba Cistanches) 15 g, *Chuan Xiong* (Rhizoma Chuanxiong) 15 g, *Zhi Gan Cao* (Radix Glycyrrhizae Preparata) 15 g, *Zhi Qiao* (Fructus Aurantii) 15 g, *Qing Xiang Zi* (Semen Celosiae) 15 g, *Fang Feng* (Radix Saposhinkoviae) 15 g, *Chuan Huang Lian* (Rhizoma Coptidis) 15 g, *Wu Xi Jiao* (Cornu Rhinocerotis) 15 g, *Ling Yang Jiao* (Cornu Saigae Tataricae) 15 g.

Explanation:

Tian Dong, Mai Dong, Shu Di, Sheng Di, Wu Wei Zi and *Shi Hu:* Promoting the production of body fluids and tonifying blood.

Tu Si Zi, Gou Qi Zi, Niu Xi and *Rou Cong Rong:* Replenishing *Yin* and reinforcing the kidney.

Ren Shen, Fu Ling, Gan Cao and *Shan Yao:* Invigorating the spleen and supplementing the lung.

Zhi Qiao, Chuan Xiong, Ju Hua, Xing Ren, Fang Feng, Cao Jue Ming, Ji Li and *Qing Xiang Zi:* Dispersing pathogenic wind—heat.

Huang Lian, Xi Jiao and *Ling Yang Jiao*: Suppressing the hyperactivities of the liver, purging heart—fire, removing pathogenic heat from blood.

Effect: Calming the liver to stop wind, nourishing *Yin* to improve eyesight.

Indications: Eye disorders due to up—flaring of fire caused by *Yin*—deficiency of the liver and kidey, marked by platycoria, blurred vision, photophobia, lacrimation, dizziness, vertigo, and internal oculópathy; including such disorders with the above symptoms as glaucoma and cataracta.

Administration: All the ingredients are ground into powder and sifted and made with honey into boluses, each of which weighs 10 g, 1 bolus is taken with slightly salty boiled water each time, twice daily, in the morning and evening.

8.24   The Prescription of *Bufei Ejiao Tang*

Name: Ass--hide Glue Decoction for Invigorating the Lung
Source: The book *Xiao Er Yao Zheng Zhi Jue*
Ingredients:

E Jiao (Colla Corii Asini) 45 g, *Niu Bang Zi* (Fructus Arctii) 7.5 g, *Zhi Gan Cao* (Radix Glycyrrhizae Preparata) 7.5 g, *Ma Dou Ling* (Fructus Aristolochiae) 15 g, *Chao Xing Ren* (stir—fried Semen Armeniacae Amarum) 6 g, *Chao Nuo Mi* (stir—fried Semen Oryzae Glutinosae) 30 g.

Explanation:

E Jiao: The principal drug, being sweet in flavor and neutral in nature, nourishing *Yin* and tonifying the lung, enriching blood to arrest bleeding.

Niu Bang Zi: Dispersing pathogenic wind—heat, benefiting the throat and chest.

Ma Dou Ling: Clearing away heat pathogen in the lung, re-solving phlegm, relieving cough.

Xing Ren: Moisturizing the lung to relieve cough.

Nuo Mi and *Gan Cao:* Being sweet in flavor, nourishing the spleen *Yin,* moisturizing and tonifying the lung.

Effect: Nourishing *Yin,* tonifying the lung, relieving cough, arresting bleeding.

Indications: Syndrome due to deficiency of the lung and exuberance of pathogenic heat, marked by cough, dyspnea, dry throat, expectoration with little or blood—stained sputum, floating thready rapid pulse, and reddened tongue with little coating; including such diseases with the above symptoms as pulmonary tuberculosis and bronchiectasis complicated by hemoptysis.

Administration: The ingredients are ground into powder, 3—6 g of which is decocted in water and taken warm. Or the ingredients are decocted in water for the decoction, to which *E Jiao* that has been melted in boiling water is added. The decoction is taken 3 times.

8.25   The Prescription of *Guilu Erxian Jiao*

Name: Glue of the Two Ingredients Tortoise Plastron and Antler

Source: The book *Yi Fang Kao*

Ingredients:

Lu Jiao (Cornu Cervi) 5000 g, *Gui Ban* (Carapax et Plastrum Testudinis) 2500 g, *Gou Qi Zi* (Fructus Lycii) 1500 g, *Ren Shen* (Radix Ginseng) 500 g.

Explanation:

Lu Jiao: Promoting the flow of *Qi* through the *Du* channels to support *Yang*.

Gui Ban: Activating the flow of *Qi* through the *Ren* channels to replenish *Yin* .

Ren Shen: Invigorating the primordial *Qi*.

Gou Qi: Nourish the kidney—*Yin*.

Effect: Supplementing kidney—essence and marrow,invigorating *Qi,* strengthening *Yang*.

Indications:

Syndrome due to deficiency of both *Yin* and *Yang* in the kidney and weakness of both essence and blood in the *Ren* and *Du* Channels, marked by emaciation, nocturnal emission, impotence, blurred vision, soreness and weakness of the loins and knees; including such diseases with the above symptoms as various kinds of anemia and impotence.

Administration: *Lu Jiao* is sawed into pieces and scraped clean and steeped in water. *Gui Ban* and the processed *Lu Jiao* are boiled into glue. *Ren Shen* and *Gou Qi* are decocted and condensed into an extract. The glue and the extract are mixed together into *Guilu Erxian Jiao*. 3 g of it is dissolved in liquor and taken with slightly salty boiled water every morning.

8.26   The Prescription of *Qibao Meiran Dan*

Name: Bolus for Promoting the Growth of Hair and Beard with Seven Noble Ingredients.

Source: The book *Yi Fang Ji Jie*

Ingredients:

He Shou Wu (Radix Polygoni Multiflori) 300 g, *Bai Fu Ling* (Poria) 150 g, *Huai Niu Xi* (Radix Achyran this Bidentatae) 150 g, *Dang Gui* (Radix Angelicae Sinensis) 150 g, *Gou Qi* (Fructus Lycii) 120 g, *Tu Si Zi* (Semen Cuscutae) 120 g, *Po Gu Zhi* (Fructus Psoraleae) 120 g.

Explanation:

He Shou Wu: The principal drug, being sweet, bitter and astringent in taste and slightly warm in nature, moisturizing and tonifying the liver and kidney, strengthening the tendons and bones, arresting emission.

Gou Qi, Tu Si Zi and *Zhi Ma:* Tonifying the liver and kidney, consolidate kidney—essence, relieving nocturnal emission.

Niu Xi: Tonifying the liver and kidney, strengthening the tendons and bones, enhancing the loins and knees.

Dang Gui: Nourishing blood to supplement the liver.

Effect: Nourishing the kidney—water and enriching the liver—blood.

Indications: Syndrome due to insufficiency of both the liver and kidney, marked by preceded greying of the beard and hair, unsteady teeth, nocturnal emission and spermatorrhea, weakness and soreness of the loins and knees, including such disorders with the above symptoms as early greying of hair and neurosism.

Administration: All the ingredients are parched with sesame seeds and ground into fine powder and made with honey into boluses, each of which weighs 10 g. 1 bolus is taken with slightly salty boiled water each time, twice daily, in the morning and evening.

8.27   The prescription of *Er Zhi Wan*

Name: Two Solstices Pill

Source: The book *Yi Fang Ji Jie*

Ingredients:

Nü Zhen Zi (Fructus Ligustri Lucidi) adequate amount

Han Lian Cao (Herba Ecliptae) adequate amount

Explanation:

Nü Zhen Zi: Being sweet and bitter in taste and cold in nature, nourishing the kidney and tonifying the liver.

Han Lian Cao: Being sweet and sour in taste and cold in nature, nourishing *Yin* and supplementing vital essence, cooling blood to stop bleeding.

Effect: Tonifying the kidney and nourishing the liver.

Indications: Syndrome due to *Yin* deficiency of the liver and kidney, marked by bitter taste in the mouth, dry throat, dizziness and vertigo, insomnia, dreaminess, soreness and weakness of the loins, flaccidity of the lower limbs, nocturnal emission, and early greying of the hair; including such diseases with the above symptoms as neurosism and early greying of the beard and hair.

Administration: *Nü Zhen Zi* is steamed until it is done, dried in the air, ground into fine powder, and sifted. *Han Lian Cao* is decocted in water 3 times for the decoctions, which is condensed into liquid extract, into which an adequate amount of honey is added and stirred evenly. The extract and the powder of *Nü Zhen Zi* are mixed together into boluses, each of which weighs 15 g. 1 bolus is taken with boiled water each time, twice daily, in the morning and evening.

8.28   Prescriptions for Invigorating *Yang*

This kind of prescriptions are mainly made up of drugs with the action of invigorating *Yang*. They are suitable for the syndrome due to insufficiency of the kidney—*Yang*, marked by soreness of the loins and knees, cool and weak limbs, cold pain and straining sensation in the lower abdomen, dysuria or frequent urination, impotence, premature ejaculation, general debility and emaciation, polydipsia, deep thready pulse or deep hidden cubit pulse. Drugs such as

Fu Zi (Radix Aconiti Lateralis Preparata), *Rou Gui* (Cortex Cinnamomi), *Du Zhong* (Cortex Eucommiae), *Ba Ji Tian* (Radix Morindae Officinalis), *Bu Gu Zhi* (Fructus Psoraleae), are commonly used in these prescriptions, whose representatives are *Shenqi Wan* and *Yougui Wan*.

8.29   The Prescription of *Shenqi Wan*

Name: Bolus for Invigorating the Kidney−*Yang*
Source: The book *Jin Gui Yao Lue*
Ingredients:

Gan Di Huang (Radix Rehmanniae) 240 g, *Shan Yao* (Rhizoma Dioscoreae) 120 g, *Shan Zhu Yu* (Fructus Corni) 120 g, *Ze Xie* (Rhizoma Alismatis) 90 g, *Fu Ling* (Poria) 90 g, *Mu Dan Pi* (Cortex Moutan) 90 g, *Gui Zhi* (Ramulus Cinnamomi) 30 g, *Fu Zi* (Radix Aconiti Lateralis Preparata) 30 g.

Explanation:

Gan Di Huang: Nourishing and tonifying the kidney−*Yin*.

Shan Zhu Yu and *Shan Yao:* Being able not only to nourish the liver and spleen but also to supplement the kidney−*Yin*.

Gui Zhi and *Fu Zi:* Warming up the kidney−*Yang*.

Ze Xie and *Fu Ling:* Promoting water matebolism and inducing diuresis.

Dan Pi: Dispersing and purging the liver−fire.

Effect: Warming up and tonifying the kidney−*Yang*.

Indications:

Syndrome due to insufficiency of the kidney−*Yang*, marked by lumbago, flaccidity of the feet, cold sensation in the lower part of the body, tension in the lower abdomen, dysuria or polyuria, pale and puffy tongue with thin whitish moisture coating, and deep thready cubit pulse, or syndromes of beriberi, phlegm retention, diabetes, and dysuria with lower abdominal colic; including such diseases with the above symptoms as coronary heart disease, toxemia of pregnancy, chronic nephritis, prostatitis, lupus sebaceus, addisonian syndrome, mucous edema, chronic bronchitis, etc.

Case Study:

6 cases of chronic nephritis were clinically treated with modified *Shenqi Wan* of *Xue's*, whose ingredients were:

Shu Di (Radix Rehmanniae Preparata) 12 g, *Shan Yao* (Rhizoma Dioscoreae) 3 g, *Shan Zhu Yu* (Fructus Corni) 3 g, *Ze Xie* (Rhizoma Alismatis) 3 g, *Dan Pi* (Cortex Moutan) 3 g, *Rou Gui* (Cortex Cinnamomi) 3 g, *Che Qian Zi* (Semen Plantaginis) 3 g, *Niu Xi* (Radix Achyranthis) 3 g, *Fu Ling* (Poria) 9 g, *Fu Zi* (Radix Aconiti Lateralis Preparata) 1.5 g.

The treatment result was: The patient's edema and urinary protein were gradually reduced or completely eliminated with the volume of their urine increased. Their renal functions ,appetite and physical strength were improved and their blood pressure was lowered. No side—effects was found and satisfactory curative effects was obtained.

284 cases, who were treated with this method for half a month to 9 years and a half, of senile cataract not complicated by diabetes, nephritis, outstanding disorders of the anterior chamber and fundus of the eyes were sucessfully treated with *Shenqi Wan* with 568 diseased eyes improved, the total effective rate being 81.4%. This showed that this prescription has remarkable effects in relieving the senile cataract and in preventing its further development.

8.30 The Prescription of *Yougui Wan*

Name: Bolus for Reinforcing the Kidney—*Yang*

Source: The book *Jing Yue Quan Shu*

Ingredients:

Shu Di (Radix Rehmanniae Preparata) 240 g, *Shan Yao* (stir-fried Rhizoma Dioscoreae) 120 g, *Shan Zhu Yu* (slightly stir-fried Fructus Corni) 90 g, *Gou Qi* (slightly stir-fried Fructus Lycii) 120 g, *Lu Jiao Jiao* (stir-fried Colla Cornus Cervi) 120 g, *Tu Si Zi* (Semen Cuscutae Preparata) 120 g, *Du Zhong* (stir-fried Cortex Eucommiae) 120 g, *Dang Gui* (Radix Angelicae Sinensis) 90 g, *Rou Gui* (Cortex Cinnamomi) 60–120 g, *Fu Zi* (Radix Aconiti Lateralis Preparata) 60–180 g.

Explanation:

Rou Gui, Fu Zi and *Lu Jiao Jiao:* Warming up and tonifying the kidney–*Yang,* supplementing the vital essence, enriching the marrow.

Shu Di, Shan Zhu Yu, Shan Yao, Tu Si Zi, Gou Qi and *Du Zhong:* Nourishing *Yin,* benefiting the kidney, tonifying the liver and invigorating the spleen.

Dang Gui: Enriching blood to tonifying the liver.

Effect: Warming up the kidney–*Yang,* supplementing essence, enriching blood.

Indications: Syndrome due to insufficiency of the kidney–*Yang* and decline of fire from *Mingmen,* marked by lassitude resulting from prolonged disease, aversion to cold and cold limbs, or impotence and emission, or sterility caused by impotence, or loose stools and even diarrhea with undigested food, or enuresis, or soreness and weakness of the loins and knees, and edema of the lower limbs; including such diseases with the above symptoms as coronary heart disease, toxemia of pregnancy, chronic nephritis, primary hypertension, prostatitis, lupus sebaceus, Addison's disease syndrome, mucous edema, chronic bronchitis, and Sheehan's syndrome.

Administration: All the ingredients are ground into fine powder and made with honey into boluses, each of which weighs 15 g. 1 bolus is taken with boiled water each time, twice daily, in the morning and evening. (Taken also in the form of decoction with the dosage of the ingredients increased or reduced according to the proportions in the original prescription).

Case Study: Modified *Yougui Wan* was clinically employed to treat 1 case of hereditary cerebellar ataxia, a syndrome due to deficiency of the kidney—*Qi,* marked by staggering along, dizziness, tinnitus, hypomnesis, aversion to cold, cold limbs, weakness of the loins and knees, pale tongue with thin coating, and thready and Chi—weak pulse. The ingredients of the modified prescription were:

Fu Zi (Radix Aconiti Lateralis Praeparata) 6 g, *Rou Gui* (Cortex Cinnamomi) 4 g. *Lu Jiao Shuang* (Cornu Cervi Degelatinatum) 9 g, *Du Zhong* (Cortex Eucommiae) 9 g, *Shan Yao* (Rhizoma Dioscoreae) 9 g, *Niu Xi* (Radix Achyranthis Badentatae) 9 g, *Dang Gui* (Radix Angelicae Sinensis) 9 g, *Tu Si Zi* (Semen Cuscutae) 12 g, *Gui Ban* (Carapax et Plastrum Testudinis) 12 g, *Gou Qi* (Fructus Lycii) 12 g, *Shu Di.*(Radix Rehmanniae Preparata) 12 g, *Zhi Shu Wu* (Radix Polygoni Multiflori Preparata) 12 g.

The symptoms and signs were relieved after 20 doses were taken. Remarkable improvement of the disease condition resulted after another 50 doses in each of which 12 g, of *Sheng Di* (Radix Rehmanniae) was added were taken.

9 Prescriptions for Tranquilizing the Mind

9.1 Prescriptions for Tranquilizing the Mind

Prescriptions of this kind consist of heavy materials or nourishing drugs for tranquilizing the mind. Being sedative, they are used to treat mental disorders. Mental disorders result from many causes. As far as the mental disorders treated with prescriptions for tranquilizing the mind are concerned, they are divided into two groups. The first group involves exogenous fear, and pathogenic fire due to the stagnated liver—Qi attacking the mind from the interior, both of which usually result in excessive syndromes marked by fear, unusual joy or anger, irritability, etc. They should be treated with the method of "tranquilizing the mind with heavy materials" so as to calm the mind through relieving palpitation and removing heat and restlessness. The second group involves over—anxiety, blood deficiency of the heart and liver, malnutrition of the mind or Yin—insufficiency of the heart, and disturbance of the fire of deficiency type in the interior, all of which usually result in syndromes of deficiency type marked by palpitation, amnesia, restlessness, and insomnia. They should be treated with the method of "tranquilizing the mind with nourishing drugs" so as to calm the mind through replenishing Yin, dispersing fire and enriching blood. According to the deficient or excessive nature of a mental syndrome, prescriptions for tranquilizing the mind are classified as the following two: those with weighty sedatives and those with tonic sedatives. Besides, treatment of the mental disorders due to heat or phlegm pathogen is to be stated in the introduction to "prescriptions for removing heat" and "prescriptions for eliminating phlegm".

Most of the weighty sedatives in prescriptions for tranquilizing the mind are minerals, metals or shells. It is not advisable to take them regularly. Or else the normal function of the spleen and stomach will be affected. If used to treat a patient with weak spleen and stomach, such weighty sedatives should be administered together with drugs with the action of strengthening the spleen and regulating the function of the stomach.

9.2 Prescriptions for Tranquilizing the Mind with Weighty Sedatives

This kind of prescriptions are mainly made up of drugs from minerals, metals or shells and with the action of calming the mind. They are suitable for the syndrome due to *Yang* exuberance of the heart and liver, marked by vexation, vertigo, insomnia, palpitation or even severe palpitation. Drugs such as

Zhu Sha (Cinnabaris), *Ci Shi* (Magnetitum), *Long Chi* (Dens Draconi), *Zhen Zhu Mu* (Concha Margaritifera Usta),
are usually used in these prescriptions, whose representatives are *Zhusha Anshen Wan, Zhen Zhumu Wan* and *Cizhu Wan*.

9.3 The Prescription of *Zhu sha Anshen Wan*

Name: Cinnabaris Sedative Bolus
Source: The book *Yi Xue Fa Ming*
Ingredients:

Zhu Sha (Cinnabaris) 15 g, *Huang Lian* (Rhizoma Coptidis) 18 g, *Zhi Gan Cao* (Radix Glycyrrhizae Preparata) 16 g, *Sheng Di Huang* (Radix Rehmanniae) 8 g, *Dang Gui* (Radix Angelicae Sinensis) 8 g.

Explanation:

Zhu Sha: One of the principal drugs, being sweet in taste and cold and heavy in nature, tranquilizing the mind.

Huang Lian: The other principal drug, being bitter in taste and cold in nature, clearing away heat to relieve vexation.

Dang Gui: Nourishing blood.

Sheng Di: Replenishing *Yin*.

Gan Cao: Tempering the actions of all the ingredients.

Effect: Purging pathogenic heat and nourishing *Yin* to tranquilize the mind.

Indications: Syndrome due to exuberance of the heart—fire and insufficiency of *Yin*—blood, marked by vexation, insomnia, dreaminess, palpitation or even severe palpitation, burning sensation in the chest, reddened tongue, and thready rapid pulse; including such diseases with the above symptoms as neurosism, myocarditis and mental depression.

Administration: The ingredients are ground into fine powder and made into pills. 6—9 g of the pills is taken with boiled water before sleep in the night. This prescription may also be used in the form of decoction. In so doing, the doses of the drugs should be re—adjusted according to the proportions of the drugs in the original prescription. *Zhu Sha* is refined with water and taken with the decoction. Since *Zhu Sha* has toxicity, this prescription should not be used regularly, and *Zhu Sha* should be used in smaller dose.

Case Study: *Zhusha Anshen Wan* and *Cizhu Wan* were clinically used to treat 1 case of night–walking, a syndrome due to interior intense heat disturbing the mind, marked by: The patient usually got up suddenly while dreaming in the night and opened the door and went out. He wandered and wandered until falling down in the wilds, remaining sleeping soundly. When he was examined, he looked in the usual manner. But he complained of fidgets, tinnitus, unconsciousness of the night–walking, dreaminess and inclination to be frightened. His tongue was reddish with yellowish coating, and his pulse was taut and rapid. The ingredients of the combined prescription were:

Sheng Di (Radix Rehmanniae) 60 g, *Huang Lian* (Rhizoma Coptidis) 18 g, *Dang Gui* (Radix Angelicae Sinensis) 30 g, *Gan Cao* (Radix Glycyrrhizae) 15 g, *Duan Ci Shi* (Magnetitum Preparata) 30 g, *Jian Qu* (Massa Medicata Fermentata) 18 g, *Zhu Sha* (Cinnabaris) 9 g.

The first 6 ingredients were ground into powder, which was made into pills with honey. The honeyed pills were coated with *Zhu Sha* which had been refined with water. 30 g of the pills, each as big as a soybean, was taken each time, twice daily, in the morning and evening. After 2 doses were taken, the patient was cured.

9.4 The Prescription of *Zhenzhumu Wan*

Name: Concha Margoritifera Usta Pill
Source: The book *Pu Ji Ben Shi Fang*
Ingredients:

Zhen Zhu Mu (Concha Margaritifera Usta) 22.5 g, *Dang Gui* (Radix Angelicae Sinensis) 45 g, *Shu Di* (Radix Rehmanniae Preparata) 45 g, *Ren Shen* (Radix Ginseng) 30 g, *Suan Zao Ren*

(Semen Ziziphi Spinosae) 30 g, *Bai Zi Ren* (Semen Platycladi) 30 g, *Xi Jiao* (Cornu Rhinoceri) 15 g, *Fu Shen* (Poria cum Ligno Hospite) 15 g, *Chen Xiang* (Lignum Aquilariae Resinatum) 15 g, *Long Chi* (Dens Darconis) 15 g, *Jin Yin Hua* (Flos Lonicerae) adequate amount, *Bo He* (Herba Menthae) adequate amount.

Explanation:

Zhen Zhu Mu: The principal drug, being salty in taste and cold in nature, calming the liver and suppressing the hyperactivities of the liver—*Yang*.

Long Chi: Tranquilizing the mind.

Zao Ren, Bai Zi Ren and *Fu Shen*: Relieving mental distress and restlessness to induce sleep.

Ren Shen, Dang Gui and *Shu Di*: Nourishing blood and *Yin*, invigorating *Qi* to promote the production of blood.

Xi Jiao: Removing pathogenic heat from the liver and calming the mind.

Chen Xiang: Suppressing the floating *Yang*.

Zhu Sha: Stopping panic to calm the mind.

Jin Yin Hua and *Bo He:* Clearing away heat from the liver.

Effect: Nourishing *Yin* and tonifying blood, tranquilizing the mind and relieving mental distress and restlessness.

Indications: Syndrome due to hyperactivity of the liver—*Yang* and insufficiency of *Yin*—blood, marked by mental distress and restlessness, insomnia, intermittent palpitation, dizziness, vertigo, and thready taut pulse; including such diseases with the above symptoms as neurosism and schizophrenia.

Administration: The ingredients are ground into powder and made with honey into pills, each as big as a seed of Chinese parasol. The pills are coated with *Zhu Sha* which has been refined with water. 40—50 pills are taken with the decoction of *Jin Yin Hua* and *Bo He* before going to bed at noon or night.

9.5 The Prescription of *Cizhu Wan*

Name: Medicated Leaven Pill

Source: The book *Bei Ji Qian Jin Yao Fang*

Ingredients:

Ci Shi (Magnetitum) 60 g, *Zhu Sha* (Cinnabaris) 30 g, *Shen Qu* (Massa Medicata Fermentata) 120 g.

Explanation:

Ci Shi: Being salty in flavor and cold in nature, enhancing *Yin* and suppressing the hyperactivity of *Yang*, calming the mind through the strong tranquilizing action.

Zhu Sha: Being sweet in flavor and cold in nature, tranquilizing the mind.

Shen Qu: Strengthening the function of the spleen and stomach, protecting the stomach from being injured by heavy materials, working together with honey to supplement the *Qi* of the middle—*Jiao* and regulate the stomach.

Effect: Tranquilizing the mind, suppressing the hyperactivity of *Yang*, improving acuity of vision.

Indications: Syndrome due to breakdown of the normal physiological coordination between the heart and the kidney, marked by palpitation, insomnia, tinnitus, deafness, and blurred vision; including such diseases with the above symptoms as neurosis and epilepsy.

Administration: The ingredients are ground into fine powder and made with honey into pills, each as big as a seed of Chinese parasol. 6 g of the pills is taken with boiled water each time, twice daily.

Case Study: 7 cases of auditory hallucination, a prominent or a remanent symptom of schizophrenia, were treated with *Cizhu Wan*. 1 course of treatment involved 1 month. 6—10 g of the pills was taken each time, 1—2 times daily. The result was that among the 7 cases, 6 with the symptom of incoordination between the heart and the kidney were effectively treated, 3 being remarkably improved and the other 3 being improved, while the 1 case without the symptom of incoordination between the heart and the kidney showed no improvement.

Cizhu Wan was also administered to treat 2 cases of platycoria, of which the case with complications was cured by over 20 doses or more, and the other without complications by mere 6 doses, which is equivalent to 43 g of the pills.

9.6 Prescriptions for Tranquilizing the Mind with Tonic Sedatives

Prescriptions of this kind are mainly made up of drugs with the action of nourishing and calming the mind. They are applicable to the syndrome due to insufficiency of *Yin*—blood and hyperactivities of *Yang*, marked by restlessness of deficiency type, insomnia, palpitation, night sweat, nocturnal emission, amnesia, and reddened tongue with little coating. The commonly used drugs are:

Sheng Di (Radix Rehmanniae), *Mai Dong* (Radix Ophiopogonis), *Suan Zao Ren* (Semen Ziziphi Spinosae), *Bai Zi Ren* (Semen Platycladi).

The representative prescriptions are *Suanzaoren Tang*, *Tianwang Buxin Dan* and *Ganmai Dazao Tang*.

9.7　The Prescription of *Suanzaoren Tang*

Name: Wild Jujube Seed Decoction

Source: The book *Jin Gui Yao Lue*

Ingredients:

Suan Zao Ren (Semen Ziziphi Spinosae stir–fried) 15–18 g, *Gan Cao* (Radix Glycyrrhizae) 3 g, *Zhi Mu* (Rhizoma Anemarrhenae) 8–10 g, *Fu Ling* (Poria) 10 g, *Chuan Xiong* (Rhizoma Chuanxiong) 3–5 g.

Explanation:

Suan Zao Ren: The principal drug, being sweet and sour in taste and neutral in nature, nourishing the liver–blood and calming the mind.

Chuan Xiong: Regulating and nourishing the liver–blood.

Fu Ling: Relieving mental stress.

Zhi Mu: Being moist in nature, clearing away heat and purging fire.

Gan Cao: Removing pathogenic heat and tempering the actions of all the other ingredients.

Effect: Nourishing blood to tranquilize the mind, clearing away pathogenic heat to relieve restlessness.

Indications: Syndrome of insomnia due to restlessness of deficiency type or consumption, marked by palpitation, night sweat, dizziness, vertigo, dry mouth and throat, and thready rapid pulse; including neurosism, etc. with the above symptoms.

Administration: *Suan Zao Ren* is decocted first and then the other ingredients are added for the decoction to be taken 3 times.

Case Study: Compound Decoction of *Suanzaoren Tang* was clinically used to treat 209 cases of neurosism, a syndrome due to consumption of the kidney—*Yin*, flaring fire caused by *Yin* deficiency, incoordination between the heart and the kidney, insufficiency of the liver—blood, and unsteadiness of the heart—*Qi*, marked by palpitation, insomnia, amnesia, etc. with the total effective rate reaching 90%.

The experimental results showed that Compound Decoction of *Suanzaoren Tang* does have the effects of sedation and hypnotism. It can inhibit hyperactivities and over excitement of the nerve cells, offer the opportunity for the cortical cells under the condition of tension and disturbance to have a rest and to be readjusted, thus promoting the restoration of the functions of the organs involved in balancing the excitement and inhibition.

9.8   The Prescription of *Tianwang Buxin Dan*

Name: Cardiotonic Pill
Source: The book *She Sheng Mi Yao*
Ingredients:
Sheng Di (Radix Rehmanniae cleaned with liquor) 120 g, *Ren Shen* (Radix Ginseng) 15 g, *Dan Shen* (slightly stir—fried Radix Salviae Miltiorrhizae) 15 g, *Yuan Shen* (slightly stir—fried Radix Scrophulariae) 15 g, *Fu Ling* (Poria) 15 g, *Wu Wei Zi* (baked Fructus Schisandrae) 15 g, *Yuan Zhi* (stir—fried Radix Polygalae) 15 g, *Jie Geng* (Radix Platycodi) 15 g, *Dang Gui* (Radix Angelicae Sinensis cleaned with water) 60 g, *Tian Men Dong* (Radix Asparagi) 60 g, *Mai Men Dong* (Radix Ophiopogonis) 60 g, *Bai Zi Ren* (parched Semen Platycladi) 60 g, *Suan Zao Ren* (Semen Ziziphi Spinosae) 60 g, *Zhu Sha* (Cinnabaris) 12 g.
Explanation:

Sheng Di: The principal drug, being sweet and bitter in taste and cold in nature, nourishing *Yin* and enriching blood.

Xuan Shen, Tian Dong and *Mai Dong:* Being sweet in taste and cold and moist in nature, clearing away fire of deficiency type.

Dan Shen and *Dang Gui:* Nourishing blood to calm the mind.

Ren Shen and *Fu Ling:* Invigorating *Qi* to relieve restlessness.

Suan Zao Ren and *Wu Wei Zi:* Astringing the heart—*Qi* to tranquilize the mind.

Bai Zi Ren, Yuan Zhi and *Zhu Sha:* Replenishing the heart to calm the mind.

Jie Geng: Guiding the actions of the other ingredients to the upper part of the body.

Effect: Nourishing *Yin* and enriching blood, replenishing the heart to tranquilize the mind.

Indications: Syndrome due to *Yin* depletion and blood insufficiency, and *Yin*—deficiency of both the heart and the kidney, marked by restlessness of deficiency type, insomnia, palpitation, low spirit, nocturnal emission, amnesia, dry stools, oral ulcer, reddened tongue with little coating, and thready rapid pulse; including such diseases with the above symptoms as neurosism, menopausal syndrome and myocarditis.

Administration: The ingredients are ground into powder and made with honey into pills, which are then coated with *Zhu Sha*. 9 g of the pills is taken each time with warm boiled water. (This prescription may also be taken in the form of decoction with the amounts of the ingredients reduced according to the proportions in the original prescription).

Case Study: Modified *Tianwang Buxin Dan,* which was prescribed in the convalescence after the therapeutic methods of emesis and purgation had been used, was clinically employed to treat 62 cases of psychosis. If the cases were weak, it was used to regulate and tonify them before and after the two methods had been used. All the 62 cases were cured. But some of them subjected relapse. They continued to be treated in the same way as the above and were cured again.

Modified *Tianwang Buxin Dan* was used to treat 1 case of chronic conjunctivitis,the result of uncured acute conjunctivitis and working under the lamp—light for about 20 days, marked by reddened eyes with dry sensation and photophobia and blurred vision, vexation in the afternoon, and nightmare—disturbed sleep. After failing to respond to Western medicine and therapeutic methods of TCM such as "removing heat from the heart", "cooling the liver", "promoting the circulation of blood", and "nourishing the kidney—*Yin*", the case began to be treated with the prescription of *Tianwang Buxin Dan* which was modified according to different symptoms. All the symptoms and signs disappeared after 10 doses in the form of decoction were taken. The pills form were, then, taken for the purpose of consolidation.

The ingredients of Modified *Buxin Dan:*

Ren Shen (Radix Ginseng) 15 g, *Mai Dong* (Radix Ophiopogonis) 30 g, *Wu Wei Zi* (Fructus Schisandrae) 30 g, *Xuan Shen* (Radix Scrophulariae) 15 g, *Pao Fu Zi* (Radix Aconiti Lateralis Preparata) 15 g, *Yuan Zhi* (Radix Polygalae) 15 g, *Ding Xiang* (Flos Caryophylli) 15 g, *Gan Cao* (Radix Glycyrrhizae) 15 g, *Dan Shen* (Radix Salviae Miltiorrhizae) 30 g, *Fu Shen* (Poria cum Ligno Hospite) 30 g, *Zao Ren* (Semen Ziziphi

Spinosae) 30 g, *Tian Dong* (Radix Asparagi) 30 g, *Bai Zi Ren* (Semen Platycladi) 30 g, *Hong Hua* (Flos Carthami) 30 g, *Dang Gui* (Radix Angelicae Sinensis) 30 g, *Sheng Di* (Radix Rehmanniae) 120 g, *Pu Huang* (Pollen Typhae) 18 g.

were decocted in water for the decoction with 100% concentration. The decoction, an experimental results showed, has evident antigonism on experimental cardiac infarction induced by isoproterenol in healthy male mice. It can not only prevent the ischemic ECG change and the pathological myocardial damage, both due to isoproterenol, but also has better effect on the biochemical metabolism of the ischemic cardiac muscle, that is, promoting the energy conversion of mitochodrion and the excitation contraction coupling of the cardiac muscle by improving activation of succinate dehydrogenase and ATP−ase, the inspiration of cell mitochondrions and the electron transport system. This decoction also has the action of improving the unspecific defensive function of the animals as well as their stress state.

9.9 The Prescription of *Gancao Xiao mai Dazao Tang*

Name: Decoction of Licorice, Wheat and Date
Source:
The book *Jin Gui Yao Lue*
Ingredients:
Gan Cao (Radix Glycyrrhizae) 9 g, *Xiao Mai* (Fructus Tritici Levis) 9−15 g, *Da Zao* (Fructus Jujubae) 5−7 dates.
Explanation:
Gan Cao: The principal drug, being sweet in taste and neu-

tral in nature, regulating the function of the middle—*Jiao,* nourishing the heart, relieving mental stress.

Xiao Mai: Tonifying the heart to calm the mind.

Da Zao: Invigorating the spleen—*Qi,* relieving the liver depression, treating deficiency of the heart.

Effect: Tonifying the heart to calm the mind, regulating the function of the middle—*Jiao* to relieve depression.

Indications: Syndrome of *Zang Zao* due to deficiency of the heart—*Qi* and depression of the liver—*Qi,* marked by trance, sorrow, inclination of weep, disturbed—sleep, unusual behavior, frequent yawning, reddened tongue with little coating; including such diseases with the above symptoms as neurosism, hysteria, and mild schizophrenia.

Administration: Decocted in water for oral dose to be taken 3 times.

Case Study: 79 cases of schizophrenia, which had a long course and almost completely failed to respond to long—term administration of antipsychotics, were clinically treated with *Gancao Xiaomai Dazao Tang* plus *Long Gu* and *Mu Li,* whose main ingredients were:

Zhi Gan Cao (Radix Glycyrrhizae Preparata) 10 g, *Huai Xiao Mai* (Fructus Tritici Levis) 30 g, *Long Gu* (Os Draconis Fossila) 30 g, *Mu Li* (Concha Ostreae) 30 g, *Da Zao* (Fructus Jujubae) 5 dates.

In case of prominent psychomotor excitement, drugs added were:

Ci Shi (Magnetitum), *Zhi Da Huang* (Radix et Rhizoma Rhei Preparata).

In case of prominent hallucination, pills prescribed also were:

Pill of *Cizhu Wan,* Pill of *Liuwei Dihuang Wan.*

In case of prominent delusion, drugs added were:

Shi Chang Pu (Rhizoma Acori Tatarinowii), Dan Nan Xing (Arisaema cum Bile), Xuan Cao (Herba Hemerocallis).

In case of severe insomnia, drugs added were:

Suan Zao Ren (Semen Ziziphi Spinosae), He Huan Pi (Cortex Albiziae), Ye Jiao Teng (Caulis Polygoni Multiflori).

The treatment result was that 5 cases were cured, 23 remarkedly improved, 34 improved, 17 unimproved.

28 cases of infantile enuresis were treated with modified Gancao Xiaomai Dazao Tang, whose ingredients were:

Zhi Gan Cao (Radix Glycyrrhizae Preparata) 20–25 g, Xiao Mai (Fructus Tritici Levis) 18 g, Sang Piao Xiao (Oötheca Mantidis Preparata) 9 g, Yi Zhi Ren (Fructus Alpiniae Oxyphyllae parched) 9 g, Tu Si Zi (Semen Cuscutae) 9 g, Da Zao (Fructus Jujubae) 8 dates.

After the treatment, 13 cases were remarkedly improved, 15 improved.

10 Prescriptions for Inducing Resuscitation

10.1 Prescriptions for Inducing Resuscitation

Prescriptions of this kind are composed of drugs aromatic in nature and with the action of inducing resuscitation. Being capable of causing resuscitation and easing mental stress, they are used to restore life or consciousness after collapse or apparant death. The syndrome of coma or unconsciousness is usually due to excessive pathogens lording it over the heart−Qi. It falls into two types: the heat one and the cold one. The former is due to warm or heat pathogens invading the pericardium, while the latter due to cold or dampness pathogens or phlegm confusing the heart−Qi. The former is treated by removing heat to make an unconscious patient come to, while the latter by warming the heart and promoting free flow of the hear−Qi to wake up a patient from coma.

Prescriptions for inducing resuscitation either by removing heat or by warming the heart are only suitable for the treatment of the excess syndrome of stroke marked by trismus, clenched fists and forceful pulse. They are contraindicated for the prostration syndrome marked by profuse sweating, cold limbs, shortness of breath, incontinence of urine, opening of mouth and closing of eyes, even if it is complicated by coma. Apart from that, they are not applicable to *Yangming Fu* excess syndrome with the symptoms of coma and delirium, which should be treated through purgation with drugs of cold nature. When *Yangming Fu* excess syndrome associated with the syndrome of lingering of pathogenic factors in the pericardium is to be treated, a prescription for inducing resuscitation and a prescription for purgating with drugs of cold nature will be both prescribed. But which should be prescribed first or when they are both prescribed must be determined according to the mild or severe and slow or critical nature of a disease. Because drgus aromatic in nature used in the prescriptions for inducing resuscitation are apt to have their action disperse, they should be taken not in the form of decoction, but in the form of pills, powders or injections. Or else their volatile nature will affect curative effects. In addition, regular intake of them will damage the primordial *Qi,* and they are rarely prescribed clinically except for first aid. When they have to be used, their administration should not be stopped till the diseases change better, prolonged taking of them being avoided.

10.2 Prescriptions for Inducing Resuscitation with Drugs Cold in Nature

This kind of prescriptions are mainly made up of drugs aromatic and cold in nature and with the actions of restoring consciousness and removing heat and toxic material. They are suitable for the treatment of the excess syndrome due to lingering of warm—heat pathogens in the pericardium, marked by high fever, coma, delirium or even convulsion, or for other syndromes complicated by heat—symptoms such as apoplexy, convulsion caused by phlegm, attack by epidemic pathogenic factors, and sudden coma without consciousness. Drugs aromatic in nature and with the action of restoring consciousness such as

She Xiang (Moschus)

Bing Pian (Borneolum Syntheticum)

Yu Jin (Radix Curcumae)

are usually used together with drugs having the action of removing heat and toxins such as Nin Huang (Calculus Bovis) Xijiao (Cornu Rhinocerotis) Huang Lian (Rhizoma Coptidis) Shi Gao (Gypsum Fibrosum), etc. in these prescriptions, whose representatives are Angong Niuhuang Wan, Zixue Dan, Zhibao Dan and Huichun Dan.

10.3 The Prescription of Angong Niuhuang Wan

Name: Bezoar Bolus for Resurrection

Source: The book Wen Bing Tiao Bian

Ingredients:

Niu Huang (Calculus Bovis) 30 g, Yu Jin (Radix Curcumae) 30 g, Xi Jiao (Cornu Rhinocerotis) 30 g, Huang Qin(Radix Scutellariae) 30 g, Huang Lian (Rhizoma Coptidis) 30 g, Xiong Huang (Realgar) 30 g, Shan Zhi (Fructus Gardeniae) 30 g, Zhu Sha (Cinnabaris) 30 g, Bing Pian (Bornelum Synthetium) 7.5 g, She Xiang (Moschus) 7.5 g, Zhen Zhu (Margarita) 15 g, Jin Bo (Gold foil) appropriate amount.

Explanation:

Niu Huang: One of the principal drugs, being bitter and sweet in taste and cool in nature, removing heat pathogen from the heart, eliminating toxic material, clearing away phlegm for resuscitation.

She Xiang: The other principal drug, being pungent in flavor and warm in nature, restoring consciousness.

Xi Jiao: Clearing away heat from the heart and blood to dispel toxic material.

Huang Lian, Huang Qin and *Shan Zhi:* Removing heat, purging fire, clearing away toxic material, assisting *Niu Huang* to expel fire from the pericardium.

Bing Pian and *Yu Jin:* Being aromatic in nature, clearing away epidemic pathogenic factors, causing resuscitation, strengthening *She Xiang's* action of restoring consciousness.

Zhu Sha and *Zhen Zhu:* Calming the mind through their heavy property to drive away dysphoria.

Xiong Huang: Aiding *Niu Huang* in eliminating phlegm and toxic material for resuscitation.

Feng Mi: Normalizing the function of the stomach and spleen.

Jin Bo: Calming the mind through its heavy nature.

Effect: Removing heat for resuscitation, eliminating phlegm and toxic material.

Indications: Excess syndromes of stroke due to warm and heat pathogens such as lingering of heat pathogen in the pericardium, phlegm and heat pathogens confusing the heart, coma caused by apoplexy, and infantile convulsion, marked by high fever, dysphoria, coma and delirium; including such diseases with the above symptoms as encephalitis B, hepatic coma, coma due to acute cerebral hemorrhage, epidemic cerebrospinal meningitis, toxic dysentery, uremia and toxic hepatitis.

Administration: The ingredients except *Jin Bo* are ground into very fine powder. The powder is made with honey into boluses, each weighing 3 g. The boluses are coated with *Jin Bo* and then enclosed with wax. 1 bolus is taken each time daily, 2−3times daily for an adult with a severe disorder and a constitution of excess type. An infantile patient takes half a bolus each time. If it doesn't work, he / she may take the other half.

Case Study: 16 cases of coma due to acute cerebral hemorrhage were clinically treated with the therapy of acupuncture and moxibustion and the drug *Angong Niuhuang Wan*. While the acupoints Ren Zhong (DU26), etc. were punctured with gentle and rapid manipulation, *Angong Niuhuang Wan* was given by nasal feeding, 1−4 boluses each day with the dosage modified according to the symptoms. After the treatment, 9 cases regained lives, 3 of whom recovered completely.

10.4   The Prescription of *Zixue Dan*

Name: Purpled Snow Pill
Source: The book *Wai Tai Mi Yao*
Ingredients:
Shi Gao (Gypsum Fibrosum) 1500 g, *Han Shui Shi* (Calcitum) 1500 g, *Hua Shi* (Talcum) 1500 g, *Ci Shi* (Magnetitum) 1500 g, *Xi Jiao* (Cornu Rhinocerotis) 150 g, *Ling Yang Jiao* (Cornu Saigae Tataricae) 150 g, *Mu Xiang* (Radix Aucklandiae) 150 g, *Chen Xiang* (Lignum Aquilariae Resinatum) 150 g, *Xuan Shen* (Radix Scrophulariae) 500 g, *Sheng Ma* (Rhizoma Cimicifugae) 500 g, *Zhi Gan Cao* (Radix Glycyrrhizae Preparata) 240 g, *Ding Xiang* (Flos Caryophylli) 30 g, *Pu Xiao* (Natrii Sulfas) 5000 g, *Xiao Shi* (Nitrum) 96 g, *She Xiang* (Moschus) 1.5 g, *Zhu Sha* (Cinnabaris) 90 g, *Huang Jin* (gold) 3000 g.

Explanation:

Shi Gao, Han Shui Shi and *Hua Shi:* Being sweet in flavor and cold in nature, clearing away heat pathogen.

Ling Yang Jiao: Removing heat from the liver, calming endopathogenic wind to relieve convulsion.

Xi Jiao: Removing heat from the heart to get rid of heat poisons.

She Xiang: Being aromatic in flavor, promoting restoration of consciousness.

The above drugs are the main ingredients.

Xuan Shen, Sheng Ma and *Gan Cao:* Removing heat and toxic material, *Xuan Shen* has the action of nourishing *Yin* and promoting the production of body fluid.

Zhu Sha, Ci Shi and *Huang Jin:* Calming the mind through their heavy nature.

Mu Xiang, Ding Xiang and *Chen Xiang:* Promoting the free flow of *Qi* throughout the body.

Po Xiao and *Xiao Shi:* Clearing away heat and resolving stagnations.

Effect: Removing heat for resuscitation, relieving convulsion, tranquilizing the mind.

Indications: Syndromes due to warm and heat pathogens, such as lingering of heat pathogen in the pericardium and infantile convulsion caused by excessive heat, marked by high fever, dysphoria, coma, delirium, convulsion, thirst, dark and dry lips, deep-colored urine, constipation; including such diseases with the above symptoms as encephalitis B, epidemic cerebrospinal meningitis, scarlet fever, infantile measles, infantile high fever and convulsion, and hepatic coma.

Administration: *Shi Gao, Han Shui Shi, Hua Shi* and *Ci Shi* are pounded into small pieces. The small pieces are put into the water in which *Huang Jin* has been steeped and boiled to get the water. The same thing is done to get the same kind of water. The water got at 2 times is mixed together. *Xuan Shen, Mu Xiang, Chen Xiang, Sheng Ma, Gan Cao* and *Ding Xiang* are placed into the water and boiled to get the decoction. The same thing is done another 2 times. The decoction got at 3 times is mixed together and decocted to condense it into a paste. The powder of *Po Xiao* and *Xiao Shi* is put into the paste to get a mixture, which is stirred until it is even. The mixture is dried and ground into fine powder (powder 1). *Xi Jiao* and *Ling Yang Jiao* are ground into fine powder (powder 2). *Zhu Sha* is refined with water or ground into fine powder (powder 3). *She Xiang* is ground into fine powder (powder 4). All the 4 kinds of powder are mixed and ground together and sieved and made even. Thus *Zixue Dan* is at last obtained. 1.5–3 g of it is taken each time, twice daily. The dosage for children is reduced properly.

10.5   The Prescription of *Zhibao Dan*

Name: Treasured Bolus

Source: The book *Tai Ping Hui Min He Ji Ju Fang*

Ingredients:

Xi Jiao (Cornu Rhinocerotis) 30 g, *Dai Mao* (Carapax Eretmochelydis) 30 g, *Hu Po* (Succinum) 30 g, *Zhu Sha* (Cinnabaris) 30 g, *Xiong Huang* (Realgar) 30 g, *Long Nao* (Resina Dryobalanops Aromaticae) 7.5 g, *She Xiang* (Moschus) 7.5 g, *Niu Huang* (Calculus Bovis) 15 g, *An Xi Xiang* (Benzoinum) 45 g, *Jin Bo* (gold foil) 50 pieces, *Yin Bo* (silver foil) 50 pieces.

Indications: Sunstroke, apoplexy, infantile convulsion and excess syndrome of stroke due to phlegm and heat pathogens in epidemic febrile disease, marked by coma, delirium, fever, dysphoria, excess phlegm, shortness of breath, reddened tongue with yellowish thick greasy coating, and slippery rapid pulse; including such diseases with the above symptoms as cerebrovascular accident, hepatic coma, encephalitis B and epilepsy.

Administration: *Xi Jiao, Dai Mao, Hu Po, Long Nao, Niu Huang* and *Yin Bo* are separately ground into powder. *Zhu Sha* and *Xiong Huang* are ground into powder and refined with water separately. *An Xi Xiang* is ground into powder and refined with limeless wine and filtered into about 30 g of it, which is heated on gentle fire into a paste. Half of the gold foil is used to make the medicine (The rest is used to coat the boluses.). All the ingredients are mixed and ground together and made into boluses, each weighing 3 g. 1 bolus is ground and taken with boiled water each time for an adult, half a bolus for a child. It is ordered in the original prescription that this bolus is melted in ginseng decoction and taken. Ginseng has the action of replenishing *Qi* and consolidating the constitution. It is compatible with pungent and aromatic natured drugs with the action of restoring consciousness to exert the action of clearing the mind, strengthening the constitution and removing pathogenic factors. So, taking *Zhibao Dan* with ginseng decoction is suggested for the patients with complex and complicated disorder, weak vital *Qi* and pulse of deficiency type.

10.6   The Prescription of *Xiaoer Huichun Dan*

Name: Pill for Treating Infantile Convulsion
Source: *Jing Xiu Tang Yao Shuo*
Ingredients:

Chuan Bai Mu (Bulbus Fritillariae Cirrhosae) 37.5 g, *Chen Pi* (Pericarpium Citri Reticulatae) 37.5 g, *Mu Xiang* (Radix Aucklandiae) 37.5 g, *Bai Dou Kou* (Fructus Amomi Rotundus) 37.5 g, *Zhi Qiao* (Fructus Aurantii) 37.5 g, *Fa Ban Xia* (Rhizoma Pinelliae Preparata) 37.5 g, *Chen Xiang* (Lignum Aquilariae Resinatum) 37.5 g, *Tian Zhu Huang* (Concretio Silicea Bambusae) 37.5 g, *Jiang Can* (Bombyx Batryticatus) 37.5 g, *Quan Xie* (Scorpio) 37.5 g, *Tan Xiang* (Lignum Santali Albi) 37.5 g, *Niu Huang* (Calculus Bovis) 12 g, *She Xiang* (Moschus) 12 g, *Dan Nan Xing* (Arisaema cum Bile) 60 g, *Gou Teng* (Ramulus Uncariae cum Uncis) 240 g, *Da Huang* (Radix et Rhizoma Rhei) 60 g, *Tian Ma* (Rahizoma Gastrodiae) 37.5 g, *Gan Cao* (Radix Glycyrrhizae) 26 g, *Zhu Sha* (Cinnabaris) proper amount.

Explanation:

Niu Huang: Clearing away heat and toxic material, removing phlegm for resuscitation, calming endopathogenic wind and relieving convulsion.

She Xiang: Being aromatic in nature, restoring consciousness.

Chuan Bei Mu, Tian Zhu Huang, Dan Nan Xing and *Fa Ban Xia:* Removing heat and resolving phlegm.

Gou Teng, Tian Ma, Quan Xie and *Jiang Can:* Dispelling pathogenic wind, relieving convulsion and spasm.

Zhu Sha: Tranquilizing the mind through its heavy nature.

Da Huang: Clearing away heat and purging fire, eliminating stagnations to discharge phlegm and heat pathogens from the digestive tract.

Zhi Qiao, Mu Xiang, Chen Pi, Chen Xiang, Bai Dou Kou and *Tan Xiang:* Regulating the flow of *Qi* to remove phlegm, taking away the conditions for phlegm to be produced in the interior.

Gan Cao: Tempering the actions of all the other ingredients

Effect: Restoring consciousness, relieving convulsion, removing heat, resolving phlegm.

Indications: Syndrome of acute infantile convulsion due to phlegm and heat pathogens lording it over the heart—*Qi,* marked by fever, dysphoria, coma, convulsion, or nausea, vomiting, night crying, vomiting of milk, cough with sputum, asthma, abdominal pain, and diarrhea; including infantile high fever and convulsion with the above symptoms.

Contraindication: Chronic infantile convulsion due to deficiency cold of the spleen and kidney.

Administration: All the ingredients are ground into fine powder, which is then made into pills, each weighing 0.09 g. 1 pill is taken orally by children below 1 year old each time, 2 pills by children between 1—2 years old, 2—3 times daily.

10.7 Prescriptions for Inducing Resuscitation with Drugs Warm in Nature

Prescriptions of this kind are mainly made up of aromatic—pungent—warm natured drugs with the action promoting the circulation of *Qi* and restoring consciousness. They are suitable for the syndromes of apoplexy, syncope due to pathogenic cold, convulsion due to phlegm and excess syndrome due to cold pathogens, marked by sudden loss of consciousness, lock—jaw, coma, dysphasia, whitish tongue coating, and slow pulse. The commonly used drugs aromatic in nature and with the action of restoring consciousness are:

Su He Xiang (Styrax), She Xiang (Moschus), Bing Pian (Borneolum Syntheticum).

The commonly used drugs pungent in flavor and warm in nature and with the action of promoting the circulation of Qi are:

Chen Xiang (Lignum Aquilariae Resinatum)

Ding Xiang (Flos Caryophylli), etc.

The two kinds of drugs are compatible with each other in these prescriptions, whose representatives are Suhexiang Wan, Zijin Ding, etc.

10.8   The Prescription of Suhexiang Wan

Name: Storax Pill

Source: The book Tai Ping Hui Min He Ji Ju Fang

Ingredients:

Bai Zhu (Rhizoma Atractylodis Macrocephalae) 60 g, Mu Xiang (Radix Aucklandiae) 60 g, Xi Jiao (Cornu Rhinocerotis) 60 g, Xiang Fu (Rhizoma Cyperi) 60 g, Zhu Sha (Cinnabaris) 60 g, He Zi (Fructus Chebulae) 60 g, Tan Xiang (Lignum Santali Albi) 60 g, An Xi Xiang (Benzoium) 60 g, Chen Xiang (Lignum Aquilariae Resinatum) 60 g, She Xiang (Moschus) 60 g, Ding Xiang (Flos Caryophylli) 60 g, Bi Bo (Fructus Piperis Longi) 60 g, Long Nao (Resina Dryobalanops Aromaticae) 30 g, Su He Xiang You (Styrax Oleum) 30 g, Ru Xiang (Resina Olibani) 30 g.

Explanation:

Su He Xiang, She Xiang, Bing Pian and *An Xi Xing:* The principal drugs, being aromatic in nature, restoring consciousness.

Mu Xiang, Tan Xiang, Chen Xiang, Ru Xiang, Ding Xiang and *Xiang Fu:* Promoting the circulation of *Qi* to remove stasis, expelling cold and turbid pathogens, eliminating the stagnation of *Qi* and blood in the *Zang—Fu* organs.

Bi Bo: Expelling cold and stasis.

*Xi Jiao :*Detoxidating.

Zhu Sha: Calming the mind through its heavy nature.

Bai Zhu: Invigorating *Qi* and strengthening the spleen, drying dampness and getting rid of turbid pathogen.

He Zi: Astringing *Qi,* tempering the actions of the drugs pungent and aromatic in nature.

Effect: Restoring consciousness by means of the aromatic nature, promoting the circulation of *Qi* to relieve pain.

Indications: Syndromes of apoplexy, affection of pestilent factors or epidemic pestilential pathogens, marked by sudden loss of consciousness, lock—jaw, whitish tongue coating, and slow pulse, or *Qi* controlled only in the interior due to pathogenic cold, sudden pain in the heart and abdomen, and syncope in severe case, or sudden loss of consciousness resulting from *Qi* stagnated due to excess phlegm; including such disorders with the above symptoms as hysteria, angina pectoris due to coranary heart disease, food poisoning and epilepsy.

Contraindication: This prescription is contraindicated for pregnant women, for quite a number of drugs in it are aromatics which tend to impair the original *Qi* of fetus.

Administration: All the ingredients are ground into powder

with *Zhu Sha, An Xi Xiang, Ru Xiang* ground separately. Before grinding, *Xiang Fu* is parched with its hair removed, *He Zi* is baked with its peel eliminated. After grinding, the powder of *Zhu Sha* is refined with water, the powder of *An Xi Xiang* is made into paste with one litre of limeless wine, and, then, *Su He Xiang You* is put into the paste of *An Xi Xiang*. Finally, the fine powders are made into pills with the mixture of the paste of *An Xi Xiang* and honey, each pill weighing 3 g. 1 pill is taken with warm boiled water each time, 1—2 times daily. The dosage for children is properly reduced.

Case Study: *Suhexiang Wan* in combination with western medicines was clinically used to treat 5 cases of acute myocardiac infarction, whose main symptom was precordialgia. The precordialgia had been relieved with morphinic drugs with the side effects of morphinism and inhibition of breath. After *Suhexiang Wan* was taken, 4 cases were remarkedly improved. Of the 4 cases, 1, who had been suffering from posterior myocardial infarction, felt the disappearance of the precordialgia half an hour later after the pill was taken, no side effects being found.

Suhexiang Wan was used to save and treat 2 cases of manihot poisoning, marked by chills, dizziness, fullness in the chest, vomiting, cold limbs in severe case, mild convulsion of hands and feet, pallor of face and lips, nasal flaring, shortness of breath, half coma, and indistinct pulse. After 1 pill was ground in warm boiled water and fed, the 2 cases were both cured.

10.9 The Prescription of *Tongguan San*

Name: Powder for Restoring Consciousness
Source: The book *Dan Xi Xin Fa Fu Yu*

Ingredients:

Zhu Ya Zao (Fructus Gleditsiae Abnormalis), *Xi Xin* (Herba Asari).

The 2 ingredients are in the same amount.

Explanation

Zhu Ya Zao: Being pungent in flavor and warm in nature, removing phlegm for resuscitation.

Xi Xin: Being pungent in flavor and warm in nature, inducing resuscitation through dispersing.

Effect: Restoring consciousness and inducing resuscitation.

Indications: Excess syndrome of stroke due to convulsive seizure resulting from attack by pestilent factors or due to convulsion caused by phlegm retention, marked by trismus, obstruction of breath, coma, lock-jaw, and profuse sputum and saliva; including such diseases with the above symptoms as epilepsy, cerebrovascular accident and craniocerebral trauma.

Administration: The 2 ingredients are ground into fine powder and mixed evenly. Small amount of it is blown into the nose to induce sneezing.

This prescription is used externally for first aid. After the patient comes to, his disease should be differentiated and treated with other prescriptions.

10.10   The Prescription of *Zijin Ding*

Name: Knoxia and Moleplant Loxenge

Source: The book *Pian Yu Xin Shu*

Ingredients:

Shan Ci Gu (Pseudobulbus Cremastrae seu Pleiones) 90 g, *Hong Da Ji* (Radix Knoxiae) 45 g, *Qian Jin Zi* (Semen

Euphorbiae) 30 g, *Wu Bei Zi* (Galla Chinensis) 90 g, *She Xiang* (Moschus) 9 g, *Xiong Huang* (Realgar) 30 g, *Zhu Sha* (Cinnabaris) 30 g, *Nuo Mi* (Semen Oryzae Glutinosae) proper amount.

Explanation:

She Xiang: Being aromatic in nature, inducing resuscitation, promoting the circulation of *Qi* and relieving pain.

Shan Ci Gu: Dispelling heat to subdue swelling.

Xiong Huang: Expelling pathogenic factors and toxic material.

Qian Jin Zi and *Hong Da Ji:* Eliminating phlegm and subduing swelling.

Zhu Sha: Calming the mind through its heavy nature.

Wu Bei Zi: Drying the intestines to alleviate diarrhea.

Effect: Taken orally, it has the action of causing resuscitation, resolving phlegm, getting rid of pestilent pathogenic factors and toxic material, purgating slowly, and descending the adverse flow of *Qi*. Applied externally, it functions in subduing swelling and dispersing masses.

Indications: Syndrome due to attack of pestilent pathogenic factors and phlegm retention, marked by distending full painful sensation in the stomach and intestines, vomiting, diarrhea, and skin and external diseases; including such diseases with the above symptoms as food poisoning, furuncle, boil and swelling.

Administration: The ingredients are ground into powder and made into lozenges with the paste of *Nuo Mi*. 0.6−1.5 g of the lozenge is taken orally each time, twice daily. When applied externally, it is ground in vinegar and applied on the affected area. Because *Qian Jin Zi* and *Hong Da Ji* are both poisoning, the dosage for children should be reduced. Meanwhile, it is contraindicated for pregnant women, for *She Xiang* in it is aromatic and apt to drift off its channel.

11 Prescriptions for Inducing Astringency

11.1 Prescriptions for Inducing Astringency

Prescriptions mainly composed of astringents, having the action of inducing astringency, and used to arrest discharge of *Qi*, blood, semen or body fluid are all known as "prescription for inducing astringency". The discharge of *Qi*, blood, semen or body fluids, a morbid condition,   is in such different ways according to different disease causes and locations as spontaneous sweating, night sweating, prolonged cough due to deficiency of the lung, emission, spermatorrhoea, incontinence of urine, chronic diarrhea, prolonged dysentery, metrorrhagia or metrostaxis, and leukorrhagia.   As a result, prescriptions of this kind are classified as the following five: those for consolidating the superficies to stop sweating, those for astringing the lung to arrest cough, those for relieving diarrhea with astringents, those for astringing spontaneous emission, and those for curing metrorrhagia and leukorrhagia.

This kind of prescriptions are too potent to be suitable for such disorders due to pathogenic factors of excess type as spontaneous sweating, night sweating, prolonged cough, emission, spermatorrhoea, incontinence of urine, chronic diarrhea or dysentery, metrorrhagia or metrostaxis, and leukorrhagia.

11.2 Prescriptions for Consolidating the Superficies to Stop Sweating

Prescriptions of this kind are mainly made up of drugs with the action of consolidating the superficies of the body to stop sweating. They are suitale for the syndrome of spontaneous sweating and night sweating due to incompact superficies and *Yin*-deficiency. The commonly used drugs are:

Huang Qi (Radix Astragali), *Mu Li* (Concha Ostreae), *Ma Huang Gen* (Radix Ephedrae), *Fu Xiao Mai* (Fructus Tritici Levis).

The representative prescriptions are *Muli San, Yupingfeng San,* etc.

11.3 The Prescription of *Yupingfeng San*

Name: Jadescreen Powder

Source: The book *Dan Xi Xin Fa*

Ingredients:

Fang Feng (Radix Saposhinkoviae) 30 g, *Huang Qi* (Radix Astragali) 30 g, *Bai Zhu* (Rhizoma Atractylodis Macrocephalae) 60 g.

Explanation:

Huang Qi: Replenishing *Qi* to consolidate the supericial resistance.

Bai Zhu: Strengthening the spleen to invigorate *Qi,* working together with *Huang Qi* to ensure the flourish of *Qi* and the consolidation of the superficial resistance, thus preventing excessive perspiration and invasion of exogenous pathogens.

Fang Feng: Being pungent in flavor and warm in nature, dispelling pathogenic wind, working together with *Huang Qi* to consolidate the superficies with pathogens expelled and expell pathogenic factors with vital *Qi* unhurt.

Effect: Replenishing *Qi,* consolidating the superficial resistance, arresting spontaneous sweating.

Indications: Syndrome of spontaneous sweating due to deficiency of the superficies, marked by aversion to wind, puffy and pale complexion, pale tongue with thin whitish coating, and floating weak pulse; including such diseases with the above symptoms as chronic rhinitis. allergic rhinitis and respiratory tract infection.

Administration: All the ingredients are ground into fine powder. 6–9 g of the powder is taken each time, twice daily. (Taken also in the form of decoction with the amounts of the ingredients reduced properly according to a patient's condition and the proportions of the drugs in the original prescription).

Case Study: *Yupingfeng San* was clinically used to treat 32 children who were with weak constitutions and often attacked by common cold, bronchitis or pneumonia.The powder was given in 15 days in a month. The treatment lasted three and a half months, during which no attack of any of the three diseases occurred in 11 cases, only one time of common cold took place in 13 cases, two times of common cold were seen in 7 cases, ineffectiveness was found in 1 case who had not taken the powder on time.

16 cases of postoperative spontaneous sweating complicated by aversion to wind were treated with *Yupingfeng San*. All of them were cured, the average doses for each case to take being 5.

11.4   The Prescription of *Muli San*

Name: Oyster Shell Powder

Source: The book *Tai Ping Hui Min He Ji Ju Fang*

Ingredients:

Huang Qi (Radix Astragali) 30 g, *Ma Huang Gen* (Radix Ephedrae) 30 g, *Mu Li* (Concha Ostreae) 30 g, *Xiao Mai* (Fructus Tritici Levis) 30 g.

Explanation:

Mu Li: The principal drug, replenishing *Yin*, suppressing the hyperactivities of *Yang*, relieving restlessness and astringing sweating.

Huang Qi: Invigorating *Qi* to consolidate the superficial resistance.

Ma Huang Gen: Arresting perspiration specially.

Xiao Mai: Invigorating the heart–*Qi*, replenishing the heart–*Yin*, stopping sweating.

Effect: Consolidating the superficial resistance and stopping sweating.

Indications: Syndrome of spontaneous sweating due to floating of *Yang*, marked by frequent perspiration, severe night sweating lasting longer, palpitation, inclination to be frightened, pale tongue with whitish coating, and thready weak pulse; including such diseases with the above symptoms as spontaneous sweating and night sweating due to disturbance of the vegetative nerve function and night sweating due to tuberculosis.

Administration: The first 3 ingredients are ground into coarse powder. 9 g of the powder is taken with the decoction of 30 g of *Xiao Mai* each time, twice daily. Or the first 3 ingredients are properly reduced and decocted in water with 30 g of *Xiao Mai* for the decoction to be taken orally.

Case Study: *Muli San* was clinically adopted to treat 28 cases, of whom 15 were suffering from night sweating, 6 spontaneous sweating, 7 both spontaneous and night sweating. The treatment result was that 20 cases were cured, 5 basically cured, 1 improved, 2 unimproved. 2—5 doses were taken by each of the 18 cases, 6—10 by each of the 5, more than 10 by each of the 5.

11.5 Prescriptions for Astringing the Lung to Arrest Cough

This kind of prescriptions are mainly made up of drugs with the action of astringing the lung and stopping cough. They are applicable to the syndromes of deficiency of the lung due to intractable cough, consumption of *Qi* and *Yin,* shortness of breath and spontaneous sweating, and weak rapid pulse. Drugs such as

Wu Wei Zi (Fructus Schisandrae), *Ying Su Qiao* (Pericarpium Papaveris), *Wu Mei* (Fructus Mume), *Ren Shen* (Radix Ginseng), *E Jiao* (Colla Corii Asini), etc.,

are usually used in these prescriptions, whose representative is *Jiuxian San.*

11.6 The Prescription of *Jiuxian San*

Name: Nine Noble Ingredients Powder
Source: The book *Yi Xue Zheng Zhuan*
Ingredients:

Ren Shen (Radix Ginseng) 2 g, *Kuan Dong Hua* (Flos Farfarae) 2 g, *Jie Geng* (Radix Platycodi) 2 g, *Sang Bai Pi*

(Cortex Mori) 2 g, *Wu Wei Zi* (Fructus Schisandrae) 2 g, *E Jiao* (Colla Corii Asini) 2 g, *Bei Mu* (Bulbus Fritillariae) 2 g, *Wu Mei* (Fructus Mume) 6 g, *Ying Su Qiao* (Pericarpium Papaveris) 6 g, *Sheng Jiang* (Rhizoma Zingiberis Recens) 1 piece, *Da Zao* (Fructus Jujubae) 1 date.

Explanation:

Ying Su Qiao: One of the principal drugs, astringing the lung to arrest cough.

Ren Shen: The other principal drug, invigorating *Qi* and benefiting the lung.

E Jiao: Nourishing *Yin* and benefiting the lung.

Wu Wei Zi and *Wu Mei:* Astringing the lung to arrest cough.

Kuan Dong Hua and *Bei Mu:* Arresting cough, resolving phlegm, descending the adverse flow of the lung–*Qi* to relieve dyspnea.

Sang Bai Pi: Removing pathogenic heat from the lung to arrest cough.

Jie Geng: Arresting cough and resolving phlegm.

Effect: Astringing the lung to arrest cough, invigorating *Qi* and nourishing *Yin*.

Indications: Syndrome due to deficiency of the lung and insufficiency of *Qi*, marked by protracted cough which even leads to dyspnea and spontaneous when severe, pale tongue with whitish coating, and weak rapid pulse; including such diseases with the above symptoms as chronic bronchitis, bronchial asthma, pleurisy and pneumonia in the convalescence.

Administration: All the ingredients except the last two are ground into fine powder. The powder is decocted in water with *Sheng Jiang* and *Da Zao* for the decoction to be taken twice.

Contraindication: Because this prescription is very strong in astringing the lung and stopping cough, it should not be administered to treat patients with protracted cough complicated by profuse expectoration, or with exterior syndrome due to exogeneous pathogens for fear that the disease be prolonged or worsened.

11.7 Prescriptions for Relieving Diarrhea with Astringents

Prescriptions of this kind are mainly composed of drugs with the action of astringing the intestines to relieve diarrhea. They are suitable for the syndrome of intractable diarrhea due to deficiency—cold of the spleen and kidney. The commonly used drugs are:

Chi Shi Zhi (Halloysitum Rubrum), *Rou Dou Kou* (Semen Myristicae), *He Zi* (Fructus Chebulae), *Wu Wei Zi* (Fructus Schisandrae), *Bu Gu Zhi* (Fructus Psoraleae), *Rou Gui* (Cortex Cinnamomi), *Ren Shen* (Radix Ginseng), *Bai Zhu* (Rhizoma Atractylodis Macrocephalae).

The representative prescriptions are *Zhenren Yangzang Tang*, *Sishen Wan* and *Taohua Tang*.

11.8 The Prescription of *Zhenren Yangzang Tang*

Name: Decoction for Nourishing *Zang*—organs
Source: The book *Tai Ping Hui Min He Ji Ju Fang*
Ingredients:

Ren Shen (Radix Ginseng) 6 g, *Gan Cao* (Radix Glycyrrhizae) 6 g, *Dang Gui* (Radix Angelicae Sinensis) 9 g, *Mu Xiang* (Radix Aucklandiae) 9 g, *Bai Zhu* (Rhizoma Atractylodis Macrocephalae) 12 g, *Rou Dou Kou* (Semen Myristicae) 12 g, *He*

Zi (Fructus Chebulae) 12 g, *Bai Shao* (Radix Paeoniae Alba) 15 g, *Ying Su Qiao* (Pericaupium Papaveris) 20 g, *Rou Gui* (Cortex Cinnamomi) 3 g.

Explanation:

Ying Su Qiao: One of the principal drugs, astringing the intestines to stop diarrhea.

Rou Gui: The other principal drug, warming the kidney and spleen .

Ren Shen and *Bai Zhu:*Invigorating *Qi* and strengthening the spleen.

Dang Gui and *Bai Shao:* Enriching blood and coordinating *Ying.*

Mu Xiang: Regulating the flow of *Qi* to relieve pain.

Gan Cao: Tempering the actions of all the other ingredients, relieving spasm and pain.

Effect: Astringing the intestines to stop diarrhea, warming and tonifying the kidney and spleen.

Indications: Syndrome due to deficiency–cold of the spleen and kidney, marked by protracted diarrhea and dysentery, incontinence of defecation, abdominal pain relieved by pressing and warming, or frequent diarrhea with pus and blood, lassitude and anorexia, pale tongue with whitish coating, and deep slow pulse; including such diseases with the above symptoms as chronic enteritis, chronic bacillary dysentery, and intestinal tuberculosis.

Administration: Decocted in water for oral dose to be taken twice.

Case Study: 13 cases of infantile diarrhea of deficiency–cold type were clinically treated with modified *Zhenren Yangzang*

Tang. In case of retained food, drugs added to the prescription of *Zhenren Yangzang Tang* were:

Shen Qu (Massa Medicata Fermentata)

Shan Zha (Rhizoma Crataegi).

In case of fecal incontinence, drugs added were:

Shi Liu Pi (Pericarpium Granati)

Shi Di (Calyx Kaki).

In case of oliguria, drugs added were:

Che Qian Zi (Semen Plantaginis)

Mu Tong (Caulis Akebiae)

Fu Ling (Poria).

The treatment cured all the cases.

11.9 The Prescription of *Sishen Wan*

Name: Pill of Four Miraculous Drugs

Source: The book *Zheng Zhi Zhun Sheng*

Ingredients:

Rou Dou Kou (Semen Myristicae) 60 g, *Wu Wei Zi* (Fructus Schisandrae) 60 g, *Bu Gu Zhi* (Fructus Psoraleae) 120 g, *Wu Zhu Yu* (Fructus Evodiae) 30 g, *Sheng Jiang* (Rhizoma Zingiberis Recens) 24 g, *Da Zao* (Fructus Jujubae) 100 dates.

Explanation:

Bu Gu Zhi: The principal drug, warming and tonifying the kiendy–*Yang.*

Rou Dou Kou: Warming the spleen to arrest diarrhea, promoting the flow of *Qi* and removing stagnated food.

Wu Zhu Yu and *Sheng Jiang:* Warming the middle–*Jiao* to expel pathogenic cold.

Wu Wei Zi: Astringing the intestines to arrest diarrhea.

Da Zao: Tonifying the spleen and benefiting the stomach.

Effect: Warming and tonifying the spleen and kidney, astringing the intestines to arrest diarrhea.

Indications: Syndrome due to cold—deficiency of the spleen and kidney, marked by diarrhea before dawn, loss of appetite, abdominal pain, soreness of the loins, cold limbs, listlessness, lassitude, pale tongue with thin whitish coating, and deep slow weak pulse; including such diseases with the above symptoms as chronic colitis, allergic colitis and intestinal tuberculosis.

Administration: *Da Zao* without the cores is boiled up to being done. The other ingredients are ground into fine powder, which is mixed with the boiled *Da Zao* into pills. 6—9 g of the pills is taken each time, twice daily. Or all the ingredients are decocted in water for oral dose after the amounts of the drugs are reduced according to the proportions in the original prescription.

Case Study: 20 cases of diarrhea before dawn were clinically treated with *Sishen Wan* with 16 cases cured and 4 remarkably improved.

Sishen Wan was also employed to treat 1 case of allergic colitis with a history of 9 years, marked by abdominal pain and 3—5 times of laxation every day. 20 days later after *Sishen Wan* was taken, the stools took form and only 1—2 times of laxation occurred each day. The taking of *Sishen Wan* was continued for another 10 days and all the symptoms disappeared. Then 1 month of observation without giving *Sishen Wan* turned out that the curative effects had been maintained.

Experimental results showed that *Sishen Wan* can inhibit the spontaneous movements of the intestines and the intestinal spasm induced by acetylcholine or by parium chloride.

11.10 The Prescription of *Taohua Tang*

Name: Pink Decoction

Source: The book *Shang Han Lun*

Ingredients:

Chi Shi Zhi (Halloysitum Rebrum) 30 g, *Jing Mi* (Semen Oryzae Sativae) 30 g, *Gan Jiang* (Rhizoma Zingiberis) 9 g.

Explanation:

Chi Shi Zhi: The principal drug, being heavy and warm in nature, astringing the intestines to relieve diarrhea.

Gan Jiang: Warming the middle—*Jiao* to expel pathogenic cold.

Jing Mi: Nourishing the stomach and regulating the function of the middle—*Jiao*.

Effect: Warming up the middle—*Jiao* to astringe the intestines.

Indications: Syndrome due to deficiency—cold of the spleen and stomach, marked by protracted dysentery, deep—colored stools with pus and blood, dysuria, abdominal pain alleviated by warming and pressing, pale tongue with whitish coating, and feeble thready pulse; including such diseases with the above symptoms as amebic dysentery, chronic bacillary dysentery and chronic enteritis.

Administration: Decocted in water for oral dose to be taken twice.

Case Study: 4 cases of chronic amebic dysentery, whose course was from half a year to 2 years, were clinically treated with *Taohua Tang* plus:

Yu Yu Liang (Limonitum), *Chao Di Yu* (Radix Sanguisorbae

stir–fried), *Shan Yao* (Rhizoma Dioscoreae), *Qin Pi* (Cortex Fraxini), *Long Gu* (Os Draconis Fossilia), *Mu Li* (Concha Ostreae).

3–5 doses were taken by each of the cases and effectiveness resulted in all of them. Then in the following 7 days, the cases were treated with the therapeutic method of strengthening the spleen and regulating the stomach and they were all cured.

11.11 Prescriptions for Astringing Spontaneous Emission

This kind of prescriptions are mainly made up of drugs with the action of reinforcing the kidney to astringe emission. They are indicated for the syndrome of enuresis or emission due to the inability of the weak kidney to store and control the discharge of urine and sperm, or enuresis and frequent urination due to the inability of the weak kidney to control the opening–closing function of the bladder. The commonly used drugs are:

Sha Yuan (Semen Astragali Complanati), *Ji Li* (Fructus Tribuli), *Lian Xu* (Stamen Nelumbinis), *Qian Shi* (Semen Euryales), *Sang Piao Xiao* (Oötheca Mantidis), *Yi Zhi Ren* (Fructus Alpiniae Oxyphyllae), etc.

The representative prescriptions are *Jinsuo Gujing Wan*, *Sangpiaoxiao San* and *Suoquan Wan*.

11.12 The Prescription of *Jinsuo Gujing Wan*

Name: Golden Lock Pill for Keeping the Kidney Essence
Source: The book *Yi Fang Ji Jie*
Ingredients:
Sha Yuan (Semen Astragali Complanati) 60 g, *Ji Li* (Fructus

Tribuli) 60 g, *Qian Shi* (Semen Euryales) 60 g, *Lian Xu* (Stamen Nelumbinis) 60 g, *Long Gu* (Os Draconis) 30 g, *Mu Li* (Concha Ostreae) 30 g.

Explanation:

Sha Yuan and *Ji Li:* The principal drugs, reinforcing the kidney to astringe emission.

Lian Zi: Clearing away the heart—fire and easing mental anxiety.

Long Gu, Mu Li, Lian Xu and *Qian Shi:* Astringing emission and enuresis.

Effect: Reinforcing the kidney and astringing emission.

Indications: Syndrome due to deficiency of the kidney and depletion of the vital essence, marked by nocturnal emission, spermatorrhea, listlessness, lassitude, soreness and weakness of the limbs, lumbar aching, tinnitus, pale tongue with whitish coating, and thready weak pulse; including such diseases with the above symptoms as functional disturbance of the vegetative nerves and myasthenia gravis.

Administration: All the ingredients are ground into powder, the powder is made into pills with the paste of *Lian Zi Rou* (Semen Nelumbinis). 9 g of the pills is taken each time with slightly salty water or boiled water, 3 times daily. Or the ingredients are properly reduced according to the original proportions and decocted in water with an adequate amount of *Lian Zi Rou* for the decoction to be taken orally.

Case Study: *Jinsuo Gujing Wan* was clinically used to treat 1 case of myasthenia gravis marked by complete ptosis of the right upper eyelid, weakness of the limbs, keeping bedrid with the legs drawn up, difficulty in chewing, dyspnea, shortness of breath, nocturnal emission, spermatorrhea, cold pain in the loins and knees. 12 g of *Jinsuo Gujing Wan* was taken each time, 3 times daily. 2 weeks later, the disease condition was remarkably improved. Several months later, the case was cured. A six—year follow—up found no relapse.

11.13 The Prescription of *Sangpiaoxiao San*

Name: Mantis Egg—case Powder

Source: The book *Ben Cao Yan Yi*

Ingredients:

Sang Piao Xiao (Oötheca Mantidis) 30 g, *Yuan Zhi* (Radix Polygalae) 30 g, *Chang Pu* (Rhizoma Acori Graminei) 30 g, *Long Gu* (Os Draconis Fossilia) 30 g, *Ren Shen* (Radix Ginseng) 30 g, *Fu Shen* (Poria cum Ligno Hospite) 30 g, *Dang Gui* (Radix Angelicae Sinensis) 30 g, *Gui Ban* (Carapax et Plastrum Testudinis) 30 g.

Explanation:

Sang Piao Xiao: The principal drug, reinforcing the kidney to replenish vital essence and arrest emission.

Long Gu and *Gui Ban:* Nourishing the kidney to strengthen its astringing function.

Ren Shen, Dang Gui and *Fu Shen:* Replenishing *Qi* and nourishing blood.

Chang Pu and *Yuan Zhi:* Tranquilizing the mind to relieve anxiety, promoting the coordination between the heart and kidney.

Effect: Tonifying and regulating the heart and kidney to astringe emission and enuresis.

Indication: Syndrome due to deficiency of both the heart and kidney, marked by frequent urination, or ricewashed—water like urine, enuresis, spermatorrhea, trance, amnesia, poor appetite, pale tongue with whitish coating, and thready weak pulse; including such diseases with the above symptoms as diabetes insipidus, diabetes mellitus, neurosism and neurogenic frequency of urination.

Administration: The ingredients are guound into fine powder. 6 g, of the powder is taken with the decoction of *Ren Shen* before going to bed. or, the ingredients are properly reduced according to the original proportions and decocted in water for the decoction to be taken orally.

Case Study: Modified *Sangpiaoxiao San* was clinically employed to treat the cases of hysteroptosis complicated by frequent urination and hyperexudation of the cervical orifice with remarkable effectiveness. A case with 8—year hysteroptosis marked by dizziness, shortness of breath, listlessness, lassitude, frequent urination, intermittent yellowish discharge from the cervical orifice, pale tongue with whitish coating, and weak feeble pulse was treated with modified *Sangpiaoxiao San,* whose ingredients were:

those of the prescription of *Sangpiaoxiao San*

Huang Qi (Radix Astragali), *Chai Hu* (Radix Bupleuri), *Sheng Ma* (Rhizoma Cimicifugae).

Prolapse of the uterus was noticeably retracted after 4 doses were taken. Another 3 doses taken, the case was cured.

11.14 The Prescription of *Suoquan Wan*

Name: Pill for Reducing Urination
Source: The book *Fu Ren Liang Fang*

Ingredients:

Wu Yao (Radix Linderae), *Yi Zhi Ren* (Fructus Alpiniae Oxyphyllae).

The 2 ingredients are in the same amount.

Explanation:

Yi Zhi Ren: The principal drug, warming up the kidney to strengthening its function in governing the reception of air, warming the spleen to arrest spermatorrhea and astringing urination.

Wu Yao: Warming up the kidney and expelling cold.

Shan Yao: Strengthening the spleen and reinforcing the kidney.

Effect: Warming up the kidney to disperse pathogenic cold, astringe urine and arrest spontaneous emission.

Indications: Syndrome due to deficiency and cold in the lower—*Jiao,* marked by frequent urination, infantile enuresis, pale tongue with whitish coating, and deep slow pulse; including such diseases with the above symptoms as neurogenic frequency of urination, diabetes insipidus and medullitis.

Administration: The ingredients are ground into fine powder. An adequate amount of *Shan Yao* (Rhizoma Dioscoreae) is broken into small pieces and decocted in liquor into a paste. The powder and paste are mixed together into pills. 6 g of the pills is taken each time, twice daily. Or, the ingredients are reduced according to the original proportions and decocted in water for the decoction to be taken orally.

This prescription is weak in potency. Given the syndromes to be treated are more severe, drugs with the action of warming, tonifying and astringing should be added adequately in order that its curative effects can be enhanced.

Case Study: 1 case of obstinate constipation marked by constipation which, milder in summer and more serious in winter, lasted 30 years, soreness of the loins, frequent urination, anal pain, deep—colored tongue with little coating, and deep thready slow pulse was treated with the prescription of *Suoquan Wan* plus:

Mu Li (Concha Ostreae), *Gou Qi* (Fructus Lycii), *Shu Di* (Radix Rehmanniae Preparata), *Zhi Fu Zi* (Radix Aconiti Lateralis Preparata), *Tao Ren* (Semen Persicae), *Gan Cao* (Radix Glycyrrhizae).20 doses cured the case with all the symptoms driven away.

11.15 Prescriptions for Curing Metrorrhagia and Leukorrhagia

Prescriptions of this kind are mainly made up of such drugs with the action of arresting metrorrhagia and leukorrhagia as
Chun Gen Pi (Cortex Ailanthi), *Hei Jing Jie* (Herba Schizonepetae), *Chi Shi Zhi* (Halloysitum Rubrum), etc.
The representative prescriptions are *Gu Jing Wan, Wandai Tang,* etc., which are used to cure metrorrhagia and leukorrhagia.

11.16 The Prescription of *Gujing Wan*

Name: Pill for Arresting Metrorrhagia
Source: The book *Yi Xue Ru Men*
Ingredients:

Huang Qin (Radix Scutellariae) 30 g, *Bai Shao* (Radix Paeoniae Alba) 30 g, *Gui Ban* (Carapax et Plastrum Testudinis) 30 g, *Chun Gen Pi* (Cortex Ailanthi) 21 g, *Huang Bai* (Cortex Phellodendri) 9 g, *Xiang Fu* (Rhizoma Cyperi) 7.5 g.

Explanation:

Gui Ban: Benefiting the kidney through nourishing *Yin* to purge fire.

Bai Shao: Astringing *Yin* and enriching blood to nourish the liver.

Huang Qin and *Huang Bai:* Clearing away heat and purging fire to arrest bleeding.

Chun Gen Pi: Strengthening the channels to arrest leukorrhagia, eliminating dampness and heat.

Xiang Fu: Regulating the flow of *Qi* to remove stasis and coordinate blood.

Effect: Nourishing *Yin,* clearing away pathogenic heat, arresting bleeding, and consolidating the channels.

Indications: Syndrome of pathogenic heat in the interior due to *Yin*—deficiency, marked by prolonged menstruation, metrorrhagia or metrostaxis, deep—colored blood being mixed with dark purple clots, dysphoria and feverish sensation in the chest and epigastric region, abdominal pain, dark urine, reddened tongue, and taut rapid pulse; including such diseases with the above symptoms as menoxenia and dysfunctional uterine bleeding, etc., all secondary to the inflammation of the reproductive system.

Administration: All the ingredients are ground into powder. The powder is mixed with liquor into pills. 9 g of the pills is taken each time, twice daily. Or, the ingredients are properly reduced according to the original proportions and decocted in water for the decoction to be taken orally.

11.17 The Prescription of *Zhenling Dan*

Name: Pill for Removing Blood Stasis and Arresting Bleeding.

Source: The book *Tai Ping Hui Min He Ji Ju Fang*

Ingredients:

Yu Yu Liang (Limonitum) 200 g, *Zi Shi Ying* (Fluoritum) 200 g, *Chi Shi Zhi* (Halloysitum Rubrum) 200 g, *Dai Zhe Shi* (Haematitum) 200 g, *Ru Xiang* (Resina Olibani) 100 g, *Wu Ling Zhi* (Faeces Trogopterori) 200 g, *Mo Yao* (Myrrha) 100 g, *Zhu Sha* (Cinnabaris) 50 g, *Nuo Mi* (Semen Oryzae Glutinosae) 200 g.

Explanation:

Chi Shi Zhi, Yu Yu Liang, Zi Shi Ying and *Zhe Shi:* Warming up the uterus to control menstruation, nourishing blood to arresting metrorrhagia.

Ru Xiang, Mo Yao and *Wu Ling Zhi:* Promoting the circulation of blood to remove blood stasis, activating the flow of *Qi* to relieve pain.

Nuo Mi: Reinforcing the lung, strengthening the spleen, invigorating *Qi,* warming up the middle—*Jiao.*

Effect: Removing blood stasis and arresting bleeding.

Indications: Syndrome due to deficiency—cold of the *Chong* and *Ren* channels and obstruction of the uterus by blood stasis, marked by metrorrhgia or metrostaxis, purplish red or dark purple blood with clots, pain in the lower abdomen aggravated by pressing,   dark purplish tongue, and deep thready taut pulse; including such diseases with the above symptoms as dysfunctional uterine bleeding and postpartum profuse loss of blood.

Administration: All the ingredients except *Nuo Mi* and *Zhu Sha* are ground together into fine powder *Nuo Mi* is ground and stir—fried until done. The two powders are mixed together and made with water into pills. The pills are coated with *Zhu Sha*. 6 g, of the pills is taken each time, twice daily.

Contraindication: Because drugs for astringing are compatible with drugs for removing blood stasis in this prescription, it should not be used to treat the syndrome of "weakness and depletion of the kidney not complicated by blood stasis".

11.18　The Prescription of *Wandai Tang*

Name: Decoction for Morbid Leukorrhea
Source: The book *Fu Qing Zhu Nü Ke*
Ingredients:

Bai Zhu (Rhizoma Atractylodis Macrocephalae) 30 g, *Shan Yao* (Rhizoma Dioscoreae) 30 g, *Che Qian Zi* (Semen Plantaginis) 9 g, *Cang Zhu* (Rhizoma Atractylodis) 9 g, *Bai Shao* (Radix Paeoniae Alba) 15 g, *Ren Shen* (Radix Ginseng) 6 g, *Chen Pi* (Pericarpium Citri Reticulatae) 1.5 g, *Hei Jie Sui* (Spica Schizonepetae) 1.5 g, *Chai Hu* (Radix Bupleuri) 1.8 g, *Gan Cao* (Radix Glycyrrhizae) 3 g.

Explanation

Bai Zhu, Cang Zhu, Ren Shen, Shan Yao and *Gan Cao:* Invigorating *Qi,* strengthening the spleen, removing dampness, arresting leukorrhagia.

Bai Shao, Chen Pi and *Chai Hu:* Nourishing the liver and elevating the clear *Yang.*

Che Qian Zi: Removing pathogenic dampness by inducing diuresis.

· 278 ·

Hei Jie Sui: Dispelling pathogenic wind—dampness to cure morbid leukorrhea.

Effect: Tonifying the middle—*Jiao* to strengthen the spleen, removing dampness to arrest leukorrhagia

Indications: Syndrome due to deficiency of the spleen, depression of the liver—*Qi* and dampness flowing downward, marked by clear odorless whitish or light—yellowish leukorrhea, puffy and pale complexion, lassitude, loose stools, pale tongue with whitish coating, slow or soft weak pulse; including leukorrhagia with the above symptoms caused by chronic inflammation of the reproductive system.

Administration: Decocted in water for oral dose to be taken twice.

Case Study: 100 cases of leukorrhagia were clinically treated with *Wandai Tang* plus:

Nü Zhen Zi (Fructus Ligustri Lucidi) 9 g.

All the cases were remarkably improved and follow—up didn't find out any relapse.

Clinical experience found out that amenorrhea and irregular menstruation as well as leukorrhagia might be treated with *Wandai Tang* plus:

He Huan Pi (Cortex Albiziae), *Nü Zhen Zi* (Fructus Ligustri Lucidi), *Dang Gui*(Radix Angelicae Sinensis), *Huang Bai* (Cortex Phellodendri), *Hei Da Dou* (Semen Sojae Nigrum).

12　Prescriptions for Regulating the Flow of Qi

12.1　Prescriptions for Regulating the Flow of Qi

Prescriptions mainly consisting of drugs for regulating Qi, having the effect of promoting the circulation, and checking the upward adverse flow of Qi, and being suitable for the syndrome of stagnation, or adverse flow, of Qi are all known as "prescription for regulating the flow of Qi". As the commander of all the activities of the body, Qi flows throughout the body by its ascending, descending, out−going and in−coming movements, thus warming up and tonifying the whole body. Whenever exogenous pathogens attack the body, the descending and ascending movements of Qi will be disturbed, which will result in the syndrome of "stagnation of Qi" or "the upward adverse flow of Qi". The syndrome of stagnation of Qi should be treated with the prescription for promoting the circulation of Qi in order that the stagnation or accumulation of Qi can be eliminated. As for the syndrome of the upward adverse flow of Qi, it should be treated with the prescription for descending Qi in order that the upward adverse flow of Qi can be checked. From the above, we can see that the disorders of Qi are different and the prescriptions used to treat them are also different. Based on this, prescriptions for regulating the flow of Qi are classified as the following two: those for removing stagnancy of Qi and those for checking the upward adverse flow of *Qi*.

Most drugs with the action of regulating the flow of *Qi* are aromatic, pungent and dry in nature. They tend to impair body fluid and exhaust *Qi*. Therefore, they should be used in adequate amount and for proper duration. Overdose of them should be avoided and they should not be administered any longer once their effectiveness appear. When they are used to treat the old, the debilitated, the pregnant or the patients suffering from metrorrhagia, metrostaxis or epistaxis, great caution is needed.

12.2 Prescriptions for Removing Stagnancy of *Qi*

Prescriptions of this kind are mainly made up of drugs with the action of promoting the flow of *Qi* and drugs of relieving the depressed liver. They are suitable for such syndromes due to stagnation of *Qi* as gastrointestinal distention with eructation and regurgitation of sour fluid, distending pain in the chest and hypochondria, pain due to hernia, irregular menstruation and dysmenorrhea. Drugs such as

Chen Pi (Pericarpium Citri Reticulatae), *Hou Po* (Cortex Megnoliae Officinalis), *Mu Xiang* (Radix Aucklandiae), *Zhi Shi* (Fructus Aurantii Immaturus), *Chuan Lian Zi* (Fructus Toosendan), *Wu Yao* (Radix Linderae), *Xiang Fu* (Rhizoma Cyperi), *Xiao Hui Xiang* (Fructus Foeniculi), *Ju He* (Semen Citri Reticulatae), are usually used in these prescriptions, whose representatives are *Yueju Wan, Jinlingzi San, Banxia Houpo Tang, Zhi shi, Xiebai Guizhi Tang, Juhe Wan, Tiantai Wuyao San, Nuangan Jian* and *Houpo Wenzhong Tang*.

12.3 The Prescription of *Yueju Wan*

Name: Pill for Relieving Stagnancy

Source: The book *Dan Xi Xin Fa*

Ingredients (in the same amount):

Cang Zhu (Rhizoma Atractylodis), *Xiang Fu* (Rhizoma Cyperi), *Chuan Xiong* (Rhizoma Chuanxiong), *Shen Qu* (Massa Medicata Fermentata), *Zhi Zi* (Fructus Gardeniae).

Explanation:

Xiang Fu: The principal drug, promoting the circulation of *Qi* to treat stagnation of *Qi*.

Chuan Xiong: Activating the flow of blood to treat blood stasis.

Zhi Zi: Clearing away heat and fire to treat stagnation of fire.

Cang Zhu: Drying dampness and promoting the transporting function of the spleen to treat accumulation of dampness.

Shen Qu: Promoting digestion and removing stagnated food to treat indigestion.

Effect: Promoting the circulation of *Qi* and removing stagnancy of *Qi* .

Indications: Syndrome due to stagnancy of *Qi,* marked by fullness distention in the chest and abdomen, eructation with foul odor, regurgitation of sour fluid, nausea, vomiting, indigestion, including such diseases with the above symptoms as chronic gastritis, gastroneurosis, gastroduodenal ulcer, hepatitis, cholicystitis and intercostal neuralgia, etc.

Administration: All the ingredients are ground into fine powder. The powder is made in to pills with water. 6−9 g of the pills is taken each time, twice daily. Or the ingredients are adequately reduced according to the original proportions and decocted in water for the decoction to be taken orally.

Case Study: Modified *Yueju Wan* was clinically employed to treat 1 case of volvulus of stomach marked by gastrointestinal fullness and distention, vague pain, nausea, loss of appetite, and loose stools. 10 doses taken, all the symptoms vanished and the volvulus was corrected as shown in barium meal examination.

4 cases of psychosis diagnosed as a syndrome due to stagnation of *Qi* were also successfully treated with modified *Yueju Wan*.

12.4 The Prescription of *Jinlingzi San*

Name: Sichuan Chinaberry Powder
Source: The book *Su Wen Bing Ji Qi Yi Bao Ming Ji*
Ingredients:

Jin Ling Zi (Fructus Meliae Toosendan) 30 g, *Yan Hu Suo* (Rhizoma Corydalis) 30 g.

Explanation:

Jin Ling Zi: The principal drug, soothing the liver and regulating the circulation of *Qi,* purging the liver of pathogenic fire.

Yan Hu Suo: Promoting the flow of both *Qi* and blood.

Effect: Promoting the circulation of *Qi* to soothe the liver, activating the flow of blood to arrest pain.

Indications: Syndrome of intense heat due to stagnation of the liver—*Qi,* marked by intermittent pain in the chest, abdomen and hypochondriac region, bitter taste in the mouth, reddened tongue with yellowish coating, and taut rapid pulse; including such diseases with the above symptoms as gastroduodenal ulcer, chronic gastritis, and virus hepatitis.

Administration: The two ingredients are ground into fine powder. 9 g of the powder is taken each time, twice daily. Or the ingredients are decocted in water for oral dose with their amounts properly modified.

Case Study: Modified *Jinlingzi San* was clinically used to treat 15 cases of stomachache due to stagnation of pathogenic fire, indigestion caused by over—intake of liquor and meat, or liver—Qi attacking the stomach. The pain was relieved by 1 dose. All the cases were cured, each taking 2 doses.

12.5 The Prescription of *Banxia Houpo Tang*

Name: Decoction of Pinellia and Magnolia Bark
Source: The book *Jin Gui Yao Lue*
Ingredients:
Ban Xia (Rhizoma Pinelliae) 12 g, *Fu Ling* (Poria) 12 g, *Hou Po* (Cortex Magnoliae Officinalis) 9 g, *Sheng Jiang* (Rhizoma Zingiberis Recens) 9 g, *Su Ye* (Folium Perillae) 6 g.
Explanation:
Ban Xia: The principal drug, dissolving phlegm and dispersing accumulation of pathogens, keeping the adverse *Qi* flowing downward and regulating the stomach.

Hou Po: Inducing *Qi* to flow downward and relieving distention.

Fu Ling: Being sweet and tasteless in flavor, inducing diuresis.

Sheng Jiang: Being pungent in taste and warm in nature, dispersing accumulation of pathogens, regulating the stomach to arrest vomiting.

Su Ye: Being aromatic in taste, promoting the flow of *Qi,* regulating the lung, soothing the liver.

Effect: Promoting the circulation of *Qi* and dispersing accumulation of pathogens, making the adverse *Qi* flow downward to dissolve phlegm.

Indications: Syndrome of globus hystericus marked by a sensation of something stuck in the throat which is difficult to vomit out or swallow, fullness in the chest and hypochondrium, whitish moist tongue coating, and taut slow pulse; including such diseases with the above symptoms as hysteria, gastroneurosis, esophageal spasm and chronic pharyngitis.

Administration: Decocted in water for oral dose to be taken twice.

Case Study: 19 cases of globus hystericus whose courses were different from half a day to half a year were successfully treated with *Banxia Houpo Tang*.

Modified *Banxia Houpo Tang* was used to treat 2 cases of chronic pharyngitis with a course of 2 years. Either of them was cured by taking 20 or more doses.

12.6 The Prescription of *Zhishi Xiebai Guizhi Tang*

Name: Decoction of Immature Bitter Orange, Macrostem Onion and Cinnamon Twigs

Source: The book *Jin Gui Yao Lue*

Ingredients:

Zhi Shi (Fructus Aurantii Immaturus) 12 g, *Hou Po* (Cortex Magnoliae Officinalis) 12 g, *Gua Lou* (Fructus Trichosanthis) 12 g, *Xie Bai* (Bulbus Allii Macrostemi) 9 g, *Gui Zhi* (Ramulus

Cinnamomi) 6 g.

Explanation:

Zhi Shi: Inducing downward flow of *Qi* to disperse stagnation of *Qi,* relieving fullness and distention.

Xie Bai: Being pungent in taste and warm in nature, promoting the circulation of *Yang—Qi,* relieving stuffiness in the chest and dissolving masses.

Gui Zhi: Reinforcing *Yang—Qi* and promoting its circulation to dispel pathogenic cold, keeping upward adverse flow of *Qi* going downward.

Gua Lou: Removing phlegm and dissolving masses.

Hou Po: Promoting the downward flow of *Qi* to relieve fullness.

Effect: Promoting the circulation of *Yang—Qi* and resolving masses, removing phlegm and inducing *Qi* to flow downward.

Indications: Syndrome due to obstruction of *Qi* in the chest, marked by choking pain in the chest which even refers to the back, dyspnea, cough, shortness of breath, whitish greasy tongue coating, and deep taut or tense pulse; including such diseases with the above symptoms as coronary heart disease, angina pectoris, intercostal neuralgia and costal chondritis.

Administration: Decocted in water for oral dose to be taken twice.

Case Study: *Zhishi Xiebai Guizhi Tang* in combination with *Gualou Xiebai Baiju Tang* and modified *Gualou Xiebai Banxia Tang* was clinically used to cases of non—supurative costochondritis. The symptoms were relieved or removed in a short time in most cases after the decoction was taken, relapse was seldom.

12.7 The Prescription of *Juhe Wan*

Name: Tangerine Seed Pill

Source: The book *Ji Sheng Fang*

Ingredients:

Ju He (Semen Citri Reticulatae) 30 g, *Hai Zao* (Sargassum) 30 g, *Kun Bu* (Thallus Echloniae) 30 g, *Hai Dai* (Thallus Laminariae) 30 g, *Chuan Lian Zi* (Fructus Toosendan). 30 g, *Tao Ren* (Semen Persicae) 30 g, *Hou Po* (Cortex Magnoliae Officinalis) 15 g, *Mu Tong* (Caulis Aristolochiae Manshuriensis) 15 g, *Zhi Shi* (Fructus Aurantii Immaturus) 15 g, *Yan Hu Suo* (Rhizoma Corydalis) 15 g, *Gui Xin* (Lignum Cinnamomi) 15 g, *Mu Xiang* (Radix Aucklandiae) 15 g.

Explanation:

Ju He: The principal drug, promoting the circulation of *Qi* to treat hernia.

Mu Xiang and *Chuan Lian Zi:* Promoting the flow of *Qi* to relieve pain.

Tao Ren and *Yan Hu Suo:* Activating the circulation of blood to remove obstruction in the channels.

Gui Xin: Warming up the liver and kidney to dispel pathogenic cold.

Zhi Shi and *Hou Po:* Drastically promoting the circulation of *Qi* to eliminate stagnancy of *Qi*.

Mu Tong: Promoting the flow of blood through the vessels and getting rid of dampness.

Hai Zao, Kun Bu and *Hai Dai:* Softening and dispersing hard masses.

Effect: Promoting the flow of *Qi* to relieve pain, softening and dispersing hard masses.

Indications: Hernia due to cold—damp pathogen, marked by swollen and distending scrotum with bearing—down sensation, or scrotum as hard as stone, or pain of the testicle radiating to the umbilical or abdominal region, pale tongue with whitish coating, and deep taut pulse; including such diseases with the above symptoms as hydrocele testis, testitis and epididymitis.

Administration: All the ingredients are ground into powder and made with liquor into pills. 9 g of the pills is taken each time,twice daily. Or the ingredients are decocted in water for oral dose, their amounts being properly modified according to the original proportions.

Case Study: Cases of testical dropsy were clinically treated with modified *Juhe Wan* with noticeable results. In general, the dropsy was relieved after 6 doses were taken. Further taking of the pills brought about complete recovery, the doses taken averaging 20—28.

12.8　The Prescription of *Tiantai Wuyao San*

Name: Linderae Powder

Source: The book *Yi Xue Fa Ming*

Ingredients:

Wu Yao (Radix Linderae) 12 g, *Chuan Lian Zi* (Fructus Toosendan) 12 g, *Gao Liang Jiang* (Rhizoma Alpiniae Officinarum) 9 g, *Bing Lang* (Semen Arecae) 9 g, *Mu Xiang* (Radix Aucklandiae) 6 g, *Xiao Hui Xiang* (Fructus Foeniculi) 6 g, *Qing Pi* (Pericarpium Citri Reticulatae Viride) 6 g, *Ba Dou* (Semen Crotonis) 70 particles.

Explanation:

Wu Yao: The principal drug, promoting the circulation of *Qi* to soothe the liver, dispersing pathogenic cold to alleviate pain.

Mu Xiang, Xiao Hui Xiang, Qing Pi and *Gao Liang Jiang:* Promoting the flow of *Qi* and resolving masses, dispelling pathogenic cold and dampness.

Bing Lang: Acting directely on the lower—*Jiao* to promote the circulation of *Qi,* thus removing stagnancy and resolving masses.

Chuan Lian Zi and *Ba Dou:* Being stir—fried together so as to restrain the cold nature, and enhance the potency of promoting the flow of *Qi* to eliminate stagnancy, of *Chuan Lian Zi.*

Effect: Promoting the flow of *Qi* to soothe the liver, expelling pathogenic cold to relieve pain.

Indications: *Shan* syndrome of cold—type due to stagnation of *Qi,* marked by hernia of the small intestines, pain in the lower abdomen referring to the testis, pale tongue with whitish coating, and deep slow or taut pulse; including such diseases with the above symtoms as external abdominal hernia, dysmenorrhea, and disorder of the testis.

Administration: *Chuan Lian Zi* and *Ba Dou* are parched until they look dark, and *Ba Dou* is removed to get *Chuan Lian Zi.* All the ingredients except *Ba Dou* are decocted in water for the decoction. The decoction is taken twice daily with adequate amount of millet wine.

Case Study: Modified *Tiantai Wuyao San* was clinically adopted to treat the syndrome of stagnation of *Qi* due to accumulation of cold and transverse invasion of the depressed liver—*Qi,* marked by hernia, abdominal pain, stomachache, pain due to ascaris and dysmenorrhea with satisfactory results.

12.9   The Prescription of *Nuangan Jian*

Name: Decoction for Warming the Liver Channel

Source: The book *Jing Yue Quan Shu*

Ingredients:

Dang Gui (Radix Angelicae Sinensis) 6–9 g, *Rou Gui* (Cortex Cinnamomi) 3–6 g, *Gou Qi* (Fructus Lycii) 9 g, *Xiao Hui Xiang* (Fructus Foeniculi) 6 g, *Wu Yao* (Radix Linderae) 6 g, *Fu Ling* (Poria) 6 g, *Chen Xiang* (Lignum Aquilariae Resinatum) 3 g, *Sheng Jiang* (Rhizoma Zingiberis Recens)3 pieces.

Explanation:

Dang Gui and *Gou Qi:* Warming and reinforcing the liver and kidney.

Rou Gui and *Xiao Hui Xiang:* Warming up the kidney and dispelling pathogenic cold.

Wu Yao and *Chen Xiang:* Regulating the flow of *Qi* to relieve pain.

Fu Ling: Inducing diuresis to strengthen the spleen.

Sheng Jiang: Expelling pathogenic cold and regulating the function of the stomach.

Effect: Warming up the liver and kidney, promoting the circulation of *Qi* to relieve pain.

Indications: Syndrome due to *Yin*–cold of the liver and kidney, marked by pain in the lower abdomen, hernia, pale tongue with whitish coating, and deep taut pulse; including external abdominal hernia, abdominal pain and sterility with the above symptoms.

Administration: Decocted in water for oral dose to be taken twice.

Case Study: Modified *Nuangan Jian* was clinically used to treat 1 case of 5–year sterility with the symptoms of vague pain in the lower abdomen, cold and damp testis which became retracted in the cold. The lab sperm count was 30,000,000 / ml, of which 50% were abnormal and only 30% kept alive within 2 hours. Aftre 10 doses were taken, the symptoms were relieved. 1 month later, the sperm count reached 50,000,000 / ml, of which only 20% were abnormal and over 60% kept alive within 2 hours, and all the symptoms were removed. His wife got pregnant at last.

Modified *Nuangan Jian* was also used to treat 1 case of penis–retraction manifested by pevis retracting with severe pain, disappearance of the penis in appearance, and lower abdominal pain referring to the scrotum. The symptoms were relieved after 3 doses were taken and removed after 15 doses.

12.10   The Prescription of *Houpo Wenzhong Tang*

Name: Magnolia Decoction for Warming the Middle–*Jiao*
Source: The book *Nei Wai Shang Bian Huo Lun*
Ingredients:

Hou Po (Cortex Magnoliae Officinalis) 30 g, *Chen Pi* (Pericarpium Citri Reticulatae) 30 g, *Fu Ling* (Poria) 15 g, *Cao Kou Ren* (Semen Alpiniae Katsumadai) 15 g, *Mu Xiang* (Radix Aucklandiae) 15 g, *Gan Cao* (Radix Glycyrrhizae) 15 g, *Gan Jiang* (Rhizoma Zingiberis) 2 g.

Explanation:

Hou Po: The principal drug, promoting the flow of *Qi* to subdue distention, drying dampness and removing fullness.

Cao Kou Ren: Warming up the middle–*Jiao* to expel

pathogenic cold, drying dampness to reduce phlegm.

Chen Pi and *Mu Xiang:* Promoting the circulation of *Qi* to benefit the middle—*Jiao.*

Gan Jiang: Warming the spleen and stomach and dispersing pathogenic cold.

Fu Ling and *Gan Cao:* Inducing diuresis, strengthening the spleen and regulating the function of the middle—*Jiao.*

Effect: Warming up the middle—*Jiao* to promote the circulation of *Qi,* drying dampness and removing fullness.

Indications: Syndrome of the spleen impaired by cold—dampness, marked by distention or pain in the epigastric region and abdomen, loss of appetite, weary limbs, pale tongue with whitish greasy coating, and deep slow pulse; including such diseases with the above symptoms as acute and chronic enteritis, gastritis and gastroduodenal ulcer.

Administration: Decocted in water with 3 pieces of *Sheng Jiang* (Rhizoma Zingiberis Recens) added for oral dose to be taken twice. When used, the dosages of the ingredients may be modified according to their original proportions.

12.11 Prescriptions for Checking the Upward Adverse Flow of *Qi*

Prescriptions of this kind are mainly composed of drugs with the action of descending *Qi* and suitable for the syndrome due to the upward adverse flow of the lung—*Qi* and the stomach—*Qi,* marked by cough, dyspnea, vomiting, eructation and hiccup. Drugs such as

Su Zi (Fructus Perillae), *Xing Ren* (Semen Armeniacae Amarum), *Chen Xiang* (Lignum Aquilariae Resinatum), *Xuan Fu*

Hua (Flos Inulae), *Dai Zhe Shi* (Ochra Haematitum), *Chen Pi* (Pericarpium Citri Reticulatae), *Ding Xiang* (Flos Caryophlli), *Shi Di* (Calyx Kaki) are commonly used in these prescriptions, whose representatives are *Suzi Jiangqi Tang, Dingchuan Tang, Xuanfu Daizhe Tang, Jupi Zhuru Tang* and *Dingxiang Shidi San.*

12.12   The Prescription of *Suzi Jiangqi Tang*

Name: Decoction of Perilla Seed for Descending *Qi*

Source: The book *Tai Ping Hui Min He Ji Ju Fang*

Ingredients:

Su Zi (Fructus Perillae) 9 g, *Ban Xia* (Rhizoma Pinelliae) 9 g, *Dang Gui* (Radix Angelicae Sinensis) 6 g, *Hou Po* (Cortex Magnoliae Officinalis) 6 g, *Qian Hu* (Radix Peucedani) 6 g, *Zhi Gan Cao* (Radix Glycyrrhizae Preparata) 6 g, *Rou Gui* (Cortex Cinnamomi) 3 g, *Sheng Jiang* (Rhizoma Zingiberis Recens) 2 pieces, *Da Zao* (Fructus Jujubae) 1 dates, *Su Ye* (Folium Perillae) 2 g.

Explanation:

Su Zi: The principal drug, descending *Qi*, dissolving phlegm, arresting cough and relieving dyspnea.

Ban Xia, Hou Po and *Qian Hu:* Arresting cough and relieving dyspnea.

Rou Gui: Warming the kidney to enhance its function of receiving air.

Dang Gui: Nourishing blood, tonifying the liver, relieving cough and shortness of breath.

Sheng Jiang and *Su Ye:* Dispelling pathogenic cold and facilitating the flow of the lung—*Qi*.

Gan Cao and *Da Zao;* Regulating the function of the

middle—*Jiao,* tempering the actions of all the other ingredients.

Effect: Checking the upward adverse flow of the lung—*Qi* to relieve dyspnea, removing phlegm and arresting cough.

Indications: Syndrome due to accumulation of phlegm as well as excessiveness in the upper and insufficiency in the lower, marked by dyspneic cough, shortness of breath, fullness and distention in the chest and epigastric region, or lumbago and weakness of the feet,or swelling of the limbs, pale tongue with whitish slippery coating, and deep pulse; including such diseases with the above symptoms as bronchial asthma, chronic bronchitis, pulmonary emphysema, and pulmonary heart disease.

Administration: Decocted in water for oral dose to be taken twice.

Case Study: 10 cases of bronchial asthma were clinically treated with *Suzi Jiangqi Tang* plus:

Chen Xiang (Lignum Aquilariae Resinatum)

Bai Guo (Semen Ginkgo)

Xing Ren (Semen Armeniacae Amarum)

Wu Wei Zi (Fructus Schisandrae).

5 cases were remarkedly improved and the rest improved.

Cases of bronchiectasis were also treated with *Suzi Jiangqi Tang* minus:

Rou Gui (Cortex Cinnamomi), *Sheng Jiang* (Rhizoma Zingiberis Recens).

Dang Gui (Radix Angelicae Sinensis) but plus:

Ting Li Zi (Semen Lepidii seu Descurainiae), *Huang Qin* (Radix Scutellariae), *Da Huang* (Radix et Rhizoma Rhei).

After 3 doses were taken, the hemoptysis was stopped and the cough relieved. Then the treatment was continued with *Pipa*

Gao and the cases were cured at last.

12.13   The Prescription of *Dingchuan Tang*

Name: Asthma—relieving Decoction
Source: The book *She Sheng Zhong Miao Fang*
Ingredients:

Bai Guo (Semen Ginkgo) 9 g, *Ma Huang* (Herba Ephedrae) 9 g, *Kuan Dong Hua* (Flos Farfarae) 9 g, *Xing Ren* (Semen Armeniacae Amarum) 9 g, *Sang Bai Pi* (Cortex Mori) 9 g, *Ban Xia* (Rhizoma Pinelliae) 9 g, *Su Zi* (Fructus Perillae) 6 g, *Huang Qin* (Radix Scutellariae) 6 g, *Gan Cao* (Radix Glycyrrhizae) 3 g.

Explanation:

Ma Huang: One of the principal drugs, facilitating the flow of the lung—*Qi* to dispel pathogenic factors and relieve asthma.

Bai Guo: The other principal drug, astringing the lung to stop asthma and remove phlegm.

Su Zi, Xing Ren, Ban Xia and *Kuan Dong Hua:* Descending the lung—*Qi* to alleviate asthma, relieve cough and eliminate phlegm.

Sang Bai Pi and *Huang Qin:* Clearing away the lung—heat to relieve cough and asthma.

Gan Cao: Tempering the actions of all the other ingredients.

Effect: Facilitating the flow of the lung—*Qi* to descend its upward flow, eliminating phlegm and relieving asthma.

Indications: Syndrome due to wind—cold in the exterior and retention of phlegm—heat in the interior, marked by massive viscid yellowish sputum, dyspnea, asthma, cough, pale tongue with yellowish greasy coating, and slippery rapid pulse; including such diseases with the above symptoms as chronic bronchitis and bronchial asthma.

Administration: Decocted in water for oral dose to be taken twice.

Case Study: Modified *Dingchuan Tang* was clinically used to treat 30 cases of infantile acute bronchiolitis. The wheeze disappeared in all the cases within 3 days, the dyspnea was relieved remarkedly in 28 cases, and all the cases were cured. The time for the cases in this group to stay in the hospital averaged 4 days, shorter than the cases in the group treated with mere western medicines who stayed for 7 days on the average.

100 cases of chronic asthmatic bronchitis were also treated with *Dingchuan Tang*. Remarkable improvement was obtained in 83% of the cases with the total effective rate being 97%.

12.14 The Prescription of *Simo Tang*

Name: Decoction of Four Powdered Drugs

Source: The book *Ji Sheng Fang*

Ingredients:

Ren Shen (Radix Ginseng) 3 g, *Chen Xiang* (Lignum Aquilariae Resinatum) 3 g, *Bing Lang* (Semen Arecae) 9 g, *Tian Tai Wu Yao* (Radix Linderae) 9 g.

Explanation:

Wu Yao: Promoting the flow of *Qi* and soothing the liver so as to remove stagnancy.

Chen Xiang: Checking upward adverse flow of the lung—*Qi* to relieve asthma.

Bing Lang: Promoting the flow of *Qi* and removing stagnated food to alleviate fullness.

Ren Shen: Invigorating *Qi* and supporting the body resistance.

Effect: Promoting the flow of *Qi* and checking its upward flow, facilitating the flow of *Qi* throughout the chest and removing stagnancy.

Indications: Syndrome due to depression of the liver—*Qi*, marked by restlessness in the chest, dyspnea, fullness in the epigastric region, poor appetite, pale tongue with whitish coating, and deep taut pulse; including such diseases with the above symptoms as hepatitis, cholecystitis, periarthritis of shoulder and mastitis.

Administration: Decocted in water for oral dose to be taken twice.

Case Study: 1 case of mastitis due to retention of milk, marked by distending pain of the breast with egg—like hard masses which was complicated by dry cough, chest pain, dysphoria, irritability, bitter taste in the mouth, anorexia, and taut slippery pulse, was clinically treated with *Simo Tang* minus:

Ren Shen (Radix Ginseng).

Bing Lang (Semen Arecae) but plus:

Qing Pi (Pericarpium Citri Reticulatae Viride), *Chi Shao* (Radix Paeoniae Rubra), *Gong Ying* (Herba Taraxaci), *Sha Shen* (Radix Adenophorae strictae), *Bai Hua She Cao* (Herba Oldenlandiae Diffusae).

The case was cured by taking 6 doses of the decoction.

12.15   The Prescription of *Xuanfu Daizhe Tang*

Name: Decoction of Inula and Hematitum

Source: The book *Shang Han Lun*

Ingredients:

Xuan Fu Hua (Flos Inulae) 9 g, *Dai Zhe Shi* (Hematitum) 9 g, *Ban Xia* (Rhizoma Pinelliae) 9 g, *Ren Shen* (Radix Ginseng) 6 g, *Gan Cao* (Radix Glycyrrhizae Praeparata) 6 g, *Sheng Jiang* (Rhizoma Zingiberis Recens) 10 g, *Da Zao* (Fructus Jujubae) 12 dates.

Explanation:

Xuan Fu Hua: The principal drug, descending the adverse flow of Qi to remove phlegm and stop hiccup.

Dai Zhe Shi: Checking the adverse flow of Qi by its heavy nature.

Ren Shen: Invigorating Qi and strengthening the body resistance.

Zhi Gan Cao: Warming and tonifying the Qi of the middle—Jiao.

Da Zao: Nourishing the stomach and reinforcing the spleen.

Sheng Jiang: Warming up the stomach to dissolve phlegm, dispelling pathogenic cold to arrest vomiting.

Ban Xia: Eliminating phlegm, removing masses, keep the upward adverse flow of Qi going downward and regulating the function of the stomach.

Effect: Descending the upward adverse flow of Qi and dissolving phlegm, invigorating Qi and regulating the function of the stomach.

Indications: Syndrome due to weakness of the stomach—Qi and retention of phlegm in the interior, marked by fullness and rigidity in the epigastric region, incessive belching, whitish slippery tongue coating, and taut weak pulse; including such diseases with the above symptoms as gastrointestinal neurosis, gastric dilatation, incomplete pylorochesis and peptic ulcer.

Administration: Decocted in water for oral dose to be taken twice.

Case Study:

Xuanfu Daizhe Tang was clinically employed to treat 50 cases of dizziness and vomiting, which derived from gastritis or gastric ulcer in 6 cases, from neurosis in 11 cases, from hypertention in 1 case, from Meniere's disease in 1 case, from hysteria in 1 case, and from sequel of meningitis in 1 case. The treatment result was that the dizziness and vomiting were removed in 34 cases, relieved in 14 cases, remained the same in 2 cases.

12.16　The Prescription of *Jupi Zhuru Tang*

Name: Tangerine Peel and Bamboo Shavings Decoction
Source: The book *Jin Gui Yao Lue*
Ingredients:

Ju Pi (Pericarpium Citri Reticulatae) 12 g, *Zhu Ru* (Caulis Bambusae in Taeniam) 12 g, *Ren Shen* (Radix Ginseng) 3 g, *Sheng Jiang* (Rhizoma Zingiberis Recens) 9 g, *Gan Cao* (Radix Glycyrrhizae) 6 g, *Da Zao* (Fructus Jujubae) 5 dates.

Explanation:

Ju Pi: The principal drug, regulating the flow of *Qi* and the function of the stomach, checking upward adverse flow of *Qi* to arrest vomiting.

Zhu Ru: The other principal drug, clearing heat from the stomach to arrest vomiting.

Ren Shen: Invigorating *Qi* to. Streng then the body resistance.

Sheng Jiang: Regulating the stomach to arrest vomiting.

Gan Cao and *Da Zao:* Invigorating *Qi* to regulate the stomach, tempering the actions of all the other ingredients.

Effect: Checking upward adverse flow of *Qi* to arrest vomiting, invigorating *Qi* and clearing away pathogenic heat.

Indications: Syndrome of pathogenic heat due to deficiency of the stomach and upward adverse flow of the stomach—*Qi*, marked by hiccup or retching, reddened tongue with thin yellowish coating, and weak rapid pulse; including such diseases with the above symptoms as vomiting of pregnancy, imcomplete pylorochesis and postoperative belching.

Administration: Decocted in water for oral dose to be taken twice.

Case Study: Modified *Jupi Zhuru Tang* was clinically used to treat 1 case of obstinate hiccup with a history of more than 10 years, marked by frequent hiccup, eructation, nausea, intermittent frothy vomiting, bad sleep, anorexia, constipation, and deep-colored urine. 6 doses cured the case, 4-month follow-up found no relapse.

12.17   The Prescription of *Dingxiang Shidi Tang*

Name: Cloves and Kaki Calyx Decoction

Source: The book *Zheng Yin Mai Zhi*

Ingredients:

Ding Xiang (Flos Caryophylli) 6 g, *Sheng Jiang* (Rhizoma Zingiberis Recens) 6 g, *Shi Di* (Calyx Kaki) 9 g, *Ren Shen* (Radix Ginseng) 3 g.

Explanation:

Ding Xiang: Warming the stomach, dispelling pathogenic cold, checking the upward adverse flow of *Qi,* and arresting hiccup.

Shi Di: Checking the upward adverse flow of *Qi,* arresting hiccup.

Ren Shen: Invigorating *Qi,* strengthening the body resistance.

Sheng Jiang: Warming the stomach, checking the upward adverse flow of *Qi.*

Effect: Warming the stomach, invigorating *Qi,* checking the upward adverse flow of *Qi,* arresting hiccup.

Indications: Syndrome due to deficiency—cold of the stomach—*Qi,* marked by incessant hiccup, fullness in the chest, and slow pulse; including such diseases with the above symptoms as phrenospasm and nervous hiccup.

Administration: Decocted in water for oral dose to be taken twice.

Case Study: *Dingxiang Shidi Tang* was clinically used to treat 2 cases of obstinate hiccup with both of them cured.

1 case of cardiospasm was clinically treated with *Dingxiang Shidi San* in combination with *Xuanfu Daizhe Tang* and the modification of *Gualou Xiebai Tang.*1 month of treatment cured the case.

13 Prescriptions for Treating Blood Disorders

13.1 Prescriptions for Treating Blood Disorders

All the prescriptions which have the following three characteristics are known as "prescription for treating blood disorders": 1, being composed of drugs with the action of regulating blood; 2, having the effect of promoting blood circulation, tonifying blood or stopping bleeding; 3, being used to treat the syndrome of blood stasis or hemorrhage. Under normal physiological condition, blood keeps circulating through the vessels, tonifying the five—*Zang* and six—*Fu* organs and nourishing the limbs, bones and skeleton of the body. Inhibited blood circulation or blood flow out of the vessels due to one cause or another will result in blood stasis or hemorrhage. According to these two major blood disorders, prescriptions of this kind fall into two: those for promoting blood circulation to remove blood stasis and those for stopping bleeding.

13.2 Prescriptions for Promoting Blood Circulation to Remove Blood Stasis

This kind of prescriptions are mainly made up of drugs with the action of activating the flow of blood to eliminate blood stasis. They are suitable for the syndrome of blood retention or stasis, including the following disorders: swelling and pain due to blood stasis, blood stasis and swelling due to trauma, hemiparalysis due to blood stasis in the channels, pain of various kinds in the chest and abdomen due to blood retention in the interior, amenia, dysmenorrhea, and puerperal lochiostasis. Drugs such as

Chuan Xiong(Rhizoma Chuanxiong), *Tao Ren*(Semen Persicae), *Hong Hua* (Flos Carthami), *Dan Shen*(Radix Salviae Miltiorrhizae), are commonly used in these prescriptions, whose representatives are *Taohe Chengqi Tang*, *Xuefu Zhuyu Tang* and *Fuyuan Huoxue Tang*.

As the name indicates, "prescriptions for promoting blood circulation to remove blood stasis" function in activating the flow of blood and removing blood stasis. Therefore, they tend to result in abortion. When they are prescribed for pregnant women or women who are suffering from the disorder of profuse menstruation, caution should be taken.

13.3 The Prescription of *Taohe Chengqi Tang*

Name: Decoction of Peach Kernel for Activating *Qi*

Source: The book *Shang Han Lun*

Ingredients:

Tao Ren(Semen Persicae)12g, *Da Huang* (Radix et Rhizoma Rhei)12g, *Gui Zhi*(Ramulus Cinnamomi)6g, *Mang Xiao*(Natrii Sulfas)6g, *Gan Cao*(Radix Glycyrrhizae)6g.

Explanation:

Tao Ren: One of the principal drugs, removing blood stasis.

Da Huang: The other principal drug, dispersing blood stasis and pathogenic heat.

Gui Zhi: Promoting the circulation of blood and assisting

Tao Ren in removing blood stasis.

Mang Xiao: Clearing away heat to resolve masses, assisting *Da Huang* in removing blood stasis and dispersing heat.

Gan Cao: Invigorating *Qi* to regulate the middle—*Jiao,* tempering the actions of all the other ingredients.

Effect:Promoting the flow of blood to remove blood stasis Indications:Syndrome due to blood retention in the lower—*Jiao,* marked by rigidity and masses in the lower abdomen, frequent free urination, delirium, restlessness, thirst, fever during night followed by irritability, dark tongue, and deep solid or unsmooth pulse; including such diseases with the above symptoms as pelvic inflammation, adnexitis and intestinal obstruction.

Administration: Decocted in water for oral dose to be taken twice Case Study: *Taohe Chengqi Tang* was clinically used to treat 22 cases of acute necrotic enteritis, among whom 19 were cured, 2 died, 1 was transferred to surgery for treatment.

Taohe Chengqi Tang plus:

Huang Qin(Radix Scutellariae), *Huang Lian*(Rhizoma Coptidis), *Mu Xiang*(Radix Aucklandiae), *Ma Chi Xian*(Herba Portulacae), was prescribed to treat 26 cases of fulminating dysentery, among whom 22 were cured, 2 died, 2 were unimproved.

13.4 The Prescription of *Xuefu Zhuyu Tang*

Name: Decoction for Removing Blood Stasis in the Chest Source: The book *Yi Lin Gai Cuo*

Ingredients:

Tao Ren (Semen Persicae)12g, *Hong Hua* (Flos Carthami)9g, *Dang Gui* (Radix Angelicae Sinensis)9g, *Sheng Di* (Radix Rehmanniae)9g, *Niu Xi* (Radix Achyranthis Bidentatae)9g, *Chi*

Shao (Radix Paeoniae Rubra)6g, *Zhi Qiao*(Fructus Aurantii)6g, *Chuan Xiong* (Rhizoma Chuanxiong)5g, *Jie Geng*(Radix Platycodi)5g, *Chai Hu* (Radix Bupleuri)3g, *Gan Cao*(Radix Glycyrrhizae)3g.

Explanation:

Tao Ren, Hong Hua, Chi Shao, Chuan Xiong and *Dang Gui:* Promoting the circulation of blood to remove blood stasis.

Niu Xi: Eliminating blood stasis to activate blood circulation, inducing blood to go downward.

Chai Hu: Soothing the liver and regulating the circulation of *Qi.*

Jie Geng and *Zhi Qiao:* Promoting the flow of *Qi* throughout the chest.

Sheng Di: Dispelling heat from blood, nourishing blood and moistening dryness.

Gan Cao: Tempering the actions of all the other ingredients.

Effect: Promoting the circulation of blood to remove blood stasis, activating the flow of *Qi* to relieve pain.

Indications: Syndrome due to *Qi* stagnation and blood stasis, marked by prolonged prickle fixative headache, restlessness, irritability, high fever starting in the evening, or prolonged hiccup, palpitation, deep red tongue, and uneven or taut tight pulse; including such diseases with the above symptoms as coronary heart disease, hypertension, neurosis and sequel due to concussion of brain.

Administration: Decocted in water for oral dose to be taken twice Case Study: *Xuefu Zhuyu Tang* plus *Gao Ben* (Rhizoma et Radix Ligustici) was clinically prescribed to treat 31 cases of hypertension manifested as headache, dizziness, congestion of eyelids, etc. All the cases were cured. In general, a case would have his / her symptoms and signs abated after taking 2–5 doses. 2–3 times of follow–up found no relapse.

Xuefu Zhuyu Tang was used to treat 22 cases of acute diseminated intravascular coagulation, bleeding existed in 19 cases, shock in 16. The result was that 16 cases were cured, 1 improved, 4 unimproved, 1 died.

13.5 The Prescription of *Fuyuan Huoxue Tang*

Name: Decoction for Recovery and Activating Blood Circulation

Source: The book *Yi Lin Gai Cuo*

Ingredients:

Da Huang (Radix et Rhizoma Rhei)30g, *Chai Hu* (Radix Bupleuri)15g, *Gua Lou Gen* (Radix Trichosanthis)9g, *Dang Gui* (Radix Angelicae Sinensis)9g, *Tao Ren* (Semen Persicae)9g, *Hong Hua* (Flos Carthami)6g, *Chuan Shan Jia* (Squama Manitis)6g, *Gan Cao* (Radix Glycyrrhizae)6g.

Explanation:

Da Huang: One of the principal drugs in larger dosage, clearing away blood retention and stasis.

Chai Hu: The other principal drug. soothing the liver and regulating the circulation of *Qi*.

Dang Gui, Tao Ren and *Hong Hua:* Activating blood flow to remove blood stasis, subduing swelling and relieving pain.

Chuan Shan Jia: Removing blood stasis in the channels.

Gua Lou Gen: Removing blood stasis and lumps, clearing away heat and moistening dryness.

Gan Cao: Relieving spasm and pain, tempering the actions of all the other ingredients.

Effect: Promoting the circulation of blood to remove blood stasis, soothing the liver and eliminating obstruction in the channels.

Indications: Traumatic stasis of blood, marked by blood stasis retained under the hypochondrium with severe pain due to traumatic injury, deep red tongue and taut uneven pulse; including such diseases with the above symptoms as intercostal neuralgia, costal chondritis and injury of soft tissues.

Administration: Decocted in water for oral dose to be taken twice.

Case Study: *Fuyuan Huoxue Tang* was clinically used to treat 9 cases of costal chondritis with a history of 1−6 weeks. Any of the cases had his / her swelling and pain remarkedly relieved by taking 1−2 doses and had his / her disorder basically cured by taking 5−7 doses.

Fuyuan Huoxue Tang was used to treat several hundred cases of traumatic injury with better curative effects obtained.

13.6   The Prescription of *Qili San*

Name: Anti−bruise Powder

Source: The book *Liang Fang Ji Ye*

Ingredients:

Xue Jie (Resina Draconis)30g, *She Xiang* (Moschus)0.4g, *Bing Pian* (Borneolum Syntheticum)0.4g, *Ru Xiang* (Resina Olibani)5g, *Mo Yao* (Myrrha)5g, *Hong Hua* (Flos Carthami)5g, *Zhu Sha* (Cinnabaris)4g, *Er Cha* (Catechu)7.5g.

Explanation:

Xue Jie and *Hong Hua*: Promoting the circulation of blood to remove blood stasis.

Ru Xiang and *Mo Yao:* Eliminating blood stasis, activating the flow of *Qi,* subduing swelling and relieving pain.

She Xiang and *Bing Pian:* Promoting the flow of *Qi* and blood through the channels.

Zhu Sha: Calming the mind.

Er Cha: Removing heat and stopping bleeding.

Effect: Promoting the circulation of blood to disperse blood stasis, relieving pain and stopping bleeding.

Indications: Stasis of blood with swelling and pain due to fractures of tendons and bones, or bleeding due to incised wound; including burn, scald, herpes zoster, coronary heart diseases and myocarditis.

Administration: All the ingredients are ground into fine powder and taken with yellow rice wine or warm boiled water, 0.22—0.15 g each time, twice daily when externally applied on the affected part, proper amout of the powder is mixed with liquor.

Case Study: Modified *Qili San* was clinically used to treat 11 cases of herpes zoster. The pain was generally relieved after 1—2 doses were taken, the maculopapules began to subside after 2—3, the vesicopustules became dry and scabbed after 4—6. All the cases were cured, the treatment course averaging 4.6 days.

Modified *Qili San* was used to treat 100 cases of coronary heart disease, among which 76 were accompanied by angina pectoris, 13 by remote myocardial infarction with angina pectoris, 3 by remote myocardial infarction, 8 by latent coronary pain. The treatment result was that 14 cases were remarkably improved, 49 improved, 24 unimproved, 3 deteriorated.

13.7 The Prescription of *Buyang Huanwu Tang*

Name: Decoction Invigorating *Yang* for Recuperation

Source: The book *Yi Lin Gai Cuo*

Ingredients:

Huang Qi (Radix Astragali)120g, *Dang Gui* (Radix Angelicae Sinensis)6g, *Chi Shao* (Radix Paeoniae Rubra)6g, *Di Long* (Lumbricus)3g, *Chuan Xiong* (Rhizoma Chuanxiong)3g, *Hong Hua* (Flos Carthami)3g, *Tao Ren* (Semen Persicae)3g.

Explanation:

Huang Qi: The principal drug in larger dose, invigorating primordial *Qi* to activate the circulation of blood.

Dang Gui, Chuan Xiong, Chi Shao, Tao Ren, Hong Hua and *Di Long:* Promoting the flow of blood through the channels.

Effect: Invigorating *Qi*, promoting the circulation of blood, removing obstruction in the channels.

Indications: Sequel of apoplexy, marked by hemiparalysis, distortion of the face, dysphasia, salivation due to paralytic lips, flaccidity of the lower limbs, frequent urination or enuresis, whitish tongue coating and slow pulse; including such diseases with the above symptoms as sequel of cerebrovascular accident and sequel of poliomyelitis.

Administration: Decocted in water for oral dose to be taken twice Case Study: *Buyang Huanwu Tang* was clinically used to treat 12 cases of hemiparalysis with satisfactory effects. 5 cases were cured within 7−18 days, 7 within 24−90 days.

Buyang Huanwu Tang was prescribed to treat 100 cases of sciatica with 89 cases cured, 7 remarkedly improved and 2 improved.

13.8   The Prescription of *Shixiao San*

Name: Wonderful Powder for Relieving Blood Stagnation

Source: The book *Tai Ping Hui Min He Ji Ju Fang*

Ingredients (with the same dosage):

Wu Ling Zhi(Faeces Trogopterori), *Pu Huang* (Pollen Typhae).

Explanation: The ingredients complement each other to promote blood circulation, remove blood stasis and relieve pain.

Effect: Activating blood flow to disperse blood stasis, removing obstruction to relieve pain.

Indications: Syndrome due to blood stasis, marked by megalgia in the chest and abdomen, or puerperal lochiorrhea or irregular menstruation, imperative pain in the lower abdomen, deep red tongue and uneven pulse; including such diseases with the above symptoms as angina pectoris and ectopic pregnancy.

Administration: The two ingredients are ground into fine powder and taken with yellow rice wine or vinegar, 6 g each time, twice daily. Their amounts reduced according to their original proportions, they may be decocted in water for oral dose. Vinegar or yellow rice wine used in taking this powder will enhance the drugs'potency of promoting the circulation of blood and relieving pain.

Case Study: *Shixiao San* and *Jiaoai Siwu Tang* were clinically used as the main remedy to treat 18 cases of ectopic pregnancy, among which 16 were old ones, 2 were subacute. Any of the cases took 10−20 doses and they were all cured.

Modified *Shixiao San* was used to treat 46 cases of coronary heart disease. 1 course of treatment involved 1 month. The result was: of the 44 cases with angina pectoris, 12 were remarkedly improved, 27 improved, 5 unimproved, no case was deteriorated.

13.9　The Prescription of *Danshen Yin*

Name: Red Sage Drink

Source: The book *Shi Fang Ge Kuo*

Ingredients:

Dan Shen (Radix Salviae Miltiorrhizae)30g, *Tan Xiang* (Lignum Santali Albi)5g, *Sha Ren* (Fructus Amomi)5g.

Explanation:

Dan Shen: The principal drug in larger dosage, promoting blood circulation and dispelling blood stasis.

Tan Xiang and *Sha Ren:* Working together to regulate the *Qi* of the middle—*Jiao* and alleviate pain.

Effect: Promoting blood circulation to remove blood stasis, alleviating the flow of *Qi* to relieve pain.

Indications: Syndrome of blood stasis due to stagnation of *Qi*, marked by pain in the chest and stomach, deep red tongue and taut uneven pulse; including such diseases with the above symptoms as chronic gastritis, peptic ulcer and chronic pancreatitis.

Administration: Decocted in water for oral dose to be taken twice.

Case Study: The prescription of *Danshen Yin* plus:

Yan Hu Suo (Rhizoma Corydalis), *Su Ye* (Folium Perillae), *Bai Zhu* (Rhizoma Atractylodis Macrocephalae), *Hou Po* (Cortex Magnoliae Officinalis),

was clinically used to treat stomachache and diseases with the symptom of upper abdominal pain such as hepatitis, cholecystitis and pancreatitis. Successful curative effects were obtained.

13.10   The Prescription of *Wenjing Tang*

Name: Decoction for Warming Channels

Source: The book *Jin Gui Yao Lue*

Ingredients:

Wu Zhu Yu (Fructus Euodiae)9g, *Dang Gui* (Radix Angelicae Sinensis)9g, *E Jiao* (Colla Corii Asini)9g, *Mai Dong* (Radix Ophiopogonis)9g, *Shao Yao* (Radix Paeoniae)6g, *Chuan Xiong* (Rhizoma Chuanxiong)6g, *Ren Shen* (Radix Ginseng)6g, *Gui Zhi* (Ramulus Cinnamomi)6g, *Dan Pi* (Cortex Moutan Ridicis)6g, *Ban Xia* (Rhizoma Pinelliae)6g, *Sheng Jiang* (Rhizoma Zingiberis Recens)6g, *Gan Cao* (Radix Glycyrrhizae)6g.

Explanation:

Wu Zhu Yu and *Gui Zhi:* Warming up the channels to dispel cold and promoting blood circulation.

Dang Gui and *Chuan Xiong:* Activating blood circulation to remove blood stasis and nourishing blood to regulate the channels.

E Jiao, Shao Yao and *Mai Dong:* Nourishing blood and replenishing *Yin*.

Dan Pi: Eliminating blood stasis in the channels and reducing heat of deficiency type.

Ren Shen, Gan Cao, Sheng Jiang and *Ban Xia:* Invigorating *Qi* and regulating the stomach to enhance the digestive function.

Effect: Warming up the channels, clearing away cold, removing blood stasis and nourishing blood.

Indications: Syndrome of blood stasis due to deficiency—cold in *Chong* and *Ren* channels, marked by irregular menstruation, metrostaxis, fever in the dusk, heat sensation in the palms, contraction of genital organ or intractable infertility, deep red tongue and deep thready or uneven pulse; including such diseases with the above symptoms as dysfunctional uterine bleeding and chronic pelvic inflammation.

Administration: Decocted in water for oral dose to be taken twice.

Case Study: Modified *Wenjing Tang* was clinically used to treat 1 case of oophoritic cyst, manifested as delayed menstruation with less amount of dark blood, pain in the right lower abdomen, a mass in the right vault. The symptoms and signs were alleviated after 10 doses were taken, and eliminated after another several doses, the case being cured.

13.11　The Prescription of *Shenghua Tang*

Name: Decoction for Postpartum Troubles

Source: The book *Fu Qing Zhu Nü Ke*

Ingredients:

Dang Gui (Radix Angelicae Sinensis)25g, *Chuan Xiong* (Rhizoma Chuanxiong)9g, *Tao Ren* (Semen Persicae)6g, *Gan Jiang* (Rhizoma Zingiberis)2g, *Gan Cao* (Radix Glycyrrhizae)2g.

Explanation:

Dang Gui: The principal drug in larger dose, tonifying blood, promoting blood circulation by means of removing blood stasis.

Chuan Xiong: Promoting blood circulation and activating the flow of *Qi*.

Tao Ren: Activating blood circulation to remove blood stasis.

Gan Jiang: Removing cold from the blood to warm the

channels and relieve pain.

yellow rice wine: Being warm and disperse in nature, enhancing the potency of all the other ingredients.

Gan Cao: Tempering the actions of all the other ingredients.

Effect: Promoting blood circulation to remove blood stasis, warming the channels to relieve pain.

Indications: Syndrome due to attack by cold in the state of postpartum blood—deficiency, marked by retention of lochia, cold pain in the lower abdomen, pale tongue or tongue with ecchymosis, deep slow or uneven pulse; including such diseases with the above symptoms as endometrial inflammation, retention of placenta and metrypertrophia.

Administration: Decocted in water (appropriate amount of yellow rice wine may be added) for oral dose to be taken twice.

Case Study: The prescription of *Wenjing Tang* plus:

Dan Pi (Cortex Moutan), *Shu Di* (Radix Rehmanniae Preparata), *Hong Hua* (Flos Carthami), *Ai Ye* (Folium Artemisiae Argyi), roasted ginger
was clinically used to treat 22 cases of retention of placenta due to abortion. 2—6 doses taken by each of the cases, the retained placenta was discharged out in any of them.

The prescription of *Wenjing Tang* plus:

Jie Zi (Semen Sinapis), *Yi Mu Cao* (Herba Leonuri),
was prescribed to treat 15 cases of metrypertrophis with a history of 3—9 years. The smallest womb was 7.5 × 6 cm, the largest 12 × 10 cm. 1 course of treatment lasted 30 days. The result was that 7 cases were cured, 4 improved, 4 unimproved.

13.12　The Prescription of *Huoluo Xiaoling Dan*

Name: Bolus for Activating Enery Flow in the Channels and Collaterals

Source: The book *Yi Xue Zhong Zhong Can Xi Lu*

Ingredients: *Dang Gui* (Radix Angelicae Sinensis)15g, *Dan Shen* (Radix Salviae Miltiorrhizae)15g, *Ru Xiang* (Resina Olibani)15g, *Mo Yao* (Myrrha)15g.

Explanation: *Dang Gui:* Promoting blood circulation and nourishing blood.

Dan Shen: Promoting blood circulation and removing blood stasis.

Ru Xiang and *Mo Yao:* Promoting the circulation of blood to remove blood stasis, activating the flow of *Qi* to relieve pain.

Effect: Promoting blood circulation to eliminate blood stasis, removing obstruction in the channels to relieve pain.

Indications: Syndrome due to stagnation of blood and *Qi* , marked by pain in the chest and abdomen, sore limbs, stasis and swelling due to traumatic injury, ulcer, skin and external disorders, mass in the abdomen, deep red tongue, and taut uneven pulse; including such diseases with the above symptoms as angina pectoris, ectopic pregnancy, cerebral thrombosis and sciatica.

Administration: Decocted in water for oral dose to be taken twice.

Case Study: Modification of *Huoluo Xiaoling Dan* and *Hongteng Jian* was clinically used to treat 1 case of appendiceal abscess manifested as mass in the right lower abdomen which progessively became larger and severe tenderness, listlessness, lassitude and poor appetite. All the symptoms vanished and the case was cured after 12 doses were taken.

13.13   The Prescription of *Guizhi Fuling Wan*

Name: Cinnamon Twig and Poria Pill

Source: The book *Jin Gui Yao Lue*

Ingredients: *Gui Zhi* (Ramulus Cinnamomi)9g, *Fu Ling* (Poria)9g, *Dan Pi* (Cortex Moutan Ridicis)9g, *Tao Ren* (Semen Persicae)9g, *Shao Yao* (Radix Paeoniae)9g.

Explanation:

Gui Zhi: One of the principal drugs, warming and clearing the channels.

Fu Ling: The other principal drug, promoting water metabolism and reinforcing the *Qi* of the heart and spleen, helping remove blood stasis and prevent miscarriage.

Dan Pi, Shao Yao and *Tao Ren:* Removing blood stasis and clearing away heat.

honey: Moderating the actions of all the other ingredients.

Effect: Promoting blood circulation to remove blood stasis, subduing mass.

Indications: Blood stasis in the uterus, marked by threatened abortion, metrostaxis, tender abdominal pain, deep red tongue and uneven pulse; including such diseases with the above symptoms as irregular menstruation, dysmenorrhea, prostatic hyperplasia and schizophrenia.

Administration: All the ingredients are ground in to fine powder and made with honey into pills. 3—5 g of the pills is taken each time, twice daily. Or, the ingredients are decocted in water for oral dose with their dosage modified according to their proportions in the original prescription.

Case Study: The Prescription of *Guizhi Fuling Wan* plus:

Hong Hua (Flos Carthami), *Da Huang* (Radix et Rhizoma Rhei), *Niu Xi* (Radix Achyrantis Bidentatae), *Ze Lan* (Herba Lycopi), *Yi Mu Cao* (Herba Leonuri),

was clinically prescribed to treat 5 cases of prostatic hyperplasia. Each of the cases took 10 doses. Disappearance of the symptoms and free urination were seen in 4 cases but not in the rest 1 after the treatment.

13.14　The Prescription of *Dahuang Zhechong Wan*

Name: Rhubark Ground—beetle Pill

Source: The book *Jin Gui Yao Lue*

Ingredients: *Da Huang* (Radix et Rhizoma Rhei)300g, *Gan Di Huang* (Radix Rehmanniae)300g, *Huang Qin* (Radix Scutellariae)60g, *Tao Ren* (Semen Persicae)60g, *Xing Ren* (Semen Armeniacae Amarum)60g, *Shui Zhi* (Hirudo)60g, *Meng Chong* (Tabanus Bivittatus)60g, *Qi Cao* (Grub)60g, *Zhe Chong* (Eupolyphaga seu Steleophaga)30g, *Gan Qi* (Resina Toxicodendri)30g, *Shao Yao* (Radix Paeoniae) 120g, *Gan Cao* (Radix Glycyrrhizae)90g.

Explanation:

Da Huang: One of the principal drugs, removing blood stasis through invigorating blood circulation and purgating, clearing away heat from blood.

Zhe Chong: The other principal drug, removing blood stasis through purgation.

Gan Qi, Tao Ren, Qi Cao, Shui Zhi and *Meng Chong:* Promoting blood circulation and clearing obstruction from the channels, removing extravasated blood by catharsis.

Huang Qin: Assisting *Da Huang* in removing blood stasis and heat.

Xing Ren: Aiding *Tao Ren* in moistening mass due to dryness, activating blood flow and descending *Qi.*

Sheng Di and *Shao Yao:* Nourishing blood and *Yin.*

Gan Cao: Regulating the stomach and supplementing the body resistance, tempering the actions of all the other ingredients.

Effect: Promoting blood circulation by removing blood stasis.

Indications: Syndrome due to five kinds of impairments caused by overstrain, marked by emaciation, fullness in the stomach which leads to poor appetite, dry skin and nails, dark eyes, deep red tongue and sinking thready uneven pulse; including traumatic injury, swelling and pain due to blood stasis, and cirrhosis.

Administration: All the ingredients are ground into fine powder and made with honey into pills. 3 g of the pills is taken each time, twice daily. With the amounts properly modified according to the original proportions, the ingredients may be decocted in water for oral use.

Case Study: *Dahuang Zhechong Wan* was clinically administered to treat 1 case of arthralgia—syndrome manifested as severe prickle pain with burning sensation around the acupoint of Huantiao which was more severe in the night and made walking difficult. The pain was relieved in the night after 3 pills were taken. After another 20 pills or so were taken, the case was cured.

13.15　Prescriptions for Stopping Bleeding

Prescriptions of this kind are mainly made up of drugs with the action of stopping bleeding. They are indicated for various kinds of hemorrhage due to blood flowing out of the channels such as hematemesis, epistaxis, hemoptysis, hematochezia, metrorrhagia and metrostaxis. The commonly used drugs are:

Ce Bai Ye (Cacumen Platycladi), Xiao Ji (Herba Cirsii), Huai Hua (Flos Sophorae), Zao Xin Tu (ignited yellow earth), Ai Ye (Folium Artemisiae Argyi).

The representative prescriptions are Shihui San, Sisheng Wan, Xiaoji Yinzi, Huaihua San, Huangtu Tang and Jiaoai Tang.

13.16　The Prescription of Shihui San

Name: Powder Made of Ashes of Ten Drugs
Source: The book Shi Yao Shen Shu
Ingredients (with the same dosage):

Da Ji (Radix Cirsii Japonici), Xiao Ji (Herba Cirsii), He Ye (Folium Nelumbinis), Ce Bai Ye (Cacumen Platycladi), Mao Gen (Rhizoma Imperatae), Qian Cao Gen (Radix Rubiae), Mu Dan Pi (Cortex Moutan), Zong Lü Pi (Petiolus Trachycarpi), Shan Zhi (Fructus Gardeniae), Da Huang (Radix et Rhizoma Rhei).

Explanation:

Da Ji, Xiao Ji, He Ye, Qian Cao Gen, Ce Bai Ye and Bai Mao Gen: Removing heat from blood and stopping bleeding.

Zong Lü Pi: Stopping bleeding by astringing.

Zhi Zi: Dispelling heat and purging fire.

Da Huang: Inducing heat to go downward.

Dan Pi: Eliminating heat from blood and removing blood

stasis, stopping bleeding without blood retained.

Effect: Removing heat from blood and stopping bleeding.

Indications: Bleeding due to blood—heat, marked by hematemesis, hemoptysis, reddened tongue and rapid pulse; including such diseases with the above symptoms as pulmonary tuberculosis, bronchiectasis and gastric ulcer.

Administration: Each of ingredients is burned with its nature maintained and then ground into powder. A Chinese ink stick is properly ground in an adequate amount of juice of lotus rhizome or carrot. 9 g of the powder is taken with the juice containing Chinese ink each time, twice daily. The drugs are burned with their nature maintained so as to enhance their action of astringing and stopping bleeding. The powder is taken with the juice so as to strengthen its action of removing heat from blood and stopping bleeding.

Case Study: *Shihui San* was clinically used to treat 27 cases of pulmonary tuberculosis with 20 remarkedly improved, 2 improved and 5 unimproved. The bleeding was usually stopped at the 4th—6th day after the powder began to be taken, the course from the time of the powder to be taken to the time of the bleeding to be stopped averaging 5 days.

13.17 The Prescription of *Sisheng Wan*

Name: Bolus of Four Fresh Drugs

Source: The book *Fu Ren Liang Fang*

Ingredients:

Sheng He Ye (fresh Folium Nelumbinis)9g, *Sheng Ai Ye* (fresh Folium Artemisiae Argyi)9g, *Sheng Bai Ye* (fresh Folium Biotae)12g, *Sheng Di Huang* (fresh Radix Rehmanniae)15g.

Explanation:

Ce Bai Ye: The principal drug, removing heat from blood to stop bleeding.

Sheng Di: Clearing away heat from blood to stop bleeding, nourishing *Yin* and promoting the production of body fluids.

He Ye and *Ai Ye:* Stopping bleeding and removing blood stasis.

Effect: Removing blood heat and stopping bleeding.

Indications: Bleeding due to blood–heat, marked by hematemesis and epistaxis with bright red blood, dry mouth and throat, reddish or deep red tongue and taut rapid pulse; including such diseases with the above symptoms as pulmonary tuberculosis and bronchiectasis with the symptom of hemoptysis and gastric ulcer with the symptom of hematemesis.

Administration: Decocted in water for oral dose to be taken twice.

13.18   The Prescription of *Kexue Fang*

Name: Prescription for Treating Hemoptysis
Source: The book *Dan Xi Xin Fa*
Ingredients:

Qing Dai (Indigo Naturalis)6g, *He Zi* (Fructus Chebulae)6g, *Gua Lou Ren* (Semen Trichosanthis)9g, *Hai Shi* (Os Costaziae)9g, *Zhi Zi* (Fructus Gardeniae)9g.

Explanation:

Qing Dai and *Zhi Zi:* The principal drugs, purging fire in the liver and clearing away heat from blood.

Gua Lou Ren and *Hai Shi:* Removing heat and fire pathogens, moistening dryness and resolving phlegm.

He Zi: Astringing the lung—*Qi* to relieve cough.

Effect: Eliminating fire pathogen, resolving phlegm, astringing the lung—*Qi* and relieving cough.

Indications: Syndrome due to attack of the lung by the liver—fire, marked by cough, thick sputum with blood streak, difficulty in expectoration, or dysphoria, irritability, prickle pain in the chest and hypochondrium, reddened cheeks, constipation, reddish tongue with yellowish coating, and taut rapid pulse; including such diseases with the above symptoms as bronchiectasis and pulmonary tuberculosis with the symptom of hemoptysis.

Administration: Decocted in water for oral dose to be taken twice.

13.19   The Prescription of *Huaihua San*

Name: Sophora Powder

Source: The book *Ben Shi Fang*

Ingredients:

Huai Hua (Flos Sophorae)12g, *Bai Ye* (Cacumen Platycladi)12g, *Jing Jie* (Herba Schizonepetae)6g, *Zhi Qiao* (Fructus Aurantii)6g.

Explanation: *Huai Hua:* The principal drug, removing dampness and heat in the large intestines and dispersing heat from blood to stop bleeding.

Bai Ye: Helping *Huai Hua* to remove heat from blood and stop bleeding.

Jing Jie: Dispelling wind pathogen, stopping bleeding.

Zhi Qiao: Keeping upward adverse flow of *Qi* going downward and relieving stuffiness of the intestines.

Effect: Removing pathogenic factors in the intestines, stopping bleeding, dispelling wind pathogen and keeping upward adverse flow of *Qi* going downward.

Indications: Syndrome of bloody stools due to toxic heat in the stomach and intestines, marked by hematochezia before or after defecation, or stool with blood, or bleeding due to hemorrhoid, the blood being bright or dark red, reddish tongue with whitish or thin yellowish coating, and rapid pulse; including such diseases with the above symptoms as hemorrhoid, amebic dysentery and peptic ulcer.

Administration: Decocted in water for oral dose to be taken twice.

13.20   The Prescription of *Xiaoji Yinzi*

Name: Small Thistle Decoction
Source: The book *Ji Sheng Fang*
Ingredients:

Di Huang (Radix Rehmanniae)30g, *Xiao Ji* (Herba Cirsii)15g, *Hua Shi* (Talcum)15g, *Mu Tong* (Caulis Aristolochiae Manshuriensis)9g, *Pu Huang* (Pollen Typhae)9g, *Ou Jie* (Nodus Nelumbinis Rhizomatis)9g, *Dan Zhu Ye* (Herba Lophatheri)9g, *Shan Zhi Zi* (Fructus Gardeniae)9g, *Dang Gui* (Radix Angelicae Sinensis)6g, *Zhi Gan Cao* (Radix Glycyrrhizae Preparata)6g.

Explanation:

Xiao Ji: The principal drug, removing heat from blood and stopping bleeding.

Ou Jie and *Pu Huang:* Removing heat from blood, stopping bleeding and eliminating blood stasis.

Hua Shi: Removing heat pathogens, promoting water metabolism and inducing diuresis.

Mu Tong, Zhu Ye and *Zhi Zi:* Removing and purging heat from the heart, lung and tri—*Jiao.*

Sheng Di: Nourishing *Yin* and removing heat, removing heat from blood and stopping bleeding.

Dang Gui: Nourishing and regulating blood.

Gan Cao: Tempering the actions of all the other ingredients.

Effect: Removing heat from blood, stopping bleeding, promoting water metabolism and inducing diuresis.

Indications: Syndrome due to retention of heat in the lower—*Jiao,* marked by painful and dribbling and frequent urination with scanty and deep—colored and bloody urine, reddened tongue and rapid pulse; including such diseases with the above symptoms as urinary infection and stone in the urinary system.

Administration: Decocted in water for oral dose to be taken twice.

Case Study: Modified *Xiaoji Yinzi* was clinically used to treat 2 cases of acute nephritis manifested an edema of the face, dysuria, scanty and deep—colored urine, restlessness, thirst, reddened tongue tip with little coating, and floating rapid pulse. Either of the cases was cured after 9—20 doses were taken by either of them.

13.21   The Prescription of *Huangtu Tang*

Name: Decoction of Baked Yellow Earth

Source: The book *Jin Gui Yao Lue*

Ingredients:

Zao Xin Tu (ignited yellow earth)30g, *Gan Di Huang* (Radix Rehmanniae)9g,   *Bai   Zhu   (Rhizoma   Atractylodis

Macrocephalae)9g, *Fu Zi* (Radix Aconiti Lateralis Preparata)9g, *E Jiao* (Colla Corii Asini)9g, *Huang Qin* (Radix Scutellariae)9g, *Gan Cao* (Radix Glycyrrhizae)9g.

Explanation:

Zao Xin Tu: The principal drug, warming the middle–*Jiao* and stopping bleeding.

Bai Zhu and *Fu Zi:* Warming the spleen–*Yang* to invigorate the *Qi* in the middle–*Jiao.*

Sheng Di and *E Jiao:* Nourishing *Yin* and blood.

Gan Cao: Tempering the actions of all the other ingredients.

Huang Qin bitter in taste and cold in nature is compatible with *Sheng Di* sweet in flavor and cold and moisture in nature so as to restrain the over–warm and over–dry nature of *Bai Zhu* and *Fu Zi.*

Effect: Warming *Yang*, strengthening the spleen, nourishing blood and stopping bleeding.

Indications: Syndrome due to insufficiency of the spleen–*Yang* and deficiency–cold of the middle–*Jiao,* marked by bloody stools, or hematemesis, epistaxis, metrorrhagia and metrostaxis, all with deep–colored blood, cold limbs, sallow complexion, pale tongue with whitish coating, and deep thready weak pulse; including such diseases with the above symptoms as chronic hemorrhage of gastrointestinal tract and dysfunctional uterine bleeding.

Administration: *Zao Xin Tu* is decocted in water for the decoction, into which the other ingredients are put and decocted. The decoction is divided into 2 portions. 1 portion is taken each time.

Case Study: 23 cases of hemorrhage of the upper digestive

tract were clinically treated with the prescription of *Huangtu Tang* plus *Dan Pi* (Cortex Moutan). 120 g of red brick was used to substitute for *Zao Xin Tu* and pounded into small pieces and steeped in water to get the clear solution, in which the other ingredients were put and decocted to get the decoction for oral dose. The treatment result was that 22 cases were cured, 1 case was unimproved.

13.22 The Prescription of *Jiaoai Tang*

Name: Ass—hide Glue and Argyi Leaf Decoction

Source: The book *Jin Gui Yao Lue*

Ingredients:

E Jiao (Colla Corii Asini)9g, *Ai Ye* (Folium Artemisiae Argyi)9g, *Dang Gui* (Radix Angelicae Sinensis)9g, *Chuan Xiong* (Rhizoma Chuanxiong)6g, *Gan Cao* (Radix Glycyrrhizae)6g, *Gan Di Huang* (Radix Rehmanniae)12g, *Shao Yao* (Radix Raeoniae)12g.

Explanation:

E Jiao: One of the principal drugs, nourishing blood and stopping bleeding.

Ai Ye: The other principal drug, warming the channels and stopping bleeding.

Di Huang, Dang Gui, Shao Yao and *Chuan Xiong:* Nourishing blood, regulating the channels and promoting blood circulation.

Gan Cao: Tempering the actions of all the other ingredients.

Effect: Nourishing blood, stopping bleeding, regulating the channels, preventing miscarriage.

Indications: Syndrome due to deficiency and impairment of

the Chong and Ren channels, marked by metrorrhagia, metrostaxis, profuse and dribbling menstruation, or incessive hemorrhage after incomplete abortion, or uterine bleeding during pregnancy, pain in the abdomen, pale tongue, and deep thready pulse; including such diseases with the above symptoms as threatened abortion and incomplete recovery of the womb after delivery.

Administration: The ingredients except *E Jiao* are decocted in water for the decoction. *E Jiao* is melted in adequate amount of liquor. The decoction and the liquor are mixed together and taken twice. The liquor here can help the ingredients to exert their actions.

Case Studey: Modified *Aijiao Tang* was clinically used to treat 41 cases of threatened abortion with 36 cured, 5 improved.

14 Prescriptions for Treating Wind Syndromes

14.1 Prescriptions for Treating Wind Syndromes

Prescriptions with the following three characteristics are all known as "prescription for treating wind syndrome": consisting of drugs pungent in flavor and disperse in nature and with the potency of expelling wind pathogen or calming wind to relieve spasm, having the action of dispersing exogenous wind or calming endogenous wind, being suitable for the syndromes due to wind pathogen. Diseases due to wind have a broad range. Their symptoms and signs vary a great deal. Their cause involves two kinds of pathogens: exogenous and endogenous. Exogenous wind refers to wind pathogen invading the body from the superficies and retaining in the superficies of the body, the channels and collaterals, the tendons, the muscles and the joints, while endogenous wind refers to wind produced in the interior due to diseases of the internal organs. When diseases due to wind are treated, exogenous wind is to be dispelled, while endogenous wind is to be calmed. As a result, prescriptions for treating wind syndromes are classified as the following two: those for dispersing exogenous wind and those for calming endogenous wind.

When prescriptions for treating wind syndromes are to be prescribed to treat a disease due to pathogenic wind, the first thing to be done is to identify which causes it: exogenous wind or endogenous wind, and what is its nature: cold or heat, deficiency or excess. If it is caused by exogenous wind, prescription for dispersing exogenous wind should be prescribed. If it is caused by endogenous wind, prescription for calming endogenous wind should be used. If the wind is complicated by cold, heat, warmth or phlegm, the way of expelling wind should be used together with that of removing cold, heat, dampness or phlegm.

14.2 Prescriptions for Dispersing Exogenous Wind

This kind of prescriptions are mainly composed of drugs pungent in flavor and disperse in nature and with the action of expelling wind pathogen. They are indicated for such disorders due to exogenous wind pathogen as headache, dizziness, rubella and eczema. Drugs such as

Fang Feng (Radix Saposhinkoviae), *Chuan Xiong* (Rhizoma Chuanxiong), *Bai Zhi* (Radix Angelicae Dahuricae), *Jing Jie* (Herba Schizonepetae), *Bai Fu Zi* (Fhizoma Typhonii),
are commonly used in the these prescriptions, whose representatives are *Da Qinjiao Tang, Xiaofeng San, Chuanxiong Chatiao San, Qianzheng San* and *Xiao Huoluo Dan.*

14.3 The Prescription of *Da Qinjiao Tang*

Name: Major Gentian Decoction
Source: The book *Su Wen Bing Ji Qi Yi Bao Ming Ji*
Ingredients:

Qin Jiao(Radix Gentianae Macrophyllae) 90 g, *Gan Cao* (Radix Glycyrrhizae) 60 g, *Chuan Xiong* (Rhizoma Chuanxiong) 60 g, *Dang Gui* (Radix Angelicae Sinensis) 60 g, *Bai Shao* (Radix

Paeoniae Alba) 60 g, *Shi Gao* (Gypsum Fibrosum) 60 g, *Du Huo* (Radix Angelicae Pubescentis) 60 g, *Qiang Huo* (Rhizoma seu Radix Notopterygii) 30 g, *Fang Feng* (Radix Saposhinkoviae) 30 g, *Huang Qin* (Radix Scutellariae) 30 g, *Bai Zhi* (Radix Angelicae Dahuricae) 30 g, *Bai Zhu* (Rhizoma Atractylodis Macrocephalae) 30 g, *Sheng Di* (Radix Rehmanniae) 30 g, *Shu Di* (Radix Rehmanniae Preparata) 30 g, *Fu Ling* (Poria) 30 g, *Xi Xin* (Herba Asari) 15 g.

Explanation:

Qin Jiao: The principal drug, expelling wind and clearing obstruction in the channels.

Qiang Huo, Du Huo, Fang Feng, Bai Zhi and *Xi Xin*:   Dispelling wind pathogen.

Dang Gui, Bai Shao and *Shu Di*:   Nourishing blood and softening the tendons.

Chuan Xiong: Promoting blood circulation and clearing away obstruction in the channels.

Huang Qin, Shi Gao and *Sheng Di*:   Removing heat from blood.

Gan Cao: Tempering the actions of all the other ingredients.

Effect: Expelling wind, dispelling heat, nourishing blood and promoting blood circulation.

Indications: Syndrome due to primary attack of the channels by wind, marked by distortion of the face, stiff tongue, inability to speak, difficulty in moving the hands and feet, whitish tongue, and floating pulse; including such diseases with the above symptoms as facial paralysis and tetanus.

Administration: All the ingredients are ground into fine powder, 30 g of the powder is decocted in water for the decoction to be taken twice daily. Or, the ingredients are decocted in water for oral dose with their amounts properly modified according to their original proportions.

Drugs pungent in flavor are more in this prescription, which tends to damage *Yin*—blood. So, attention should be paid to modify their dosages in clinical practice.

14.4　The Prescription of *Xiaofeng San*

Name:　Powder for Dispersing Pathogenic Wind
Source:　The book *Wai Ke Zheng Zong*
Ingredients:

Dang Gui(Radix Angelicae Sinensis) 3 g, *Sheng Di*(Radix Rehmanniae) 3 g, *Fang Feng* (Radix Saposhinkoviae) 3 g, *Chan Tui*(Periostracum Cicadae) 3 g, *Zhi Mu* (Rhizoma Anemarrhenae) 3 g, *Ku Shen* (Radix Sophorae Flavescentis) 3 g, *Hu Ma* (Sesamum Indicum) 3 g, *Jing Jie* (Herba Schizon epetae) 3 g, *Cang Zhu* (Rhizoma Atractylodis) 3 g, *Niu Bang Zi*(Fructus Arctii) 3 g, *Shi Gao* (Gypsum Fibrosum) 3 g, *Mu Tong* (Caulis Aristolochiae Manshuriensis) 1.5 g, *Gan Cao* (Radix Glycyrrhizae) 1.5 g.

Explanation:

Jing Jie, Fang Feng, Niu Bang Zi and *Chan Tui*:　The principal drugs, dispersing wind pathogen through the superficies of the body.

Cang Zhu:　Dispelling wind pathogen and removing dampness.

Ku Shen:　Removing heat and drying dampness.

Mu Tong:　Removing dampness and heat.

Shi Gao and *Zhi Mu*:　Removing heat and purging fire.

Dang Gui, Sheng Di and *Hu Ma*: Nourishing blood, promoting blood circulation, tonifying *Yin* and moistening dryness.

Gan Cao: Removing heat pathogen and toxic material, tempering the actions of all the other ingredients.

Effect: Dispelling wind pathogen, nourishing blood, removing dampness and heat.

Indications: Rubella and eczema, marked by red skin eruption, or spots dotted on the skin in the shape of clouds, itching, fluid produced from the diabrotic eruptions, whitish or yellowish tongue coating, and floating rapid forceful pulse; including such diseases with the above symptoms as allergic dermatitis, paddy field dermatitis, neurodermatitis and drug dermatitis.

Administration: Decocted in water for oral dose to be taken twice.

Case Study: 1 case of allergic subsepicemia with a history of 3 years during which both Chinese and western drugs had failed to control it was clinically treated with *Xiaofeng San* plus:

Huang Teng (Caulis Fibraureae) *Dan Pi* (Cortex Moutan), *Tu Fu Ling* (Rhizoma Smilacis Glabrae), *Jiang Can* (Bombyx Batryticatus), *Bei Mu* (Bulbus Fritillariae).

70 days later, the case was cured, all the symptoms and signs except for fusiform interphalangeal articulations of hand disappearing.

44 cases of eczema were treated with *Xiaofeng San* with 38 temporarily and 6 basically cured, 20 doses on an average being taken by each of them.

14.5　The Prescription of *Chuanxiong Chatiao San*

Name:　Chuanxiong Mixture

Source:　The book *Tai Ping Hui Min He Ji Ju Fang*

Ingredients:

Chuan Xiong (Rhizoma Chuanxiong) 120 g, *Jing Jie* (Herba Schizonepetae) 120 g, *Bai Zhi* (Radix Angelicae Dahuricae) 60 g, *Qiang Huo* (Rhizoma seu Radix Notopterygii) 60 g, *Gan Cao*(Radix Glycyrrhizae) 60 g, *Xi Xin* (Herba Asari) 45 g, *Fang Feng* (Radix Saposhinkoviae) 45 g, *Bo He* (Herba Menthae) 240 g.

Explanation:

Chuan Xiong, *Bai Zhi* and *Qiang Huo*:　The principal drugs, dispelling wind pathogen and relieving pain.

Xi Xin:　Removing cold to relieve pain.

Bo He:　Being used in larger dose so as to refresh the mind and dispel wind and heat pathogens.

Jing Jie and *Fang Feng*:　Being pungent in taste and disperse in nature , dispelling wind pathogen in the upper body.

Gan Cao:　Tempering the actions of all the other ingredients.

tea:　Being bitter in flavor and cold in nature, refreshing the mind, restraining the over—warm, over—dry, over—ascending and over—dispersing nature of drugs for treating wind syndromes so as to coordinate their ascending and descending nature.

Effect:　Dispelling wind pathogen and relieving pain.

Indications:　Wind syndrome of head, marked by migraine, headache, or ache in the vertex, aversion to cold, fever, dizziness, stuffy nose, thin whitish tongue coating, and floating pulse; including such diseases with the above symptoms as chronic rhinitis, nasosinusitis and neuroheadache.

Administration: All the ingredients are ground into fine powder, 6 g of which is taken with tea each time, twice daily.

Case Study: *Chuanxiong Chatiao San* was clinically used to treat 126 cases of prolonged migraine manifested as alternative ache in the left and right temples, complicated by vomiting, lethargy, vexation, lassitude and constipation. The general effective rate reached 83.3%.

14.6   The Prescription of *Qianzheng San*

Name: Powder for Treating Wry—mouth
Source: The book *Yang Shi Jia Cang Fang*
Ingredients:
Bai Fu Zi (Rhizoma Typhonii), *Jiang Can* (Bombyx Batryticatus), *Quan Xie* (Scorpio).

The above three ingredients are in the same amount.
Explanation:
Bai Fu Zi: Dispelling wind pathogen, resolving phlegm, having the special action of treating wind syndrome of the head.

Jiang Can and *Quan Xie*: Dispelling wind pathogen and relieving spasm.

These three ingredients works together to exert special and great potency.

Effect: Dispelling wind, removing phlegm and relieving spasm.

Indications: Wind syndrome manifested as facial paralysis, distortion of the face, or even convulsion of the facial muscles, whitish tongue, and floating slippery pulse; including facial neuroparalysis and prosopalgia.

Administration: The three ingredients are ground into fine powder, 3 g of which is taken each time, twice daily. The ingredients may also be decocted in water for oral dose, but, in so doing, their dosages should be modified properly according to their original proportions.

Case Study: The ingredients of modified *Qianzheng San* were ground into powder, the powder was mixed with the juice of *Sheng Jiang*(Rhizoma Zingiberis Recens) into a paste, the paste was clinically applied externally to treat 33 cases of Bell's facial paralysis.   29 cases were cured, 2 improved, 2 unimproved.

50% compound injection of *Qianzheng San,* whose ingredients were:

Bai Fu Zi (Rhizoma Typhonii), *Jiang Can* (Bombyx Batryticatus), *Quan Xie* (Scorpio), *Dang Gui*(Radix Angelicae Sinensis), *Wu Gong* (Scolopendra),

was alternatively injected at the acupoints: Dicang (ST 4), Jiache (ST 6), Yangbai (GB 14), etc. on the diseased side to treat 418 cases of facial neuroparalysis. The course of treatment lasted 7−42 days. The curative rate reached 90%.

14.7   The Prescription of *Yuzhen San*

Name: Powder with Marvellous Effect

Source: The book *Wai Ke Zheng Zong*

Ingredients (with the same amounts):

Tian Nan Xing(Rhizoma Arisaematis), *Fang Feng* (Radix Saposhinkoviae), *Bai Zhi* (Radix Angelicae Dahuricae), *Tian Ma* (Rhizoma Gastrodiae), *Qiang Huo* (Rhizoma seu Radix Notopterygii), *Bai Fu Zi*(Rhizoma Typhonii), additives: hot wine and child's urine.

Explanation:

Nan Xing and *Bai Fu Zi*: Dispelling wind pathogen, removing phlegm, relieving spasm and pain.

Qiang Huo, Fang Feng and *Bai Zhi;* Dispersing wind pathogen out of the channels and collaterals.

Tian Ma: Dispelling wind pathogen and relieving spasm.

hot wine and urine of a child: Clearing away obstruction from the channels and collaterals and promoting the circulation of *Qi* and blood.

Effect: Dispelling wind pathogen, removing phlegm and relieving spasm and pain.

Indications: Tetanus manifested as tightly clenched jaws with tightly closed mouth, rigidity of the trunk, opisthotonos, whitish tongue coating, and taut tight pulse; including such diseases with the above symptoms as tetanus, whooping cough and rabies.

Administrations: The ingredients are ground into fine powder and taken or applied externally after being infused with hot wine or a child's urine, 3 g each time for oral use or appropriate amount for external use on the affected area. Also, the ingredients may be decocted in water for oral dose with their amounts properly modified according to their original proportions.

Case Study: 3 cases of tetanus were clinically treated with *Yuzhen San,*which was internally and externally used, 9 g each time, 3 times daily. All the cases were cured, the course of treatment averaged 4.8 days.

Yuzhen San infused with wine was externally used to treat

tenosynovitis due to traumatic sprain. The swelling and pain were usually relieved within 3—5 days with the function recovered.

14.8　The Prescription of *Xiao Huoluo Dan*

Name:　Bolus for Activating Energy Flow in the Channels and Collaterals

Source:　The book *Tai Ping Hui Min He Ji Ju Fang*

Ingredients:

Chuan Wu (Radix Aconiti) 66 g, *Cao Wu* (Radix Aconiti Kusnezoffii) 66 g, *Di Long* (Lumbricus) 66 g, *Tian Nan Xing* (Rhizoma Arisaematis) 66 g, *Ru Xiang* (Resina Olibani) 66 g, *Mo Yao*(Myrrha) 66 g.

additives:　old wine and honey

Explanation:　*Chuan Wu* and *Cao Wu*: The principal drugs, dispelling wind, removing dampness, warming and clearing the channels and collaterals.

Tian Nan Xing:　Drying dampness, resolving phlegm, removing phlegm—dampness in the channels and collaterals.

Ru Xiang and *Mo Yao*:　Promoting the circulation of *Qi* and blood.

Di Long:　Clearing away obstruction from the channels and collaterals.

old wine:　Enhancing the potency of all the other ingredients.

Effect:　Dispelling wind, removing dampness, resolving phlegm. clearing obstruction in the channels and collaterals, promoting blood circulation and relieving pain.

Indications:　Syndrome due to retention of wind, cold and dampness pathogens in the channels and collaterals, marked by spasm and movable pain of the tendons, limited movement of the joints, prolonged and unhealing wind—stroke, numbness of the extremities, phlegm—dampness and retained blood in the channels and collaterals, heaviness in the loins and legs, or pain in the limbs, whitish tongue, and deep taut pulse; including such diseases with the above symptoms as sequel due to cerebral apoplexy, rheumatic arthritis and rheumatoid arthritis.

Administration: The ingredients are ground into fine powder and made into boluses with honey. 3 g of the bolus is taken with old wine or warm boiled water each time, twice daily.

14.9 Prescriptions for Calming Endogenous Wind

This kind of prescriptions are mainly made up of drugs with the action of calming or nourishing the liver to disperse wind. They are suitable for the syndrome due to wind produced in the interior. The commonly used drugs are:

Ling Yang Jiao(Cornu Saigae Tataricae), Gou Teng (Ramulus Uncariae cum Uncis), Shi Jue Ming (Concha Haliotidis), Tian Ma (Rhizoma Gastrodiae), Ju Hua(Flos Chrysanthemi), Mu Li (Concha Ostreae), Di Huang (Radix Rehmanniae), Bai Shao (Radix Paeoniae Alba), E Jiao (Colla Corii Asini), Ji Zi Huang (egg yolk), Rou Cong Rong (Herba Cistanches).

The representative prescriptions are Lingjiao Gouteng Tang, Zhengan Xifeng Tang, Da Dingfeng Zhu and Dihuang Yinzi, etc.

14.10　The Prescription of *Lingjiao Gouteng Tang*

Name:　Decoction of Antelope's Horn and Uncaria Stem

Source:　The book *Tong Su Shang Han Lun*

Ingredients:

Ling Yang Jiao(Cornu Saigae Tataricae) 4.5 g, *Sang Ye* (Folium Mori) 6 g, *Chuan Bei* (Bulbus Fritillariae Cirrhosae) 12 g, *Sheng Di* (Radix Rehmanniae) 15 g, *Zhu Ru* (Caulis Bambusae in Taeniam) 15 g, *Gou Teng* (Ramulus Uncariae cum Uncis) 9 g, *Ju Hua* (Flos Chrysanthemi) 9 g, *Fu Shen* (Poria cum Ligno Hospite) 9 g, *Bai Shao* (Radix Paeoniae Alba) 9 g, *Gan Cao* (Radix Glycyrrhizae) 2.4 g.

Explanation:

Ling Yang Jiao and *Gou Teng*:　The principal drugs, removing heat from the liver, calming wind and relieving spasm.

Sang Ye and *Ju Hua*:　Working together with *Ling Yang Jiao* and *Gou Teng* to enhance the effect of calming wind.

Bai Shao and *Sheng Di*:　Replenishing *Yin* and promoting the production of body fluids so as to nourish the liver and relax the muscles and tendons.

Bei Mu and *Zhu Ru*:　Removing heat and resolving phlegm.

Fu Shen:　Calming the liver and tranquilizing the mind.

Gan Cao:　Tempering the actions of all the other ingredients.

Effect:　Removing heat from the liver, calming wind, promoting the production of body fluid and relaxing the muscles and tendons.

Indications:　Syndrome due to wind transferred from the intense heat in the Liver Channel, marked by standing high fever, vexation, irritability, convulsion of the hands and feet, spasm, even coma, deep–colored and dry tongue and taut rapid pulse; including such diseases with the above symptoms as epidemic encephalitis B and primary hypertension.

Administration:　Decocted in water for oral dose to be taken twice.

Case Study:　*Lingjiao Gouteng Tang* was clinically used to treat 8 cases of epidemic encephalitis B, all of which were cured without any sequel.

Lingjiao Gouteng Tang plus:

Shi Jue Ming (Concha Haliotidis)

Zhen Zhu Mu (Concha Margaritifera Usta)

was prescribed to treat the syndrome of convulsion marked by convulsion of the body, lock–jaw, stiff neck and opisthotonus. The treatment resulted in satisfactory curative effects.

14.11　The Prescription of *Zhengan Xifeng Tang*

Name:　Tranquilizing Liver–wind Decoction

Source:　The book *Yi Xue Zhong Zhong Can Xi Lu*

Ingredients:

Niu Xi (Radix Achyranthis Bidentatae) 30 g, *Zhe Shi* (Haematitum) 30 g, *Long Gu* (OS Draconis) 15 g, *Mu Li* (Concha Ostreae) 15 g, *Gui Ban* (Carapax et Plastrum Testudinis) 15 g, *Bai Shao* (Radix Paeoniae Alba) 15 g, *Xuan Shen* (Radix Scrophulariae) 15 g, *Tian Dong* (Radix Asparagi) 15 g, *Chuan Lian Zi* (Fructus Toosendan) 6 g, *Mai Ya* (Fructus Hordei Germinatus) 6 g, *Yin Chen* (Herba Artemisiae Scopariae) 6 g, *Gan Cao* (Radix Glycyrrhizae) 4.5 g.

Explanation:

Niu Xi: Being used in larger dose, inducing blood to go downward, invigorating the liver and kidney.

Zhe Shi, Long Gu and *Mu Li*:   Descending the adverse flow of *Qi* , suppressing the hyperactivity of *Yang* and calming the liver—wind.

Gui Ban, Xuan Shen, Tian Dong and *Bai Shao*:

Nourishing *Yin*—fluid to suppress excess of *Yang*.

Yin Chen, Chuan Lian Zi and *Mai Ya*:   Assisting the principal drug in purging the excessive part of the liver—*Yang*, removing the stagnancy of the liver—*Qi*.

Gan Cao: Tempering the actions of all the other ingredients.

Effect: Calming the liver—wind, nourishing *Yin*.

Indications: Syndrome due to *Yin*—deficiency of the liver and kidney and hyperactivity of the liver—*Yang*, marked by dizziness, vertigo, distention of the eyes, tinnitus, heat pain in the head, vexation, limited movement of the body, gradual distortion of the mouth corner, even faint without consciousness which is freed from when the patient is moved or leaves sequel when the patient comes to, reddened tongue and taut long forceful pulse; including such diseases with the above symptoms as hypertension, pheochromocytoma and cerebrovascular accident.

Administration: Decocted in water for oral dose to be taken twice.

Case Study: *Zhengan Xifeng Tang* was clinically used to treat 66 cases of hypertension. 50 cases were secondary ones, among which 30 were remarkably improved, 9 improved, 1 unimproved. 16 cases were tertiary ones, among which 6 remarkably improved, 9 improved, 1 basically unimproved. The general effective rate reached 93.7%.

14.12   The Prescription of *Tianma Gouteng Yin*

Name: Decoction of Gastrodia and Uncaria

Source: The book *Za Bing Zheng Zhi Xin Yi*

Ingredients:

Tian Ma (Rhizoma Gastrodiae) 9 g, *Shan Zhi* (Fructus Gardeniae) 9 g, *Huang Qin* (Radix Scutellariae) 9 g, *Du Zhong* (Cortex Eucommiae 9 g, *Yi Mu Cao* (Herba Leonuri) 9 g, *Sang Ji Sheng* (Herba Taxilli) 9 g, *Ye Jiao Teng* (Caulis Polygoni Multiflori) 9 g, *Zhu Fu Shen* (Poria cum Ligno Hospite) 9 g, *Gou Teng* (Ramulus Uncariae cum Uncis) 12 g, *Niu Xi* (Radix Achyranthis Bidentatae) 12 g, *Shi Jue Ming* (Concha Haliotidis) 18 g.

Explanation:

Tian Ma, Gou Teng and *Shi Jue Ming*:   The principal drugs, calming the liver−wind.

Shan Zhi and *Huang Qin*:   Removing heat and purging fire.

Yi Mu Cao: Promoting blood circulation and inducing diuresis.

Niu Xi: Inducing blood to go downward.

Sang Ji Sheng and *Du Zhong*:   Invigorating the liver and kidney.

Ye Jiao Teng and *Zhu Fu Shen*:   Relieving mental stress.

Effect: Calming the liver−wind, removing heat and promoting blood circulation, invigorating the liver and kidney.

Indications: Syndrome due to excess of the liver−*Yang* and up−stirring of the liver−wind, marked by headache, dizziness and insomnia; including such diseases with the above symptoms as tetanus, hypertension and cerebrovascular accident.

Administration: Decocted in water for oral dose to be taken twice

Case Study: *Tianma Gouteng Yin* was clinically used to treat 2 cases of tetanus manifested as headache, stiff neck, convulsion of the limbs, opisthotonus, lock—jaw and coma. Either of the 2 cases was cured by 7—15 doses.

14.13   The Prescription of *E Jiao Jizihuang Tang*

Name: Ass—hide Glue and Yolk Decoction
Source: The book *Tong Su Shang Han Lun*
Ingredients:

E Jiao (Colla Corii Asini) 6 g, *Gou Teng* (Ramulus Uncariae cum Uncis) 6 g, *Bai Shao* (Radix Paeoniae Alba) 9 g, *Luo Shi Teng* (Caulis. Trachelospermi) 9 g, *Shi Jue Ming* (Concha Haliotidis) 15 g, *Sheng Di* (Radix Rehmanniae) 12 g, *Mu Li* (Concha Ostreae) 12 g, *Fu Shen* (Poria cum Ligno Hospite) 12 g, *Gan Cao* (Radix Glycyrrhizae) 1.8 g, *Ji Zi Huang* (egg yolk) 2 ones.

Explanation:

E Jiao and *Ji Zi Huang*: Nourishing *Yin*—blood, calming wind and suppressing hyperactive *Yang*.

Sheng Di, Shao Yao and *Gan Cao*: Being sour and sweet to the taste, nourishing *Yin*, reinforcing the liver and calming wind.

Gou Teng, Shi Jue Ming and *Mu Li*: Calming the liver and suppressing the hyperactivity of *Yang*.

Fu Shen: Soothing the liver and calming the mind.

Luo Shi Teng: Relaxing the muscles and tendons and clearing away obstructions in the channels.

Effect: Nourishing *Yin*, blood and the liver to calm wind.

Indications: Wind—syndrome due to deficiency of *Yin*, marked by rigidity of the muscles and tendons, trembling of the hands and feet like the symptom caused by apoplexy, or dizziness, vertigo, deep—colored tongue with little coating, and thready rapid pulse; including such diseases with the above symptoms as neurosism, senile tremor and hypertension.

Administration: Decocted in water for oral dose to be taken twice.

14.14 The Prescription of *Da Dingfeng Zhu*

Name: Great Pearl for Wind—syndrome

Source: The book *Wen Bing Tiao Bian*

Ingredients:

Bai Shao (Radix Paeoniae Alba) 18 g, *Di Huang* (Radix Rehmanniae) 18 g, *Mai Dong* (Radix Ophiopogonis) 18 g, *Gui Ban* Carapax et (Plastrum Testudinis) 12 g, *Mu Li* (Concha Ostreae) 12 g, *Zhi Gan Cao*(Radix Glycyrrhizae Preparate) 12 g, *Bie Jia* (Carapax Trionycis) 12 g, *E Jiao* (Colla Corii Asini) 9 g, *Ma Ren* (Fructus Cannabis) 6 g, *Wu Wei Zi* (Fructus Schisandrae) 6 g, *Ji Zi Huang* (egg yolk) 2 ones.

Explanation:

Ji Zi Huang and *E Jiao*: The principal drugs, nourishing *Yin*—fluid to calm endogenous wind.

Di Huang, Mai Dong and *Bai Shao*: Replenishing *Yin* and nourishing the liver.

Gui Ban and *Bie Jia*: Nourishing *Yin* and suppressing the hyperactivity of *Yang*.

Ma Ren: Nourishing *Yin* and moistening dryness.

Mu Li: Calming the liver and suppressing the hyperactivity of *Yang*.

Wu Wei Zi and *Zhi Gan Cao*: Being sour and sweet in taste to nourish *Yin*.

Effect: Replenishing *Yin* and calming wind.

Indications: Wind—syndrome due to impairment of *Yin* by the intense heat produced by prolonged epidemic febrile disease or consumption of *Yin*—fluid caused by mistaking drugs with the action of diaphoresis or purgation, marked by lassitude, trembling of the hands and feet, deep—colored tongue with little coating and weak pulse; including such diseases with the above symptoms as epidemic encephalitis B and typhoid fever.

Administration: The ingredients except *Ji Zi Huang* are decocted in water for the decoction, in which *Ji Zi Huang* is put. The decoction is divided into 2 portions, 1 portion is taken each time.

Case Study: *Da Dingfeng Zhu* was clinically used to treat 39 cases of epidemic encephalitis B manifested as lassitude, trembling of the extremities and weak pulse. The treatment result was that 36 cases were cured, 3 died.

14.15   The Prescription of *Dihuang Yinzi*

Name: Rehmannia Decoction
Source: The book *Huang Di Su Wen Xuan Ming Lun Fang*
Ingredients (with the same dose):

Shu Di (Radix Rehmanniae Preparata), *Ba Ji Tian* (Radix Morindae Officinalis), *Shan Zhu Yu* (Fructus Corni), *Shi Hu*

(Herba Dendrobii), *Rou Cong Rong* (Herba Cistanches), *Fu Zi* (Radix Aconiti Lateralis Preparata), *Wu Wei Zi* (Fructus Schisandrae), *Rou Gui* (Cortex Cinnamomi), *Fu Ling* (Poria), *Mai Dong* (Radix Ophiopogonis), *Chang Pu* (Rhizoma Acori Graminei), *Yuan Zhi* (Radix Polygalae), additives in appropriate amount: *Sheng Jiang* (Rhizoma Zingiberis Recens), *Da Zao* (Fructus Jujubae), *Bo He* (Herba Menthae).

Explanation:

Shu Di and *Shan Zhu Yu*: The principal drugs, replenishing the kidney—*Yin*.

Rou Cong Rong and *Ba Ji Tian*: The principal drugs, warming and strengthening the kidney—*Yang*.

Fu Zi and *Rou Gui*: Helping the principal drugs to warm and nourish the kidney—*Yang*, absorbing the floating *Yang*.

Mai Dong, Shi Hu and *Wu Wei Zi*: Replenishing *Yin*, astringing body fluids, harmonizing *Yin* and *Yang*.

Chang Pu, Yuan Zhi and *Fu Ling*: Coordinating the heart and kidney, removing phlegm for resuscitation.

Sheng Jiang, Da Zao and *Bo He*: Being the guiding drugs, regulating *Ying* and *Wei*.

Effect: Nourishing the kidney—*Yin*, tonifying the kidney—*Yang* and removing phlegm for resuscitation.

Indications: Aphasia and paralysis, marked by stiff tongue, dysphasia, inability to walk, dry mouth without desire for drinking, greasy tongue coating and deep thready weak pulse; including such diseases with the above symptoms as syringomyelia, sequel of cerebrovascular accident and hypertension.

Administration: Decocted in water for oral use with the dosages of the ingredients properly determined according to their original proportions

Case Study: The modification of *Dihuang Yinzi* was clinically prescribed to treat 5 cases of syringomyelia manifested as numbness of the muscles, myophagism with occasional spasm, difficulty in walking and speaking. The symptoms and signs were relieved to certain extent after the decoction was taken for 1 month or more. The temporary curative effects was satisfactory.

The modification of *Dihuang Yinzi* was prescribed to treat 180 cases of generalized itching, among which 103 were cured, 42 remarkably improved, 35 unimproved, the total effective rate being 80.5%.

15 Prescriptions for Treating Dryness Syndromes

15.1 Prescriptions for Treating Dryness Syndromes

Prescriptions with the following 3 characteristics are all known as "prescription for treating dryness syndrome".:   1.being composed of drugs bitter and pungent in flavor and warm and moist in nature, or sweet in taste and cold and moist in nature, 2. having the action of ventilating the lung to dispel dryness or promoting the production of body fluids to moisten dryness, 3. being used to treat dryness syndromes. There are two kinds of dryness syndromes: exogenous and endogenous. Exogenous dryness syndrome is due to the invasion of external dryness pathogen into the body. It varies with the climate. When its onset is in cool climate, it is called as cool–dryness–syndrome.When its onset is in warm climate, it is called as warm–dryness–syndrome. Endogenous dryness syndrome is due to the exhaustion of essence of life and the consumption of body fluids. According to the pathogenic positions of dryness syndromes in the body, they , both the exogenous and endogenous, are classified as the following three: upper–dryness–syndrome in the upper part of the body, middle–dryness–syndrome in the middle part of the body and lower–dryness–syndrome in the lower part of the body. Exogenous dryness syndrome is treated by way of ventilating the lung to dispel dryness, endogenous dryness syndrome by way of promoting the production of body fluids to moisten dryness cool dryness syndrome by way of warmly—ventilating the lung, warm dryness syndrome by way of coolly—ventilating the lung. From the above, it is clear that prescriptions for treating dryness syndromes are in two groups: those for treating dryness syndromes by way of ventilating the lung to dispel dryness, and those for treating dryness syndromes by way of promoting the production of body fluids to moisten dryness.

Most of the drugs in prescriptions for treating dryness syndromes are greasy in nature, which tends to worsen dampness and affect Qi.That's why they are contraindicated for those who are susceptible to damp pathogen. In addition, they sholud be cautiously used for those who loose stools due to deficiency of the spleen or have stagnated Qi or abundant expectoration in the body.

15.2   Prescriptions for Ventilating the Lung to Dispel Dryness

This kind of prescriptions are mainly made up of drugs warm and moist in nature and with the action of ventilating the lung to dispel dryness. They are suitable for the syndrome due to exogenous cool or warm dryness. The commonly used drugs are:

Su Ye (Folium Perillae), Jie Geng (Radix Platycodi), Qian Hu (Radix Peucedani), Xing Ren (Semen Armeniacae Amarum), Sang Ye (Folium Mori), Sha Shen (Radix Adenophorae Strictae), Mai Dong (Radix Ophiopogonis).

The representative prescriptions are Xing Su San, Sang Xing Tang and *Qingzao Jiufei Tang*.

15.3 The Prescription of *Xing Su San*

Name: Apricot Kernel and Perilla Powder

Source: The book *Wen Bing Tiao Bian*

Ingredients:

Su Ye (Folium Perillae) 6 g, *Ban Xia* (Rhizoma Pinelliae) 6 g, *Fu Ling* (Poria) 6 g, *Qian Hu* (Radix Peucedani) 6 g, *Jie Geng* (Radix Platycodi) 6 g, *Zhi Qiao* (Fructus Aurantii) 6 g, *Gan Cao* (Radix Glycyrrhizae) 6 g, *Sheng Jiang* (Rhizoma Zingiberis Recens) 6 g, *Ju Pi* (Pericarpium Citri Reticulatae) 6 g, *Xing Ren* (Semen Armeniacae Amarum) 6 g, *Da Zao* (Fructus Jujubae) 2 dates.

Explanation:

Su Ye and *Qian Hu*: Inducing diaphoresis to dispel pathogens.

Xing Ren and *Jie Geng*: Facilitating the flow of the lung—Qi.

Ban Xia and *Fu Ling*: Removing dampness and resolving phlegm.

Zhi Qiao and *Ju Pi*: Regulating Qi and relieving the chest stuffiness.

Sheng Jiang, Da Zao and *Gan Cao*: Regulating Ying and Wei.

Effect: Ventilating the lung to dispel dryness with drugs warm and moist in nature, facilitating the flow of the lung—Qi to remove phlegm.

Indications: Cool—dryness—syndrome manifested as mild headache, aversion to cold without sweat, cough with dilute sputum, stuffy nose, dry throat, whitish tongue coating and taut pulse; including such diseases with the above symptoms as chronic bronchitis, bronchiectasis and pulmonary emphysema.

Administration:　Decocted in water for oral dose to be taken twice.

15.4　The Prescription of *Sang Xing Tang*

Name:　Decoction of Mulberry Leaf and Apricot Kernel

Source:　The book *Wen Bing Tiao Bian*

Ingredients:

Sang Ye (Folium Mori) 3 g, *Bei Mu* (Bulbus Fritillariae) 3 g, *Dan Dou Chi* (Semen Sojae Preparatum) 3 g, *Zhi Pi* (Pericarpium Gardeniae) 3 g, *Li Pi* (Exocarpium Pyrus) 3 g, *Xing Ren* (Semen Armeniacae Amarum) 4.5 g, *Sha Shen* (Radix Adenophorae Strictae) 6 g.

Explanation:

Sang Ye and *Dan Dou Chi*:　Ventilating the lung to disperse pathogens.

Xing Ren:　Facilitating the flow of the lung—*Qi*.

Sha Shen, Bei Mu and *Li Pi*:　Moistening the lung to relieve cough.

Zhi Zi:　Removing heat from the chest and diaphragm.

Effect:　Ventilating the lung to moisten dryness.

Indications:　Syndrome of pathogenic factors in the lung due to exogenous warm—dryness, marked by mild fever, cough without sputum, dry throat, thirst, reddened tongue with thin whitish coating, and floating rapid pulse; including such diseases with the above symptoms as infection of the upper respiratory tract, measles and whooping cough.

Administration: Decocted in water for oral dose to be taken twice.

Case Study: *Sang Xing Tang* was clinically used to treat 72 cases of whooping cough, among whom 69 cases each averaged 3 doses and drove away all the symptoms, 33 case each averaged 5–10 doses and made a complete recovery.

15.5   The Prescription of *Qingzao Jiufei Tang*

Name: Decoction for Relieving Dryness of the Lung

Source: The Book *Yi Men Fa Lü*

Ingredients:

Sang Ye (Folium Mori) 9 g, *Shi Gao* (Gypsum Fibrosum) 7.5 g, *Ren Shen* (Radix Ginseng) 2 g, *Xing Ren* (Semen Armeniacae Amarum) 2 g, *Gan Cao* (Radix Glycyrrhizae) 3 g, *Hu Ma Ren* (Fructus Cannabis) 3 g, *Pi Pa Ye* (Folium Eriobotryae) 3 g, *E Jiao* (Colla Corii Asini) 2.4 g, *Mai Dong* (Radix Ophiopogonis) 3.6 g.

Explanation:

Sang Ye: The principal drug, ventilating the lung to dispel dryness.

Shi Gao: Removing heat in the Lung Channel.

Mai Dong: Removing dryness from the lung.

Xing Ren and *Pi Pa Ye*:   Facilitating the flow of the lung—*Qi*.

E Jiao and *Hu Ma Ren*:   Moistening the lung and nourishing *Yin*.

Ren Shen and *Gan Cao*:   Invigorating *Qi* and regulating the function of the middle—*Jiao*.

Effect: Removing dryness and moistening the lung.

Indications: Impairment of the lung due to warm–dryness, marked by headache, fever, dry cough without sputum, belching, dyspnea, dry throat, restlessness, thirst, dry tongue without coating, and weak large rapid pulse; including such diseases with the above symptoms as respiratory tract infection, pneumonia and pulmonary tuberculosis.

Administration: Decocted in water for oral dose to be taken twice.

Case Study: Modified *Qingzao Jiufei Tang* was clinically used to treat 1 case of hemiparalysis manifested as headache, cough, dry throat and mouth, sudden vomiting, followed by dysphasia and paralysis of the limbs. All the symptoms were eliminated after 3 doses were taken.

Qingzao Jiufei Tang was also used to treat 85 cases of aphonia with 84 cured and 1 unimproved. Among the 84 cases cured, 45 each averaged 1–3 doses, 33 each averaged 4–6 doses, 6 each averaged over 7 doses.

15.6 Prescriptions for Promoting the Production of Body Fluids to Moisten Dryness

Prescriptions of this kind are mainly made up of drugs with the action of replenishing *Yin* and moistening dryness. They are suitable for the syndrome of dryness in the interior due to insufficiency of body fluids in *Zang* and *Fu* organs. The commonly used drugs are:

Sha Shen (Radix Adenophorae Strictae), *Mai Dong* (Radix Ophiopogonis), *Sheng Di* (Radix Rehmanniae), *Xuan Shen*(Radix Scrophulariae).

The representative prescriptions are *Yangyin Qingfei Tang*,

Maimendong Tang and *Zengye Tang*.

15.7   The Prescription of *Yangyin Qingfei Tang*

Name: Decoction for Nourishing *Yin* and Clearing the Lung-heat

Source: The book *Zhong Lou Yu Yue*

Ingredients:

Sheng Di (Radix Rehmanniae) 6 g, *Mai Dong* (Radix Ophiopogonis) 5 g, *Xuan Shen* (Radix Scrophulariae) 5 g, *Gan Cao* (Radix Glycyrrhizae) 2 g, *Bo He* (Herba Menthae) 2 g, *Bei Mu* (Bulbus Fritillariae) 3 g, *Dan Pi* (Cortex Moutan) 3 g, *Chao Bai Shao* (stir-fried Radix Paeoniae Alba) 3 g.

Explanation:

Sheng Di: Nourishing the kidney—*Yin*.

Mai Dong: Nourishing the lung—*Yin*.

Xuan Shen: Dispersing fire and removing toxic material.

Dan Pi: Removing heat from blood and relieving swelling.

Bei Mu: Moistening the lung and resolving phlegm.

Bai Shao: Astringing *Yin* and purging heat.

Bo He: Dispersing pathogenic factors and benefiting the throat.

Gan Cao: Tempering the actions of all the other ingredients and removing toxic materials.

Effect: Nourishing *Yin* and removing heat from the lung.

Indications: Baihou syndrome manifested as white ulcerative spots in the throat which are hard to heal, swelling and pain in the throat, dry nose and lips, or cough or no cough, breathing with noise and difficulty, reddened tongue and rapid pulse; including such diseases with the above symptoms as tonsillitis, laryngopharyngitis and nasopharyngeal carcinoma.

Administration:　Decocted in water for oral dose to be taken twice.

Case Study:　Modified *Yangyin Qingfei Tang* was clinically used to treat 213 cases of diphtheria. The fever subsided at the 2nd day after the decoction began to be taken in most of the cases. It took 2–12 days for the tunica albuginea to vanish, averaging 5.5 days; 2–12 days for the bacilliculture to become native, averaging 6.4 days.

Among the 213 cases treated, 192 were cured, 21 cases died.

Yangyin Qingfei Tang was also employed to treat 100 cases of acute tonsillitis. The effective rate reached 95%.

15.8　The Prescription of *Baihe Gujin Tang*

Name:　Lily Decoction for Strenthening the Lung

Source:　The book *Yi Fang Ji Jie*

Ingredients:　*Sheng Di*(Radix Rehmanniae) 6 g, *Shu Di* (Radix Rehmanniae Preparata) 9 g, *Mai Dong* (Radix Ophiopogonis) 5 g, *Bai He* (Bulbus Lilii) 3 g, *Bai Shao* (Radix Paeoniae Alba) 3 g, *Dang Gui* (Radix Angelicae Sinensis) 3 g, *Bei Mu* (Bulbus Fritillariae Cirrhosae) 3 g, *Gan Cao* (Radix Glycyrrhizae) 3 g, *Xuan Shen* (Radix Scrophulariae) 3 g, *Jie Geng* (Radix Platycodi) 3 g.

Explanation:

Shu Di:　One of the principal drug, nourishing *Yin* and tonifying the kidney.

Sheng Di:　The other principal drug, removing heat from blood and stopping bleeding.

Mai Dong, Bai He and *Bei Mu*:　Moistening the lung, nourishing *Yin*, resolving phlegm and relieving cough.

Xuan Shen: Nourishing *Yin*,removing heat from blood, purging fire of deficiency type.

Dang Gui: Nourishing blood and moistening dryness.

Bai Shao: Nourishing blood and replenishing *Yin*.

Jie Geng: Ventilating the lung to relieve cough.

Gan Cao: Tempering the actions of all the other ingredients.

Effect: Nourishing *Yin*, moistening the lung, resolving phlegm and relieving cough.

Indications: Syndrome due to *Yin*—deficiency of the lung and kidney, marked by cough with bloody sputum, dry and painful throat, feverish sensation in the palms and soles, bone—heat, night sweating, reddened tongue with little coating, and thready rapid pulse; including such diseases with the above symptoms as pulmonary tuberculosis, bronchitis and bronchiectasis.

Administration: Decocted in water for oral dose to be taken twice.

Case Study: *Baihe Gujin Tang* was clinically used to treat 11 cases of spontaneous pneumothorax. Only this prescription was prescribed for milder cases, decompression air and antibiotics were added for the severe cases. All the cases were cured. It took 2—20 days for the pneumothorax to be eliminated.

Baihe Gujin Tang was also employed to treat 1 case of chronic hepatitis, marked by distention in the lower abdomen, frequent belching, abnormal liver function. After the treatment, the symptoms and signs vanished, the liver function returned to normal, and 1 year of follow—up didn't see any relapse.

15.9   The Prescription of *Maimendong Tang*

Name: Ophiopogon Decoction

Source: The book *Jin Gui Yao Lue*

Ingredients:

Mai Men Dong(Radix Ophiopogonis 60 g, *Ban Xia* (Rhizoma Pinelliae) 9 g, *Ren Shen* (Radix Ginseng) 6 g, *Jing Mi*(Semen Oryzae Sativae) 6 g, *Gan Cao* (Radix Glycyrrhizae) 4 g, *Da Zao* (Fructus Jujubae) 3 dates.

Explanation:

Mai Dong: The principal drug in larger dose, nourishing *Yin* of the lung and stomach and clearing fire of deficiency type.

Ban Xia: Checking upward adverse flow of *Qi* , regulating the function of the stomach and resolving phlegm.

Ren Shen, Jing Mi, Gan Gao and *Da Zao*:   Tonifying the spleen and regulating the stomach, invigorating *Qi* and promoting the production of body fluids.

Effect: Nourishing the lung and stomach, regulating the function of the stomach and checking upward adverse flow of *Qi*.

Indications: Syndrome due to *Yin*—deficiency of the lung and stomach, marked by cough, belching, difficulty in expectorating, or frothy expectoration ,dry mouth and throat, feverish sensation in the palms and soles, vomiting following belching, reddened tongue with little coating, and weak rapid pulse; including such diseases with the above symptoms as pulmonary tuberculosis, chronic bronchitis, pleurisy, gastric ulcer, prolapse of gastric mucosa, etc.

Administration: Decocted in water for oral dose to be taken twice.

Case Study: *Maimendong Tang* was clinically used to treat 19 cases of peptic ulcer. After the decoction was taken, the symptoms and signs, especially the pain, were remarkably relieved. 45−120 days later after the treatment began, 8 cases recheck with X−ray showed that the niche and distortion were removed in 4 cases and improved in another 4.

15.10   The Prescription of *Qiongyu Gao*

Name: Paste for Reinforcing the Lung
Source: *Hong Shi Ji Yan Fang*
Ingredients:
Ren Shen (Radix Ginseng) 750 g, *Sheng Di* (Radix Rehmanniae) 8000 g, *Fu Ling* (Poria) 1500 g, *Bai Mi* (Mel) 5000 g.
Explanation:
Sheng Di: The principal drug, nourishing *Yin* and promoting water metabolism.
Bai Mi: Nourishing the lung and moistening dryness.
Ren Shen and *Fu Ling*:   Tonifying the spleen−*Qi* besides *Fu Ling's* action of inducing diuresis and resolving phlegm.
Effect: Nourishing *Yin*,moistening the lung, invigorating *Qi* and reinforcing the spleen.
Indications: Syndrome due to consumption and impairment of the lung−*Yin*,marked by inproductive cough of deficiency and consumption type, dry throat, hemoptysis, emaciation, shortness of breath, lassitude, reddened tongue with little coating, and thready rapid pulse; including such diseases with the above symptoms as pulmonary tuberculosis, bronchiectasis, pneumonia and pleurisy.

Administration: *Ren Shen* and *Fu Ling* are ground into fine powder, *Sheng Di* is pounded to get its juice (or *Shu Di* is decocted in water for the decoction , which is used instead of the juice of *Sheng Di.*). The powder, the juice and *Feng Mi* are mixed evenly into a paste. The paste is *Qiongyu Gao*, which is stored in a porcelain pot for use. 6—9 g of the paste is taken each time, twice daily.

15.11 The Prescription of *Yuye Tang*

Name: Decoction for Regulating the Kidney and Stomach
Source: The book *Yi Xue Zhong Zhong Can Xi Lu*
Ingredients:

Shan Yao (Rhizoma Dioscoreae) 30 g, *Huang Qi* (Radix Astragali) 15 g, *Zhi Mu* (Rhizoma Anemarrhenae) 15 g, *Wu Wei Zi* (Fructus Schisandrae) 9 g, *Tian Hua Fen* (Radix Trichosanthis) 9 g, *Ji Nei Jin* (Endothelium Corneum Gigeriae Galli) 6 g, *Ge Gen* (Radix Puerariae) 4.5 g.

Explanation:

Shan Yao: Reinforcing the spleen and consolidating the kidney so as to reduce the times of urination, promoting the production of body fluids to moisten the lung and relieve thirst, the first principal drug.

Huang Qi: Elevating *Yang*,invigorating *Qi,* assisting the spleen—*Qi* in going upward to conduct its action of distributing essence to the lung, the second principal drug.

Zhi Mu, Hua Fen: Nourishing *Yin*,moistening dryness, relieving cough.

Ji Nei Jin: Assisting the spleen in transportation and transformation, promoting digestion and the production of body fluids, consolidating the kidney to control emission.

Effect: Invigorating *Qi* ,promoting the production of body fluids, moistening dryness, relieving thirst.

Indications: Syndrome due to failing to distribute body fluids adequately because of diabetes, deficiency of the kidney and dryness in the stomach, marked by thirst with strong desire for drinking, frequent urination with profuse urine, or turbid urine, sleepiness, lassitude, shortness of breath, reddened tongue with little coating, and weak thready pulse; including such diseases with the above sumptoms as diabetes and diabetes insipidus.

15.12　The Prescription of *Zengye Tang*

Name: Fluid—increasing Decoction

Source: The book *Wen Bing Tiao Bian*

Ingredients:

Xuan Shen (Radix Scrophulariae) 30 g, *Mai Dong* (Radix Ophiopogonis) 24 g, *Sheng Di* (Radix Rehmanniae) 24 g.

Explanation:

Xuan Shen: The principal drug in larger dose, nourishing *Yin,* promoting the production of body fluids, moistening dryness, removing heat.

Mai Dong: Promoting the production of body fluids to moisten dryness.

Sheng Di: Nourishing *Yin* and removing heat.

Effect: Nourishing *Yin,* removing heat, moistening dryness, inducing laxation.

Indications: Insufficiency of body fluids, constipation or reoccurrence of the following symptoms 2—3 days after defecation, all due to febrile disease of *Yangming,*marked by constipation, thirst, reddened and dry tongue, and deep feeble pulse: including such diseases with the above symptoms as intestinal tuberculosis, hemorrhoid, irritable colon, chronic pancreatitis, etc..

Administration: Decocted in water for oral dose to be taken twice.

Case Study: Modified *Zengye Tang* was clinically used to treat 120 cases of oral respondence to radiotherapy, marked by dry mouth, thirst with strong desire for drinking, reddish and swelling gingivae, reddish or leukoplakia—dotted mucous membrane of mouth which is ulcerative and great painful in severe case. After the treatment, 41 cases were cured, 65 remarkedly improved, 13 improved, 1 unimproved.

16   Prescriptions for Treating Dampness Syndromes

16.1   Prescriptions for Treating Dampness Syndromes

Prescriptions with the following three characteristics are all known as "prescriptions for treating dampness syndromes": 1. being composed of drugs with the action of eliminating dampness; 2. being able to induce diuresis so as to dispel the turbid; 3. being suitable for the syndromes due to dampness pathogen. Dampness syndromes include exogenous—dampness one and endogenous—dampness one. The former is caused by long living in a wet place, wading across a river or attacking of pathogenic dampness. It is marked by aversion to cold, fever, distention of the head, heavy sensation of the whole body, general aching, and edema of the face. The latter is caused by over—intake of raw and cold food, alcoholic drinks and cheese, which leads to the dysfunction of the spleen in transporting water and dampness. It is marked by fullness in the chest and epigastric region, nausea, vomiting, diarrhea, jaundice, turbid urine, and edema of the feet. Muscles and skin are connected with *Zang* and *Fu* organs by channels and collaterals. This is the reason that dampness in the superficies of the body may be carried inward to *Zang* and *Fu* organs, and dampness in the interior may also be delivered outward to muscles and skin. As a result, exogenous dampness may be complicated by endogenous one, and vice versa. Moreover, dampness is often accompanied by wind, cold, summer–heat or heat. This shows that dampness syndromes are usually complicated. Apart from the above, human bodies are different: deficiency or excess, fitness or weakness; pathogenic positions of dampness syndromes are different: in the upper or lower, exterior or interior, of the body; transformations of dampness syndromes are different: cold or heat. So, methods to remove dampness are, accordingly, different. Generally speaking, dampness in the upper or exterior may be eliminated by way of inducing mild diaphoresis; dampness in the interior or lower by way of administering drugs aromatic and dry in nature and bitter in taste or drugs sweet and insipid in flavor and with the action of inducing diuresis; dampness of cold–transformation by way of warming up *Yang*; dampness of heat–transformation by way of clearing away heat; dampness accompanied by general deficiency by way of strengthening the body as well as removing dampness. Therefore, prescriptions for treating dampness syndromes may fall into the following five: those by way of drying dampness and regulating the stomach, those by way of clearing away heat to remove dampness, those by way of inducing diuresis to remove dampness, those by way of heat–transformation to remove dampness, and those by way of dispelling wind to remove dampness.

Pathogenic dampness, heavy and greasy and sticky in property, is apt to disturb the activities of *Qi*.Therefore, drugs with the action of regulating *Qi* are usually used in prescriptions for treating dampness syndromes, most of which are made up of drugs pungent, aromatic, warm and dry in nature or drugs sweet and insipid in flavor and with the action of inducing diuresis. They tend to exhaust and impair body fluids and should be cautiously used when dampness to be treated is complicated by consumption of body fluids due to *Yin*-deficiency.

16.2 Prescriptions for Drying Dampness and Regulating the Stomach

This kind of prescriptions are mainly made up of drugs with the action of drying dampness and regulating the stomach. They are suitable for the syndrome due to retention of dampness and incoordination between the spleen and the stomach, marked by fullness in the abdomen, belching, regurgitation of sour fluid, vomiting, diarrhea, poor appetite and lassitude. The commonly used drugs are:

Cang Zhu (Rhizoma Atractylodis)

Chen Pi (Pericarpium Citri Reticulatae)

Huo Xiang (Herba Agastachis)

Dou Kou (Fructus Amomi Rotundus).

The representative prescriptions are *Pingwei San* and *Huoxiang Zhengqi San*.

16.3 The Prescription of *Pingwei San*

Name: Peptic Powder

Source: The book *Tai Ping Hui Min He Ji Ju Fang*

Ingredients:

Cang Zhu (Rhizoma Atratylodis) 15 g, *Huo Po* (Cortex Magnoliae Officinalis) 9 g, *Chen Pi*(Pericarpium Citri Reticulatae) 9 g, *Gan Cao* (Radix Glycyrrhizae Praeparata) 4 g, *Sheng Jiang* (Rhizoma Zingiberis Recens) 2 pieces, *Gan Zao*

(Fructus Jujubae) 2 dates.

Explanation:

Cang Zhu: The principal drug pungent, bitter in flavour and warm in nature, being good at removing dampness to promote the function of the spleen.

Hou Po: Promoting the circulation of *Qi*, resolving dampness, relieving distention and fullness in the abdomen.

Chen Pi: Regulating *Qi* to remove stagnancy.

Gan Cao: Regulating the stomach and tempering the actions of all the other ingredients.

Sheng Jiang and *Da Zao*: Regulating the function of the spleen and stomach.

Effect: Removing dampness, promoting the function of the spleen, activating the flow of *Qi* and regulating the stomach.

Indications: Syndrome due to retention of dampness in the spleen and stomach, marked by distention and fullness in the abdomen, loss of appetite, tastelessness in the mouth, vomiting, nausea, belching, regurgitation of sour fluid, heavy sensation of the body, lassitude with desire for bed, intermittent diarrhea, whitish greasy thick tongue coating, and slow pulse; including such diseases with the above symptoms as chronic gastritis, gastrointestinal neurosis, acute gastritis, infantile dyspepsia and gastroduodenal ulcer.

Administration: Decocted in water for oral dose to be taken twice (Taken originally in the form of powder).

Case Study: 1 case of gastrointestinal neurosis not complicated by peptic ulcer or gastritis and manifested as hiccup having lasted more than 5 months, pale and sallow complexion, anorexia, distention in the abdomen, lassitude, whitish greasy tongue coating, and lingering slow pulse, and having failed to respond to western medicines was clinically treated with modified *Pingwei San,* whose ingredients were:

Cang Zhu (Rhizoma Atractylodis) 9 g, *Hou Po* (Cortex Magnoliae Officinalis) 9 g, *Chen Pi* (Pericarpium Citri Reticulatae) 6 g, *Gan Cao* (Radix Glycyrrhizae) 3 g, *Ban Xia* (Rhizoma Pinelliae) 12 g, *Yin Chen* (Herba Artemisiae Scopariae) 15 g, *Fu Ling* (Poria) 12 g, *Ding* Xiang (Flos Caryophylli) 4.5 g.

The distention was eliminated and the hiccup was gradually relieved after 5 doses were taken. Then the case continued to be treated with prescriptions for strengthening the spleen with the result of being cured.

4cases of induced labor manifested as distention and fullness in the abdomen, poor appetite, lassitude, tastelessness in the mouth, loose stools, and whitish greasy thick tongue coating were treated with modified *Pingwei San,*whose ingredients were:

Chen Pi(Pericarpium Citri Reticulatae) 12 g, *Cang Zhu* (Rhizoma Atractylodis) 9 g, *Gan Cao* (Radix Glycyrrhizae) 6 g, *Xuan Ming Fen* (Natrii Sulfas Exsiccatus taken 12 g,after infused in water), *Zhi Shi* (Fructus Aurantii Immaturus) 12 g.

Sure curative effects were seen in all the 4 cases.

16.4　The Prescription of *Huoxiang Zhengqi San*

Name:　Powder of Agastachis for Restoring Health
Source:　The book *Tai Ping Hui Min He Ji Ju Fang*
Ingredients:

Da Fu Pi (Pericaupium Arecae) 6 g, *Bai Zhi* (Radix Angelicae Dahuricae) 6 g, *Zi Su* (Caulis Perillae) 6 g, *Fu Ling*

(Poria) 6 g, *Ban Xia Qu* (Rhizoma Pinelliae Preparata) 9 g, *Bai Zhu* (Rhizoma Atractylodis Macrocephalae) 9 g, *Chen Pi* (Pericarpium Citri Reticulatae) 9 g, *Hou Po* (Cortex Magnoliae Officinalis) 9 g, *Ku Jie Geng* (Radix Platycodi) 9 g, *Huo Xiang* (Herba Agastachis) 12 g, *Zhi Gan Cao* (Radix Glycyrrhizae Preparata) 4.5 g, *Sheng Jiang* (Rhizoma Zingiberis Recens) 3 g, *Da Zao* (Fructus Jujubae) 1 date.

Explanation:

Huo Xiang: The principal drug, being pungent in flavor and slightly warm in nature, not only dispersing wind—cold but also removing dampness as well as sending up the lucid *Qi* and sending down the turbid to treat cholera morbus.

Su Ye and *Bai Zhi*: Being pungent in flavor and aromatic in nature, removing dampness.

Ban Xia and *Chen Pi*: Removing dampness, regulating the stomach, checking upward adverse flow of *Qi* and relieving vomiting.

Bai Zhu and *Fu Ling*: Strengthening the spleen, removing dampness, regulating the stomach and arresting diarrhea.

Hou Po and *Fu Pi*: Promoting the circulation of *Qi* , removing dampness and regulating the middle—*Jiao* to relieve fullness in the abdomen.

Jie Geng: Facilitating the flow of the lung—*Qi* to relieve fullness. in the chest and removing exterior syndrome and dampness.

Sheng Jiang, Da Zao and *Gan Cao*: Coordinating the spleen and stomach.

Effect: Relieving exterior syndrome, removing dampness, promoting the circulation of *Qi* and regulating the function of the stomach.

Indications: Syndrome due to wind—cold in the exterior and dampness in the interior, marked by sudden and drastic vomiting and diarrhea in cholera morbus, fever, aversion to cold, headache, fullness in the chest, pain in the abdomen, and whitish greasy tongue coating; including such diseases with the above symptoms as acute gastroenteritis, food poisoning, common cold of gastrointestinal type, etc.

Administration: Decocted in water for oral dose to be taken twice (Taken originally in the form of powder).

Case Study: Modified *Huoxiang Zhengqi San* was clinically used to treat 30 cases of acute enteritis marked by mild general discomfort, slight pain around the navel, fullness in the abdomen, poor appetite, borborygmus, and 4 to 8—time—per—day diarrhea with gruel or water—like and ligh—yellow or frothy stools. In general, effectiveness or complete cure occurred in the next day after the decoction was taken.

Huoxiang Zhengqi San was employed to treat 1 case of allergic purpura of gastrointestinal type manifested as abdominal pain, black watery stools, hemorrhagic spots in the skin of the whole body especially in the limbs. After 1 dose was taken, the nausea, vomiting and abdominal pain were remarkedly relieved and the appetite was improved; after 5 doses, most of the symptoms were eliminated; after 10 doses, the case was cured.

16.5 Prescriptions for Clearing away Heat to Remove Dampness

This kind of prescriptions are mainly made up of drugs with the action of clearing away heat and removing dampness. They are indicated for the syndrome due to exogenous or endogenous dampness—heat or dampness—heat flowing downward, marked by jaundice, afternoon—fever, fullness in the chest, distention in the abdomen, or swelling and pain of the feet and knees, etc.. The commonly used drugs are:

Yin Chen (Herba Artemisiae Scopariae), *Yi Yi Ren*(Semen Coicis), *Shan Zhi* (Fructus Gardeniae), *Hua Shi* (Talcum).

The representative prescriptions are *Yinchenhao Tang*, *Sanren Tang* and *Bazheng San*.

16.6   The Prescription of *Yinchenhao Tang*

Name: Oriental Wormwood Decoction

Source: The book *Shang Han Lun*

Ingredients:

Yin Chen (Herba Artemisiae Scopariae) 30 g, *Zhi Zi*(Fructus Gardeniae) 15 g, *Da Huang* (Radix et Rhizoma Rhei) 9 g.

Explanation:

Yin Chen: The principal drug, being bitter in flavor and slightly cold in nature, having the special action of clearing away dampness—heat to treat jaundice.

Zhi Zi: Removing obstructions from the tri—*Jiao*, leading damp—heat to go downward, inducing damp—heat to be eliminated through urination.

Da Huang: Clearing away heat and stagnancy and relieving constipation.

Effect: Clearing away heat, removing dampness and treating jaundice.

Indications: Syndrome of jaundice due to damp—heat pathogen, marked by yellowish face and body surface, slight full sensation in the abdomen, thirst, disturbance in urination, yellowish greasy tongue coating, and deep rapid pulse; including such diseases with the above symptoms as acute infectious icterohepatitis, acute cholecystitis, cholelithiasis, leptospirosis, etc.

Administration: Decocted in water for oral dose to be taken 3 times.

Case Study: 115 cases of infantile acute infectious icterohepatitis marked by icteric coloration, alternate chills and fever, anorexia, lassitude, yellow urine, fire pathogen in the liver, impairment of the liver function, etc. were clinically treated with modified *Yinchenhao Tang*,whose ingredients were:

Yin Chen (Herba Artemisiae Scopariae) 15 g, *Shan Zhi* (Fructus Gardeniae) 9 g, *Huang Bai* (Cortex Phellodendri) 4.5 g, *Da Huang* (Radix et Rhizoma Rhei) 3 g, *Long Dan Cao* (Radix Gentianae) 4.5 g, *Ji Gu Cao* (Herba Abri) 30 g, *Chi Shao* (Radix Paeoniae Rubra) 9 g, *Tao Ren* (Semen Persicae) 6 g, *Chuan Lian Zi*(Fructus Toosendan) 9 g, *Mu Tong* (Caulis Clematidis Armandii) 6 g.

It took 2−22 days for the jaundice to be eliminated, 30 days or so for the disease to be cured.

65 doses of the combined prescription of *Yinchenhao Tang* and *Sijunzi Tang* plus:

Mai Ya (Fructus Hordei Germinatus), *Cang Zhu* (Rhizoma Atractylodis), *Sha Ren* (Fructus Amomi), *Chen Pi* or *Shan Yao*(Percarpium Citri Reticulatae or Rhizoma Dioscoreae). cured 1 case of biliary cirrhosis, marked by icteric coloration in the eyeballs and the skin of the whole body, discomfort in the upper abdomen, distention in the abdomen after meals, anorexia, nausea, vomiting, less amount of urine deep—colored as strong tea, listlessness, aversion to cold, dizziness, wan and sallow complexion, thin and whitish tongue coating, thready and soft pulse, etc., as it is reported.

16.7   The Prescription of *Sanren Tang*

Name: Decoction of Three Kinds of Kernels

Source: The book *Wen Bing Tiao Bian*

Ingredients:

Xing Ren (Semen Armeniacae Amarum) 15 g, *Fei Hua Shi* (refined Talcum) 18 g, *Bai Tong Cao* (Medulla Tetrapanacis) 6 g, *Bai Kou Ren* (Semen Amomi Cardamomi) 6 g, *Zhu Ye* (Herba Lophatheri) 6 g, *Hou Po* (Cortex Magnoliae Officinalis) 6 g, *Yi Yi Ren* (Semen Coicis) 18 g, *Ban Xia* (Rhizoma Pinelliae) 10 g.

Explanation:

Xing Ren: One of the principal drugs, being bitter in flavor and slightly warm in nature, facilitating the flow of the lung—*Qi* to promote the function of the upper—*Jiao*.

Bai Kou Ren: One of the principal drugs, being pungent in flavor and warm in nature, removing dampness, promoting the circulation of *Qi* to regulate the middle—*Jiao*.

Yi Yi Ren: One of the principal drugs, being insipid in flavor and slightly cold in nature, mildly inducing diuresis to remove dampness so as to dredge the lower—*Jiao*.

Ban Xia and *Hou Po*: Promoting the circulation of *Qi*,removing dampness and relieving fullness.

Hua Shi, Tong Cao and *Zhu Ye*: Inducing diuresis to remove damp—heat.

Effect: Promoting the functional activities of *Qi* and removing damp—heat.

Indications: Syndrome due to newly—formed severe dampness and mild heat pathogens, marked by headache, aversion to cold, heaviness and soreness of the body, yellowish complexion, fullness in the chest, loss of appetite, afternoon—fever, whitish tongue, no thirst, and taut thready feeble pulse; including such diseases with the above symptoms as typhoid fever, gastroenteritis, pyelonephritis, bronchopneumonia and postoperative intestinal adhesion.

Administration: Decocted in water for oral dose to be taken 3 times.

Case Study: 15 cases of pyelonephritis manifested as urinary protein and pus cells at different level, and positive midstream urine culture were clinically treated with modified *Sanren Tang*, whose ingredients were:

those in the prescription of *Sanren Tang*

Lian Qiao (Fructus Forsythiae), *Fu Ling* (Poria).

In case of high fever, the drugs added were:

Chai Hu (Radix Bupleuri), *Huang Qin*(Radix Scutellariae).

In case of urethralgia, the drugs added were:

Che Qian Zi (Semen Plantaginis), *Hu Po* (Succinum), *Huang Bai* (Cortex Phellodendri).

In case of lumbago, the drugs added were:

Mu Gua (Fructus Chaenomelis), *Du Zhong* (Cortex Eucommiae).

In case of urine always with bacteria, the drugs added were:

Ma Chi Xian (Herba Portulacae), *Jin Qian Cao* (Herba Lysimachiae), *Lian Qiao* (Fructus Forsythiae), *Ku Shen* (Radix

Sophorae Flavescentis).

The treatment result was that 12 cases were cured, 3 improved.

16.8   The Prescription of *Ganlu Xiaodu Dan*

Name: Sweet Dew Detoxication Pill

Source: The book *Wen Re Jing Wei*

Ingredients:

Fei Hua Shi (refined Talcum) 450 g, *Yin Chen* (Herba Artemisiae Scopariae) 330 g, *Huang Qin* (Radix Scutellariae) 300 g, *Shi Chang Pu*) Rhizoma Acori Tatarinowii) 180 g, *Chuan Bei Mu* (Bulbus Fritillariae Cirrhosae) 150 g, *Mu Tong* (Caulis Aristolochiae Manshuriensis) 150 g, *Huo Xiang* (Herba Agastachis) 120 g, *She Gan* (Rhizoma Belamcandae) 120 g, *Lian Qiao* (Fructus Forsythiae) 120 g, *Bo He* (Herba Menthae) 120 g, *Bai Dou Kou* (Fructus Amomi Rotundus) 120 g.

Explanation:

Huo Xiang: One of the principal drugs, being pungent in flavor and slightly warm in nature, clearing away heat, promoting diuresis, resolving dampness, activating the circulation of *Qi*.

Yin Chen: The other principal drug, being bitter in flavor and slightly cold in nature, having the same action as *Huo Xiang*.

Hua Shi: Clearing away heat, promoting diuresis, relieving summer—heat.

Mu Tong: Clearing away heat and promoting diuresis, inducing damp—heat to be eliminated along with urine.

Huang Qin: Clearing away heat and removing dampness.

Lian Qiao: Clearing away heat and toxic material.

Bei Mu and *She Gan*:   Removing intense heat from the throat and dispersing masses.

Shi Chang Pu, Bai Kou Ren and *Bo He*: Resolving dampness by their aromatic nature, promoting the flow of *Qi* and benefiting the spleen.

Effect: Inducing diuresis, resolving dampness and removing heat and toxic material.

Indications: Syndrome of damp—heat pathogen lingering in the *Qi* system due to epidemic diseases, marked by fever, sleepiness, lassitude, fullness in the chest, distention in the abdomen, soreness of the limbs, swollen throat, yellowish body surface, thirst, scanty deep—colored urine, vomiting, diarrhea, stranguria with turbid urine, pale or thick and greasy or dry and yellowish tongue coating; including such diseases with the above symptoms as typhoid fever, infectious icterochepatitis, cholecystitis, acute gastroenteritis, etc.

Administration: All the ingredients are ground into fine powder. 9 g of the powder is taken with boiled water each time, twice daily. Or the powder is made into pills with the paste of *Shen Qu* (Massa Medicata Fermentata), 9 g of the pills is taken each time. Or the ingredients are decocted in water for oral use. In doing so, their amounts should be properly reduced according to their original proportions.

Case Study: All the ingredients of the prescription of *Ganlu Xiaodu Dan* were ground into coarse powder. The powder was decocted in water for the decoction. The decoction was clinically used to treat 26 cases of infantile acute infectious hepatitis marked by anorexia, yellow urine, fever, lassitude, nausea, vomiting, cough, reddened tongue with thin whitish or whitish and yellowish coating, and taut slippery pulse. Within 2 weeks, the icteric index of 13—20 units in 9 cases returned to normal; within 3 weeks, the content of GPT in 24 cases returned to normal; within 1−5 days, the poor appetite in all the cases returned to normal; after the treatment, 1.5−2 cm of the liver was palpable in 20 cases.

Modified *Ganlu Xiaodu Dan* was used to treat 1 case of standing low fever having lased 8years, a sequela of acute gastroenteritis which had failed to respond to any treatment, marked by no other gastrointestinal abnormality except gastroduodenal ulcer found in barium meal examination, emaciation, sallow complexion, lassitude, soreness of the limbs, shortness of breath. languor, fullness in the chest and abdomen, sleepiness, drowsiness even in the time of diagnosis, intermittent anorexia, constipation, yellow turbid urine, light red tongue with yellowish thick greasy coating, taut ligering pulse, and body temperature of 37.8 C. The case was differentiated as a syndrome due to turbid damp−heat lingering in both the interior and exterior of the *Qi* system and treated with the decoction of *Ganlu Xiaodu Dan* minus *Bo He* (Herba Menthae) but plus *Su Ye*(Folium periuae). 2 doses improved and 8 doses cured the case.

16.9　The Prescription of *Lian Po Yin*

Name:　Decoction of Coptis Rhizome and Bark of Officinalis Magnolia

Source:　The book Huo Luan Lun

Ingredients:

Zhi Hou Po (Cortex Magnoliae Officinalis Preparata) 6 g, *Huang Lian* (Rhizoma Coptidis stir−fried with juice of ginger) 3 g, *Shi Chang Pu* (Rhizoma Acori Tatarinowii) 3 g, *Zhi Ban Xia* (Rhizoma Pinelliae Preparata) 3 g, *Xiang Chi* (Stir−fried Semen

Sojae Preparatum) 9 g, *Jiao Shan Zhi* (Fructus Gardeniae Preparata) 9 g, *Lu Gen* (Rhizoma Phragmitis) 60 g.

Explanation:

Hou Po: One of the principal drugs, being bitter and pungent in flavor and warm in nature, promoting the circulation of *Qi*, resolving dampness.

Huang Lian: The other principal drug, being bitter in flavor and cold in nature, clearing away heat, drying dampness.

Shan Zhi and *Dou Chi*:   Clearing away stagnated heat in the chest and epigastric region.

Chang Pu: Removing dampness through its aromatic nature so as to benefit the spleen.

Ban Xia: Drying dampness, checking upward adverse flow of *Qi* and regulating the function of the stomach.

Lu Gen: Clearing away heat and dampness, regulating the stomach to relieve vomiting.

Effect: Clearing away heat and dampness, promoting the flow of *Qi* and regulating the function of the spleen and stomach.

Indications: Syndrome of failure of descending of the stomach—*Qi* and failure of ascending of the spleen—*Qi* both due to the retention of damp—heat, marked by sudden vomiting and diarrhea in cholera morbus, fullness in the chest and epigastrium, scanty deep—colored urine, and yellowish greasy tongue coating; including such diseases with the above symptoms as typhoid fever and acute gastroenteritis.

16.10   The Prescription of *Canshi Tang*

Name: Silkworm Excrement Decoction

Source: The book *Huo Luan Lun*

Ingredients:

Wan Can Sha (Excrementum Bombycis) 15 g, *Sheng Yi Ren* (Semen Coicis) 12 g, *Da Dou Huang Juan* (Semen Sojae Germinatum) 12 g, *Chen Mu Gua* (Fructus Chaenomelis) 9 g, *Chuan Lian* (Rhizoma Coptidis) 9 g, *Zhi Ban Xia* (Rhizoma Pinelliae Preparata) 3 g, *Huang Qin* (Radix Scutellariae) 3 g, *Tong Cao* (Medulla Tetrapanacis) 3 g, *Jiao Shan Zhi* (fried Fructus Gardeniae) 5 g, *Chen Wu Yu* (Fructus Euodiae) 1 g.

Explanation:

Can Sha: The principal drug, being pungent and sweet in flavor and slightly warm in nature, regulating the stomach, treating cramp due to cholera morbus.

Mu Gua: Resolving dampness, regulating the stomach, relaxing muscles and tendons and activating the flow of *Qi* and blood in the channels and collaterals, combining with *Can Sha* to treating cramp due to cholera morbus.

Da Dou Huang Juan: Resolving dampness, ascending the clear *Qi*.

Yi Yi Ren: Inducing diuresis to descend the turbid *Qi*, and relaxing muscles and tendons.

Huang Qin, Huang Lian and *Jiao Shan Zhi*:   Clearing away heat pathogen and removing dampness.

Ban Xia: Checking upward adverse flow of *Qi* to relieve vomiting.

Tong Cao: Inducing diuresis to remove dampness, activating channels and collaterals.

Wu Zhu Yu: Assisting *Ban Xia* in checking upward adverse flow of *Qi* and aiding *Huang Lian* in purging fire to relieve vomiting.

Effect: Clearing away damp—heat, ascending the lucid *Qi* and descending the turbid one.

Indications: Syndrome of sudden vomiting, diarrhea and cramp in cholera morbus due to disturbance of the spleen and stomach by damp—heat retained in the interior, marked by sudden vomiting and diarrhea, abdominal pain, cramp, thirst, restlessness, yellowish thick and dry tongue coating, and lingering rapid pulse; including such diseases with the above symptoms as typhoid fever, acute gastroenteritis.

Administration: *Chuan Lian* is fried with ginger juice, *Huang Qi* is fried with liquor, *Wu Zhu Yu* is steeped in water for a certain time. Then all the ingredients are decocted in water for the decoction. The decoction is divided into 2 portions, 1 portion is taken each time.

16.11   The Prescription of *Bazheng San*

Name: Eight Health Restoring Powder

Source: The book *Tai Ping Hui Min He Ji Ju Fang*

Ingredients:

Che Qian Zi (Semen Plantaginis) 15 g, *Qu Mai* (Herba Dianthi) 10 g, *Bian Xu* (Rhizoma Belamcandae) 12 g, *Hua Shi* (Talcum) 18 g, *Shan Zhi Zi* (Fructus Gardeniae) 9 g, *Zhi Gan Cao* (Radix Glycyrrhizae Preparata) 4.5 g, *Mu Tong* (Caulis Akebiae) 6 g, *Da Huang* (Radix et Rhizoma Rhei) 9 g, *Deng Xin Cao* (Medulla Junci) 3 g.

Explanation:

Qu Mai and *Mu Tong*: The principal drugs, being bitter in flavor and cold in nature, clearing away heat, removing dampness and inducing diuresis, treating stranguria.

Bian Chu, Shan Zhi, Hua Shi, Che Qian Zi and *Deng Xin Cao*: Clearing away heat, removing dampness, leading pathogens to go out of the body along with urine.

Da Huang: Clearing away heat and purging fire.

Gan Cao: Tempering the actions of all the other ingredients, relieving spasm.

Effect: Clearing away heat, purging fire and promoting diuresis.

Indications: Syndrome of strangury due to heat or stranguria due to the passage of urinary stone both caused by damp—heat flowing downward, marked by turbid and deep—colored urine, difficult and painful urination, even retention of urine, distention and fullness in the lower abdomen, dry mouth and throat, yellowish and greasy tongue coating, and slippery rapid pulse; including such diseases with the above symptoms as cystitis, urethritis, acute prostatitis, stone in urine system and pyelonephritis.

Administration: *Da Huang* is coated with flour and roasted. Then all the ingredients are decocted in water for the decoction. The decoction is divided into three portions. One portion is taken each time. Originally, the ingredients were ground into powder and taken.

Case Study: *Bazheng San* was clinically used to treat 28 cases of urinary tract infection, of which 19 were acute pyelonephritis, 7 were acute attack of chronic pyelonephritis, 1 was nephritis complicated by urinary tract infection, and 1 was prostatic hyperplasia complicated by infection. All the cases except 1 case of acute attack of chronic pyelonephritis were cured with the curative rate reaching 96.4%.

32 cases of postpartum or postoperative uroschesis, a syndrome due to deficiency of the kidney or *Qi* which was accompanied by stagnation of *Qi* were treated with modified *Bazheng San*,whose ingredients were:

Bian Xu (Herba Polygoni Avicularis) 15 g, *Qu Mai* (Herba Dianthi) 15 g, *Mu Tong* (Caulis Akebiae) 15 g, *Hua Shi* (Talcum) 3 g, *Che Qian Zi* (Semen Plantaginis) 9 g, *Gan Cao Shao* (Radix Glycyrrhizae) 6 g, *Yuan Ming Fen* (Natrii Sulfas) 9—15 g.

In case of fever complicated by urinary tract infection, the drugs properly added were:

Zhi Zi (Fructus Gardeniae), *Huang Lian* (Rhizoma Coptidis), *Pu Gong Ying* (Herba Taraxaci), *Zi Di Ding* (Herba Violae), *Bai Jiang Cao* (Herba Patriniae).

In case of *Yin*—deficiency, the drugs added were:

Sheng Di (Radix Rehmanniae), *Mai Dong* (Radix Ophiopogonis), *Sha Shen*(Radix Glehniae).

4 hours after the decoction was taken, unimpeded urine was induced in 15 cases; 4—8 hours, blocked urine was induced in 17 cases, who took another 2—5 doses each and made a complete recovery.

16.12　The Prescription of *Ermiao San*

Name:　Two Wonderful Drugs Powder
Source:　The book *Dan Xi Xin Fa*
Ingredients:

Huang Bai (Cortex Phellodendri) 15 g, *Gang Zhu* (Rhizoma Atractylodis) 15 g.

Explanation:

Huang Bai: Being bitter in flavor and cold in nature, having special potency of clearing away heat.

Cang Zhu: Being bitter in flavor, warm in nature and good at removing dampness.

Effect: Clearing away heat and dampness.

Indications: Syndrome due to damp—heat flowing downward, marked by flaccidity and weakness of the lower limbs, or reddish swollen hot painful feet and knees, or morbid leukorrhea, or skin and external diseases in the lower body due to affection of dampness pathogen, scanty and yellow urine, and yellowish greasy tongue coating; including such diseases with the above symptoms as sequela of poliomyelitis, multiple neuritis, varix of lower limb, Buerger's disease, ischialgia, and rheumatic arthritis.

Administration: *Huang Bai* is fried, *Cang Zhu* is first steeped in rice—washed water and then fried. The above two are decocted in water for the decoction. The decoction is divided into portions and taken. Originally the two ingredients were ground into powder and taken.

Case Study: 1 case of flaccidity—syndrome due to damp—heat, marked by weak hands without enough strength to hold things, and weak feet without enough strength to support the body was clinically treated with modified *Ermiao San*, whose ingredients were:

Cang Zhu (Rhizoma Atractylodis) 30 g, *Huang Bai* (Cortex Phellodendri) 20 g, *Niu Xi* (Radix Achyranthis Bidentatae) 15 g, *Xu Duan* (Radix Dipsaci) 15 g, *Ji Xue Teng* (Caulis Spatholobi)

25 g, *Yin Hua* (Flos Lonicerae) 25 g, *Ban Lan Gen* (Radix Isatidis) 25 g, *Pu Gong Ying* (Herba Taxaraci) 50 g, *Lian Qiao* (Fructus Forsythiae) 15 g, *Da Qing Ye* (Folium Isatidis) 15 g, *Shi Hu* (Herba Dendrobii) 25 g, *Hua Shi* (Talcum) 20 g, *Gan Cao* (Radix Glycyrrhizae) 7.5 g.

After 4 doses were taken, the case could stand and step a few paces. After treated for another 15 days, the case was cured.

1 case of arthralgia—syndrome due to damp—heat, marked by urticae all over the body, itching, swelling of the lower limbs, pain in the joints, and difficulty in walking, all due to the taking of belladonna tablets for treating abdominal pain was treated with modified *Ermiao San*, whose ingredients were:

Cang Zhu (Rhizoma Atractylodis) 15 g, *Sheng Di* (Radix Rehmanniae) 15 g, *Chi Shao* (Radix Paeoniae Rubra) 15 g, *Fang Feng* (Radix Saposhinkoviae) 15 g, *Bai Xian Pi* (Cortex Dictamni) 15 g, *Di Fu Zi* (Fructus Kochiae) 15 g, *Di Gu Pi* (Cortex Lycii) 15 g, *Fang Ji* (Radix Stephaniae Tetrandrae) 10 g, *Qin Jiao* (Radix Gentianae Macrophyllae) 15 g, *Ren Dong Teng* (Caulis Lonicerae) 25 g, *Ji Xue Teng* (Caulis Spatholobi) 25 g, *Ye Jiao Teng* (Caulis Polygoni Multiflori) 25 g.

The case was treated with the modification of the above prescription for half a month and cured.

The decoction of *Ermiao San* was administered to treat 40 cases of infectious hepatitis. After the treatment, the main clinical symptoms and signs were eliminated and the transaminase content dropped to below 40 units in 36 cases. The transaminase content was dropped to below 80 units in 4 cases with their symptoms and signs eliminated or relieved.

16.13　Prescriptions for Inducing Diuresis to Remove Dampness

This kind of prescriptions are mainly composed of drugs with the action of removing dampness and promoting diuresis. They are indicated for the syndrome of retention of urine, stranguria with burbid urine, edema or diarrhea due to abundant water and dampness retained in the body, marked by dysuria, edema with heavy sensation of the whole body, dilute or water–like stools or dizziness, or vomiting, nausea, etc. The commonly used drgus are:

Fu Ling (Poria), Ze Xie (Rhizoma Alismatis), Zhu Ling (Polyporus), etc.

The representative prescriptions are Wuling San, Wupi San, etc.

16.14　The Prescription of Wuling San

Name:　Powder of Five Drugs with Poria

Source:　The book Shang Han Lun

Ingredients:

Zhu Ling (Polyporus) 9 g, Ze Xie (Rhizoma Alismatis) 15 g, Bai Zhu (Rhizoma Atractylodis Macrocephalae) 9 g, Fu Ling (Poria) 9 g, Gui Zhi (Ramulus Cinnamomi) 6 g.

Explanation:

Ze Xie:　The principal drug, being sweet and insipid in flavor and cold in nature, removing dampness and promoting diuresis.

Fu Ling and Zhu Ling:　Removing excessive fluid by promoting diuresis.

Bai Zhu:　Strengthening the spleen to remove dampness.

Gui Zhi:　Relieving exterior syndrome by expelling

pathogenic cold, warming the urinary bladder to promote the discharge of urine.

Effect:　Removing dampness, promoting diuresis, warming up *Yang*, enhancing the function of *Qi*.

Indications:　Syndrome due to exogenous wind—cold, endogenous dampness and retention of phlegm, marked by headache, fever, restlessness, thirst with desire for drinks, vomiting occurring as soon as water is taken, dysuria, whitish tongue coating and floating pulse, or edema, diarrhea, difficulty in urinating, vomiting, or palpitation below the umbilicus, frothy salivation, dizziness, shortness of breath and cough; including such diseases with the above symptoms as acute nephritis, infectious hepatitis, Meniere s syndrome and hydrocephalus.

Administration:　All the ingredients are ground into powder. 3—6 g of the powder is taken each time, 3 times daily. Or, the ingredients are decocted in water for oral use.

Case Study:　*Wuling San* was clinically used to treat 40 cases of more severe acute nephritis, marked by remarkable edema, high blood pressure, hematuria and renal failure. A part of the cases were complicated by hydroperitoneum and nephrogenic heart failure. The treatment was carried out like this:　9 g of the powder was given to the severe cases daily, 6 g to the moderate, 3 g to the mild. All the cases, especially their renal regions, were kept warm and low salt diet and calm rest were required. One course of treatment involved 7 days. The result was: effectiveness was seen in all the 40 cases, each of the cases averaged 164 days in the hospital.

It is reported that the diuretic action of *Wuling San* doesn't take place in healthy human beings, in mice and in rabbits; it gives its full play when metabolism has been disturbed; *Wuling San* has the potency to promote the absorption of localized edema.

An experiment shows that when the symptoms of thirst, vomiting and oliguria have been caused by the taking of antibiotics, the body resistance will be weakened. If *Wuling San* is taken at this time, the general condition will be improved and the weakened body resistance will be restored. The co—use of *Wuling San* and antibiotics will lower the body temperature and relieve the symptoms.

16.15   The Prescription of *Zhuling Tang*

Name: Umbellate Pore Decoction
Source: The book *Shang Han Lun*
Ingredients:
Zhu Ling (Polyporus) 9 g, *Fu Ling* (Poria) 9 g, *Ze Xie* (Rhizoma Alismatis) 9 g, *E Jiao* (Colla Corii Asini) 9 g, *Hua Shi* (Talcum) 9 g.

Explanation *Zhu Ling*:   The principal drug, being sweet and insipid in flavor and cold in nature, removing dampness and promoting diuresis so as to clear away heat.

Fu Ling and *Ze Xie*:   Promoting diuresis.

Hua Shi: Clearing away heat and promoting diuresis.

E Jiao: Nourishing *Yin* and moistening dryness.

Effect: Removing dampness, clearing away heat and nourishing *Yin*.

Indications: Syndrome due to accumulation of dampness and heat and impairment of *Yin* by heat pathogen, marked by dysuria, fever, thirst with desire for drinking, or restlessness, insomnia, or such symptoms are accompanied as cough, vomiting, nausea and diarrhea, or difficulty and pain in micturition, dribbling urine, fullness and pain in the lower abdomen, etc.; including such diseases with the above symptoms as infection of the urinary system, nephritis, etc..

Administration: *E Jiao* is melted and,   then, all the ingredients are decocted in water for the decoction to be taken twice.

Case Study: 107 cases of acute cystitis were clinically treated with *Zhuling Tang*, whose main ingredients were:

Zhu Ling (Polyporus) 10 g, *Fu Ling* (Poria) 18 g, *Hua Shi* (Talcum) 15 g, *E Jiao* (melted Colla Corii Asini) 6 g..
In case of scanty and dribbling urine, the drug added was:

Che Qian Zi (Semen Plantaginis).
In case of difficult and painful urination, the drugs added were:

Shi Wei (Folium Pyrrosiae), *Wu Yao* (Radix Linderae).
In case of hematuria, the drugs added were:

Bai Mao Gen (Rhizoma Imperatae), *Qian Cao Tan* (Radix Rubiae Preparata).
In case of regular *Yin*−deficiency of the kidney, the drug added was:

Yuan Shen (Radix Scrophulariae).
In case of lumbago, the drugs added were:

Sang Ji Sheng (Herba Taxilli), *Huai Niu Xi* (Radix Achyranthis B dentatae).
All the 107 cases were cured, each of them taking 1−6 doses on the average.

13 cases of shock due to epidemic hemorrhagic fever were treated with *Zhuling Tang*,whose main ingredients were:

Zhu Ling (Polyporus) 30 g, *Ze Xie* (Rhizoma Alismatis)

30 g, *Fu Ling* (Poria) 15 g, *E Jiao* (Colla Corii Asini) 30 g.
(*E Jiao* was melted water—separatedly and taken alone with sugar.)

In case of diarrhea, the drug added was:

Hua Shi (Talcum) 10 g.

The decoction was given in the early shock stage in 11 cases, 9 of which ceased to reach the later shock stage, but the other 2 entered. Another 2 cases were first treated with western medicines with no curative effects. When they entered the later shock stage, the decoction of *Zhuling Tang* was chosen to replace the western medicines. Among the 13 cases, no one died, 9 took 1 dose each, 4 took 2 doses each, the second dose was given 12 hours after the first was taken. 3 homochronous cases treated with western medicines in the control group died.

16.16 The Prescription of *Fangji Huangqi Tang*

Name : Tetrandra and Astragalus Decoction
Source: The book *Jin Gui Yao Lue*
Ingredients:

Fang Ji (Radix Stephaniae Tetrandrae) 12 g, *Huang Qi* (Radix Astragali) 15 g, *Gan Cao* (Radix Glycyrrhizae Preparata) 6 g, *Bai Zhu* (Rhizoma Atractylodis Macrocephalae) 9 g, *Sheng Jiang* (Rhizoma Zingiberis Recens) 3 g, *Da Zao* Fructus Jujubae) 1 dates.

Explanation:

Fang Ji: One of the principal drugs, being bitter and pungent in flavor and slightly cold in nature, expelling wind and removing dampness.

Huang Qi: The other principal drug, being sweet in flavor

and slightly hot in nature, invigorating *Qi* and consolidating the superfioies, removing dampness and subsiding swelling.

Bai Zhu:

In vigorating *Qi*, strengthening the spleen, promoting the function of the spleen in transportation and transformation of food material.

Gan Cao: Reinforcing the spleen and regulating the stomach, tempering the actions of all the other ingredients.

Sheng Jiang and *Da Zao*: Coordinating *Ying* and *Wei*.

Effect: Invigorating *Qi*,expelling wind, strengthening the spleen and removing dampness.

Indications: Exterior syndrome of deficiency due to wind—edema and wind—damp pathogen, marked by sweating, aversion to wind, heavy sensation of the body, dysuria, pale tongue with whitish coating, and floating pulse; including such diseases with the above symptoms as chronic nephritis, edema due to heart disease, ascites due to cirrhosis and rheumatic arthritis.

Administration: Decocted in water for oral dose to be taken twice

Case Study: 34 cases of ascites due to schistosomiasis in the late stage were clinically treated with *Fangji Huangqi Tang*, whose main ingredients were:

Fang Ji (Radix Stephaniae Tetrandrae) 9 g, *Huang Qi* (Radix Astragali) 12 g, *Bai Zhu* (Rhizoma Atractylodis Macrocephalae) 9 g, *Zhu Ling* (Polyporus) 9 g, *Fu Ling* (Poria) 12 g, *Ze Xie* (Rhizoma Alismatis) 9 g, *Che Qian Zi* (Semen Plantaginis) 12 g, *Du Chi Dou* (Semen Phaseoli) 30 g, *Chuan Jiao Mu* (Semen Zanthoxyli) 3 g, *Sheng Jiang Pi* (Cortex Zingiberis

Recens) 1.5 g.

This prescription seemed to have nothing to do with the improvements of blood picture and liver function but have much to do with the improvements of the symptoms and signs and the subsidence of jaundice. The treatment result was: effectiveness was seen in 27 cases, ineffectiveness in 5, deterioration in 2.

Fangji Huangqi Tang and Modification of *Tianxianteng San* were collectively used to treat 7 cases of swelling due to the first pregnancy in the third trimester (6th —9th month). The cases were at the age of 22—30 and had suffered from the disorder for 4—7 days. In the course of treatment, drugs such as

Gou Teng (Ramulus Uncariae cum Uncis), *Ju Hua* (Flos Chrysanthemi), *Shi Jue Ming* (Concha Haliotidis), *Huang Qin* (Radix Scutellariae), were added for the cases with hyperactivity of the liver—*Yang*,headache, dizziness and high blood pressure. The result was: it took 3 days for the swelling to subside in 4 cases; 4 days in 2 cases. The swelling was relieved in 1 case.

16.17   The Prescription of *Wupi San*

Name: Powder of Peel of Five Drugs
Source: The book *Hua Shi Zhong Cang Jing*
Ingredients:

Sheng Jiang Pi (Exocarpium Zingiberis Recens) 9 g, *Sang Bai Pi* (Cortex Mori) 9 g. *Chen Ju Pi* (Pericarpium Citri Reticulatae) 9 g, *Da Fu Pi* (Pericarpium Arecae) 9 g, *Fu Ling Pi* (Extra Poriae) 9 g,

Explanation:

Fu Ling Pi: The principal drug, being sweet and tasteless in flavor and neutral in nature, removing dampness, promoting diuresis, reinforcing the spleen to assist it in transporting and transforming food material.

Sheng Jiang Pi: Being pungent in flavor to disperse retained water.

Sang Bai Pi: Descending the lung—*Qi* to dredge water passages.

Da Fu Pi: Removing retained water to relieve distention and fullness.

Chen Ju Pi: Regulating the stomach—*Qi* and removing dampness.

Effect: Removing dampness to relieve swelling, regulating the flow of *Qi* to strengthening the spleen.

Indications: Syndrome of abundant dampness in the superficies of the body due to deficiency of the spleen, marked by edema, heavy sensation of the body, fullness in the chest and abdomen, shortness of breath, dysuria, whitish greasy tongue coating, and deep slow pulse; including such diseases with the above symptoms as renal edema, cardiac edema, pregnant edema and angioneurotic edema.

Administration: All the drugs are ground into coarse powder. 9 g of the powder is decocted in water for the decoction to be taken warm each time, twice daily. The drugs may also be directly decocted in water for oral use.

Case Study: 26 cases of chronic nephritis were clinically treated with modified *Wupi Yin* in large dose, whose main ingredients were:

Fu Ling Pi (Extra Poriae) 60 g, *Da Fu Pi* (Pericarpium Arecae) 60 g, *Sang Bai Pi* (Cortex Mori) 60 g, *Di Gu Pi* (Cortex Lycii) 30 g, *Jiang Pi* (Exocarpium Zingiberis Recens) 15 g, *Zhu*

Ling (Polyporus) 15 g.

In case of high blood pressure, the drug added was:

Du Zhong (Cortex Eucommiae).

In case of nausea, vomiting, cough and shortness of breath, the drugs added were:

Cheng Pi (Pericarpium Citri Reticulatae), *Ban Xia* (Rhizoma Pinelliae).

In case of discomfort in the epigastric region, the drug added was:

Bai Zhu (Rhizoma Atractylodis Macrocephalae).

When the symptoms and signs had been relieved but urinoscopy showed that the urine remained unusual, the drugs added were:

Rou Gui (Cortex Cinnamomi), *Dang Gui* (Radix Angelicae Sinensis), *Dang Shen* (Radix Codonopsis), *Shu Di* (Radix Rehmanniae Preparata), and, at the same time, the dosages of such drugs in the prescription were reduced by half as:

Fu Ling Pi (Extra Poriae), *Da Fu Pi* (Percarpium Arecae), *Di Gu Pi* (Cortex Lycii), *Sang Bai Pi* (Cortex Mori).

The treatment result was: cure was achieved in 5 cases, effectivement was seen in 16 cases, improvement in 4 cases, failure in 1 case.

43 cases of edema due to pregnancy were treated with *Wupi Yin* plus *Yu Mi Xu*, whose main ingredients were:

Sang Bai Pi (Cortex Mori) 15 g, *Fu Ling Pi* (Extra Poriae) 9 g, *Da Fu Pi* (Pericarpium Arecae) 12 g, *Chen Pi* (Pericarpium Citri Reticulatae) 9 g, *Sheng Jiang Pi* (Exocarpium Zingiberis Recens) 6 g, *Yu Mi Xu* (dried Stigma Maydis or the fresh one) 30 g, 60 g.

In case of severe swelling, the drugs added were:

Zhu Ling (Polyporus) 9 g, Ze Xie (Rhizoma Alismatis) 9 g.

In case of morning sickness, the drugs added were:

Zhu Ru (Caulis Bambusae in Taeniam) 9 g, Bai Zhu (Rhizoma Atractylodis Macrocephalae) 12 g, Dai Zhe Shi (Ochra Haematitum) 15 g.

In case of cough, the drugs added were:

Xing Ren (Semen Armeniacae Amarum) 6 g, Bai He (Bulbus Lilii) 9 g.

In case of dyspnea, the drug added was:

Su Zi (Fructus Perillae) 12 g.

After the treatment, satisfactory result was obtained.

16.18   Prescriptions for Warming and Removing Dampness

This kind of prescriptions are mainly made up of drugs with the action of warming and resolving dampness.They are suitable for the syndromes of retention of phlegm, edema, arthralgia and beriberi because of cold–dampness, all due to dampness coming from cold or failed to be resolved by Yang, marked by dizziness, palpitation, edema and heaviness and soreness of the limbs, cold extremities, loose stools, whitish slippery tongue coating, and deep pulse. The commonly used drugs are:

Gui Zhi (Ramulus Cinnamomi), Fu Zi (Radix Aconiti Lateralis Preparata), Bai Zhu (Rhizoma Atractylodis Macrocephalae).

The representative prescriptions are Ling Gui Zhu Gan Tang and Zhen Wu Tang.

16.19 The Prescription of *Ling Gui Zhu Gan Tang*

Name: Decoction of Poria, Bighead, Atractylodes, Cinnamom and Licorice

Source: The book *Jin Gui Yao Lue*

Ingredients:

Fu Ling (Poria) 12 g, *Gui Zhi* (Ramulus Cinnamomi) 9 g, *Bai Zhu* (Rhizoma Atractylodis Macrocephalae) 6 g, *Gan Cao* (Radix Glycyrrhizae) 6 g.

Explanation:

Fu Ling: The principal drug, being sweet and tasteless in flavor and neutral in nature, strengthening the spleen, removing dampness, dissolving phlegm.

Gui Zhi: Warming up *Yang* to induce diuresis, descending the adverse flow of *Qi*.

Bai Zhu: Strengthening the spleen and removing dampness.

Gan Cao: Invigorating *Qi* to regulate the stomach.

Effect: Warming and dissolving phlegm, strengthening the spleen, inducing diuresis.

Indications: Syndrome of retention of phlegm due to insufficiency of *Yang* of the middle–*Jiao*, marked by fullness in the chest and hypochondrium, vertigo, palpitation, or shortness of breath, cough, whitish slippery tongue coating, and taut slippery pulse; including such diseases with the above sumptoms as chronic bronchitis, bronchial asthma and chronic nephritis.

Administration: Decocted in water for oral dose to be taken 3 times.

Case Study: The ingredients of *Ling Gui Zhu Gan Tang*

plus:

Huang Qi (Radix Astragali), *Fang Ji* (Radix Stephaniae Tetrandrae), *Dan Shen* (Radix Salviae Miltiorrhizae) were clinically administered to cure 1 case of hydropericardium, a syndrome due to up—attack of abundant dampness developed by deficiency of the spleen, marked by fever having lasted half a month, cough, fullness and pain in the chest, dyspnea, edema, and deep thready pulse, 10 doses being taken.

1 case of enuresis marked by postpartum cough having lasted more than 1 month, accompanied by drop—by—drop urine and worsened in the night, 16—month disease course, regular appetite, less amount of whitish sputum, thin whitish tongue coating, and taut thready pulse was treated with *Ling Gui Zhu Gan Tang* whose ingredients were:

Fu Ling (Poria) 15 g, *Gui Zhi* (Ramulus Cinnamomi) 6 g, *Bai Zhu* (Rhizoma Atractylodis Macrocephalae) 9 g, *Gan Cao* (Radix Glycyrrhizae) 3 g.

After 3 doses were taken, the symptoms and signs were greatly relieved; after 6 doses, the cough was arrested, the enuresis was stopped.

16.20 The Prescription of *Zhen Wu Tang*

Name: Decoction for Strengthening the Spleen—Yang

Source: The book *Shang Han Lun*

Ingredients:

Fu Ling (Poria) 9 g, *Shao Yao* (Radix Paeoniae Alba) 9 g, *Bai Zhu* (Rhizoma Atractylodis Macrocephalae) 6 g, *Sheng Jiang* (Rhizoma Zingiberis Recens) 9 g, *Fu Zi* (Radix Aconiti Lateralis Preparata) 9 g.

Explanation:

Fu Zi: The principal drug, being pungent and sweet in flavor and hot in nature, warming up the kidney and spleen, supporting *Yang* to dispel cold.

Fu Ling: Strengthening the spleen, removing dampness, inducing diuresis.

Sheng Jiang: Assisting *Fu Zi* in warming up *Yang* to dispel cold, working together with *Fu Ling* to warm and remove dampness.

Bai Zhu: Strengthening the spleen and removing dampness.

Bai Shao: Inducing diuresis, relieving spasm, arresting pain.

Effect: Warming up *Yang* to remove dampness.

Indications: Syndrome of retention of dampness in the interior due to *Yang*−deficiency of the spleen and kidney, marked by dysuria, heaviness and soreness of the limbs, abdominal pain, diarrhea, edema, no thirst, whitish tongue coating, and deep pulse, or fever unrelieved after sweating, palpitation under the heart, dizziness, twitching of the body with the tendency to fall down, etc., including such diseases with the above symptoms as chronic colitis, chronic nephritis, cardiac edema, hyperaldosteronism, hypothyroidism, intestinal tuberculosis, Menier's syndrome, etc..

Administration: Decocted in water for oral dose to be taken twice.

Case Study: 15 cases of congestive heart−failure, 7 cases with 4 degree's heart function, 7 with 3 degree's and 1 with 2 degree's, 3 cases with 1 onset of heart failure, 9 with 2−3 repeated onsets and 3 with more than 4, were clinically treated with the method of resisting infection and removing wind—dampness and the prescription of *Zhen Wu Tang*,whose ingredients were:

Fu Zi (Radix Aconiti Lateralis Preparata) 9—18 g, *Fu Ling* (Poria) 15—30 g,*Bai Zhu* (Rhizoma Atractylodis Macrocephalae) 9 g, *Bai Shao* (Radix Paeonia Alba) 9 g, *Tao Ren* (Semen Persicae) 9 g, *Hu Po* (Cortex Magnoliae Officinalis) 9 g, *Sheng Jiang* (Rhizoma Zingiberis Recens) 9—15 g, *Hong Hua* (Flos Carthami) 6—9 g.

After the treatment, basic cure was seen in 1 case, remarkable effectiveness in 6, effectiveness in 5, ineffectiveness in 3.

41 cases of Meniere's disease, a syndrome due to insufficiency of the kidney—*Yang*,dysfunction of the urinary bladder, upward adverse movement of dampness and lucid *Yang* failing to rise, marked by dizziness, vertigo, tinnitus, deafness, palpitation and twitching of the muscles in part of the cases, were treated with *Zhen Wu Tang*, whose ingredients were:

Fu Zi (Radix Aconiti Lateralis Preparata) 8 g, *Bai Zhu* (Rhizoma Atractylodis Macrocephalae) 10 g, *Fu Ling* (Poria) 12 g, *Sheng Jiang* (Rhizoma Zingiberis Recens) 10 g, *Bai Shao* (Radix Paeoniae Alba) 6 g, *Xi Xin* (Herba Asari) 3 g, *Gui Zhi* (Ramulus Cinnamomi) 5 g, *Wu Wei Zi* (Fructus Schisandrae) 6 g, *Chuan Xiong* (Rhizoma Chuanxiong) 8 g.

The result was: 35 cases were cured, 6 cases were improved.

It has proved that *Zhen Wu Tang* has the effects of strengthening the heart, inducing diuresis, promoting the function of the stomach and intestines in absorbing nutrients and eliminating the remains in the body.

16.21   The Prescription of *Shipi San*

Name: Powder for Reinforcing the Spleen
Source: The book *Chong Ding Yan Shi Ji Sheng Fang*
Ingredients:

Hou Po (Cortex Magnoliae Officinalis prepared with ginger juice) 6 g, *Bai Zhu* (Rhizoma Atractylodis Macrocephalae) 6 g, *Mu Gua* (Fructus Chaenomelis) 6 g, *Mu Xiang* (Radix Aucklandiae) 6 g, *Cao Guo Ren* (Fructus Tsaoko) 6 g, *Da Fu Zi* (Semen Arecae) 6 g, *Fu Zi* (Radix Aconiti Lateralis Preparata) 6 g, *Bai Fu Ling* (Poria) 6 g, *Gan Jiang* (Prepared Rhizoma Zingiberis) 6 g, *Zhi Gan Cao* (Radix Glycyrrhizae Preparata) 3 g, *Sheng Jiang* (Rhizoma Zingiberis Recens) 3 g, *Da Zao* (Fructus Jujubae) 1 dates.

Explanation:

Fu Zi: One of the principal drugs, being pungent and sweet in flavor and greatly heat in nature, warming the spleen and kidney, promoting the functional activity of *Qi*, dispelling cold–dampness.

Gan Jiang: The other principal drug, being pungent in flavor and hot in nature, warming up the spleen–*Yang*, assisting the spleen in digesting food material, dispelling cold–dampness.

Fu Ling and *Bai Zhu*: Strengthening the spleen, removing dampness, mildly inducing diuresis.

Mu Gua: Being aromatic in nature, enlivening the spleen, removing dampness, inducing diuresis.

Hou Po, Mu Xiang, Da Fu Pi and *Cao Guo*: Desending *Qi* to eliminate stagnancy, resolving dampness, inducing diuresis.

Gan Cao, Sheng Jiang and *Da Zao*: Tempering the actions

of all the other ingredients, invigorating the spleen and regulating the stomach.

Effect: Warming up *Yang* to strengthening the spleen, promoting the circulation of *Qi*, removing dampness.

Indications: Syndrome of edema due to deficiency of *Yang*,marked by severe swelling of the lower limbs, cold hands and feet, no thirst, fullness in the chest and abdomen,loose stools, thick greasy tongue coating, and deep slow pulse; including such diseases with the above symptoms as chronic nephritis, ascites due to cirrhosis and cardiac edema.

Administration: Decocted in water for oral dose to be taken twice (Taken originally in the form of powder).

Case Study: 1 case of severe ascites due to cirrhosis , a syndrome of stagnation of *Qi* and deficiency of both the spleen and kidney, marked by distention and fullness in the abdomen, poor appetite, belching, regurgitation of sour fluid, lassitude of the limbs, difficulty in walking, etc., was clinically treated with modified *Shipi Yin*,whose ingredients were:

Dang Shen (Radix Codonopsis) 12 g, *Mu Tong* (Caulis Aristolochiae Manshuriensis) 9 g, *Ze Xie* (Rhizoma Alismatis) 9 g, *Yu Jin* (Radix Curcumae) 9 g, *Chen Pi* (Pericarpium Citri Reticulatae) 4.5 g. 5 doses taken relieved the symptoms and signs, another 40 doses taken in combination with pills of *Sijunzi* and *Guipi Wan* cured the case.

16.22 The Prescription of *Bixie Fenqing Yin*

Name: Yam Decoction for Clearing Turbid Urine
Source; The book *Dan Xi Xin Fa*
Ingredients:

Yi Zhi (Fructus Alpiniae Oxyphyllae) 10 g, *Chuan Bi Xie* (Rhizoma Dioscorea Hypoglaucae) 10 g, *Shi Chang Pu*(Rhizoma Acori Tatarinowii) 10 g, *Wu Yao* (Radix Linderae) 10 g.

Explanation:

Bi Xie: The principal drug, being bitter in flavor and cold in nature, inducing diuresis and removing dampness.

Yi Zhi: Warming up the kidney–*Yang*,astringing urination to arrest enuresis.

Wu Yao: Warming the kieney and urinary bladder, cutting down the frequency of urination.

Shi Chang Pu: Promoting diuresis to remove dampness and eliminate deficiency–cold of the urinary bladder.

Effect: Warming the kidney, inducing diuresis and removing dampness.

Indications: Syndrome due to deficiency–cold of the lower–*Jiao* and down–flowing dampness, marked by frequent urination with urine as white as rice–soup and as thick as a dilute paste; including such diseases with the above symptoms as chyluria, chronic prostatitis and chronic cystitis.

Administration: Decocted in water for oral dose to be taken twice.

Case Study: 1 case of itching and pain in the penis, a syndrome due to damp–heat flowing downward to the urinary bladder and urethra and damage of the penis, marked by imaginable itching in the penis of a child at the age of 8 with a history of 6 years, light–red tongue with thin slightly yellowish coating, and thready rapid pulse, was clinically treated with *Bixie Fenqing Yin,* whose ingredients were:

Bi Xie (Rhizoma Dioscoreae Septemlobae) 12 g, *Yi Ren*

(Semen Coicis) 12 g, *Mu Gua* (Fructus Chaenomelis) 4.5 g, *Sheng Di* (Radix Rehmanniae) 12 g, *Zhu Ye* (Herba Lophatheri) 6 g, *Chi Shao* (Radix Paeoniae Rubra) 6 g, *Dang Gui* (Radix Angelicae Sinensis) 6 g, *Yuan Shen* (Radix Scrophulariae) 9 g, *Yin Hua* (Flos Lonicerae) 12 g, *Ku Shen* (Radix Sophorae Flavescentis) 9 g, *Liu Yi San* (a kind of powder) 12 g. The itching was remarkedly relieved after 5 doses were taken, the case was cured after another 20 doses.

2 cases of renal tuberculosis complicated by hematuria marked by waist ache, frequent urination and bloody urine, were treated with *Bixie Fenqing Yin* until the urine became clear. Then the ingredients except the principal drug were omitted one by one. Finally only *Bi Xie* was administered. 9 g of it was decocted in water for oral use each day and this was kept doing for half a year to 2 years. By so doing, the symptoms and signs were relieved, the hematuria was arrested, no side effects being found.

16.23 Prescriptions for Dispelling Wind to Remove Dampness

This kind of prescriptions are mainly composed of drugs with the action of dispelling wind and removing dampness. They are indicated for arthragia due to affection of exogenous wind–dampness and beriberi due to cold–dampness, marked by headache, general ache, obstinate numbness of the loins and knees, heaviness in the limbs, or swelling and heaviness and weakness in the feet and legs, etc.. The commonly used drugs are:

Qiang Huo (Rhizoma seu Radix Notopterygii), *Du Huo* (Radix Angelicae Pubescentis), *Fang Feng* (Radix

Saposhinkoviae), *Qin Jiao* (Radix Gentianae Macrophyllae).
The representative Prescriptions are *Qianghuo Shengshi Tang* and *Duhuo Jisheng. Tang.*

16.24   The Prescription of *Qianghuo Shengshi Tang*

Name: Decoction of Notoperygium for Rheumatism
Source: The book *Nei Wai Shang Ban Huo Lun*
Ingredients:

Qiang Huo (Rhizoma seu Radix Notopterygii) 6 g, *Du Huo* (Radix Angelicae Pubescentis) 6 g, *Gao Ben* (Rhizoma Ligustici) 3 g, *Fang Feng* (Radix Saposhinkoviae) 3 g, *Zhi Gan Cao* (Radix Glycyrrhizae Preparata) 3 g, *Chuan Xiong* (Rhizoma Chuanxiong) 3 g, *Man Jing Zi* (Fructus Viticis) 2 g.

Explanation:

Qiang Huo: One of the principal drugs, being pungent and bitter in flavor and warm in nature, taking a particular role in removing wind—dampness. in the upper of the body, working together with *Du Huo* to expel wind—dampness throughout the body and the joints so as to treat arthralgia,

Du Huo: The other principal drug, being pungent and bitter in flavor and slightly warm in nature, playing an active part in removing wind—dampness in the lower of the body, working together with *Qiang Huo* to expel wind—dampness throughout the body and the joints so as to treat arthralgia.

Fang Feng, Gao Ben and *Man Jing Zi*:   Eliminating wind—dampness and relieving headache.

Chuan Xiong: Promoting the circulation of blood, removing wind, relieving pain.

Gan Cao: Tempering the actions of all the other ingredients.

Effect: Dispelling wind to remove dampness.

Indications: Syndrome due to wind—dampness in the superficies of the body, marked by pain of the shoulders and back which makes the head impossible turn backward, headache, heavy sensation of the body, or soreness of the loins and back bone which makes turning sideward impossible, whitish tongue coating, and floating pulse; including such diseases with the above symptoms as common cold, rheumatic arthritis, nervous headache, etc.

Administration: Decocted in water for oral dose to be taken twice.

16.25 The Prescription of *Duhuo Jisheng Tang*

Name: Pubescent Angelica and Loranthus Decoction

Source: The book *Bei Ji Qian Jin Yao Fang*

Ingredients:

Du Huo (Radix Angelicae Pubescentis) 9 g, *Ji Sheng* (Herba Taxilli) 18 g, *Du Zhong* (Cortex Eucommiae) 9 g, *Niu Xi* (Radix Achyrantis Bidentatae) 9 g, *Xi Xin* (Herba Asari) 3 g, *Qin Jiao* (Radix Gentianae Macrophyllae) 9 g, *Fu Ling* (Poria) 12 g, *Rou Gui Xin* (Cortex Cinnamomi) 1.5 g, *Fang Feng* (Radix Saposhinkoviae) 9 g, *Chuan Xiong* (Rhizoma Chuanxiong) 6 g, *Ren Shen* (Radix Ginseng) 10 g, *Gan Cao* (Radix Glycyrrhizae) 6 g, *Dang Gui* (Radix Angelicae Sinensis) 12 g, *Shao Yao* (Radix Paeoniae Alba) 9 g, *Gan Di Huang* (Radix Rehmanniae) 15 g.

Explanation:

Du Huo: The prinicpal drug, being pungent and bitter in

flavor and slightly warm in nature, playing an active part in removing cold—dampness in the lower—*Jiao* and the joints.

Xi Xin: Dispelling cold to relieve pain.

Fang Feng: Dispelling wind to remove dampness.

Qin Jiao: Expelling wind—dampness to relax the tendons.

Ji Sheng, Du Zhong and *Niu Xi*: Expelling wind—dampness and reinforcing the liver and kidney.

Dang Gui, Chuan Xiong, Di Huang and *Bai Shao*: Nourishing blood and promoting its circulation.

Ren Shen and *Fu Ling*: Invigorating *Qi* and strengthening the spleen.

Gui Xin: Warming and clearing the blood vessels.

Gan Cao: Tempering the actions of all the other ingredients.

Effect: Expelling wind—dampness, relieving, arresting pain due to arthralgia—syndrome, reinforcing the liver and kidney, tonifying *Qi* and blood.

Indications: Syndromes such as arthralgia due to persistent wind—cold—dampness, insufficiency of the liver and kidney, and deficiency of both *Qi* and blood, all marked by pain of the loins and knees, limited movement or numbness of the joints, aversion to cold, preference for warmth, palpitation, shortness of breath, pale tongue with whitish coating, and thready feeble pulse; including such diseases with the above symptoms as chronic arthritis, rheumatic sciatica, etc.

Administration: Decocted in water·for oral dose to be taken 3 times.

Case Study: 19 cases of sciatica were clinically treated with modified *Duhuo Jisheng Tang* ,whose main ingredients were:

Du Huo (Radix Angelicae Pubescentis) 15 g, *Sang Ji Sheng*

(Herba Taxilli) 20 g, *Qin Jiao* (Radix Gentianae Macrophyllae) 15 g, Xi Xin (Herba Asari) 5 g, *Chuan Xiong* (Rhizoma Chuanxiong) 15 g, *Fang Feng*(Radix Saposhinkoviae) 15 g, *Gou Ji* (Rhizoma Cibotii) 25 g, *Tu Si Zi* (Semen Cuscutae) 25 g, *Xu Duan* (Radix Dipsaci) 40 g, **Huang Qi** (Radix Astragali) 25 g, *Xi Xian Cao* (Herba Siegesbeckiae) 20 g, *Dang Gui* (Radix Angelicae Sinensis) 15 g, *Hong Hua* (Flos Carthami) 10 g, *Dang Shen* (Radix Codonopsis) 25 g, *Niu Xi* (Radix Achyranthis Bidentatae) 15 g, *Gan Cao* (Radix Glycyrrhizae) 10 g.

In case of severe pain due to trauma, the drugs added were:

Ru Xiang (Resina Olibani Preparata)

Mo Yao (Myrrha Preparata)

In case of heaviness in the legs, the drug added was:

Sheng Yi Ren (Semen Coicis).

In case of numbness, the drugs added were:

Mu Gua (Fructus Chaenomelis)

Hei Mu Er (Jew's ear).

In case of severe chills, the drug added was:

Gui Zhi (Ramulus Cinnamomi).

The treatment brought about satisfactory curative effects in all the 19 cases.

40 cases of dysfunction of temporomandibular joint syndrome were treated with modified *Duhuo Jisheng Tang,*whose ingredients were:

Shu Di (Radix Rehmanniae Preparata), *Niu Xi* (Radix Achyranthis Bidentatae), *Du Zhong* (Cortex Eucommiae), *Sang Ji Sheng* (Herba Taxilli), *Dang Gui* (Radix Angelicae Sinensis), *Bai Shao* (Radix Paeoniae Alba), *Chuan Xiong* (Rhizoma Chuanxiong), *Dang Shen* (Radix Codonopsis), *Fu Ling* (Poria),

Gan Cao (Radix Glycyrrhizae), *Qiang Huo* (Rhizoma seu Radix Notopterygii), *Du Huo* (Radix Angelicae Pubescentis), *Xi Xin* (Herba Asari), *Gui Xin*(Ramulus Cinnamomi), *Qin Jiao* (Radix Gentianae Macrophyllae), *Fang Feng* (Radix Saposhinkoviae).

After 3—30 doses on the average were taken by each of the 40 cases, complete cure was seen in 38 cases, remarkable effectiveness in 2.

16.26   The Prescription of *Jiming San*

Name: Cock Crowing Powder

Source: The book *Zheng Zhi Zhun Sheng*

Ingredients:

Bing Lang (Semen Arecae) 15 g, *Chen Pi* (Pericarpium Citri Reticulatae) 9 g, *Mu Gua* (Fructus Chaenomelis) 9 g, *Wu Yu* (Fructus Evodiae) 3 g, *Zi Su Ye* (Folium Perillae) 3 g, *Jie Geng* (Radix Platycodi) 5 g, *Sheng Jiang* (Rhizoma Zingiberis Recens) 5 g, *Sheng Jiang Pi* (Exocarpium Zingiberis Recens) 5 g.

Explanation:

Bing Lang: The principal drug, being Pungent and bitter in flavor and warm in nature, promoting the circulation of Qi and removing dampness.

Mu Gua: Relaxing muscles and tendons and activating the flow of *Qi* and blood in the channels and collaterals, and resolving dampness.

Chen Pi: Strengthening the spleen, removing dampness, promoting the flow of *Qi* to eliminate stagnancy.

Zi Su Ye and *Jie Geng*:   Facilitating the activity of *Qi*, dispersing pathogens in the exterior, resolving stagnancy in the interior.

Wu Zhu Yu and *Sheng Jiang*: Warming and resolving cold—dampness, checking upward adverse flow of *Qi* and relieving vomiting.

Effect: Promoting the circulation of *Qi* , descending the turbid, dispersing and resolving cold—dampness.

Indications: Beriberi due to cold—dampness, marked by swelling and heaviness and weakness and numbness and cold—pain in the feet and tibias, aversion to cold, fever, or muscles cramps, upward flow of *Qi* , even full sensation in the chest and nausea; including such diseases with the above symptoms as beriberi and filariasis.

Administration: All the drugs are decocted in water for the decoction. The decoction is taken cold on an empty stomach in the early morning.

Case Study: 12 cases of beriberi were clinically treated with *Jiming San.* 4 cases were cured after 1 dose was taken by each of them, 5 after 2, and 3 after 3.

52 cases of filariasis, most of which were included in the syndrome of cold—dampness stagnated in the channels, were treated with *Jiming San,* whose main ingredients were:

Bing Lang (Semen Arecae) 60 g, *Mu Gua* (Fructus Chaenomelis) 30 g, *Gan Jiang* (Rhizoma Zingiberis) 30 g, *Chen Pi* (Pericarpium Citri Reticulatae) 30 g, *Jie Geng* (Radix Platycodi) 30 g, *Su Ye* (Folium Perillae) 30 g, *Wu Yu* (Fructus Evodiae) 30 g, *Fu Ling (*Poria) 30 g, *Qiang Huo* (Rhizoma seu Radix Notopterygii) 30 g.

All the above were ground into fine powder, which was divided into 50 portions and wrapped in paper separately. Taking this powder was began from 1: 30 pm, 1 portion was taken each time, 1 time every 2 hours, 5 times every day, 10 days constituted 1 course of treatment. The result was: complete subsiding of the feet swelling occurred in 34 cases, half subsiding in 11, relieving in 7.

17 Prescriptions for Eliminating Phlegm

17.1 Prescriptions for Eliminating Phlegm

Prescriptions mainly composed of phlegm−eliminating drugs, having the effect of removing phlegm−retention and used for treating various diseases due to phlegm are all known as "prescriptions for eliminating phlegm". They are suitable for all the disorders due to phlegm such as cough, dyspnea, shortness of breath, dizziness, vomiting, manic−depressive psychosis, epilepsy induced by terror, subcutaneous nodule, scrofula, etc,. Based on the differences in phlegm pathogens and in the ways for treating them, prescriptions for eliminating phlegm fall into the following five: those for removing dampness to eliminate damp−phlegm, those for clearing away heat to eliminate heat−phlegm, those for moistening dryness to eliminate dry−phlegm, those for warming the cold to eliminate cold−phlegm, and those for dispelling wind to eliminate wind−phlegm.

Any of the prescriptions for eliminating phlegm consists of drugs most of which have the action of promoting the circulation of *Qi* and blood and dispersing the stagnancy of them, so prolonged use of it is not suggested. prescriptions for warming the cold or moistening dryness to eliminate phlegm should be cautiously used for a patient with the tendency of hemoptysis lest large amount of hemoptysis be induced. When cough due to exogenous pathogens and with exterior syndrome is treated, what should be first prescribed is prescriptions for ventilating the lung to relieve exterior syndrome not prescriptions for clearing away heat or moistening dryness to eliminate phlegm.

17.2　Prescriptions for Removing Dampness to Eliminate Damp−phlegm

This kind of prescriptions are mainly made up of drugs with the action of removing dampness and eliminating phlegm. They are suitable for the syndrome due to damp−phlegm, marked by cough with profuse sputum easy to expectorate, fullness in the chest and abdomen, nausea, vomiting, dizziness, palpitation, whitish slippery or whitish greasy tongue coating, and slow or taut slippery pulse. The commonly used drugs are:

Chen Pi (Pericarpium Citri Reticulatae), *Ban Xia* (Rhizoma Pinelliae), *Ju Hong* (Exocarpium Citri Rubrum), etc.

The representative prescriptions are *Erchen Tang, Wendan Tang* and *Fuling Wan.*

17.3　The Prescription of *Erchen Tang*

Name: Two Old Drugs Decoction
Source:
Tai Ping Hui Min He Ji Ju Fang
Ingredients:
Ban Xia (Rhizoma Pinelliae) 9 g, *Ju Hong* (Exocarpium Citri Rubrum) 9 g, *Fu Ling* (Poria) 6 g, *Zhi Gan Cao* (Radix Glycyrrhizae Preparata) 3 g, *Sheng Jiang* (Rhizoma Zingiberis

Recens) 3 g, *Wu Mei* (Fructus Mume) one.

Explanation:

Ban Xia: The principal drug, removing dampness, resolving phlegm, regulating the stomach, relieving vomiting.

Ju Hong: Promoting the circulation of *Qi,* removing dampness, resolving phlegm.

Fu Ling: Strengthening the spleen, inducing diuresis.

Sheng Jiang: Checking upward adverse flow of *Qi,* resolving phlegm, assisting *Ban Xia* and *Ju Hong* in promoting the circulation of *Qi* to eliminate phlegm.

Wu Mei: Astringing the lung—*Qi* so as to make it not be damaged while phlegm is eliminated.

Zhi Gan Cao: Tempering the actions of all the other ingredients.

Effect: Removing dampness, resolving phlegm, promoting the circulation of *Qi,* regulating the stomach.

Indications: Syndrome due to damp—phlegm, marked by cough with profuse whitish sputum easy to expectorate, fullness in the chest, nausea, vomiting, lassitude, or dizziness, palpitation, whitish greasy tongue coating, and slippery pulse; including such diseases with the above symptoms as chronic bronchitis, pulmonary emphysema, peptic ulcer, Meniere's disease, morning sickness during pregnancy, infantile salivation, etc.

Administration: Decocted in water for oral dose to be taken twice.

Case Study: *Erchen Tang* in combination with modified *Pingwei San* was clinically used to treat 55 cases of chronic bronchitis, 33 of which were associated with pulmonary emphysema. Effectiveness was seen in all the cases. In general, the cough and dyspnea were relieved within 1 week. Meanwhile, the time—vital—capacity and movable function of the diaphragm were also improved to certain extent.

Erchen Tang was taken in the form of powder to treat 7 cases of simple goiter with 5 cases cured, 2 improved, the course of treatment averaging 15 days.

17.4 The Prescription of *Wendan Tang*

Name: Decoction for Clearing away Gallbladder—heat

Source: The book *San Yin Ji Yi Bing Zheng Fang Lun*

Ingredients:

Ban Xia (Rhizoma Pinelliae) 6 g, *Zhu Ru* (Caulis Bambusae in Taeniam) 6 g, *Zhi Shi* (Fructus Aurantii Immaturus) 6 g, *Chen Pi* (Pericarpium Citri Reticulatae) 9 g, *Zhi Gan Cao* (Radix Glycyrrhizae Preparata) 3 g, *Fu Ling* (Poria) 5 g, *Sheng Jiang* (Rhizoma Zingiberis Recens) 3 g, *Da Zao* (Fructus Jujubae) 1 dates.

Explanation:

Ban Xia: The principal drug, checking upward adverse flow of *Qi,* regulating the stomach, removing dampness, resolving phlegm.

Zhu Ru: Clearing away heat, resolving phlegm, relieving vomiting, reducing dysphoria.

Zhi Shi: Promoting the flow of *Qi,* eliminating phlegm.

Chen Pi: Regulating the flow of *Qi,* removing dampness, resolving phlegm.

Fu Ling: Strengthening the spleen and inducing diuresis to aid in eliminating phlegm.

Sheng Jiang, Da Zao and *Zhi Gan Cao:* Replenishing the spleen, regulating the stomach, tempering the actions of all the other ingredients.

Effect: Regulating the flow of *Qi,* resolving phlegm, clearing away heat in the gallbladder, promoting the function of the stomach.

Indications: Syndrome due to incoordination between the gallbladder and stomach and disturbance of phlegm—heat in the interior, marked by vexation of deficiency type, insomnia, or vomiting, hiccup, dizziness, fullness in the chest, palpitation, nervousness, yellowish, greasy tongue coating, and slippery rapid or taut rapid pulse; including such diseases with the above symptoms as peptic ulcer, Meniere's disease, hypertension, cerebral arteriosclerosis, psychoneurosis, climacteric syndrome and coronary arteriosclerotic cardiopathy.

Administration: Decocted in water for oral dose to be taken twice.

Case Study: At a time, modified *Wendan Tang* was clinically used to treat 62 cases of Meniere's disease and 6 cases of vertebrobasilar ischemia with better curative effects.

17.5   The Prescription of *Fuling Wan*

Name: Pill of Poria

Source: The book *Zhi Mi Fang*

Ingredients:

Ban Xia (Rhizoma Pinelliae) 60 g, *Fu Ling* (Poria) 30 g, *Zhi Qiao* (Fructus Aurantii Preparata) 15 g, *Feng Hua Pu Xiao* (efflorescenced Natrii Sulfas) 7.5 g.

Explanation:

Ban Xia: The principal drug, removing dampness, resolving phlegm.

Fu Ling: Strengthening the spleen and inducing diuresis so as to promote the elimination of phlegm.

Zhi Qiao: Regulating the flow of *Qi* and relieving depression.

Pu Xiao: Softening masses and causing laxation.

Jiang Zhi: Reducing the toxicity of *Ban Xia* and resolving phlegm.

Effect: Removing dampness, promoting the circulation of *Qi,* eliminating phlegm.

Indications: Syndrome due to retention of phlegm—dampness in the interior, marked by soreness of the upper limbs or edema in the 4 limbs, or cough with profuse sputum, fullness in the chest and epigastric region, whitish greasy tongue coating, and taut slippery pulse; including such diseases with the above symptoms as peripheral neuritis, dysthyroidism, chronic bronchitis and pulmonary emphysema.

Administration: The ingredients are ground into fine powder and made with an adequate amount of ginger juice into pills. 6 g of the pills is taken with ginger—infused water or boiled water each time, twice daily.

17.6 Prescriptions for Clearing away Heat to Eliminate Heat—phlegm

This kind of prescriptions are mainly composed of drugs with the action of clearing away heat and eliminating phlegm. They are suitable for the syndrome due to heat—phlegm, marked by cough with yellowish thick sputum and difficult to expectorate, reddened tongue with yellowish greasy coating, and slippery rapid pulse.

Drugs such as:

Huang Qin (Radix Scutellariae), *Huang Lian* (Rhizoma Coptidis), *Gua Lou* (Fructus Trichosanthis), *Dan Nan Xing* (Arisaema cum Bile), *Ban Xia* (Rhizoma Pinelliae), etc..

The representative prescriptions are *Qing Qi Huatan Wan* and *Xiao Xianxiong Tang*.

17.7 The Prescriptions of *Qing Qi Huatan Wan*

Name: Bolus for Clearing Heat and Phlegm

Source: The book *Yi Fang Kao*

Ingredients:

Gua Lou Ren (Semen Trichosanthis) 30 g, *Chen Pi* (Pericarpium Citri Reticulatae) 30 g, *Huang Qin* (Radix Scutellariae) 30 g, *Xing Ren* (Semen Armeniacae Amarum) 30 g, *Zhi Shi* (Fructus Aurantii Immaturus) 30 g, *Fu Ling* (Poria) 30 g, *Dan Nan Xing* (Arisaema cum Bile) 45 g, *Zhi Ban Xia* (Rhizoma Pinelliae Preparata) 45 g.

Explanation:

Dan Nan Xing: Clearing away heat and resolving phlegm.

Gua Lou: Assisting *Dan Nan Xing* in clearing away the lung—heat so as to resolve heat—phlegm.

Zhi Shi and *Chen Pi:* Regulating the flow of *Qi,* eliminating phlegm, dispersing stagnancy.

Fu Ling: Strengthening the spleen, inducing diuresis. *Xing Ren:* Ventilating the lung and arresting cough.

Ban Xia: Removing dampness and resolving phlegm.

Effect: Clearing away heat ,resolving phlegm, regulating the flow of *Qi,* arresting cough.

Indications: Syndrome due to retention of phlegm—heat in the lung, marked by cough with yellowish thick sputum difficult to expectorate, fullness in the chest, reddened tongue with yellowish greasy coating, and slippery rapid pulse; including such diseases with the above symptoms as pneumonia, acute bronchitis, acute attack of chronic bronchitis, and bronchiectasis complicated by infection.

Administration: All the drugs are ground into fine powder. The powder is made with an adequate amount of ginger juice into boluses. 6 g of the boluses is taken with warm boiled water each time, twice daily. With their amounts reduced according to their original proportions, the drugs may be decocted in water for oral use.

17.8   The Prescription of *Xiao Xianxiong Tang*

Name: Minor Decoction for Relieving Stuffiness in the Chest

Source: The book *Shang Han Lun*

Ingredients:

Huang Lian (Rhizoma Coptidis) 6 g, *Ban Xia* (Rhizoma Pinelliae) 12 g, *Gua Lou* (Fructus Trichosanthis) 30 g.

Explanation:

Gua Lou: The principal drug, clearing away heat, resolving phlegm, relieving stuffiness in the chest, dispersing stagnancy.

Huang Lian: Clearing away heat and purging fire.

Ban Xia: Checking upward adverse flow of *Qi,* regulating the stomach, resolving phlegm.

Effect: Clearing away heat, resolving phlegm, relieving stuffiness in the chest, dispersing stagnancy.

Indications: Syndrome due to combination of phlegm and heat, marked by fullness and tenderness in the chest and epigastric region, or cough with yellowish thick sputum, yellowish greasy tongue coating, and slippery rapid or floating rapid pulse; including such diseases with the above symptoms as pleuritis, intercostal neuralgia, bronchitis, pneumonia, acute and chronic gastritis and cholecystitis.

Administration: Decocted in water for oral dose to be taken twice.

Case Study: *Xiao Xianxiong Tang* and *Guizhi Jiagui Tang* were clinically used to treat angioneuropathy headache with temporary curative effects. In general, the headache was remarkably relieved after 3—5 doses were taken.

17.9   The Prescription of *Guntan Wan*

Name: Pill for Eliminating Stubborn Phlegm
Source: The book *Dan Xi Xin Fa Fu Yu*
Ingredients:

Da Huang (Radix et Rhizoma Rhei steamed with liquor) 240 g, *Huang Qin* (Radix Scutellariae cleaned with liquor) 240 g, *Duan Meng Shi* (Lapis Micae Aureus Usta) 30 g, *Chen Xiang* (Lignum Aqailariae Resinatum) 15 g.

Explanation:

Duan Meng Shi : Sending down the flow of *Qi* to arrest

asthma, eliminating phlegm to alleviate palpitation.

Da Huang: Relaxing the bowels and purging fire.

Huang Qin: Clearing away heat in the upper—*Jiao*.

Chen Xiang: Regulating the activity of *Qi*.

Effect: Purging fire and eliminating phlegm

Indications: Syndrome due to heat of excess type and stubborn phlegm, marked by manic—depressive psychosis, palpitation due to fright, irritability, or severe palpitation leading to coma, or cough and dyspnea with thick sputum, or fullness in the chest and epigastric region, dizziness, tinnitus, constipation, reddened tongue with yellow thick greasy coating, and slippery rapid forceful pulse; including such diseases with the above symptoms as manic—depressive psychosis, epilepsia, chronic bronchitis, bronchial asthma, etc..

Administration: All the drugs are ground into fine powder and made with water into pills. 6—9 g of the pills is taken with warm boiled water each time, twice daily.

With drastic drug potency, this prescription is suitable for mere stubborn phlegm due to excess heat and strong constitution. It should be cautiously used when patients with weak constitution or pregnant women are treated.

Case Study: 30 cases of post—traumatic brain syndrome were clinically treated with *Guntan Wan* and modified *Guizhi Jiagui Tang*. The symptoms and signs were nearly eliminated in 22 cases, remarkable improvement was seen in 6 cases, improvement in 1 case.

17.10 Prescriptions for Moistening Dryness to Eliminate Dry-phlegm

This kind of prescriptions are mainly made up of drugs with the action of moistening the lung and eliminating phlegm. They are indicated for the syndrome due to dry-phlegm, marked by thick and sticky sputum difficult to expectorate, dry throat, or irritating cough with hoarse noise, etc.. The commonly used drugs. are:

Bei Mu (Bulbus Fritillariae), *Gua Lou* (Fructus Trichosanthis), etc..

The representative prescriptions are *Beimu Gualou San,* etc..

17.11 The Prescription of *Beimu Gualou San*

Name: Powder of Fritillary Bulb and Snakegourd Fruit

Source: The book *Yi Xue Xin Wu*

Ingredients:

Bei Mu (Bulbus Fritillariae) 5 g, *Gua Lou* (Fructus Trichosanthis) 3 g, *Tian Hua Fen* (Radix Trichosanthis) 2.5 g, *Fu Ling* (Poria) 2.5 g, *Ju Hong* (Exocarpium Citri Reticulatae) 2.5 g, *Jie Geng* (Radix Platycodi) 2.5 g.

Explanation:

Bei Mu: Clearing away heat, moistening the lung, resolving phlegm, arresting cough.

Gua Lou: Clearing away heat and eliminating phlegm so as to moistening dryness.

Tian Hua Fen: Clearing away heat, resolving phlegm, promoting the production of body fluids, moistening dryness.

Fu Ling: Strengthening the spleen, inducing diuresis.

Ju Hong: Regulating the flow of *Qi,* resolving phlegm.

Jie Geng: Ventilating the lung, checking upward adverse flow of *Qi,* eliminating phlegm, relieving cough.

Effect: Moistening the lung, clearing away heat, resolving phlegm, relieving cough.

Indications: Syndrome of retention of phlegm due to dryness in the lung, marked by cough, dyspnea difficulty in coughing up sputum, dry and sore throat, reddened tongue with little dry coating etc.; including such diseases with the above symptoms as chronic bronchitis, bronchial asthma, bronchiectasis, pulmonary tuberculosis and pneumosilicosis.

Administration: Decocted in water for oral dose to be taken twice.

17.12 Prescriptions for Warming the Cold to Eliminate Cold−phlegm

This kind of prescriptions are mainly made up of drugs pungent in flavor and warm in nature and drugs with the action of eliminating phlegm. They are suitable for the syndrome due to cold−phlegm, marked by cough, shortness of breath, clear watery whitish sputum, fullness in the chest, and whitish slippery or whitish greasy tongue coating. The commonly used drugs are:

Gan Jiang (Rhizoma Zingiberis), *Xi Xin* (Herba Asari), *Wu Wei Zi* (Fructus Schisandrae), *Su Zi* (Fructus Perillae), etc.

The representative prescriptions are *Ling Gan Wuwei Jiang Xin Tang* and *Sanzi Yangqin Tang.*

17.13 The Prescription of *Ling Gan Wuwei Jiang Xin Tang*

Name: Decoction of Poria, Licorice, Schisandra, Dried Ginger and Asarum

Source: The book *Jin Gui Yao Lue*

Ingredients:

Fu Ling (Poria) 12 g, *Gan Cao* (Radix Glycyrrhizae) 6 g, *Gan Jiang* (Rhizoma Zingiberis) 9 g, *Xi Xin* (Herba Asari) 6 g, *Wu Wei Zi* (Fructus Schisandrae) 6 g.

Explanation:

Gan Jiang: Being pungent in flavor and hot in nature, not only warming the lung and dispelling cold so as to eliminate retained phlegm but also warming up the spleen—*Yang* so as to removing dampness.

Xi Xin: Warming the lung to dispel cold, assisting *Gan Jiang* in eliminating retained phlegm.

Fu Ling: Strengthening the spleen and inducing diuresis so as to eliminate phlegm.

Wu Wei Zi: Astringing the lung to relieve cough.

Gan Cao: Regulating the stomach, tempering the actions of all the other ingredients.

Effect: Warming and eliminating phlegm

Indications: Syndrome due to retention of cold—phlegm in the in terior, marked by cough with profuse watery sputum, fullness in the chest, shortness of breath, whitish slippery tongue coating, and taut slippery pulse; including such diseases with the above symptoms as chronic bronchitis, pulmonary emphysema, bronchial asthma and bronchiectasis.

17.14   The Prespription of *Sanzi Yangqin Tang*

Name: Decoction of Three Kinds of Seeds for the Aged.

Source: The book *Han Shi Yi Tong*

Ingredients:

Bai Jie Zi (Semen Sinapis Albae 6 g, *Su Zi* (Fructus Perillae) 9 g, *Lai Fu Zi* (Semen Raphani) 9 g.

Explanation:

Bai Jie Zi: Warming the lung to regulate the flow of *Qi,* soothing the chest to resolve phlegm.

Su Zi: Descending the flow of *Qi* to resolve phlegm, relieving cough and asthma.

Lai Fu Zi: Promoting digestion to remove food stagnancy, activating the circulation of *Qi* to eliminate phlegm.

Effect: Resolving phlegm, promoting digestion, relieving cough and arresting asthma.

Indications: Cough and asthma due to retention of phlegm and stagnation of *Qi,* marked by cough and dyspnea with profuse whitish sputum, fullness in the chest, poor appetite, whitish greasy tongue coating, and slippery pulse; including such diseases with the above symptoms as chronic bronchitis, bronchial asthma, bronchiectasis, pulmonaryemphysema and pulmonary heart disease.

Administration: All the drugs are pounded into powder. The powder is wrapped in gauze and decocted in water for the decoction. The decoction is taken regularly.

Prolonged use of this prescription is not suggested to the

aged and the weak. If it does be needed, drugs for regulating and tonifying the spleen and lung or for strengthening the spleen and reinforcing the kidney should be added.

Case Study: *Sanzi Yangqin Tang* was clinically used together with *Gui Fu Lizhong Tang* to treat, in turn, 195 and 97 cases of chronic bronchitis, the effective reaching 88% and 85.6%. Most of the cases became stronger and less susceptible to common cold, showing that this prescription has the action of enhancing body resistance.

17.15 The Prescription of *Lengxiao Wan*

Name: Pill for Treating Asthma of Cold Type.

Source: The book *Zhang Shi Yi Tong*.

Ingredients:

Ma Huang (Herba Ephedrae) 30 g, *Sheng Chuan Wu* (Radix Aconiti) 30 g, *Xi Xin* (Herba Asari) 30 g, *Hua Jiao* (Pericarpium Zanthoxyli) 30 g, *Bai Fan* (Alumen) 30 g, *Zhi Zao Jiao* (Spina Gleditsiae Preparata) 30 g, *Ban Xia Qu* (Rhizoma Pinelliae prepared with flour and ginger juice) 30 g, *Dan Nan Xing* (Arisaema cum Bile) 30 g, *Xing Ren* (Semen Armeniacae Amarum) 30 g, *Gan Cao* (Radix Glycyrrhizae) 30 g, *Zi Wan* (Radix Asteris) 60 g, *Dong Hua*(Flos Farfarae) 60 g.

Explanation:

Ma Huang, *Chuan Wu* and *Xi Xin:* Warming the lung, resolving phlegm, ventilating the lung, relieving asthma. *Hua Jiao:* Warming up the middle—*Jiao* and removing dampness.

Bai Fan and *Zao Jiao:* Eliminating phlegm and relieving fullness.

Ban Xia Qu and *Dan Nan Xing:* Eliminating phlegm and checking upward adverse flow of *Qi.*

Xing Ren, Zi Wan and *Dong Hua:* Eliminating phlegm, arresting cough and relieving dyspnea.

Gan Cao: Tempering the actions of all the other ingredients.

Effect: Warming the lung, eliminating phlegm.

Indications: Dyspnea and cough due to wind—cold, marked by dyspnea and shortness of breath which makes it difficult to lie flat, cough with sputum occurring when it is cold, fullness in the chest, whitish slippery tongue coating, and floating slippery or taut slippery pulse; including such diseases with the above symptoms as bronchial asthma, asthmatic bronchitis, chronic bronchitis and pulmonary emphysema.

Administration: All the drugs are ground into fine powder. The powder is made with ginger juice into pills. 6 g of the pills is taken with warm boiled water each time, twice daily. Instead, the drugs may be decocted in water for oral use. In doing so, their amounts should be reduced according to their original proportions.

This prescription is used mainly when the onset of cough and dyspnea take place. Once the disease condition is controlled, prescriptions for regulating and reinforcing the spleen and lung should be used instead or as the compatible ones in order that the body resistance can be enhanced and relapse may be prevented.

17.16 Prescriptions for Dispelling Wind to Eliminate Wind—phlegm

This kind of prescriptions are mainly composed of drugs

with the action of dispelling wind pathogen or calming the liver to tranquilize the endogenous wind and the compatible drugs with the action of eliminating phlegm. They are indicated for the syndrome due to wind—phlegm. Because the syndrome due to wind—phlegm is caused either by exogenous or endogenous pathogen, prescriptions for treating it fall into two: those for dispelling exogenous wind to eliminate phlegm and those for calming endogenous wind to eliminate phlegm.

Prescriptions for dispelling exogenous wind to eliminate phlegm are suitable for the syndrome due to attack of exogenous wind pathogen on the lung, marked by aversion to wind, fever, productive cough, thin whitish tongue coating, etc.. Drugs such as:

Jing Jie (Herba Schizonepetae), *Zi Wan* (Radix Asteris), *Jie Geng* (Radix Platycodi), *Bai Bu* (Radix Stemonae), *Chen Pi* (Pericarpium Citri Reticulatae), etc.

are commonly used in these prescriptions, whose representatives are *Zhisou San* , etc.

Prescriptions for calming endogenous wind to eliminate phlegm are suitable for the syndrome due to endogenous wind pathogen and phlegm, marked by dizziness, headache, or epilepsy which even leads to coma and unconsciousness, etc.. Drugs such as:

Tian Ma (Rhizoma Gastrodiae), *Ban Xia* (Rhizoma Pinelliae), *Fu Ling* (Poria), etc.

are commonly used in these prescriptions, whose representatives are *Banxia Baizhu Tianma Tang*, *Dingxian Wan*, etc.

17.17　The Prescription of *Zhisou San*

Name: Cough Powder

Source: The book *Yi Xue Xin Wu*

Ingredients:

Jie Geng (Radix Platycodi) 1000 g, *Zi Wan* (Radix Asteris) 1000 g, *Jing Jie* (Herba Schizonepetae) 1000 g, *Bai Bu* (Radix Stemonae) 1000 g, *Bai Qian* (Rhizoma Cynanchi Stauntonii) 1000 g, *Zhi Gan Cao* (Radix Glycyrrhizae Preparata) 375 g, *Chen Pi* (Pericarpium Citri Reticulatae) 500 g.

Explanation:

Zi Wan, Bai Bu and *Bai Qian:* Arrest cough and eliminating phlegm.

Jie Geng and *Chen Pi:* Ventilating and descending the lung−*Qi*, eliminating phlegm and arresting cough.

Jing Jie: Dispelling wind to relieve exterior syndrome.

Gan Cao: Tempering the action of all the other ingredients.

Jing Jie, Jie Geng and *Gan Cao:* Working together to remove intense heat from the throat and relieve pain.

Effect: Dispelling wind, ventilating the lung, eliminating phlegm, arresting cough.

Indications:

Cough and dyspnea due to attack of wind pathogen on the lung, marked by cough, itching of the throat, expectoration, or mild aversion to cold, fever, thin whitish tongue coating, and floating pulse; including such diseases with the above symptoms as acute bronchitis, chronic bronchitis, pertussis and influenza.

Administration: All the drugs are ground into fine powder. 6

g of the powder is taken with warm boiled water each time 2–3 times daily. With the amounts reduced according to their orignal proportions, the drugs may also be decocted in water for oral use.

Case Study: 28 cases of whooping cough were clinically treated with modified *Zhisou San,* 1 dose daily. The decoction was taken regularly in small amounts. 19 cases were cured, who took 5–7 doses each, improvement showed in 6 cases, ineffectiveness in 3, one of which was complicated by pneumonia.

Modified *Zhisou San* was decocted in water to treat 290 cases of cough due to affection of exogenous pathogens, in which there were infection of the upper respiratory tract, acute bronchitis and pneumonia. The onset of the disorder in 238 cases occurred not more than 15 days ago. The result was: 273 cases (97%) were cured, they each avoraging just more than 3 doses. The curative effects was not satisfactory in 7 cases. But no side effects was found in any of the cases.

17.18   The Prescription of *Banxia Baizhu Tianma Tang*

Name: Decoction of Pinellia, Bighead Atractylodes and Gastrodia

Source: The book *Yi Xue Xin Wu*

Ingredients:

Zhi Ban Xia (Rhizoma Pinelliae Preparata) 9 g, *Tian Ma* (Rhizoma Gastrodiae) 6 g, *Fu Ling* (Poria) 6 g, *Ju Hong* (Exocarpium Citri Reticulatae) 6 g, *Bai Zhu* (Rhizoma Atractylodis Macrocephalae) 15 g, *Gan Cao* (Radix Glycyrrhizae)

4 g, *Sheng Jiang* (Rhizoma Zingiberis Recens) 1 piece, *Da Zao* (Fructus Jujubae) 2 dates.

Explanation: *Ban Xia:* Removing dampness, eliminating phlegm, checking upward adverse flow of *Qi* and arresting nausea.

Tian Ma: Soothing the liver to calm the endogenous wind, being good at relieving dizziness, often used compatibly with *Ban Xia* to treat dizziness due to wind—phlegm.

Bai Zhu and *Fu Ling:* Strengthening the spleen and inducing diuresis so as to eradicate the source of phlegm.

Ju Hong: Regulating the flow of *Qi* and eliminating phlegm.

Sheng Jiang and *Da Zao:* Regulating the function of the spleen and stomach.

Effect: Removing dampness, eliminating phlegm, calming the liver to tranquilize the endogenous wind.

Indications: Syndrome due to disturbance of wind—phlegm in the interior, marked by dizziness, headache, fullness in the chest, nausea, vomiting, whitish greasy tongue coating and taut slippery pulse; including such diseases with the above symptoms as hypertension, Meniere's disease, squela of cerebral concussion, cerebral arteriosclerosis and vestibular neuritis.

Indications: Decocted in water for oral dose to be taken twice

Case Study: Modified *Banxia Baizhu Tianma Tang* was clinically used to treat 28 cases Meniere's disease with satisfactory curative effects, controlling the onset and improving the symptoms and signs.

At a time, modified *Banxia Baizhu Tianma Tang* was employed to treat 7 cases of tuberculous meningitis with satisfactory curative effects. 5–year follow–up found out that all the cases remained in good condition, showing that this prescription has the action of lowering blood pressure, arresting nausea and stopping spasm. Tuberculous meningitis has a long disease course. So, taking the decoction was continued after the symptoms and signs were eliminated so that the curative effects was consolidated.

17.19   The Prescription of *Dingxian Wan*

Name: Pills for Relieving Epilepsy

Source: The book *Yi Xue Xin Wu*

Ingredients:

Tian Ma (Rhizoma Gastrodiae) 30 g, *Chuan Bei Mu* (Bulbus Fritillariae Cirrhosae) 30 g, *Ban Xia* (Rhizoma Pinelliae) 30 g, *Fu Ling* (Poria) 30 g, *Fu Shen* (Poria cum Ligno Hospite) 30 g, *Dan Nan Xing* (Arisaema cum Bile) 15 g, *Shi Chang Pu* (Rhizoma Acori Tatarinowii) 15 g, *Quan Xie* (Scorpio) 15 g, *Gan Cao* (Radix Glycyrrhizae) 15 g, *Jiang Can* (Bombyx Batryticatus) 15 g, *Hu Po* (Cortex Magnoliae Officinalis) 15 g, *Deng Xin Cao* (Medulla Junci) 15 g, *Chen Pi* (Pericarpium Citri Reticulatae) 22 g, *Yuan Zhi* (Radix Polygalae) 22 g, *Dan Shen* (Radix Salviae Miltiorrhizae) 60 g, *Mai Dong* (Radix Ophiopogonis) 60 g, *Zhu Sha* (Cinnabaris) 9 g.

Explanation:

Zhu Li: Clearing away heat, eliminating phlegm, relieving convulsion, calming the mind, working together with ginger juice to exert the potency of resolving phlegm to induce resuscitation.

Dan Nan Xing: Clearing away heat, resolving phlegm, tranquilizing the mind, relieving epilepsy.

Ban Xia, Chen Pi, Chuan Bei Mu, Fu Ling and *Mai Dong:* Eliminating phlegm, checking upward adverse flow of *Qi* and protecting *Yin* from being damaged.

Dan Shen and *Shi Chang Pu:* Resolving stasis for resuscitation.

Quan Xie and *Jiang Can:* Calming endogenous wind and relieving muscle spasm.

Tian Ma: Calming the liver to tranquilize endogenous wind so as to eliminate wind—phlegm.

Zhu Sha, Hu Po, Yuan Zhi, Deng Xin Cao and *Fu Shen:* Relieving convulsion, calming the mind so as to aid in relieving muscle spasm and epilepsy.

Gan Cao: Invigorating *Qi* to strengthen body resistance, tempering the actions of all the other ingredients.

Effect: Eliminating phlegm to induce resuscitation, calming endogenous wind to relieve epilepsy.

Indications: Syndrome of epilepsy and depressive psychosis due to phlegm—heat, marked by sudden loss of consciousness leading to falling down, rigidity of the muscles, convulsion and white frothy saliva or laryngeal rales, coming to within a short time, or irritability, reddened tongue with yellowish or whitish greasy coating, and taut slippery or slippery rapid pulse; including such diseases with the above symptoms as depressive psychosis, schizophrenia, manic—depressive psychosis, etc..

Administration: All the drugs are ground into fine powder Another 120 g of *Gan Cao* (Radix Glycyrrhizae) is decocted in an appropriate amount of water and condensed into a paste. The powder, the paste, 100 ml of *Zhu Li* (Succus Bambusae) and 50 ml of ginger juice are mixed evenly into pills. 6 g of the pills is taken with warm boiled water each time, twice daily. With their amounts reduced according to their proportions in the original prescription, the drugs may be decocted in water for oral use.

Case Study: 21 cases of epilepsy were clinically treated with this prescription with the total effective rate reaching 85.7%.

Dingxian Wan and modified *Fengyin Tang* were used together to treat 31 cases of epilepsy, of which 9 cases were cured and didn't see relapse in the following 2 years of follow-up, 11 cases were basically controlled, 5 cases were improved, the rest were remained the same, the total effective rate being 80.6%.

18 Prescriptions for Promoting Digestion and Removing Stagnated Food

18.1 Prescriptions for Promoting Digestion and Removing Food Stagnation

Prescriptions mainly composed of drugs with the action of removing food retention and promoting digestion, and used to eliminate stagnancy of indigested food, relieve flatulence and disintegrate masses are all known as "prescriptions for promoting digestion and removing food stagnation". In this chapter, we only deal with the following two: those for promoting digestion to remove stagnancy of indigested food and those for removing stagnation of *Qi* to disintegrate masses.

Digestion—promoting prescriptions and purgative prescriptions are the same in eliminating formalized pathogens of excess type. But they are different in clinical practice. Mild in potency, the former is used to remove retained food and gradually—developed masses in the stomach or intestines which are chronic and last longer. Drastic in potency, the latter is used to remove accumulation of tangible pathogens in the intestines and constipation which are acute and last shorter.

Although mild in potency, prescriptions for promoting digestion and removing food stagnation are, after all, those which play their part by eliminating. They, therefore, are contraindicated for the syndromes only due to deficiency not accompanied by excess. While they are used, such food difficult to digest as the raw, the cold and the greasy are avoided.

18.2 Prescriptions for Promoting Digestion to Remove Stagnancy of Indigested Food

This kind of prescriptions are mainly made up of drugs with the action of promoting digestion to remove retained food. They are suitable for the syndrome due to retention of food, marked by fullness in the epigastrium and abdomen, anorexia, hiccup with foul odor, nausea, vomiting, or abdominal pain, diarrhea, etc. The commonly used drugs are:

Shan Zha (Fructus Crataegi), Shen Qu (Massa Medicata Fermentata), Lai Fu Zi (Semen Raphani), Zhi Shi (Fructus Aurantii Immaturus), etc.

The representative prescriptions are Baohe Wan and Zhishi Daozhi Wan.

In case of weakness of the spleen and stomach, indigestion of food or impairment of the spleen and stomach due to long retention of food, drugs with the action of promoting digestion to remove retained food should be compatibly used with the action of invigorating Qi to strengthen the spleen to form prescriptions for both reinforcing and eliminating, whose reprentatives are Jianpi Wan and Zhi Zhu Wan.

18.3 The Prescription of Baohe Wan

Name: Lenitive Pill

Source: The book *Dan Xi Xin Fa*

Ingredients:

Shan Zha (Fructus Crataegi) 180 g, *Shen Qu* (Massa Medicata Fermentata) 60 g, *Ban Xia* (Rhizoma Pinelliae) 90 g, *Fu Ling* (Poria) 90 g, *Chen Pi* (Pericarpium Citri Reticulatae) 30 g, *Lian Qiao* (Fructus Forsythiae) 30 g, *Lai Fu Zi* (Semen Raphani) 30 g.

Explanation:

Shan Zha: The principal drug, promoting digestion to remove food stagnancy especially the stagnancy of greasy meat food.

Shen Qu: Promoting digestion, strengthening the spleen, playing an active part in dispelling retained spoiled food with liquor.

Lai Fu Zi: Promoting digestion, descending *Qi* flowing adversely, being good at removing stagnated grain food.

Ban Xia and *Chen Pi:* Promoting the circulation of *Qi* to remove stagnated food, regulating the function of the stomach to arrest nausea.

Fu Ling: Strengthening the spleen and inducing diuresis, regulating the stomach and relieving diarrhea.

Lian Qiao: Clearing away heat possibly produced by stagnated food and removing food stagnancy.

Effect: Promoting digestion, regulating the function of the stomach.

Indications: Syndrome due to retention of various kinds of food, marked by fullness in the epigastrium and abdomen, distending pain, foul belching, regurgitation of sour fluid, anorexia, nausea, vomiting, or loose stools, thick greasy tongue coating, and slippery pulse; including such diseases with the above symptoms as indigestion, acute or chronic gastroenteritis, chronic gastritis and chronic pancreatitis.

Administration: All the drugs are ground into fine powder. The powder is made with water into pills. 6—9 g of the pills is taken with warm boiled water each time, twice daily. With their amounts reduced according to their original proportions, the drugs may be also decocted in water for oral use.

Case Study: Modified *Baohe Wan* was clinically used to treat 69 cases of infantile indigestion included in the syndrome of food retention with 61 cases cured, 5 cases improved and 3 cases unimproved.

Modified *Baohe Wan* was also used to treat 20 cases of acute infection of biliary tract, of which 7 were simple cholecystitis, 9 were cholelithiasis complicated by cholecystitis, 4 were cholangitis. The treatment result was: remarkable effectiveness was shown in 14 cases, the signs being eliminated, recovery being shown in the laboratory report; improvement in 5 cases, the symptoms being eliminated, recovery being shown in the laboratory report, but there remaining mild signs; ineffectiveness in 1 case.

18.4   The Prescription of *Zhishi Daozhi Wan*

Name: Pill of Immature Bitter Orange for Removing Stagnancy

Source: The book *Nei Wai Shang Bian Huo Lun*

Ingredients:

Da Huang (Radix et Rhizoma Rhei) 30 g, *Zhi Shi* (Fructus

Aurantii Immaturus stir−fried with wheat bran) 15 g, *Shen Qu* (stir−fried Massa Medicata Fermentata) 15 g, *Fu Ling* (Poria) 9g, *Huang Qin* (Radix Scutellariae) 9 g, *Huang Lian* (Rhizoma Coptidis) 9 g, *Bai Zhu* (Rhizoma Atractylodis Macrocephalae) 9 g, *Ze Xie* (Rhizoma Alismatis) 6 g.

Explanation:

Da Huang: Eliminating stagnancy and purging heat by way of laxation.

Zhi Shi: Assisting *Da Huang* in promoting the circulation of *Qi,* eliminating stagnancy and relieving distention and fullness in the epigastrium and abdomen.

Huang Qin and *Huang Lian:* Being the assistant drugs in this prescription, clearing away heat, removing dampness and relieving diarrhea.

Shen Qu: Promoting digestion and regulating the function of the stomach.

Effect: Promoting digestion, removing stagnated food, clearing away heat and expelling dampness.

Indications: Syndrome due to retention of damp−heat and indigested food in the stomach and intestines, marked by distending pain in the epigastrium and abdomen, loose stools, or constipation, scanty deep−colored urine, yellowish greasy tongue coating, and slippery rapid pulse; including such diseases with the above symptoms as acute indigestion, gastroenteritis, bacterial dysentery and acute or chronic cholecystitis.

Administration: All the drugs are ground into fine powder. The powder is made with water into pills. 6−9 g or the pills is taken with warm boiled water each time, twice daily. With their amounts properly reduced according to their original proportions, the drugs may be also decocted in water for oral dose.

This prescription is for removing stagnancy. It is not suggested to prescribe it to treat diarrhea or dysentery not due to stagnated food.

18.5 The Prescription of *Muxiang Binglang Wan*

Name: Pill of Aucklandia and Areca Seed

Source: The book *Dan Xi Xin Fa*

Ingredients:

Mu Xiang (Radix Aucklandiae) 30 g, *Bing Lang* (Semen Arecae) 30 g, *Qing Pi* (Pericarpium Citri Reticulatae Viride) 30 g, *Chen Pi* (Pericarpium Citri Reticulatae) 30 g, *E Zhu* (Rhizoma Curcumae) 30 g, *Huang Lian* (Rhizoma Coptidis) 30 g, *Huang Bai* (Cortex Phellodendri) 30 g, *Da Huang* (Radix et Rhizoma Rhei) 15 g, *Zhi Xiang Fu* (Rhizoma Cyperi Preparata) 60 g, *Qian Niu Zi* (Semen Pharbitidis) 60 g.

Explanation:

Mu Xiang and *Bing Lang:* Promoting the circulation of *Qi* to remove stagnancy, relieving fullness in the epigastrium and abdomen and arresting tenesmus, acting as the principal drugs.

Qian Niu Zi and *Da Huang:* Clearing away heat, promoting bowel movement and removing stagnancy.

Qing Pi and *Chen Pi:* Promoting the flow of *Qi* to remove stagnancy.

Xiang Fu and *E Zhu:* Soothing the liver and regulating the circulation of *Qi*, harmonizing *Qi* and blood.

Zhi Qiao: Promoting the flow of *Qi,* removing stagnancy, strengthening the stomach to activate the digestive function.

Huang Lian and *Huang Bai:* Clearing away heat, removing dampness and arrest diarrhea.

Effect: Promoting the circulation of *Qi,* removing stagnancy, eliminating stagnated food and clearing away heat.

Indications: Syndrome due to indigested food and damp—heat retained in the interior, marked by fullness and distending pain in the epigastrium and abdomen, stools with blood and pus, tenesmus, or constipation, yellowish greasy tongue coating, and deep replete pulse; including such diseases with the above symptoms as acute gastroenteritis, bacterial dysentery and ulcerative colitis.

Administration: All the drugs are ground into fine powder. The powder is made with water into small pills. 3—6 g of the pills is taken with warm boiled water each time, twice daily.

In clinical practice, constipation, diarrhea or dysentery may be all treated with this prescription as long as they are, proved through differentiation and analysis of TCM, due to food retention and not complicated by exterior syndrome and deficiency of vital *Qi.* But they should be cautiously used when weak patients with deficiency of vital *Qi.*

18.6   The Prescription of *Zhi Zhu Wan*

Name: Pill of Immature Bitter Orange and Bighead Atractylodes

Source: The book *Pi Wei Lun*

Ingredients:

Chao Zhi Shi (stir-fried Fructus Aurantii Immaturus) 30 g, *Bai Zhu* (Rhizoma Atractylodis Macrocephalae) 60 g.

Explanation:

Bai Zhu: Strengthening the spleen, removing dampness so as to assist the spleen in transporting and transforming of food material, being administered in the amount 1 time more than *Zhi Shi* in order that its action of invigorating the pleen—*Qi* can be enhanced.

Zhi Shi: Promoting the circulation of *Qi,* removing food stagnancy and fullness.

Effect: Strengthening the spleen and removing fullness.

Indications: Syndrome due to deficiency of the spleen, stagnancy of *Qi* and retention of food, marked by fullness or distending pain in the epigastrium and abdomen, poor appetite, or borborygmus, pale tongue with whitish slippery coating, and weak pulse; including such diseases with the above symptoms as gastroptosis, chronic gastritis, gastric neurosis and indigestion.

Administration: The drugs are ground into fine powder. The powder is made with water into pills. 6—9 g of the pills is taken with warm boiled water each time, twice daily. With their amounts properly reduced according to their original proportions, the drugs may be decocted in water for oral use.

Case Study: At a time, *Zhi Zhu Wan* and modified *Shengxian Tang* were clinically used together to treat gastroptosis, hysteroptosis and proctoptosis with better curative effects.

18.7 The Prescription of *Jianpi Wan*

Name: Pill for Invigorating the Spleen.

Source: The book *Zheng Zhi Zhun Sheng*

Ingredients:

Bai Zhu (Rhizoma Atractylodis Macrocephalae stir—fried with wheat bran) 75 g, *Mu Xiang* (Radix Aucklandiae) 22 g, *Huang Lian* (Rhizoma Coptidis) 22 g, *Gan Cao* (Radix Glycyrrhizae) 22 g, *Fu Ling* (Poria) 60 g, *Ren Shen* (Radix Ginseng) 45 g, *Chao Shen Qu* (stir—fried Massa Medicata Fermentata) 30 g, *Chen Pi* (Pericarpium Citri Reticulatae) 30 g, *Sha Ren* (Fructus Amomi) 30 g, *Chao Mai Ya* (stir—fried Fructus Hordei Germinatus) 30 g, *Shan Zha* (Fructus Crataegi) 30 g, *Shan Yao* (Rhizoma Dioscoreae) 30 g, *Wei Rou Dou Kou* (roasted Semen Myristicae) 30 g.

Explanation:

Ren Shen, Bai Zhu, Fu Ling and *Gan Cao:* Invigorating *Qi* and strengthening the spleen.

Shan Zha, Shen Qu and *Mai Ya:* Promoting digestion to remove stagnated food.

Mu Xiang, Sha Ren and *Chen Pi:* Regulating the activity of *Qi* to promote the function of the stomach.

Shan Yao and *Rou Dou Kou:* Strengthening the spleen and arresting diarrhea.

Huang Lian: Clearing away heat and removing dampness.

Effect: Strengthening the spleen and promoting digestion

Indications: Syndrome of retention of food in the interior due to weakness of the spleen and stomach, marked by poor appetite, indigestion, fullness in the epigastrium and abdomen, loose stools, greasy thin yellowish tongue coating, and weak pulse; indigestion, chronic gastroenteritis, gastric neurosis, irritable colon and intestinal tuberculosis.

Administration: All the drugs are ground into fine powder. The powder is made with water into pills. 6–9 g of the pills is taken with warm boiled water each time, twice daily. With their amounts properly reduced according to their original proportions, the drugs may be decocted in water for oral use.

Case Study:

Jianpi Wan together with *Fuzi Lizhong Wan* was clinically used to treat 24 cases of chronic diarrhea due to deficiency of the kidney–*Yang* occurred before dawn, after abdominal pain and borborygmus, followed by comfort, and complicated by aversion to cold, soreness and weakness of the loins and knees, etc. 1 bolus of *Jianpi Wan* being honeyed and weighing 3 g was taken after meal each time, 3 times daily, and 1 bolus of *Fuzi Lizhong Wan* was taken each time, twice daily. The course of treatment was 8 days to 1 month. The result was: 22 cases were cured, 2 cases didn't carry the treatment through to the end, stopping taking the boluses because the effectiveness was not seen.

18.8 Prescriptions for Removing Stagnation of *Qi* to Disintegrate Masses

This kind of prescriptions are composed of drugs with the action of promoting digestion to remove stagnated food, activating the flow of *Qi* and blood, and disintegrating and eliminating masses. They are suitable for the syndrome due to masses in the abdomen, marked by masses palpable below the hypochondrium (hepatomegaly and Splenomegaly), or distention and fullness and pain in the epigastrium and abdomen, poor appetite, emaciation, etc., The commonly used drugs are:

Zhi Shi (Fructus Aurantii Immaturus), Hou Po (Cortex Magnoliae Officinalis), Ban Xia (Rhizoma Pinelliae), Bie Jia (Carapax Trionycis), Shao Yao (Radix Paeoniae Alba), Dan Pi (Cortex Moutan), Tao Ren (Semen Persicae), etc.

The representative prescriptions are Zhishi Xiaopi Wan, Biejia Jian Wan, etc.

18.9　The Prescription of Zhishi Xiaopi Wan

Name: Pill of Immature Bitter Orange for Relieving Stuffiness.

Source: The book Lan Shi Mi Cang

Ingredients: Gan Jiang (Rhizoma Zingiberis) 3 g, Zhi Gan Cao (Radix Glycyrrhizae Preparata) 6 g, Chao Mai Ya (Parched Fructus Hordei Germinatus) 6 g, Fu Ling (Poria) 6 g, Bai Zhu (Rhizoma Atractylodis Macrocephalae) 6 g, Ban Xia Qu (Massa Pinelliae Fermentatae) 9 g, Ren Shen (Radix Ginseng) 9 g, Hou Po (Cortex Magnoliae Officinalis) 12 g, Zhi Shi (Fructus Aurantii Immaturus) 15 g, Huang Lian (Rhizoma Coptidis) 15 g.

Explanation: Zhi Shi: The principal drug, promoting the flow of Qi, disintegrating masses and relieving fullness.

Hou Po: Promoting the flow of Qi to relieve distention.

Huang Lian: Clearing away heat and removing dampness.

Ban Xia Qu: Promoting digestion, regulating the function of the stomach and disintegrating masses.

Gan Jiang: Being pungent in flavor and disperse in nature, warming up the middle—Jiao and dispelling cold.

Huang Lian, Ban Xia Qu and Gan Jiang: Being the drugs pungent for dispersion and bitter for purgation, regulating the activity of *Qi,* acting together to assist *Zhi Shi* and *Hou Po* in promoting the flow of *Qi* and disintegrating masses.

Ren Shen, Bai Zhu, Fu Ling and *Gan Cao:* Invigorating *Qi* to strengthen the spleen.

Mai Ya: Promoting digestion and regulating the function of the stomach.

Effect: Disintegrating masses, relieving fullness, strengthening the spleen and regulating the function of the stomach.

Indications: Syndrome due to deficiency of the spleen, stagnation of *Qi* and combination of cold and heat, marked. by masses and fullness in the epigastrium and abdomen, loss of appetite, lassitude, or distending pain in the abdomen, constipation or diarrhea, pale tongue with whitish coating, and taut pulse; including such diseases with the above symptoms as indigestion, chronic gastritis, chronic enteritis, chronic pancreatitis and chronic cholecystitis.

Administration: All the drugs are ground into fine powder. The powder is made with water into pills. 6—9 g of the pills is taken with warm boiled water each time, 3 times daily. With their amounts properly reduced according to their original proportions, the drugs may be decocted in water for oral use.

18.10   The Prescription of *Biejia Jian Wan*

Name: Decocted Turtle Shell Pill
Source: The book *Jin Gui Yao Lue*
Ingredients:
Bie Jia (Carapax Trionycis) 90 g, *She Gan* (Rhizoma Belamcandae) 22.5 g, *Huang Qin* (Radix Scutellariae) 22.5 g,

Chao Shu Fu (stir—fried Armadillidium Vulgare) 22.5 g, *Gan Jiang* (Rhizoma Zingiberis) 22.5 g, *Da Huang* (Radix et Rhizoma Rhei) 22.5 g, *Gui Zhi* (Ramulus Cinnamomi) 22.5 g, *Shi Wei* (Folium Pyrrosiae) 22.5 g, *Hou Po* (Cortex Magnoliae Officinalis) 22.5 g, *Qu Mai* (Herba Dianthi) 22.5 g, *Zi Wei* (Radix Campsis) 22.5 g, *E Jiao* (Colla Corii Asini) 22.5 g, *Chai Hu* (Radix Bupleuri) 45 g, *Chao Zhang Lang* (stir—fried Blatla seu Periplaneta) 45 g, *Shao Yao* (Radix Paeoniae Alba) 37 g, *Dan Pi* (Cortex Moutan) 37 g, *Chao Zhe Chong* (Stir—fried Eupolyphaga seu Stelephaga) 37 g, *Zhi Feng Chao* (Nedus Vespar Preparata) 30 g, *Chi Xiao* (Natrii Sulfas) 90 g, *Tao Ren* (Semen Persicae) 15 g, *Ren Shen* (Radix Ginseng) 7.5 g, *Ban Xia* (Rhizoma Pinelliae) 7.5 g, *Ting Li Zi* (Semen Lepidii) 7.5 g.

Explanation:

Bie Jia: Softening and disintegrating masses.

Huang Jiu (millet wine): Promoting the circulation of blood through the channels.

Chi Xiao, Da Huang, Zhe Chong, Zhang Lang and *Shu Fu:* Promoting the circulation of blood, removing blood stasis and disintegrating masses.

Chai Hu, Huang Qin and *Bai Shao:* Regulating the activity of the liver—*Qi*.

Hou Po, She Gan, Ting Li Zi and *Ban Xia:* Regulating the activity of *Qi*, dispersing stagnancy and eliminating phlegm.

Gan Jiang and *Gui Zhi:* Warming up the middle—*Jiao*, disintegrating masses.

Ren Shen and *E Jiao:* Invigorating *Qi*, nourishing blood and enhancing vital *Qi*.

Tao Ren, Dan Pi, Zi Wei and *Feng Chao:* Promoting the circulation of blood to remove blood stasis.

Qu Mai and *Shi Wei:* Inducing diuresis to remove dampness.

Effect: Disintegrating masses and removing stagnancy.

Indications: Syndrome due to various masses, marked by masses below the hypochondriums or in the abdomen, abdominal pain, emaciation, poor appetite, intermittent chills and fever, or amenorrhea, tongue fur purple in color or with ecchymosis, and uneven pulse; including such diseases with the above symptoms as malaria, chronic hepatitis, cirrhosis and schistosomiasis.

Administration: 1.5 kg of plant ash is steeped in 5 kg of millet wine and then the ash is filtered out to get the decoction, in which *Bie Jia* is decocted into a gum. All the other drugs are ground into fine powder. The gum and the powder are made with honey into pills. 3 g of the pills is taken with warm boiled water each time, 3 times daily.

Case Study: At a time, *Biejia Jian Wan* was clinically used to treat 251 cases of hepatosplenomegaly due to schistosomiasis in the late stage. After the treatment, both the liver and the spleen became smaller to different extent. The effective rate reached 100%, the consolidating rate being 80%.

19 Prescriptions for Expelling Intestinal Parasites

19.1 Prescriptions for Expelling Intestinal Parasites

Prescriptions with drugs having the action of expelling worms as their main ingredients, with expelling intestinal parasites, removing food stagnancy and relieving pain as their effects, and with parasitosis as their indications are all known as "prescriptions for expelling intestinal parasites". Parasites in the body are of many kinds, the common ones in the digestive canal are ascaris, pinworm, ancylostoma and cestode, which enter the body along with dirty food with ova on and cause parasitosis marked by intermittent pain around the navel and in the abdomen which does not reduce appetite, complexion sallow or blue or pale in color or with pityriasis simplex, or discomfort in the stomach, vomiting of clear water, tongue with exfoliative coating, and alternate large and small pulse. Prolonged parasitosis may be also marked by emaciation, larger belly on which blue veins are releaved, and even malnutrition. In addition, red and white spots on the inner line of the lips is a sign of ascariasis, pruritus and is a sign of oxyuriasis, white prolottis in stools is a sign of cestodiasis, addiction to eating non–food material, sallow complexion and puffiness is a sign of hookworm disease. Prescriptions of this kind are indicated for all the above parasites and parasitoses. Before they are prescribed, however, what kind of the worm to be killed shoud be identified in order that the prescription which the worm is most susceptible to is selected. Meanwhile, drugs for clearing away heat, for warming the interior, for promoting digestion or for tonification should be compatibly used in this kind of pre-scriptions according to deficiency or excess of vital Qi and cold or hot nature of accompanying syndromes. Drugs such as:

Wu Mei (Fructus Mume)

Ku Lian Gen Pi (Cortex Meliae)

Shi Jun Zi (Fructus Quisqualis)

Fei Zi (Radix Aconiti Lateralis Preparata)

Bing Lang (Semen Arecae), etc. are commonly used in these prescriptions, whose reprentatives are *Wumei Wan* , etc.

All the drugs for expelling worms should be taken on an empty stomach. Greasy food should be avoided when some of them are taken. The spleen and stomach should be regulated after the worms are expelled. Drugs for expelling worms should be cau-tiously used for the old, the weak and pregnant women. Their amounts should be properly controlled, for overdose will impair vital Qi or lead to poisning and too small dose will fail to expel the worms.

19.2   The Prescription of *Wumei Wan*

Name: Black Plum Pill

Source: The book *Shang Han Lun*

Ingredients:

Wu Mei(Fructus Mume) 480 g, *Xi Xin* (Herba Asari) 180 g,

Gan Jiang (Rhizoma Zingiberis) 300 g, *Huang Lian* (Rhizoma Coptidis) 480 g, *Dang Gui* (Radix Angelicae Sinensis) 120 g, *Fu Zi* (Radix Aconiti Lateralis Preparata) 180 g, *Chao Shu Jiao* (stir-fried Pericarpium Zanthoxyli) 120 g, *Gui Zhi* (Ramulus Cinnamomi) 180 g, *Ren Shen* (Radix Ginseng) 180 g, *Huang Bai* (Cortex Phellodendri) 180 g.

Explanation:

Wu Mei: The principal drug, being sour in flavor and neutral in nature, calming roundworms to restrain their movement so as to arrest pain.

Shu Jiao and *Xi Xin:* Being pungent in flavor to expel roundworms, being warm in nature to warm the internal organs and dispel cold.

Gui Zhi, Fu Zi and *Gan Jiang:* Helping warm the internal organs and dispel cold.

Ren Shen and *Dang Gui:* Invigorating *Qi* and nourishing blood.

Huang Lian and *Huang Bai:* Being bitter in flavor to expel roundworms, being cold in nature to remove heat in the upper, controlling the over-warm nature of all the other drugs lest *Yin* be damaged.

Effect: Warming the internal organs and calming roundworms.

Indications: Colic caused by ascaris, prolonged dysentery or diarrhea due to deficiency of vital *Qi* resulting from chills and fever, marked by intermittent fidgets and vomiting, vomiting of roundworms after eating, cold limbs, abdominal pain, or prolonged dysentery and long-lasting diarrhea; including such diseases with the above symptoms as biliary ascariasis, chronic dysentery and chronic enteritis.

Administration: *Wu Mei* is steeped in 50% vinegar for one night and then taken out. It is pounded into pieces after the core is removed. All the other drugs are also pounded into pieces. The two kinds of pieces are mixed and dried in the sun and finally ground into powder. The powder is made with honey into pills each as big as a seed of Chinese parasol. 9 g of the pills is taken on an empty stomach with warm boiled water each time, 1–3 times daily. With their amounts properly reduced according to their original proportions, the drugs may be also decocted in water for oral use.

Case Study: *Wumei Wan* was clinically used to treat 225 cases of biliary ascariasis, including the type inclining to cold, the type of alternate cold and heat and the type inclining to heat. Drugs used to treat biliary ascariasis of the type inclining to cold were:

Wu Mei (Fructus Mume) 15–30 g, *Bing Lang* (Semen Arecae) 15 g, *Chuan Lian Zi* (Fructus Toosendan) 15 g, *Hua Jiao* (Pericarpium Zanthoxyli) 6 g, *Gui Zhi* (Ramulus Cinnamomi) 6 g, *Shu Fu Zi* (Radix Aconiti Lateralis Preparata) 6 g, *Xi Xin* (Herba Asari) 3 g, *Gan Jiang* (Rhizoma Zingiberis) 3 g.

Drugs used to treat the type of alternate cold and heat were:

all of the above

Huang Bai (Cortex Phellodendri) 9 g, *Huang Lian* (Rhizoma Coptidis) 6 g.

Drugs used to treat the type inclining to heat were:

all of the above minus:

Gui Zhi (Ramulus Cinnamomi), *Gan Jiang* (Rhizoma Zingiberis), *Fu Zi* (Radix Aconiti Lateralis Preparata), *Xi Xin*

(Herba Asari).

The curative rate reached 97.6%, the effective rate 100%.

19.3 The Prescription of *Feier Wan*

Name: Fattening Baby Pill

Source: The book *Tai Ping Hui Min He Ji Ju Fang*

Ingredients:

Chao Shen Qu (stir-fried Massa Medicata Fermentata) 300g, *Huang Lian* (Rhizoma Coptidis) 300 g, *Rou Dou Kou* (Semen Myristicae coated with flour and roasted) 150 g, *Shi Jun Zi* (Fructus Quisqualis with the peel removed) 150 g, *Chao Mai Ya* (stir-fried Fructus Hordei Germinatus) 150 g, *Bing Lang* (Semen Arecae) 120 g, *Mu Xiang* (Radix Aucklandiae)60 g.

Explanation:

Shi Jun Zi: One of the principal drugs, being sweet in taste and warm in nature, killing worms and eliminating stagnated food.

Bing Lang: The other principal drug, being pungent and bitter in taste and warm in nature, killing worms and eliminating stagnated food.

Shen Qu and *Mai Ya:* Strengthening the spleen, regulating the function of the stomach and eliminating stagnated food.

Huang Lian: Clearing away retained heat.

Rou Dou Kou: Reinforcing the stomach and arresting diarrhea.

Mu Xiang: Regulating the activity of the stomach-*Qi* to relieve abdominal pain.

Zhu Dan Zhi: Clearing away heat in the liver and stomach.

Effect: Killing worms, eliminating stagnated food, strengthening the spleen and clearing away heat.

Indications: Abdominal pain due to enterositosis and indigestion, marked by sallow complexion, emaciation, anorexia, distention and fullness in the abdomen, intermittent pain around the navel, fever, foul odor in the mouth, and loose stools; including such diseases with the above symptoms as infantile ascariasis, infantile chronic indigestion and infantile malnutrition.

Administration: All the drugs are ground into fine powder. The powder is made with pig bile into pills, each as big as a millet. 3 g of the pills is for a child at the age of 3 each time, twice daily, more for the older and less for the younger.

19.4 The Prescription of *Huachong Wan*

Name: Pill for Treating Parasitic Infestation.

Source: The book *Tai Ping Hui Min He Ji Ju Fang*

Ingredients:

Hu Fen (lead powder) 1500 g, *He Shi* (Fructus Carpesii) 1500g, *Bing Lang*(Semen Arecae) 1500g, *Ku Lian Gen* (Radix Meliae) 1500 g, *Bai Fan* (Alumen) 370 g.

Explanation:

He Shi: Being bitter and pungent to the taste and neutral in nature, having slight toxicity, expelling and killing roundworms.

Ku Lian Gen Pi: Being bitter to the taste, cold in nature and poisnous, not only expelling and killing roundworms but also relieving abdominal pain.

Bing Lang: Expelling roundworms, promoting the flow of *Qi,* relieving diarrhea and helping discharge the killed worms.

Ku Fan: Detoxicating and killing worms.

Qian Fen: Being poisonous to kill worms.

Effect: Expelling and killing various of worms in the intestines.

Indications: Syndrome due to various kinds of worms in the intestines, marked by terrible abdominal pain going up and down at the onset, vomiting of clear water or roundworms.

Administration: All the drugs are ground into fine powder. The powder is made with water into pills, each as big as a hemp seed, and taken on an empty stomach with millet soup, 5 pills for an infant at the age of 1 year old.

Drastic and poisonous, this prescription should be used properly. When it is stopped, the spleen and stomach should be regulated and tonified. If continual use of it is needed to expel the remained worms, it should be one week later.

20 Preseriptions for Causing Vomiting

20.1 Prescriptions for Causing Vomiting

Prescriptions with the following three characteristics are all known as " prescriptions for causing vomiting" : 1. being composed of drugs with the action of promoting emesis, 2. having the effect of causing vomiting of sputum, saliva, indigested food and toxic material retained in the throat, chest, diaphram and stomach. 3. being suitable for the syndrome of syncope. They are usually used to eliminate abundant expectoration in apoplexy, manic−depressive psychosis and inflammation of the throat, food and toxic material stagnated in the stomach, and to promote emesis which refuses to occur but need to be reduced due to the critical disease condition. The commonly used drugs are:

Gua Di (Pedicellus Melo), Zao Jiao (Spina Gleditsiae).

The representative prescriptions are Guadi San and Jiuji Xixian San, etc.

Prescriptions for causing vomiting, quick and drastic in nature, tend to impair the stomach−Qi. They should not be used any longer when their effectiveness has been seen. When they are used to treat those infirm with age and pregnant women, caution should be taken. Over−vomiting induced by them may be stopped by taking small amount of ginger juice, cold gruel or cold boiled water. If this dosen't work, certain drugs should be chosen according to the prescription taken. For instance, 0.03–0.06g of *She Xiang* (Moschus) of 0.3–0.6g of *Ding Xiang* (Flos Caryophylli) may be taken to stop vomiting induced by *Guadi San*: prescriptions for regulating the stomach and checking upward adverse flow of *Qi* may be used to eructation following vomiting; touching of the throat with a piece of feather or a finger may be conducted to promote emesis when it does not occur after a prescription for causing vomiting is taken, or drinking more boiled water is carried out instead. Exposure to wind must be avoided so as to prevent affection by exopathogen after vomiting has been induced. In addition, the spleen and stomach need to be regulated with thin gruel. Quick intake of greasy and hard–to–digest food is inhibited lest the stomach–*Qi* be impaired again.

20.2 The Prescription of *Guadi San*

Name: Powder of Musk–melon Pedicel
Source: The book *Shang Han Lun*
Ingredients:
Gua Di (Pedicellus Melo) 4 g, *Chi Xiao Dou* (Semen Phaseoli) 4 g, *Dan Dou Chi* (Semen Sojae Preparatum) 9 g.
Explanation:
Gua Di: The Pricipal drug, being bitter in flavor and cold in nature, playing an active part in causing vomiting of sputum, saliva and stagnated food.

Chi Xiao Dou: Being sour in flavor, removing dampness, restlessness and fullness, working together with *Gua Di* to combine the sour and bitter tastes and cause vomiting.

Dou Chi: Taken in the form of decoction to expel pathogenic factors in the chest, working compatibly with *Chi Xiao Dou* to regulate the stomach—*Qi* and protect vital *Qi* from being impaired.

Effect: Causing vomiting of phlegm, saliva and stagnated food.

Indications: Syndrome due to retention of phlegm, saliva and indigested food in the chest and epigastrium, marked by fullness in the chest, heartburn, nervousness, attack of upward flow of *Qi* on the throat which leads to difficult breathing, and slight floating of *Cun* pulse; inculding such disorders with the above symptoms as mis—taking toxic material, retention of indigested food in the stomach, etc.

Administration: *Gua Di* is decocted until it looks yellow and then dried and ground together with *Chi Xiao Dou* into fine powder. 9 g of *Dou Chi* is decocted in water for the decoction. 1—3 g of the powder is taken with the decoction each time.

Because *Gua Di* is bitter, cold and poisonous, this prescription is not allowed to be used for the weak. When stagnated food has entered the intestines or phlegm and saliva are not in the chest and diaphram, this prescription is also inhibited.

20.3   The Prescription of *Juiji Xixian San*

Name: Powder for Diluting Phlegm

Source: The book *Sheng Ji Zong Lun*

Ingredients: *Zhu Ya Zao Jiao* (Fructus Gleditsiae Abnormalis) 15 g, *Bai Fan* (Alumen) 30 g.

Explanation:

Zao Jiao: The principal drug, being pungent and salty in taste and warm in nature, reducing resuscitation because of its pungent taste, softening masses because of its salty taste. eliminating turbid and sticky sputum.

Bai Fan: Being sour and bitter in flavor, resolving stubborn phlegm, reducing resuscitation to promote emesis.

Effect: Inducing resuscitation and promoting emesis.

Indications: Excess syndrome of stroke, marked by sputum in the noisy throat, difficult breathing, restlessness in the chest, blurred vision, or loosing consciousness and falling down, or face seeming to distort, and slippery replete forceful pulse; including such diseases with the above symptoms as cerebral thrombosis and chronic pharyngitis.

Administration: The drugs are ground into fine powder. 2—3g of the powder is taken with warm boiled water each time.

The usage of this prescription should be stopped and other ones are chosen instead according to the symptoms and signs as soon as the sputum becomes thin, the breathing returns to normal and the diarrhea is arrested, for this prescription is one for causing vomiting.

21 Prescriptions for Treating Carbuncles and Abscess

21.1 Prescriptions for Treating Carbuncles and abscess

Prescriptions with the following three characteristics are all known as "prescriptions for treating carbuncles and abscess": 1. being composed of drugs with the action of relieving carbuncles and abscess, 2. having the effect of removing toxic material, subduing swelling, draining pus, and promoting tissue regeneration and wound healing, 3. being used to treat skin and external disorders such as carbuncle, cellulitis, deep–rooted carbuncle, furuncle, erysipelas, multiple abscess, goiter, tumor and scrofula, and abscess in the internal organs. When skin and external disorders are treated, the local symptoms and signs manifested in the superficies of the body should be differentiated together with the general condition of the whole body in order that the *Yin* and *Yang*, the deficiency and excess, the benignancy and malignancy, and the deteriorating or favorable nature of the case can be identified. Circumscribed high–raised swelling with restrained root, deep–red skin and calor is included in *Yang* syndrome. Uncircumscribed, flat and hard or soft swelling with normal skin is included in *Yin* syndrome. When abscess in the internal organs such as pulmonary abscess, periappendicular abscess, etc. is treated, the cold and heat, the deficiency and excess, the suppuration and non–suppuration should be differentiated clearly. There are two kinds of therapeutic methods for treating carbuncle and abscess in the superficies of the body: internal and external. Prescriptions used in internal method are mainly introduced in the subject Pharmacology of Traditional Chinese Medical formulae. Internal method is subdivided into three: resolving, expelling from within and tonifying. Resolving, used in the early stage of non–suppuration, refers to relieving exterior syndrome, removing obstruction in the interior, clearing away heat, warming the channels, eliminating phlegm, activating the flow of *Qi* and promoting the circulation of blood to dispel blood stasis. Expelling from within, used in the intermediate stage, may cause the internal toxin to shift to the superficies of the body, the pus to be expelled easily, the wound to be healed soon. It fals into two; internal expelling and tonifying expelling. The former is to resolve masses and expel pus accompanied by strengthening the body resistance. The latter is both to strengthen the body resistance and expel pus. Tonifying, used in the late stage when a wound with clear watery pus is hard to heal due to deficiency of both *Qi* and blood, may enhance *Qi* and blood by means of tonification so as to promote tissue regeneration and wound healing or activate festering in undiabrosis cases. Abscess in the internal organs is treated mainly by way of clearing away heat and toxic material, removing stasis, expelling pus, resolving masses and subduing swelling. The prescriptions for this may make the wound heal easily. Drugs such as:

Shuang Hua (Flos Lonicerae), *Lian Qiao* (Fructus Forsythiae), *Chuan Shan Jia* (Squama Manitis), *Zao Ci* (Spina

Gleditsiae), *Ru Xiang* (Olibanum), *Mo Yao* (Myrrha), *Huang Qi* (Radix Astragali), *Yi Yi Ren* (Semen Coicis).

are commonly used in the prescriptions for treating abscess in the internal organs, whose representatives are *Xian fang Huoming Yin, Wuwei Xiaodu Yin, Simiao Yongan Tang, Dahuang Mudan Tang* and *Yanghe Tang.*

In clinical practice, prescriptions for treating carbuncles and abscess should be modified according to the change of disease condition. If resolving method is sticked to when carbuncle or abscess is formed, *Qi* and *blood* tend to be impaired so that festering and healing are made difficult. If expelling method is used when pus is abundant, attention should be paid to clear away the toxin completely lest the remains of it should not be eliminated. If suppuration occurs slowly, expelling should be enhanced so that toxin can be discharged along with pus, avoiding its sinking to the interior. When carbuncles with fire—toxin in the superficies of the body prevail, warmly—tonifying method is contraindicated. When the remains of toxin has not been completely eliminated, pure tonification is contraindicated.

21.2   The Prescription of *Xianfang Huoming Yin*

Name: Fairy Decoction for Treating Cutaneous Infections
Source: The book *Jiao Zhu Fu Ren Liang Fang*
Ingredients:
Bai Zhi (Radix Angelicae Dahuricae) 3 g, *Bei Mu* (Bulbus Fritillariae) 3 g, *Fang Feng* (Radix Saposhinkoviae) 3 g, *Chi Shao* (Radix Paeoniae Rubra) 3 g, *Dang Gui Wei* (Radix Angelicae Sinensis) 3 g, *Gan Cao Jie* (Radix Glycyrrhizae9 3 g, *Zao Jiao Ci* (Parched Spina Gleditsiae) 3 g, *Chuan Shan Jia* (Squama Manitis

Preparata) 3 g, *Tian Hua Fen* (Radix Trichosanthis) 3 g, *Ru Xiang* (Olibanum) 3 g, *Mo Yao* (Myrrha) 3 g, *Jin Yin Hua* (Flos Lonicerae) 9 g, *Chen Pi* (Pericarpium Citri Reticulatae) 9 g.

Explanation:

Jin Yin Hua: The principal drug, being sweet in taste and cold in nature, clearing away heat and toxic material.

Fang Feng and *Bai Zhi:* Dispelling exopathogens, expelling toxic heat through the superficies of the body.

Gui Wei, Chi Shao, Ru Xiang and *Mo Yao* Promoting blood circulation to remove blood stasis, alleviating swelling and pain.

Bei Mu and *Hua Fen:* Clearing away heat and resolving masses.

Shan Jia and *Zao Ci:* Activating the flow of *Qi* and blood in the channels and collaterals, expelling pus and promoting festering.

Chen Pi: Regulating the activity of *Qi*.

Gan Cao: Removing toxic material, regulating the stomach.

Effect: Clearing away heat and toxic material, subduing swelling, promoting festering, activating the circulation of blood and arresting pain.

Indications: Syndrome due to heat—toxin accumulation, *Qi* stagnancy and blood stasis in the early stage of carbuncle and pyogenic infection, marked by red, swelling, heat and pain of large carbuncle, or fever, slight aversion to cold, thin whitish or yellowish tongue coating, and rapid forceful pulse: including such diseases with the above symptoms as phlegmon, mammitis and purulent tonsillitis.

Administration: Decocted in water or in the same amount of liquor and water for oral dose to be taken twice.

Case Study: 30 cases of appendiceal abscess were clinically treated with *Xianfang Huoming Yin,* whose ingredients were:

Jin Yin Hua (Flos Lonicerae), *Lian Qiao* (Fructus Forsythiae), *Hua Fen* (Radix Trichosanthis), *Bei Mu* (Bulbus Fritillariae), *Zao Ci* (Spina Gleditsiae), *Sheng Di* (Radix Rehmanniae), *Dan Pi* (Cortex Moutan), *Chi Shao* (Radix Paeoniae Rubra), *Gui Wei* (Radix Angelicae Sinensis), *Gan Cao* (Radix Glycyrrhizae), *Pu Gong Ying* (Herba Taraxaci), *Ru Xiang* (Resina Olibani), *Mo Yao* (Myrrha).

After the treatment. 27 cases were cured, 3 cases were referred to surgery, No one died the rate of success was 90%. They averaged 14 days in the hospital. Follow—up of 7 cases didn't find any relapse.

Modified *Xianfang Huoming Yin* was used to treat 129 cases of carbuncle, drugs for clearing away heat and toxic material were added for the type of toxic heat, *Bazhen Tang* was added for the type of vital—*Qi* deficiency, *Liuwei Dihuang Tang* was added for the type of *Yin* —deficiency. 82 cases were treated with mere herbal medicines, 47 cases were treated with herbal medicines plus 7—day administration of western medicines, antibiofics. 14 cases were treated for 15—20 days, 20 cases for 21—30 days, 17 cases for 31—40 days, 29 cases for 41—50 days, 21 cases for 51—60 days, 28 cases for over 60 days. 127 cases (98.5%) were cured, 2 cases (1.5%) died, one of whom died of septicemia, the other renal failure due to purpuric nephritis resulting from infirmity with age. Most of the 129 cases were treated with antibiotics without any effects before admitted to hospital.

The decoction of *Xianfang Huoming Yin* in vitro, an experiment has shown, is highly resistant to streptococcus C, and so to staphylococcus. But it can not restrain Bacillus coli and Pseudomonas aeruginosa.

21.3 The Prescription of *Wuwei Xiaodu Yin*

Name: Antiphlogistic Decoction of Five Drugs
Source: The book *Yi Zong Jin Jian*
Ingredients:

Jin Yin Hua (Flos Lonicerae) 20 g, *Ye Ju Hua* (Flos Chrysanthemi) 15 g, *Pu Gong Ying* (Herba Taraxaci) 15 g, *Zi Hua Di Ding* (Herba Violae) 15 g, *Tian Kui Zi* (Radix Semiaquilegiae) 15 g.

Explanation:

Jin Yin Hua: The principal drug, being sweet in flavor and cold in nature, clearing away heat and toxic material.

Di Ding, Tian Kui, Pu Gong Ying and *Ye Ju Hua:* Clearing away heat and toxic material, removing heat from blood, resolving masses, thus subduing swelling.

Effect: Clearing heat and toxic material, expelling nail'like boil and furuncle.

Indications: Carbuncle, sore, furuncle and swelling due to fire—toxin, marked by local red, swelling, heat and pain in the early stage, or fever, chills, or deep—rooted furuncle as big as a grain and as hard as a nail, reddened tongue with yellowish coating, and rapid pulse; including such diseases with the above symptoms and signs as phlegmon, mastadenitis, suppurative tonsillitis, lymphnoditis and parotitis.

Administration: Decocted in water for oral dose to be taken twice.

Case Study: The decoction of *Wuwei Xiaodu Yin* was taken

and drugs for external use were applied externally to treat 20 cases of nail–like boil on the face in clinical practice. The boils were manifested as local heat, red, swelling and pain, pus spot as big as a grain in the centre, numbness, itching and ache, all accompanied by chills, fever, restlessness, thirst, nausea, vomiting, poor appetite, constipation, whitish greasy or yellowish greasy tongue coating, and deep replete or taut forceful pulse. The treatment gave rise to satisfactory effects.

7 cases of chronic osteomyelitis, marked by local swelling, distending and pain, pus–discharge and hard–healing after festering so that fistula was formed and long–unhealing or festering again and again resulted, were treated with modified *Wuwei Xiaodu Yin,* whose main ingredients were:

Yin Hua (Flos Lonicerae), *Pu Gong Ying* (Herba Taraxaci), *Zi Hua Di ding* (Herba Violae), *Niu Xi* (Radix Achyranthis Bidentatae), *Bai Zhi* (Radix Angelicae Dahuricae), *Jia Zhu* (Margarita), *Wu Gong* (Scolopendra), *Quan Chong* (Scorpio), and proper drugs for external use. After the treatment. all the cases were cured.

21.4 The Prescription of *Simiao Yongan Tang*

Name: Decoction of Four Wonderful Drugs for Quick Restoration of Health.

Source: The book *Yan Fang* Xin Bian

Ingredients:

Jin Yin Hua (Flod Lonicerae) 90 g, *Xuan Shen* (Radix Scrophulariae) 90 g, *Dang Gui* (Radix Angelicae Sinensis) 30 g, *Gan Cao* (Radix Glycyrrhizae) 15 g.

Explanation:

Jin Yin Hua: The principal drug, being sweet in flavor and cold in nature, clearing away heat and toxic material.

Xuan Shen: Purging fire to remove toxic material.

Dang Gui: Promoting the circulation of blood to remove blood stasis.

Gan Cao: Removing toxic material and relieving pain.

Effect: Clearing away heat and toxic material, promoting the circulation of blood to arrest pain.

Indications: Gangrene of finger or toe due to abundant heat-toxin, marked by red, swelling, burning, ulceration, putrefactive odor and terrible pain of the affected limbs, or fever, thirst, reddened tongue and rapid pulse; including such diseases with the above symptoms and signs as thromboangiitis obliterans and embolic phlebitis.

Administration: Decocted in water for oral dose to be taken twice.

Case Study: Modified *Simiao Yongan Tang* was clinically used to treat 25 cases of thromboangiitis obliterans with the foci ail in the lower limbs. Drugs such as:

Fu Zi (Radix Aconiti Lateralis Preparata), *Gan Jiang* (Rhizoma Zingiberis), *Gui Zhi* (Ramulus Cinnamomi), *Ji Xue Teng* (Caulis Spatholobi), *Huang Qi* (Radix Astragali), were added for the type of cold-deficiency. Drugs such as:

Hong Hua (Flos Carthami), *Tao Ren,* (Semen Persicae), *Ze Lan* (Herba Lycopi), *Wang Bu Liu Xing* (Semen Vaccariae).

were added for the type of *Qi*-stagnancy and blood-stasis. Drugs such as:

Pu Gong Ying (Herba Taraxaci), *Di Ding* (Herba Violae), *Huang Qin* (Radix Scutellariae), *Huang Bai* (Cortex

Phellodendri), were added for the type of heat—toxin. Drugs such as:

Dang Shen (Radix Codonopsis), Huang Qi (Radix Astragali), Bai Zhu (Rhizoma Atractylodis Macrocephalae), were added and:

Xuan Shen (Radix Scrophulariae), Jin Yin Hua (Flos Lonicerae), were omitted for the type of deficiency of both Qi and blood. After the treatment, 10 cases were cured, 11 improved, 4 unimproved, the total effective rate reaching 84%.

33 cases of chronic hepatitis with a long history, bad long—term follow—up result and persistent positive HBsAg, of which 12 cases belonged to chronic persisting type and 21 the "chronic active" type, were treated with modified Simiao Yongan Tan, whose main ingredients were:

Xuan Shen (Radix Scrophulariae) 30 g, Huang Qi (Radix Astragali) 30 g, Fu Ling (Poria) 30 g, Dang Gui (Radix Angelicae Sinensis) 15 g, Sheng Ma (Rhizoma Cimicifugae) 15 g, Ren Dong Teng (Caulis Lonicerae) 60 g, Bai Mao Gen (Rhizoma Imperatae) 60 g, Gan Cao (Radix glycyrrhizae) 10 g.

In case of jaundice, the drugs added were:

Yin Chen (herba Artemisiae Scopariae), Ku Shen (Radix Sophorae Flavescentis).

In case of splenomegaly, the drugs added were:

Ji Nei Jin (Endothelium Corneum Gigeriae Galli), Pao Shan Jia (Squama Manitis Preparata).

In case of the spleen troubled by cold—dampness, the drugs added were:

Gan Jiang (Rhizoma Zingiberis), Cang Zhu (Rhizoma Atractylodis), Bai Zhu (Rhizoma Atractylodis Macrocephalae).

In case of blood stasis, the drugs added were:

Dan Shen (Radix codonopsis), *Chuan Xiong* (Rhizoma Chuanxiong).

In case of severe bleeding, the drugs added were:

Xian He Cao (Herba Agrimoniae), *Shen San Qi* (Radix Notoginseng).

Taking 30 doses was referred to as 1 course of treatment. Vitamins were compatible used for all the cases, coenzyme Q10 for 2 cases. the result was: Remarkable effectiveness was shown in 25 cases, effectiveness in 6 cases, ineffectiveness in 2 cases, the total effective rate being 94%.

21.5   The Prescription of *Xihuang Wan*

Name: Pill of Cow—bezoare

Source: The book *Wai Ke Quan Sheng Ji*

Ingredients:

Xi Huang (Calculus Bovis) 3 g, *She Xiang* (Moschus) 15 g, *Ru Xiang* (Resina Olibani) 100 g, *Mo Yao* (Myrrha) 100 g, *Huang Mi Fan* (cooked glutinous millet) 100 g.

Explanation:

Niu Huang: The principal drug, being sweet and bitter in flavor and cold in nature, clearing away heat and toxic material, eliminating phlegm and dispelling masses.

She Xiang : Being pungent in taste and disperse in nature, not only promoting the circulation of blood and dispelling masses but also clearing and activating the channels and collaterals.

Ru Xiang and *Mo Yao:* Promoting the circulation of blood to remove blood stasis, subduing swelling and relieving pain.

Huang Mi Fan: Regulating and nourishing the stomach—*Qi*.

Effect: Removing toxins, subduing swelling, resolving phlegm, dispelling masses, promoting the circulation of blood to eliminate blood stasis.

Indications: Breast carcinoma, swelling of a lymph node in the groin caused by veneral diseases, scrofula, subcutaneous nodule, multiple abscess, pulmonary abscess and small intestinal abscess, all due to accumulation of fire, phlegm and heat—toxin, marked by local large and small swollen masses as hard as stone and difficult to heal after festering, emaciation, or diffusing swollen pain, normal skin, or non—fixed faci, etc.

Administration: The first four ingredients are removed of oil and ground into fine powder. The powder and *Huang Mi Fan* are mixed together and pounded into pills. 9 g of the pills is taken each time, 3times daily.

Prolonged use of this prescription is not suggested and pregnant women are not allowed to taken it, for most of the drugs in it are pungent in flavor and disperse in nature.

Case Study: 1 case of tuberculosis of lymph nodes having failed to respond to antiphthisic drugs, manifested as infection and festering after being punctured, yellow water—like pus with something like residue from beans, was clinically treated with modified *Xihuang Wan,* whose main ingredients were:

Kun Bu (Thallus Laminariae), *Hai Zao* (Sargassum), *Xia Ku Cao* (Spica Prunellae), *Mu Li* (Concha Ostreae).

Meanwhile, *Wuxing Dan* and *Taohua Wubao Dan* were externally applied. Better curative effects were attained, the skin was not scarry and looked as normal as before.

21.6　The Prescription of *Niubang Jieji Tang*

Name: Decoction of burdock Fruit for Expelling Pathogenic Factors from the Muscles

Source: The book *Yang Ke Xin De Ji*

Ingredients:

Niu Bang Zi (Fructus Arctii) 10 g, *Bo He* (Herba Menthae) 6 g, *Jing Jie* (Herba Schizonepetae) 6 g, *Lian Qiao* (Fructus Forsythiae) 10 g, *Shan Zhi* (Fructus Gardeniae) 10 g, *Dan Pi* (Cortex Moutan) 10 g, *Shi Hu* (Herba Dendrobii) 12 g, *Xuan Shen* (Radix Scrophulariae) 10 g, *Xia Ku Cao* (Spica Prunellae) 12 g.

Explanation:

Niu Bang Zi: The principal drug, being pungent and bitter in flavor and cold in nature, dispersing wind—heat in the head.

Bo He and *Jing Jie:* Relieving exterior syndrome by means of diaphoresis.

Lian Qiao: Clearing away heat and toxic material, dispelling masses and subduing swelling.

Dan Pi, Shan Zhi and *Xia Ku Cao:* Purging fire pathogen from blood.

Xuan Shen: Purging fire to remove toxins, working together with *Shi Hu* to nourish *Yin* and clear away heat.

Effect: Dispelling wind, clearing away heat, cooling blood and subduing swelling.

Indications: Carbuncle and swelling complicated by exterior syndrome due to wind—heat, marked by burning, red, swelling and pain caused by carbuncle on the skin, mild chills and high fever, little of sweating, thirst, deep—colored urine, or toothache, whitish or yellowish tongue, and floating rapid pulse; including such diseases with the above symptoms and signs as cervical lymphadenitis, periodontitis and influenza.

Administration: Decocted in water for oral dose to be taken twice.

21.7 The Prescription of *Haizao Yuhu Tang*

Name: Decoction of Seaweed for Resolving Hard Masses.
Source: The book *Yi Zong Jin Jian*
Ingredients:

Hai Zao (Sargassum) 3 g, *Kun Bu* (Thallus Laminariae) 3 g, *Ban Xia* (Rhizoma Pinelliae Preparata) 3 g, *Chen Pi* (Pericarpium Citri Reticulatae) 3 g, *Qing Pi* (Pericarpium Citri Reticulatae Viride) 3 g, *Lian Qiao* (Fructus Forsythiae) 3 g, *Bei Mu* (Bulbus Fritillariae) 3 g, *Dang Gui* (Radix Angelicae Sinensis) 3 g, *Chuan Xiong* (Rhizoma Chuanxiong) 3 g, *Du Huo* (Radix Angelicae Pubescentis) 3 g, *Gan Cao* (Radix Glycyrrhizae) 3 g, *Hai Dai* (kelp0 1.5 g,

Explanation:

Hai Zao, Kun Bu and *Hai Dai:* The principal drugs, being salty in flavor and cold in nature, resolving phlegm and softening masses.

Qing Pi and *Chen Pi:* Soothing the liver and activating the activity of *Qi.*

Dang Gui, Chuan Xiong and *Du Huo:* Promoting the circulation of blood to clear the channels so as to help dispel goiter.

Bei Mu and *Lian Qiao:* Dispelling masses and subduing swelling.

Gan Cao: Tempering the actions of all the other ingredients.

Effect: Resolving phlegm, softening masses and dispersing goiter.

Indications: *Qi*—stagnancy and phlegm—accumulation due to incoordination between the liver and the spleen, marked by fixed goiter as hard as stone and with normal skin in the neck; including such disorders with the above symptoms and signs as cervical carcinoma, thyroid adenoma and thyroid enlargement.

Administration: Decocted in water for oral dose to be taken twice.

21.8   The Prescription of *Tounong San*

Name: Powder for Expelling Pus
Source: The book *Wai Ke Zheng Zong*
Ingredients:
Huang Qi (Radix Astragali) 12 g, *Dang Gui* (Radix Angelicae Sinensis) 6 g, *Chuan Shan Jia* (Squama Manitis) 3 g, *Zao Jiao Ci* (Spina Gleditsiae) 5 g, *Chuan Xiong* (Rhizoma Chuanxiong) 9 g.

Explanation:

Huang Qi: The principal drug, being sweet in flavor and slightly warm in nature, invigorating *Qi* and expelling pus.

Dang Gui and *Chuan Xiong:* Nourishing blood and promoting its circulation.

Chuan Shan Jia and *Zao Jiao Ci:* Clearing away heat and promoting the flow of *Qi*, softening masses and expelling pus.

small amount of liquor: Helping promote the flow of blood.

Effect: Expelling toxins and pus.

Indications: Syndrome due to inability to expel pus resulting from deficiency of vital—*Qi,* marked by swollen and painful carbuncle of abscess with pus formed and without festering and pus–spot or with severe distention and burning–pain; including various kinds of pyogenic infections with the above symptoms and signs.

Administration: All the ingredients are decocted in water for the decoction. The decoction is divided into 2 portions. 1 portion is taken, or mixed with a small cup of liquor and then taken, each time.

21.9   The Prescription of *Yanghe Tang*

Name: Yang–activating Decoction
Source: The book *Wai Ke Quan Sheng Ji*
Ingredients:

Shu Di (Radix Rehmanniae Preparata) 30 g, *Rou Gui* (Cortex Cinnamomi) 3 g, *Ma Huang* (Herba Ephedrae) 2 g, *Lu Jiao Jiao* (Colla Cornus Cervi) 9 g, *Bai Jie Zi* (Semen Sinapis Albae) 6 g, *Jiang Tan* (Rhizoma Zingiberis Preparata) 2 g, *Gan Cao* (Radix Glycyrrhizae) 3 g.

Explanation:

Shu Di: The principal drug, being sweet in flavor and slightly warm in nature, tonifying *Ying* and nourishing blood.

Lu Jiao Jiao: Replenishing essence, supplementing marrow, strengthening the muscles and tendons, helping *Shu Di* to nourish blood.

Pao Jiang and *Rou Gui:* Warming the channels to promote the flow of *Qi* and dispel cold.

Ma Huang: Inducing diaphoresis to expel pathogenic factors in the superficies of the body.

Bai Jie Zi: Removing obstructed phlegm.

Gan Cao: Clearing away toxins and tempering the actions of all the other ingredients.

Effect: Warming up *Yang*, enriching blood, bispelling cold and removing stagnancy.

Indications: *Yin*—phlegmon resulting from cold—stasis due to *Yang* deficiency, marked by painful diffuse swelling without pus spot and burning sensation and with normal color of the skin, no thirst, pale tongue with whitish coating, and deep thready pulse including such diseases with the above symptoms and signs as bone tuberculosis, chronic osteomyelitis, rheumatoid arthritis and thromboangiitis obliterans.

Administration: Decocted in water for oral dose to be taken twice.

Case Study: 60 cases of bone tuberculosis were clinically treated with *Yanghe Tang* and *Xihuang Wan* with the former as the principal prescription in which *Rou Gui*, *Pao Jiang* and *Bai Jie Zi* were used in large dose for *Yang*—deficiency. Both internal and external treatment were conducted for 5 months. X—ray proved that complete heal of bone and disappearance of clinical symptoms and signs were seen in 19 cases; stopping of bone destruction, partial bone absorption and relieving of clinical symptoms and signs were seen in 8 cases. Relieving of clinical symptoms and signs was seen in the other 33 cases, in which X—ray re—check was not carried out.

30 cases of ischiatitis were treated with modified *Yanghe Tang* for 10—20 days. Warm sensation, perspiration and relief of pain were usually seen after 1—2 doses were taken, remarkable relief of pain after 5—8 doses. The shorter the disease course and the severer the pain, the shorter the treating course the better the curative effects; the longer the disease and the milder the pain, the

longer the treatment course and the worse the curative effects. During the treatment, no adverse reaction was found.

21.10 The Prescription of *Neibu Huangqi Tang*

Name: Decoction of astragalus for Internal Tonification
Source: The book *Wai Ke Fa Hui*
Ingredients:

Huang Qi (Radix Astragali) 10 g, *Mai Dong* (Radix Ophiopogonis) 10 g, *Shu Di Huang* (Radix Rehmanniae Preparata) 10 g, *Ren Shen* (Radix Ginseng) 10 g, *Fu Ling* (Poria) 10 g, *Gan Cao* (Radix Glycyrrhizae Preparata) 5 g, *Bai Shao* (Radix Paeoniae Alba) 5 g, *Yuan Zhi* (Radix Polygalae) 5 g, *Chuan Xiong* (Rhizoma Chuanxiong) 5 g, *Guan Gui* (Cortex Cinnamomi) 5 g, *Dang Gui* (Radix Angelicae Sinensis) 5 g, *Sheng Jiang* (Rhizoma Zingiberis Recens) 3 pieces, *Da Zao* (Fructus Jujubae) 1 dates.

Explanation:

Huang Qi: The principal drug, being sweet in flavor and slightly warm in nature, invigorating *Qi* and promoting muscle regeneration.

Ren Shen, Fu Ling and *Gan Cao:* Strengthening the spleen and invigorating *Qi*.

Dang Gui, Shu Di, Bai Shao and *Chuan Xiong:* Nourishing blood and tonifying the liver.

Rou Gui: Warming and supporting *Yang–Qi*.

Mai Dong: Nourishing *Yin* and reinforcing the heart.

Yuan Zhi: Relieving mental stress.

Effect: Invigorating *Qi* and blood, nourishing *Yin* and promoting muscle regeneration.

Indications: Syndrome due to deficiency of both *Qi* and blood after carbuncle festering, marked by paining at the site of festering, lassitude, languor, poor appetite, mild insomnia, spontaneous sweating, dry mouth, or persistent fever, pale tongue with thin coating, and thready weak pulse; including such diseases with the above symptoms and signs as chronic ulcer and chronic osteomyelitis.

Administration: *Shu Di Huang* and *Dang Gui* are mixed with small amount of liquor, *Bai Shao* and *Yuan Zhi* are stir-fried separately. *Huang Qi* is parched with salt water. Then all the drugs are decocted in water for the decoction to be taken twice.

21.11   The Prescription of *Weijing Tang*

Name: Reed Stem Decoction
Source: The book *Bei Ji Qian Jin Yao Fang*
Ingredients:
Wei Jing (Rhizoma Phragmitis) 30 g, *Yi Yi Ren* (Semen Coicis) 30 g, *Dong Gua Ren* (Semen Benincasae) 24 g, *Tao Ren* (Semen Persicae) 9 g.
Explanation:
Wei Jing: The principal drug, being sweet in flavor and cold in nature, clearing away heat form the lung.

Dong Gua Ren and *Yi Yi Ren:* Clearing and resolving phlegm-heat, removing dampness and expelling pus.

Tao Ren: Promoting the circulation of blood to remove its stasis, moistening the intestines to induce bowel movement.

Effect: Clearing away heat form the lung to resolving phlegm, removing stasis and expelling pus.

Indications: Syndrome due to accumulation of heat-toxin in

the lung and combination of phlegm and stasis, marked by pulmonary abscess, cough, low fever, viscid and fish—stench sputum in severe case, dull pain in the chest,squamous and dry skin, reddened tongue with yellowish greasy coating, and slippery rapid pulse; including such diseases with the above symptoms and signs as pulmonary abscess, lobar pneumonia, bronchiectasis and pulmonary emphysema.

Administration: Decocted in water for oral dose to be taken twice.

Case Study: *Weijing Tang* and modified *Jiegeng Tang* was clinically used to treat 12 cases of pulmonary abscess with all the cases cured except the one who did not carry the treatment through to the end. The length of treatment was 6—16 days, averaging 9.5 days.

200 cases of infantile acute bronchitis, of which 138 were mild ones, 62 were severe, the disease course averaging 1—2 days, were treated with modified *Weijing Tang*, Whose Main ingredients were:

Xian Lu Geng (fresh Rhizoma Phragmitis) 30 g, *Dong Gua Ren* (Semen Benincasae) 12 g, *Yi Yi Ren* (Semen Coicis) 12 g, *Tao Ren* (Semen Persicae) 4.5 g, *Xing Ren* (Semen Armeniacae Amarum) 4.5 g, *Qian Hu* (Radix Peucedani) 4.5 g, *Bai Qian* (Rhizoma Cynanchi Stauntonii) 4.5 g, *Su Zi* (Fructus Perillae) 6 g, *Lai Fu Zi* (Semen Raphani) 6 g, *Yu Hu Die* (Semen Oroxyli) 6 g, Dan Nan Xing (Arisaema cum Bile)3g.

The drugs were decocted in water for the decoction, The decoction was divided into 3—4 portions, 1 of which was taken warm each time, 3—4 times daily. For a big child, there was no need to divide the decoction into portions, he / she might take it at a draught. The result was: 169 cases were cured, 31 unimproved, the curative rate being 84.5%.

21.12　The Prescription of *Dahuang Mudan Tang*

Name: Rhubarb Moutan Decoction.
Source: The book *Jin Gui Yao Lue*
Ubgreduebts:

Da Huang (Radix et Rhizoma Rhei) 18 g, *Mu Dan Pi* (Cortex Moutan) 9 g, *Tao Ren* (Semen Persicae) 12 g, *Dong Gua Zi* (Semen Benincasae) 30 g, *Mang Xiao* (Natrii Sulfas) 9 g.

Explanation:

Da Huang: One of the principal drugs, removing accumulated heat from the intestines, clearing away heat and toxic material.

Dan Pi: The other principal drug, being bitter and pungent in flavor and cold in nature, clearing away heat in the blood.

Mang Xiao: Softening masses, dispersing stagnancy, assisting *Da Huang* in purging heat in the intestines.

Tao Ren: Being drastic in removing blood stasis, helping *Mu Dan Pi* and *Da Huang* to promote blood circulation and disperse blood stasis, and inducing bowel movement.

Dong Gua Ren: Clearing away damp–heat, expelling pus, resolving masses, relieving carbuncle.

Effect: Clearing away heat to remove blood stasis, resolving masses to subdue swelling.

Indications: Syndrome due to accumulation of damp–heat in the early stage of periappendicular abscess, marked by pain and tenderness in the right lower abdomen in which there are masses in severe case, scanty urine, intermittent fever, spontaneous sweating, aversion to cold, or crooked right foot which cannot be extended, and slippery rapid pulse; including such diseases with the above symptoms and signs as acute appendicitis, adnexitis, pelvic inflammation and infection after vasoligation.

Administration: Decocted in water for the decoction which is taken at a draught.

Case Study: *Dahuang Mudan Tang* was clinically used in this modified form to treat 100 cases of acute appendicitis, of which 9 cases were appendiceal perforation complicated by peritonitis, 7 cases were appendix mass. Antibiotics were added in 18 cases. All the cases were cured except one who was referred to surgery due to the critical condition of the diseases. The treatment course averaged 6.5 days.

Dahuang Mudan Tang plus:

Cang Zhu (Rhizoma Atractylodis), *Yi Yi Ren* (Semen Coicis), *Gan Cao* (Radix Glycyrrhizae),
was prescribed to treat 74 cases of local infection after vasoligation, marked by enlargement of testis, thick and hard spermatic cord which led to distending pain in the lower abdomen and discomfort in the loins, or dizziness, poor appetite, deep—colored and scanty urine, constipation, or the infection being mild only with local pain and discomfort. After the treatment, all the cases were cured.

An experiment on rabbits with *Dahuang Mudan Tang* plus:

Dang Gui (Radix Angelicae Sinensis), *Yin Hua* (Flos Lonicerae), *Lian Qiao* (Fructus Forsythiae), *Zhi Qiao* (Fructus Aurantii), *Jie Geng* (Radix Platycodi), *Gan Cao* (Radix Glycyrrhizae), has indicated that the decoction of above drugs can enhance the defentive ability of the reticuloendothelial system in the local part of the body or throughout the body.

21.13   The Prescription of *Yiyi Fuzi Baijiang San*

Name: Powder of Coix Seed, Mankshood and Patrinia

Source: The book *Jin Gui Yao Lue*

Ingredients: *Yi Yi Ren* (Semen Coicis) 30 g, *Fu Zi* (Radix Aconiti Lateralis Preparata) 6 g, *Bai Jiang Cao* (Herba Patriniae) 15 g.

Explanation:

Yi Yi Ren: The principal drug, being sweet and tasteless in flavor and slightly cold in nature, removing dampness and subduing swelling.

Bai Jiang Cao: Expelling pus and removing toxin.

Fu Zi: Being pungent in flavor and warm in nature, assisting *Yi Yi Ren* in removing cold–dampness and promoting the flow of *Qi*.

Effect: Expelling pus and subduing swelling.

Indications: Syndrome of accumulation of cold–dampness and stagnated blood due to periappendicular abscess, marked by suppurative periappendicular abscess no fever, squamous and dry skin, swollen and feeling soft abdominal skin, and rapid pulse, including such diseases with the above symptoms and signs as acute appendicitis complicated by suppuration, appendicular abscess and chronic appendicitis.

Administration: Decocted in water for oral dose to be taken twice (Taken originally in the form of powder).

Case Study: Modified *Yiyi Fuzi Baijiang San* and antibiotics were clinically used to treat 36 cases of appendicular abscess with the former as the main remedy, whose main ingredients were:

Shu Fu Zi (Radix Aconiti Lateralis Preparata) 1.5 g, *Yi Yi Ren* (Semen Coicis) 30 g, *Bai Jiang Cao* (Herba Patriniae) 30 g, *Tao Ren* (Semen Persicae) 9 g, *Hong Hua* (Flos Carthami) 9 g, *Guang Mu Xiang* (Radix Aucklandiae) 9 g.

In the first 3 days, 2 doses were used each day, 1 dose was taken 2 times. From the fourth day, 1 dose was taken each day and 2 times. While the decoction was taken, penicillin intramuscular injection of 800,000 units was conducted each day, 200,000 units each time. 35 cases in this group had their abscess eliminated, each averaging 5 days in the hospital. The rest 1 was operated on due to recurrent peritonitis, drainage being done.

3
方　剂　学

序

《英汉实用中医药大全》即将问世，吾为之高兴。

歧黄之道，历经沧桑，永盛不衰。吾中华民族之强盛，由之。世界医学之丰富和发展，亦由之。然而，世界民族之差异，国别之不同，语言之障碍，使中医中药的传播和交流受到了严重束缚。当前，世界各国人民学习、研究、运用中医药的热潮方兴未艾。为使吾中华民族优秀文化遗产之一的歧黄之道走向世界，光大其业，为世界人民造福，徐象才君集省内外精英于一堂，主持编译了《英汉实用中医药大全》。是书之问世将使海内外同道欢呼雀跃。

世界医学发展之日，当是歧黄之道光大之时。

吾欣然序之。

中华人民共和国卫生部副部长
兼国家中医药管理局局长
世界针灸学会联合会主席
中国科学技术协会委员
中华全国中医学会副会长
中国针灸学会会长

胡熙明

1989 年 12 月

序

　　中华民族有同疾病长期作斗争的光辉历程，故而有自己的传统医学——中国医药学。中国医药学有一套完整的从理论到实践的独特科学体系。几千年来，它不但被完好地保存下来，而且得到了发扬光大。它具有疗效显著、副作用小等优点，是人们防病治病，强身健体的有效工具。

　　任何一个国家在医学进步中所取得的成就，都是人类共同的财富，是没有国界的。医学成果的交流比任何其他科学成果的交流都应进行得更及时，更准确。我从事中医工作 30 多年来，一直盼望着有朝一日中国医药学能全面走向世界，为全人类解除病痛疾苦做出其应有的贡献。但由于用外语表达中医难度较大，中国医药学对外传播的速度一直不能令人满意。

　　山东中医学院的徐象才老师发起并主持了大型系列丛书《英汉实用中医药大全》的编译工作。这个工作是一项巨大工程，是一种大型科研活动，是一个大胆的尝试，是一件新事物。对徐象才老师及与其合作的全体编译者夜以继日地长期工作所付出的艰苦劳动，克服重重困难所表现出的坚韧不拔的毅力，以及因此而取得的重大成绩，我甚为敬佩。作为一个中医界的领导者，对他们的工作给予全力支持是我应尽的责任。

　　我相信《英汉实用中医药大全》无疑会在中国医学史和世界科学技术史上找到它应有的位置。

中华全国中医学会常务理事
山东省卫生厅副厅长

张奇文
1990 年 3 月

出 版 前 言

  中国医药学是我中华民族优秀文化遗产之一，建国以来由于党和国家对待中医药采取了正确的政策，使中医药理论宝库不断得到了发掘整理，取得了巨大的成绩。当前，世界各国人民对中国医药学的学习和研究热潮日益高涨，为促进这一热潮更加蓬勃的发展，为使中国医药学能更好地为全人类解除病痛服务，就必须促进中医中药在世界范围内的传播和交流，而要使这一传播和交流进行得更及时、更准确，就必须首先排除语言障碍。因此，编译一套英汉对照的中医药基本知识的书籍，供国内外学习、研究中医药时使用，已成为国内外医药学界和医药学教育界许多人士的迫切需要。

  多年来，在卫生部门的号召下，在"中医英语表达研究"方面，已经作出了一些可喜的成绩。本书《英汉实用中医药大全》的编辑出版就是在调查上述研究工作的历史和现状的基础上，继续对中医药英语表达作较系统、较全面的研究，以适应中国医药学对外传播交流的需要。

  这部"大全"的版本为英汉对照，共有 21 个分册，一个分册介绍论述中国医药学的一个分科。在编著上注意了中医药汉文稿的编写特色，在内容上注意了科学性、实用性、全面性和简明易读。汉文稿的执笔撰写者主要是有 20 年以上实践经验的教授、副教授、主任医师和副主任医师。各分册汉文稿撰写成后，均经各学科专家逐一审订。各分册英文主译、主审主要是国内既懂中医又懂英语的权威人士，还有许多中医院校的英语教师及医药卫生部门的专业翻译人员。英译稿脱稿后，经过了复审、终审，有些译稿还召开全国 22 所院校和单位人员参加的英译稿统稿定稿研讨会，对英译稿进行细致的研讨和推敲，对如何较全面、较系统、较准确地用英语表达中国医药学进行了探讨，从而推动整个译文达到较高水平，因此，这部"大全"可供中医院校高年级学生作为泛读教材使用。

这部"大全"的编纂得到了国家教育委员会、国家中医药管理局、山东省教育委员会、山东省卫生厅等各部门有关领导的支持。在国家教委高等教育司的指导下，成立了《英汉实用中医药大全》编译领导委员会。还得到了全国许多中医院校和中药生产厂家领导的支持。

希望这部"大全"的出版，对中医院校加强中医英语教学，对国内卫生界培养外向型中医药人才，以及在推动世界各国人民对中医药的学习和研究方面，都将产生良好的影响。

高等教育出版社

1990 年 3 月

前　言

　　《英汉实用中医药大全》是一部以中医基本理论为基础，以中医临床为重点，较为全面系统、简明扼要、易读实用的中级英汉学术性著作。它的主要读者是：中医药院校高年级学生和中青年教师，中医院的中青年医生和中医药科研单位的科研人员，从事中医对外函授工作的人员和出国讲学或行医的中医人员，西学中人员，来华学习中医的外国留学生和各类进修人员。

　　由于中国医药学为我中华民族之独有，因此，英译便成了本《大全》编译工作的重点。为确保译文能准确表达中医的确切含义，我们邀集熟悉中医的英语人员、医学专业翻译人员、懂英语的中医药人员乃至医古文人员于一堂，共同翻译、共同对译文进行研讨推敲的集体翻译法，这样，就把众人之长融进了译文质量之中。然而，即使这样，也难确保译文都能尽如人意。汉文稿虽反映了中国医药学的精髓和概貌，但也难能十全十美。我衷心地盼望读者能提出批评和建议，以便《大全》再版时修改。

　　参加本《大全》编、译、审工作的人员达 200 余名，他们来自全国 28 个单位，其中有山东、北京、上海、天津、南京、浙江、安徽、河南、湖北、广西、贵阳、甘肃、成都、山西、长春等 15 所中医学院，还有中国中医研究院，山东省中医药研究所等中医药科研单位。

　　山东省教育委员会把本《大全》的编译列入了科研计划并拨发了科研经费，山东省卫生厅和一些中药生产厂家也给了很大支持，济南中药厂的资助为编译工作的开端提供了条件。

　　本《大全》的编译成功是全体编译审者集体劳动的结晶，是各有关单位主管领导支持的结果。在《大全》各分册即将陆续出版之际，我诚挚地感谢全体编译审者的真诚合作，感谢许多专家、教授、各级领导和生产厂家的热情支持。

愿本《大全》的出版能在培养通晓英语的中医人才和使中医早日全面走向世界方面起到我所期望的作用。

主编　徐象才

于山东中医学院

1990 年 3 月

目　录

说　明

　　《方剂学》一书是《英汉实用中医药大全》的第 3 分册。

　　本分册分上、下两篇。上篇总论介绍了方剂与治法的关系、常用治法、方剂分类、组方原则、不同剂型的用法等方剂学基本知识。下篇各论按解表、泻下、和解、清热等 21 类介绍了 233 首基础方和常用方的出典、组成、用法、方解、功效、主治、临床应用，及部分方剂的现代药理研究成果。

　　本书既吸收了前人的经验，又精选了现代临床应用成果，并以词条的形式编写，具有重点突出、简明易读、理论联系实际、实用性强等特点，适于国内外各类临床医师和医科学生。

　　山东大学的吴正和副教授帮助校对过部分中药的拉丁学名。刘强、曹会来、张赭、郭静、孔健等帮助核对过英文稿中的部分中医术语。

编　　者

上篇 总 论

1 方剂学

是阐明和研究方剂配伍规律及临床运用的一门学科，是临床各科的基础学科之一。

2 方剂与治法的关系

方剂是理、法、方、药的组成部分，是体现和完成治法的主要手段；治法是指导组方的原则。两者的关系是十分密切的。如症见恶寒发热，头痛身疼，无汗而喘，舌苔薄白，脉浮紧的风寒表实证。在确立辛温解表的治法之后，选择体现治法原则的麻黄汤方，即可说明方剂与治法的关系。

3 常用的治法

中医学的治法是丰富多彩的，早在《内经》里已载有许多治法。至汉末，张仲景又总结出一整套中医辨证论治的方法，对治法的理论和方法作了进一步的充实和发展。历代医学家根据丰富的治法内容，结合各自的临床应用，对治法进行了特点不同的分类，其中，清代的程钟龄提出的"汗、和、下、消、吐、清、温、补"八法，简明实用，切合临床，所以，这八法仍是现在临床上的常用治法。

4 汗法

是通过宣发肺气，调畅营卫，开泄腠理等作用，促进发汗，以达到通畅气血，调和营卫，透邪于表，祛除外邪的一种治法。

汗法，除主要治疗外感六淫之邪的表证之外，还可用于麻疹初起、疹点隐隐不透、水肿病腰以上肿甚、疮疡初起而有寒热表证，以及病邪由里出表，需要透邪外达，或需先除表证者。

由于病证有寒热，邪气有兼夹，体质有强弱，故汗法又分辛温、辛凉两大类，以及与补法、消法等相结合的治法。

5 吐法

是通过引起呕吐，使停留于咽喉、胸膈、胃脘等部位的痰涎、宿食或毒物从口中排出的一种治法。吐法适用于咽喉痰涎壅阻，或顽痰停滞胸膈，或宿食留滞胃脘，或误食毒物尚在胃中等。吐法虽有一定疗效，但因刺激咽喉、胃脘引起呕吐，最容易耗损正气；又因患者多不愿意接受吐法治疗，所以后世医学家只在患者病情剧急，病位在上，急须迅速吐出实邪的情况下采用吐法.除此，则很少应用.

6 下法

是通过荡涤肠胃，泻下大便或积水，使停留于肠胃的宿食、燥屎、实热、冷积、瘀血、痰结、停水等从下窍而去，以解除疾病的一种治法。下法适用于大便不通，燥屎内结，热结便秘，停痰留饮，瘀血内蓄等邪在肠胃而邪正俱实之证。

由于病证有寒热，正气有虚实，病邪有兼夹，所以下法又有寒下、温下、润下、逐水、攻补兼施之别，以及与其他治法的配合运用。

7 和法

是通过和解或调和作用，以达到消除病邪的一种治法。和解是指和里解表之意，调和是指协调人体阴阳和调整脏腑功能之意。所以，伤寒邪在少阳的半表半里之证、肝脾不和、肝胃不和、气血不和、营卫不和等均可使用和法。和法所分具体治法，以和解少阳，调和肝脾，调和肝胃等治法为临床常用。

8 温法

是通过温阳、祛寒、回阳、通络等作用，使寒邪去，阳气复、经络通、血脉和，用于治疗里寒证的一种治法。温法，或用于外寒直入于里，或用于药误损伤阳气，或用于元阳不足而内生寒邪。所以，温法在分类上有温中祛寒，回阳救逆和温经散寒的区别。虚与寒常常并存，故温法又多与补法配合运用。

9 清法

是通过清解热邪的作用，以治里热证的一种治法。清法适用于里热证，尤其在温病中常用。根据里热证中有热在气分、营分、血分，热甚成毒，以及热在脏腑之分，因而清法又有清气分热，清营凉血，气血两清，清热解毒，以及清脏腑热等不同。

由于火热之邪易于伤津耗液，大热又能伤气，所以在清热药中常配伍生津、益气之品。若温病后期，热灼阴伤，或久病阴虚而热伏于里的，又当清法与滋阴并用。

10 消法

是通过消食导滞和消坚散结作用，对气、血、痰、食、水、虫等积聚而成的有形之结，使之渐消缓散的一种治法。从广义来讲，祛痰法、祛湿法、驱虫法、理气法和理血法等都属于消法的范畴。但目前常用的消法，一般指消食导滞和消痞散积，多用于治疗饮食积滞和气血积聚之症瘕痞块等证。

11 补法

是针对人体气血阴阳，或某一脏腑的虚损，给以滋养和补益的一种治法。补法的作用，在于补益人体气血阴阳的不足，协调阴阳的偏胜，使之归于平衡。在正气虚弱不能抗邪或祛除余邪时，亦可用补法扶助正气，达到扶正祛邪的目的。根据虚衰的不同，补法有补阴，补阳，补气，补血，补心，补肝，补脾，补肺，补肾等分类。但常用的补法，以补气，补血，补阴，补阳，以及阴阳并补，气血双补为主。

12　方剂的分类

　　方剂的分类方法很多，其中主要有"七方"说、"十剂"说，按病证分，按临床各科分，按脏腑分，按治法分和综合分类等。"七方"说始于《内经》，主要是根据病情，病位，病势，药味等不同情况，作为方剂分类的依据，把方剂分为大、小、缓、急、奇、偶、复七类。"十剂"说始于北齐徐之才，是按药物功用归类的一种方法，具体内容分"宣"，"通"，"补"，"泄"，"轻"，"重"，"滑"，"涩"，"燥"，"湿"十种。后经宋代赵佶添以"剂"字，称为"十剂"。按病证分类方剂的代表著作有《五十二病方》、《太平圣惠方》、《普济方》等。按临床各科分类方剂的代表著作有《妇人婴儿方》等。按脏腑分类方剂的代表著作有《千金备急要方》、《外台秘要》、《三因病证极一方论》等。按治法分类方剂的见于《景岳全书·古方八阵》。按综合法分类方剂的见于清代汪昂著的《医方考》，分为补养，发表，涌吐，攻里，表里，和解，理气，理血，祛风，祛寒，清暑，利湿，润燥，泻火，除痰，消导，收涩，杀虫，明目，痈疡，经产，救急等二十二剂。这种分类，既有治法，又有病因，并照顾到方治有专科，概念比较清楚，切合临床应用，现在大多借鉴汪氏分类法。本书根据全国中医学院中医专业教材的分类，将在下篇各论中，按解表，泻下，和解，清热，祛暑，温里，表里双解，补益，安神，开窍，固涩，理气，理血，治风，治燥，祛湿，祛痰，消导化积，驱虫，涌吐，痈疡等二十一剂，进行简明扼要地介绍，以便学习、掌握和应用。

13 方剂的组成

是在单方专药治病经验的基础上，根据辨证论治的原则和治法的需要，将药物有机地配合而组成的。其目的首先在于增强或综合药物的作用，以提高原有的疗效；其次，随证合药，以扩大治疗范围。此外，还可以监制药物的烈性或毒性，以消除对人体的不良作用。

14 组方原则

古人将组方原则归纳并简称为"君、臣、佐、使"，今人则改称为"主、辅、佐、使"，这是对组方原则具体、生动的表述。

主药，是针对病因或主证而起主要治疗作用的药物。辅药，是协助主药以加强治疗病因或主证，并针对相兼病因或兼证起主要治疗作用的药物。佐药，即配合主、辅药以加强治疗作用，或直接治疗次要症状；用以消除或减弱主、辅药的毒性，或制约主、辅药峻烈之性。因病重邪甚，可能拒药时，配用与主药性味相反而又能在治疗中起相成作用的药物。使药，是引方中诸药至病所，或调和方中诸药的药物。

15 组方的变化

方剂的组成，虽有一定的原则，但在临床应用时，须根据病情的缓急，体质的强弱，年龄的大小，气候的寒温，水土的宜忌等不同，予以灵活地加减化裁。临床上，依照治法选用成方，又根据具体病情化裁，大致有药味加减、药量加减和剂型更换三种变化形式。

16 药味加减的变化

临床上选用成方之后，尚须根据病情增加或减少药物，其目的是使之更加适于对病情的治疗。由于方中药味的加减，可出现以下三种变化。一是在主药、主证不变的情况下，根据次要症状或兼症的不同，加减方中的次要药味，以适应新的病情需要。例如，桂枝汤主治表现为发热、恶风寒、头痛、脉浮缓等的风寒表虚证，若兼有喘咳者，则加厚朴、杏仁，名为桂枝加厚朴杏子汤，兼以降逆平喘；若因误下而兼见脉促、胸满者，则减去性凉阴柔的芍药，宜阳气上升外达，名为桂枝去芍药汤，以消除胸满，并有利于解肌散邪。二是由于加减方中的药味，主药、主治发生了改变，方名亦随之改变。例如，桂枝汤去生姜，加当归、细辛、通草，主药变为当归、芍药，方名则为当归四逆汤，主治亦改变为治厥阴伤寒的手足厥寒、脉细欲绝之证。三是方剂的主药不变，而配伍药改变，其主治功效也随之改变。例如，苦寒清热的黄连，配伍辛温降逆的吴茱萸，名左金丸，主治肝经郁火的胁肋胀痛，若黄连配伍行气止痛的木香，名香连丸，则主治湿热痢疾。

17　药量加减的变化

方中药物不变，只增减药量，可改变方剂的主药、主治和方剂的药力，以及扩大其治疗范围。由于方中药量的加减，可出现以下三种变化。一是改变主药和主治，如小承气汤与厚朴三物汤，方中均用大黄、枳实、厚朴，但小承气汤治阳明腑实证，病机是热结阳明，所以用大黄12克（主药），枳实9克，厚朴6克；厚朴三物汤主治大便秘结，腹满而痛，病机是气闭不通，所以用厚朴24克（主药），枳实15克，大黄12克。两方相比，厚朴用量相差为1：4，大黄用量虽同，但小承气汤煎分2次服，厚朴三物汤煎分3次服，每次实际服量亦有差别。二是改变药力，如四逆汤与通脉四逆汤均用附子、干姜、炙甘草，但前方干姜、附子用量比较小，主治阴盛阳微而致四肢厥逆，恶寒蜷卧，下利，脉微细或沉迟细弱的证候，有回阳救逆的功用；后方干姜、附子用量大，主治阴盛格阳于外而致四肢厥逆，身反不恶寒，下利清谷，脉微欲绝的证候，有回阳逐阴，通脉救逆的功用。三是扩大治疗范围，如桂枝加芍药汤，其主药仍是桂枝，倍加芍药以缓急止痛，主治桂枝汤证兼腹满时痛。

18 方剂的剂型

剂型是根据临床使用中草药治疗各种疾病的不同需要，将药物制成一定大小和不同形状的制剂，以更好地发挥药效。中药剂型是我国历代医药家长期和疾病作斗争不断积累经验的结果，如《内经》十三方中，就有汤、丸、散、膏、酒等剂型。继《内经》之后，剂型又有了发展，如出现了饮、露、锭、饼、条、线，还有熏烟、熏洗、滴耳、灌肠、灌鼻、坐药等剂型。目前中药制剂的制作方法，既保留了传统的好方法，又吸取了现代制作的方法，制成了许多新的剂型，如针剂、片剂、糖浆剂、浸膏、流浸膏、冲剂、以后橡皮膏等，以满足临床各科治疗的需要。

19 剂型更换的变化

根据病情的需要，将同一个方剂的剂型改变，其治疗作用也会随之而发生变化。例如，理中丸由干姜、白术、人参、甘草各90克组成，炼蜜为丸如鸡子黄大，治中焦虚寒，腹泻不止，呕吐腹痛，舌淡苔白，脉沉迟少力者。若治上焦阳虚而致的胸痹，症见心中痞闷，胸满，胁下有气上逆抢心，四肢不温，少气懒言，脉沉细等，即用上四味各9克煎汤分3次服。这是根据病位有中上之别，病势有轻重之异，一取丸剂缓治，一取汤剂急治。

20 汤剂

把药物配齐后，加水浸透，煎煮一定时间后，去滓取汁，称为汤剂。一般作内服用，如麻黄汤、大承气汤等。汤剂的特点是吸收快，能迅速发挥疗效，而且便于加减使用，能较全面、灵活地照顾到每一个病人或各种病证的特殊性，是中医过去和现在临床使用最广泛的一种剂型。

21　散剂

是将药物碾研，成为均匀混合的干燥粉末，有内服和外用两种。内服散剂末细量少，可直接冲服，如七厘散；亦有研成粗末，临用时加水煮沸取汁服，如香苏散等。外用散剂一般作为外敷、掺撒疮面或患病部位，如生肌散、金黄散等；亦有作点眼、吹喉等外用的，如冰硼散等。散剂有制作简便，便于服用携带，吸收较快，节省药材，不易变质等优点。

22　丸剂

是将药物研成细末，以蜜、水或米糊、面糊、酒、醋、药汁等作为赋型剂制成的圆形固体剂型。丸剂吸收缓慢，药力持久，体积小，服用、携带、贮存都比较方便，也是一种常用的剂型。丸剂一般适用于慢性、虚弱性疾病，如归脾丸、人参养荣丸等；亦有用于急救，因方中含有芳香药物，不宜加热煎煮，如安宫牛黄丸、苏合香丸等。某些有毒或峻猛药品，为了使其缓和地发挥药效，亦做成丸剂。

临床常用的丸剂有蜜丸、水丸、糊丸、浓缩丸。蜜丸性质柔润，作用缓和，并能矫味，且具有补益作用，适用于慢性病。水丸吸收快，丸粒小，易于吞服，适用于多种疾病。糊丸内服后在体内缓慢吸收，即可延长药效，又能减少某些刺激性强的药物对胃肠道的刺激，故毒性较大、刺激性强的药物宜制糊丸。浓缩丸有效成分高，体积小，剂量少，易于服用，适用于治疗各种疾病。

23　膏剂

是将药物用水或植物油煎熬浓缩而成的剂型。有内服和外用两种，内服膏有流浸膏、浸膏、煎膏3种；外用膏有软膏和硬膏两种。

流浸膏，一般 1mL 的有效成分相当于 1 克药材，有效成分含量较酊剂高，溶媒的副作用小，剂量亦小，如甘草流浸膏、益母草流浸膏等。浸膏，每 1 克浸膏约相当 2～5 克药材，不含溶媒，没有溶媒的副作用，浓度高，体小，剂量小。半固体的软浸膏，如毛冬青浸膏等，多供制片或制丸用，干燥细粉为干浸膏，如紫珠草浸膏、龙胆草浸膏等，可直接冲服或装入胶囊服用。煎膏，又称膏滋，体积小，便于服用，又含有大量蜂蜜或糖，味甜而营养丰富，有润补作用，适合久病体虚者服用，如参芪膏、枇杷膏等。软膏，又称药膏，是常温下半固体外用制剂，有一定的粘稠性，涂于皮肤或粘膜能渐渐软化或溶化，有效成分可被缓慢吸收，适用于外科疮痈肿疖等病，如三黄散软膏、穿心莲软膏等。硬膏，又称膏药，常温时呈固体状态，用法简单，携带、贮藏方便，在 36～37℃ 时则溶化，外敷可起到局部或全身的治疗作用，同时亦有机械性保护作用，适用于跌打损伤、风湿痹痛和疮疡等疾病，如风湿跌打止痛膏、狗皮膏等。

24 丹剂

多指用含汞、硫黄等矿物经过加热升华而成的剂量小、作用大的一种化合制剂。有内服和外用两种，一般多外用，供外科使用，如红升丹、白降丹等。某些较贵重的药物，或用特殊功效的药物剂型，习惯上亦称为丹。所以丹没有固定的剂型，如黑锡丹、至宝丹等，此类多供内服。

25 酒剂

酒作溶媒用。一般以白酒或黄酒浸制药物，或加温同煮，去滓取液，供内服或外用。此剂多用于体虚补养、风湿疼痛或跌打扭伤等，如十全大补酒、风湿药酒。

26　灸剂

是将艾叶捣碎如绒状，捻成一定大小的形状后，置于体表的某些俞穴或患部，点燃熏灼，使之发生温热或灼痛感觉，以达到预防或治疗作用的一种外用剂型。

27　冲服剂

是将中药提炼成稠膏，加入适量糖粉及其他辅料（淀粉、山药粉、糊精等）充分拌匀，揉搓成团状，通过 10～12 目筛，制成颗粒，再将颗粒置于 40～60℃ 温度中干燥，干燥后过 8～14 目筛，使其均匀，一般用塑料袋包装避潮。冲服剂作用迅速，体积小，重量轻，易于携带，服用简便，适用于多种疾病，如咳露冲剂、感冒冲剂等。

28　煎药的方法

正确地煎药方法，可使药物充分地发挥药效。煎药用具不宜有锡、铁锅等金属器皿煎煮，宜选用陶瓷砂锅，以避免药物发生沉淀、降低溶解度和产生副作用。煎药用水，除处方中有特殊规定外，一般以水质纯净为原则，如自来水、蒸馏水或甜井水等。用水量，一般以水面漫过药物 3cm 左右为宜。煎药用火的急慢，称为火候，急火煎之谓武火，慢火煎之谓文火，一般先用武火，煎沸后改用文火。

煎药的具体方法和步骤，是在煎药前，先将药物放入容器内，加冷水漫过药面，浸透后再煎煮，则有效成分易于煎出。煎药时不宜频频打开锅盖，以尽量防止气味走失，减少挥发成分外溢。煮沸后宜改用微火，以免药液溢出及过快熬干。对解表、清热、芳香类药，宜武火急煎，以免药性挥发，药效降低或改变。厚味滋补药，宜文火久煎，使药效尽出。若将药物煎糊，必须弃去，不可加水再煎服。某些煎法较为特殊的药物，在处方中须注明，介壳类、矿石类药物、因质坚而难煎，应打碎先煎，如龟板、鳖甲、代赭石、石决明、生牡蛎、生龙骨、生石膏等，应先煮沸约10~20分钟，再下其他药；气味芳香类药易于挥发有效成分，宜在其他药物煎好前5分钟左右投入，以防药效走散，如薄荷、砂仁等。为防止药液混浊及减少对消化道、咽喉的不良刺激，某些药需用薄布将药包好，再放入锅内煎煮，如赤石脂、滑石、旋复花等。某些贵重药，为了减少同煎时被其他药物吸收，可另炖或另煎，如人参，应切成小片，另炖1小时以上。胶质、粘性大而且易溶的药物，同煎则易粘锅煮焦，且粘附他药而影响药效，用时应单独加沸水溶化，或加入去滓的药液中微煮溶解，如阿胶、鹿角胶、饴糖等。散剂、丹剂、小丸、自然汁，以及某些芳香或贵重药物，需要冲服，如牛黄、麝香、沉香末、田三七等。

29 服药的方法

　　包括服药时间和服药方法。服药时间，一般宜在饭前约1小时服，对胃肠有刺激的宜在饭后服，滋腻补益药宜空腹服，治疟药物宜在发作前2小时服，安神药宜在睡前服，急证不拘时间，慢性病服丸、散、膏、酒者应定时。

　　服药方法，一般1日1剂，分2次服或3次服。病情急的一次顿服。恶逆、呕吐或吞咽困难者，宜量少而频服。根据病情也可1日连服2剂，以增强药力。汤剂一般多宜温服。解表药服后须温覆避风，使身体出微汗。热证用寒药，宜热服，但有寒热错杂时，服药后可出现呕吐，如系真寒假热，则宜热药冷服；如系真热假寒，则宜寒药热服。服药呕吐，一般宜加入少许姜汁，或用鲜生姜擦舌，或嚼少许陈皮，然后再服汤药；或用冷服，少量频饮的方法。如遇昏迷病人，吞咽困难者，可用鼻饲法给药。使用峻烈或毒性药，宜先进小量，逐渐增加，有效即止，慎勿过量，以免发生中毒。

下篇 各 论

第1章 解表剂

1.1 解表剂

由解表药为主组成，具有发汗、解肌、透疹等作用，以治疗表证的方剂，统称解表剂。六淫之邪侵入肌表，所致恶寒，发热，头痛，身疼，脉浮，以及麻疹、疮疡、水肿等初期见有表证者，均可选用解表剂。六淫有寒热之异，人体有虚实之别，因而解表剂可分为辛温解表、辛凉解表和扶正解表3类，分别适用于表寒证、表热证和体虚感邪而致的表证。

解表剂多为辛散之品，不宜久煎。用药后宜避风寒，以保暖取微汗为佳，但不宜过汗。气候炎热、老幼、体弱者用量宜轻。兼里证者，可用表里双解，或先表后里。单纯里证，不可用解表剂；服药期间宜禁用生冷、油腻之品。

1.2 辛温解表剂

是以辛温解表的药物为主组成的方剂。适用于外感风寒表证。症见恶寒发热，头项强痛，肢体酸疼，口不渴，无汗或有汗，舌苔薄白，脉浮紧或浮缓等。常用的药有麻黄、桂枝、荆芥、防风、苏叶等。代表方剂有麻黄汤、桂枝汤、小青龙汤、九味羌活汤等。

1.3 麻黄汤

出自《伤寒论》。由麻黄6克，桂枝4克，杏仁9克，炙甘草3克组成。水煎分2次服。方中麻黄味苦辛性温，发汗解表，宣肺平喘，为主药。桂枝发汗解肌，温经散寒，既助麻黄发汗解表，又除肢体疼痛。杏仁宣畅肺气，助麻黄平喘，炙甘草调和诸药。共奏发汗解表，宣肺平喘之功。主治风寒表实证。症见恶寒发热，无汗而喘，头痛身疼，舌苔薄白，脉浮紧。现常用于感冒、流行性感冒、支气管炎、支气管哮喘等病具有上述症状者。本方是发汗峻剂，凡气、血、津、液偏虚者，皆当禁用。临床曾应用麻黄汤治疗青年矿工流行性感冒，症见恶寒发热，寒热俱甚，头痛身疼，鼻塞流涕，无汗，脉浮紧等，一般服2～3剂，汗出热退而愈；曾运用麻黄汤合四物汤加减治疗儿童银屑病10例，分别服4～49剂，平均19剂，2例痊愈，5例基本痊愈，2例显著进步，1例进步。

1.4 桂枝汤

出自《伤寒论》。由桂枝9克，芍药9克，炙甘草6克，生姜9克，大枣3枚组成。水煎分3次服，服后宜饮热稀粥或开水，复被取微汗。方中桂枝味辛甘性温，解肌发表，温经散寒，为主药。芍药益阴敛营，与桂枝相合，可使营卫调和，生姜辛温，既助桂枝解肌，又暖胃止呕，大枣甘平，益气补中，滋脾生津，炙甘草益气和中，合桂枝以解肌，配芍药以益阴，且调和诸药。共奏解肌发表，调和营卫之功。主治风寒表虚证。症见头痛发热，汗出恶风，鼻鸣干呕，苔白不渴，脉浮缓。现常用于感冒、风湿性关节炎、心脏病、肾炎等病具有上述症状者。本方禁用生冷油腻之品。临床应用桂枝汤治疗发烧20余日/例，症见发热（体温38℃），汗出，困倦，纳差，头昏，口不渴，苔白，脉浮。用本方1剂则热退病愈。运用桂枝汤加葶苈、蝉脱治疗过敏性鼻炎 20 例，除 2 例疗效不显和 4 例复发外，其余 14 例均愈，最少服 2 剂，最多服 14 剂。

1.5　九味羌活汤

引自《此事难知》。由羌活 5 克，防风 5 克，苍术 5 克，细辛 1 克，川芎 3 克，白芷 3 克，生地黄 3 克，黄芩 3 克，甘草 3 克组成。水煎分 2 次服。方中羌活味辛苦性温，上行发散，可除肌表的风寒湿邪，为主药。防风、苍术发汗祛湿，助羌活解表，细辛、川芎、白芷散风寒，宣湿痹，行气血，黄芩泄气分之热，生地泄血分之热，既治兼证之热，又制辛温之燥。甘草调和诸药。共奏发汗祛湿，兼清里热之功。主治外感风寒湿邪，内兼里热之证。症见恶寒发热，肌表无汗，头痛项强，肢体酸楚疼痛，口苦而渴。现常用于感冒、流行性感冒、风湿性关节炎等病具有上述症状者。临床应用九味羌活汤加减治疗感冒 120 例，症见恶寒发热，寒多热少，头痛，肢体酸痛，有效者 112 例，占93.33%。运用九味羌活汤加减治疗急性荨麻疹 152 例，对风寒型、风热型伴湿邪者皆有效。基本方由羌活 10 克，防风 6 克，炒苍术 6 克，细辛 1.5 克，川芎 6 克，白芷 6 克，生地黄 10克，炒黄芩 6 克，甘草 6 克，生姜 2 片，葱白 3 枚组成。其中119 例服 3 剂痊愈，15 例服 5 剂痊愈，10 例服 7 剂痊愈，6 例反复发作者，服 10 剂症状好转，2 例无效。

1.6　小青龙汤

出自《伤寒论》。由麻黄、芍药、细辛、干姜、炙甘草、桂枝、五味子、半夏各 9 克组成。水煎分 3 次服。方中麻黄、桂枝发汗解表，宣肺平喘，均为主药。干姜、细辛温肺化饮，兼助麻黄、桂枝解表，五味子敛气，芍药养血，半夏祛痰和胃而降逆，炙甘草益气和中，调和诸药。共奏解表蠲饮，止咳平喘之功。主治风寒容表，水饮内停。症见恶寒发热，无汗，喘咳，痰多而稀，不得平卧，或身体疼重，头面四肢浮肿，舌苔白滑，脉浮。现常用于慢性气管炎、支气管哮喘、老年性肺气肿等病具有上述症状者。本方辛燥，若干咳无痰，或痰稠而黄，口燥咽干者不宜使用。临床应用重剂小青龙汤治疗顽固性过敏性支气管哮喘 6例，证属外寒内饮，长期服用氨茶碱、舒喘灵、强的松、地塞米松等均无效。基本方由炙麻黄 15 克，桂枝 9 克，五味子 9 克，干姜 9 克，制半夏 30 克，白芍 30 克，细辛 6~9 克，甘草 9~15 克组成。6 例服本方半小时至 2 小时内哮喘即平，听诊两肺哮鸣音大减或基本消失，服完 2、3 剂病情趋向稳定，逐渐减本方剂量，经治疗后体症消失，6 例哮喘基本控制。运用小青龙汤加猪苓、茯苓、泽泻、附子、款冬、白术等品，治疗全身浮肿，胸满气喘，舌淡苔白，脉弦滑而患病多年的病例，经服药 30 余剂而愈。

小青龙汤加减煎液注射，对麻醉猫的支气管痉挛有明显的解痉作用。

1.7 大青龙汤

出自《伤寒论》。由麻黄 12 克，桂枝 4 克，炙甘草 5 克，杏仁 6 克，石膏 12 克，生姜 9 克，大枣 3 枚组成。水煎分 3 次服。方中麻黄味苦辛性温，发散风寒，为主药。桂枝解肌发表，助麻黄发汗。石膏辛寒，既助麻黄辛散外邪，又能清里热。杏仁润肺止咳，姜枣既助宣发，又培中气。甘草和中，调和诸药。共奏发汗解表，清热除烦之功。主治风寒表实兼有里热之证。症见发热恶寒，寒热俱重，身疼痛，无汗而烦燥，脉浮紧。现常用于重感冒、急性支气管炎、支气管肺炎、大叶性肺炎等病具有上述症状者。本方是发汗峻剂，得汗宜止后服；凡自汗表虚者，宜禁用。临床应用大青龙汤治疗外感所致的发烧 1 例，症见恶寒，高热 39.5℃，无汗烦燥，咳嗽，头、身疼痛，舌苔薄白，脉浮数，服 1 剂后寒热即退；服 2 剂而病愈。

1.8　辛凉解表剂

是以辛凉解表药物为主组成的方剂。适用于外感风热表证。症见发热，有汗，微恶风寒，头痛，口渴，咽痛，或咳嗽，舌苔薄白或微黄，脉浮数等。常用的药有薄荷、牛蒡子、桑叶、菊花、葛根等。代表方剂有桑菊饮、银翘散、麻黄杏仁甘草石膏汤等。

1.9　桑菊饮

出自《温病条辨》。由桑叶 7.5 克，菊花 3 克，杏仁 6 克，连翘 5 克，薄荷 2.5 克，桔梗 6 克，甘草 2.5 克，苇根 6 克组成。水煎分 2 次服。方中桑叶味苦甘性寒，清透肺络之热，菊花味辛甘苦，性微寒，清散上焦风热，均为主药。薄荷助散上焦风热，桔梗、杏仁一升一降，宣降肺气以止咳。连翘清透膈上之热。苇根清热生津止渴，甘草调和诸药。共奏疏风清热，宣肺止咳之功。主治风温初起。症见咳嗽，身热不甚，口微渴。现常用于流行性感冒、急性支气管炎、急性扁桃体炎、流行性结膜炎等病具有上述症状者。临床应用桑菊饮加减治疗流行性感冒 50 例，症见发热恶寒，头痛，鼻塞流涕，咳嗽，食欲不振等。86.5%病例服药 2 天即完全退热，一般症状减轻，绝大部分病例 4 天内痊愈。用桑菊饮加减治疗百日咳 11 例，发病最短者 10 天，最长者 34 天，平均为 18.6 天，经服药后均治愈，最少服 8 剂，最多服 14 剂，平均为 10.2 剂。

1.10　银翘散

出自《温病条辨》。由连翘 9 克，银花 9 克，苦桔梗 6 克，薄荷 6 克，竹叶 4 克，生甘草 5 克，荆芥穗 5 克，淡豆豉 5 克，牛蒡子 9 克，鲜苇根 18 克组成。水煎分 2 次服（原作散剂）。方中银花味甘性寒，连翘味苦性微寒，两药既轻宣透表，又清热解毒，均为主药。荆芥穗、豆豉辛温，助银花、连翘开皮毛而逐表邪。牛蒡子，桔梗宣肺利咽，甘草清热解毒，竹叶清上焦热，芦根清热生津。共奏辛凉透表，清热解毒之功。主治温病初起，风热表证。症见发热，微恶风寒，口渴，舌红苔薄白，脉浮数。现常用于麻疹、流行性感冒、急性化脓性扁桃体炎、乙型脑炎、腮腺炎等病具有上述症状者。临床应用银翘散袋泡剂治疗急性上呼吸道感染25例，银翘散袋泡剂含生药2克，入有盖杯中开水浸泡3～5分钟后服用，每次2～4包，日3次，25例中合并妊娠2例，风心病、心衰1例。症见发热畏寒，头身痛，喉咽痛，苔薄白，脉浮数，临床治愈23例，占90.2%，退热时间8～72小时，平均35小时；运用银翘散加味治疗爆发性剧烈风疹400例，在400例患者中，除5例因并发腮腺炎、牙周围炎、脑膜炎、心肌炎等无效外，其余服2～5剂而全部治愈。

1.11　麻黄杏仁甘草石膏汤

出自《伤寒论》。由麻黄5克，杏仁9克，炙甘草6克，石膏18克组成。水煎分2次服。方中麻黄味苦辛性温，宣肺平喘，为主药。石膏辛甘大寒，且用量倍于麻黄，使宣肺而不助热，清肺而不留邪。杏仁降肺气，助麻黄、石膏清肺平喘。炙甘草既益气和中，又合石膏而生津止渴，尚能调和寒温宣降。共奏辛凉宣泄、清肺平喘之功。主治风热袭肺，或风寒郁而化热，热壅于肺之证。症见身热不解，咳逆气急鼻煽，口渴，有汗或无汗，舌苔薄白或黄，脉滑而数。现常用于急性气管炎、大叶性肺炎、小儿支气管肺炎、猩红热、荨麻疹、慢性气管炎、支气管哮喘等病具有上述症状者。临床应用加味麻杏石甘汤治疗小儿肺风痰喘178例，基本方由葱白、豆豉、麻黄、石膏、甘草、桑白皮、浙贝母、川朴、瓜蒌、连翘、赤豆组成。其中治愈149例，占总人数83.7%，有效20例，占总人数11.2%，无效9例，占总人数5.1%。运用麻杏甘石汤治疗小儿肺炎30例，症见发热，气喘咳嗽，咽痛等，其中治愈 26 例，显效 1 例，病情好转 3 例，有效率 100%。

1.12　升麻葛根汤

出自《闫氏小儿方论》。由升麻 3 克，葛根 3 克，芍药 6 克，炙甘草 3 克组成。水煎分 3 次服。方中升麻味辛甘性微寒，解肌透疹而解毒，为主药。葛根助升麻解肌透疹，并能生津。芍药和营泄热，甘草益气解毒。共奏解肌透疹之功。主治麻疹未发，或发而未透之证。症见发热恶风，头痛，肢体痛，喷嚏，咳嗽，目赤流泪，口渴，舌红苔干，脉浮数。现常用于麻疹、风疹、药疹、过敏性紫癜等病具有上述症状者。临床应用升麻葛根汤加紫草治疗带状疱疹 20 余例，症见局部疱疹瘙痒疼痛，时有渗液，并伴有发冷发热，日夜不能安眠，经服本方治疗，20 余例均获捷效。运用加味升麻葛根汤治疗银屑病 162 例，经治疗临床治愈 77 例，有效 76 例，无效 9 例。

1.13　柴葛解肌汤

出自《伤寒六书》。由柴胡 6 克，葛根 9 克，甘草 3 克，黄芩 6 克，羌活 3 克，白芷 3 克，芍药 6 克，桔梗 3 克，生姜 3 片，大枣 2 枚，石膏 5 克组成。水煎分 2 次服。方中葛根味辛甘性凉，柴胡味苦辛性微寒，两药解肌清热，均为主药。羌活、白芷助柴葛解肌发表，并除诸痛。黄芩、石膏清郁热，桔梗宣肺气，芍药、甘草和营泄热，生姜、大枣调和营卫。共奏解肌清热之功。主治外感风寒，郁而化热之证。症见恶寒渐轻，身热增盛，无汗头痛，目疼鼻干，心烦不眠，眼眶痛，脉浮微洪。现常用于流行性感冒、三叉神经痛、牙周炎等病具有上述症状者。临床应用柴葛解肌汤治疗小儿病毒性上感的高热 62 例，年龄为 3 个月～13 岁，体温从 38～40℃以上，肺部 X 线检查 13 例肺纹理增强，治疗结果有效 56 例。

1.14 扶正解表剂

是以扶正和解表的药物为主组成的方剂。适用于体质素虚而又感受外邪的表证。症见乏力，汗出，口渴，恶风寒，脉浮而无力或沉等。常用扶正药人参、玉竹、附子配伍解表药羌活、葱白等，代表方剂有败毒散、麻黄细辛附子汤、加减葳蕤汤等。

1.15 败毒散

出自《小儿药证直诀》。由柴胡、前胡、川芎、枳壳、羌活、独活、茯苓、桔梗、人参各 9 克，甘草 4.5 克，生姜 3 克，薄荷 3 克组成。水煎分 2 次服（原作散剂）。方中羌活、独活味辛苦性温，两药治一身上下之风寒湿邪，均为主药。川芎行血祛风，柴胡辛散解肌，助羌活和独活祛外邪、止疼痛。枳壳降气，桔梗开肺气，前胡祛痰，茯苓渗湿。甘草调和诸药，益气和中。生姜、薄荷发散风邪，人参补气，使正气足则可鼓邪外出。共奏益气解表、散风祛湿之功。主治正气不足而外感风寒湿之证。症见憎寒壮热，头项强痛，肢体酸痛，无汗，鼻塞声重，咳嗽有痰，胸膈痞满，舌苔白腻，脉浮而重取无力。现常用于流行性感冒、麻疹、风湿性关节炎、痢疾等病具有上述症状者。临床应用败毒散治疗痢疾 2 例，症见憎寒壮热，无汗，胸腹微觉满痛，里急后重，下痢赤白相杂，昼夜 20～30 次不等，舌苔白滑，脉浮紧，均属暑湿风寒杂感于外，饮食生冷积滞于内之证，服 1 剂后汗出，外证悉解，下痢次数亦减，又服 2 剂后均愈。运用败毒散加减治疗狂犬病 2 例，1 剂症状减轻，2 剂后均愈，且无副作用。

1.16 麻黄细辛附子汤

出自《伤寒论》。由麻黄 6 克，细辛 6 克，炮附子 9 克组成。水煎分 3 次服。方中麻黄解表散寒，附子温经助阳，细辛既助麻黄解表，又助附子温经。共奏助阳解表之功。主治阳虚感寒之证。症见恶寒甚，发热轻，脉沉。现常用于慢性支气管炎、慢性肾炎、风湿性关节炎、类风湿性关节炎等病具有上述症状者。临床应用麻黄附子细辛汤治疗久咳 30 余例，证属素体阳虚而复感风寒，经本方治疗，均获满意效果。运用麻黄附子细辛汤治疗嗜睡症 1 例，证属心阳不振，症见头晕头胀，精神不振，每日早晨昏睡不起，呼之不易醒，舌质胖，苔薄，脉小而缓。用本方加味 9 剂而获显效。

1.17　加减葳蕤汤

出自《重订通俗伤寒论》。由生葳蕤（玉竹）9 克，生葱白 6 克，桔梗 5 克，白薇 3 克，淡豆豉 12 克，薄荷 5 克，炙甘草 2 克，红枣 2 枚组成。水煎分 2 次服。方中葳蕤味甘性微寒，滋阴润肺而资汗源，为主药。葱白、豆豉、薄荷、桔梗解表宣肺，止咳利咽，白薇凉血清热而除烦渴，甘草、红枣甘润滋脾。共奏滋阴清热，发汗解表之功。主治阴虚而感外邪之证。症见头痛身热，微恶风寒，无汗或有汗不多，咳嗽，心烦，口渴，咽干，舌赤，脉数。现常用于感冒，干燥综合征等病具有上述症状者。

第2章 泻下剂

2.1 泻下剂

由泻下药为主组成。具有通导大便，排除肠胃积滞，荡涤实热，攻逐水饮、寒积等作用，以治疗里实证的方剂，统称泻下剂。胃肠积滞，实热内结，大便不通，寒积，蓄水等证，均可选用泻下剂。人体素质有虚实之异，证候表现有热结、寒结、燥结、水结之别，因而泻下剂可分为寒下、温下、润下、逐水和攻补兼施5类，分别适用于里热积滞实证、里寒实证、体虚便秘证、水饮壅盛的里实证和里实正虚而大便秘结证。

泻下剂是为里实证而设，若表证未解，里未成实，不宜用泻下剂。表证未解而里实已具，宜先解表，后治里，或表里双解。老年体虚，新产血亏、病后津伤等，虽有大便秘结，均应慎用，必要时，可攻补兼施，或先攻后补。泻下剂易耗损胃气，得效即止。病愈后，对油腻及不易消化的食物，不宜早进，以防重伤胃气。

2.2 寒下剂

是以寒下的药物为主组成的方剂。适用于里热积滞实证。症见大便秘结，腹部或满或胀或痛，甚或潮热，苔黄，脉实等。常用的药有大黄、芒硝等，代表方剂有大承气汤、大陷胸汤等。

2.3 大承气汤

出自《伤寒论》。由大黄12克，厚朴15克，枳实15克，芒硝9克组成。水煎分2次服。方中大黄味苦性寒，泄热通便，荡涤肠胃，为主药。芒硝咸寒泻热，软坚润燥，厚朴、枳实行气散结，消痞除满，助芒硝、大黄推荡积滞以排泄热结。共奏峻下热结之功。主治里热实证。症见大便不通，频转矢气，脘腹痞满，腹痛拒按，按之硬，甚或潮热谵语，手足濈然汗出，舌苔黄燥起刺，或焦黑燥裂，脉沉实。或下利清水，色纯青，脐腹疼痛，按之坚硬有块，口舌干燥，脉滑实。现常用于急性单纯性肠梗阻、粘连性肠梗阻、蛔虫性肠梗阻、急性胆囊炎、急性阑尾炎、急性菌痢、中毒性痢疾、精神分裂症等病具有上述症状者。本方为峻下剂，中病即止。孕妇禁用；芒硝、大黄煎煮时间短，可增强泻下作用。临床应用大承气汤加味治疗急重病实热证，治黄疸加黄柏、栀子、金钱草、川楝子等治疗 12 例，服药 5 天后治愈 7例，病情好转 2 例。治肠痈加蒲公英、金银花、三叶鬼针草等治疗 15 例，服药 3～5 天治愈 13 例。治湿热痢加黄连、白芍等治疗 36 例，29 例治愈，5 例好转，2 例无效。运用大承气汤去厚朴，加山楂、红藤、败酱草治疗急性胰腺炎 56 例，症见心下剧痛拒按，痛引胁部，恶心呕吐，嗳腐，腹胀，发热，舌苔腻或黄，脉小弦滑，结果 54 例痊愈，2 例体征缓解消失，3 例复发。

2.4 大陷胸汤

出自《伤寒论》。由大黄 10 克，芒硝 10 克，甘遂 1 克组成。水煎分 2 次服（溶芒硝，冲甘遂末）。方中甘遂味苦性寒，善泻水逐饮，泄热散结，大黄长于荡涤邪热，两药泻水热互结之邪，均为主药。芒硝泻热软坚，助甘遂、大黄以破除积结。共奏泻热逐水散结之功。主治水饮与邪热结于胸腹之证。症见不大便 5～6 日，从心下至少腹硬满而痛不可近，日晡小有潮热，或短气躁烦，舌上燥而渴，脉沉紧而按之有力。现常用于渗出性胸膜炎、肠梗阻、腹膜炎等病具有上述症状者。本方为泻热逐水散结之峻剂，中病即止。若平素虚弱，或病后不任攻伐者，宜禁用本方。临床应用大陷胸汤治疗结核性渗出性胸膜炎 6 例，症见发烧，胸痛，气短，烦躁，头痛，恶寒，胸水少量者 4 例，达第 5

肋骨者 1 例，达第 3 肋骨者 1 例。药用大黄 9 克，芒硝 9 克，甘遂 3 克，水煎服，4 例少量胸水患者服 1～3 剂后，胸水消失，余 2 例服 6～9 剂胸水消失，其他症状也随之消失。运用大陷胸汤和大承气汤加减治疗急性胰腺炎 20 例，证属太阳阳明合病，治疗过程中不禁食，不补液，不用抗菌素，单用中药治疗，服药后腹痛开始缓解，时间最短者 2 小时，最长者 48 小时，平均 19.5 小时，完全消失腹痛时间最短 24 小时，最长 96 小时，平均 68 小时。

2.5 温下剂

是以泻下和温里的药物为主组成的方剂。适用于脏腑间寒冷积滞实证。症见大便秘结，脘腹胀满，腹痛喜温，手足不温，甚或厥冷，脉沉紧等。常用泻下药大黄、巴豆配伍温里药附子、干姜等，代表方剂有大黄附子汤、三物备急丸等。

2.6 大黄附子汤

出自《金匮要略》。由大黄 9 克，炮附子 9 克，细辛 3 克组成。水煎分 3 次服。方中附子味辛甘性大热，温阳祛寒，为主药。细辛除寒散结，大黄荡涤肠胃，泻除积滞。共奏温阳散寒，泻结行滞之功。主治寒积里实之证。症见腹痛便秘，胁下偏痛，发热，手足厥逆，舌苔白腻，脉紧弦。现常用于慢性痢疾、尿毒症、溃疡性结肠炎、急性肠梗阻等病具有上述症状者。本方是温下剂，大黄用量不宜超过附子。临床应用大黄附子汤加味治疗胆道蛔虫 1 例，证属寒实内结、阳虚厥逆，症见突发胸胁疼痛，右胁下阵发性绞痛，痛引肩背，冷汗淋漓，四肢厥逆，不呕不渴，大便 2 日未解，舌胖淡苔白，脉沉紧。药用大黄 10 克，附子（先煎）30 克，细辛 5 克，乌梅 40 克，槟榔 30 克，1 剂顿服，疼痛消除。运用大黄附子汤治疗过敏性紫癜、顽固性湿疹、药物过敏性皮炎、传染性湿疹各 1 例，4 例均为肢冷畏寒，小便清，大便干结，脉紧等寒实内结之证，经本方治疗均获愈。

2.7 温脾汤

出自《备急千金要方》。由大黄12克，附子9克，干姜6克，人参9克，甘草3克组成。水煎分3次服。方中人参味甘微苦性平，补益脾气，干姜味辛性温，温脾散寒，两药温补脾阳，均为主药。附子助干姜温阳祛寒，大黄荡涤积滞，甘草益气和中，调和诸药。共奏温补脾阳，攻下冷积之功。主治脾阳不足，寒凝积滞之证。症见冷积便秘，或久痢赤白，腹痛，手足不温，舌苔白滑，脉沉弦。现常用于慢性痢疾、溃疡性结肠炎、蛔虫病、肝硬化腹水等病具有上述症状者。临床应用温脾汤治疗肝硬化腹水1例、小儿消化不良1例、蛔虫病2例，均有腹痛便秘，证属脾胃阳虚、寒凝积滞之证，服本方后均获满意的效果。运用温脾汤加味治疗痢疾1例，证属脾胃寒湿、肠胃积滞，并兼有表证，症见泻下脓便，红白粘液，每天6～7次，少腹绞痛，肛门重坠，苔白，脉右缓迟，左细涩，本方加减服7剂而愈。

2.8 三物备急丸

出自《金匮要略》。由大黄30克，干姜30克，巴豆（去油）30克组成。研末，每服0.6～1.5克，服后不泻，可酌情再服（原亦作蜜丸）。方中巴豆味辛性热，峻下开塞，攻逐寒积，为主药。干姜温阳，助巴豆祛寒，大黄荡涤肠胃积滞，并能监制巴豆之毒。共奏攻逐寒积之功。主治寒实冷积之证。症见卒然心腹胀痛，痛如锥刺，气急口噤，大便不通，苔白，脉沉紧。现常用于食物中毒，急性单纯性肠梗阻等病具有上述症状者。本方是峻下剂，巴豆毒性剧烈，对于胃肠的刺激极强，须慎重使用。怀孕、年老体弱，以及温暑热邪所致的暴急腹痛之症，不能使用。如服后泻下不止，可吃冷粥止泻。临床应用三物备急丸（装入胶囊内）治疗肠阻梗35例，发病时间最短1小时，最长3天，平均为 10 小时左右，服药后 30 分钟左右肠鸣活跃；最快 1 小时排便，一般 3 小时排便，治愈 27 例，占 77.1%，27 例中有 5 例为寒证，其余皆有热证，8 例经本方治疗无效改行手术。

三物备急丸具有加强肠管收缩的明显作用，其作用又常与药物浓度不同而异。

2.9 润下剂

是以滋润和泻下的药物为主组成的方剂。适用于体虚便秘之证。症见大便燥结，秘塞不通等。常用滋润药麻子仁、杏仁、芍药配伍泻下药大黄等，代表方剂有麻子仁丸、济川煎等。

2.10 麻子仁丸

出自《伤寒论》。由麻子仁 500 克，芍药 250 克，枳实 250 克，大黄 500 克，厚朴 250 克，杏仁 250 克组成。上药为末，炼蜜为丸，每次 9 克，日 2 次（可按原量比例酌减，作汤剂服）。方中火麻仁味甘性平，润肠通便，为主药。杏仁降气润肠，芍药养阴和里，大黄通便泄热，枳实、厚朴下气破结，蜂蜜润燥滑肠。共奏润肠泄热，行气通便之功。主治肠胃燥热，津液不足之证。症见大便干结，小便频数。现常用于习惯性便秘，痔疮患者便秘等病具有上述症状者。本方对血少津亏的便秘，则不适宜。孕妇忌用。临床应用加味麻仁汤治疗蛔虫性肠梗阻 47 例。一般服第 1 次煎液后 1~2 小时腹痛即可缓解，服药后 6~12 小时均可通便排虫，多数病例排虫团。在通便排虫后，临床症状和体征完全消失，治疗中未发现任何毒性反应或副作用。运用麻子仁丸治疗肛门疾病手术后 500 例，以防止术后等 1 次排便时，由于大便干燥所引起的疼痛出血，服药后大便变软，成条状易于排出者为有效，以服药后大便干燥或 2~3 天排便 1 次为无效，500 例中有效者 479 例，占 95.8%，无效例中属习惯性便秘者 16 例。

2.11　济川煎

　　出自《景岳全书》。由当归 12 克，牛膝 6 克，肉苁蓉 7.5 克，泽泻 4.5 克，升麻 2 克，枳壳 3 克组成。水煎分 2 次服。方中肉苁蓉味甘咸性温，温肾益精，润肠通便，为主药。当归养血和血，润肠通便，牛膝补肾强腰，性善下行，枳壳下气宽肠而助通便，泽泻性向下而泄肾浊，升麻升清阳以达降浊阴。共奏温肾益精，润肠通便之功。主治肾虚便秘。症见大便秘结，小便清长，头目眩晕，腰膝酸软。现常用于老年体虚便秘、结核病患者体虚便秘、肿瘤病患者体虚便秘等病具有上述症状者。

2.12　逐水剂

　　是以逐水的药物为主组成的方剂。适用于水饮停聚的里实证。症见身肿，腹肿，胸闷，咳唾胸胁引痛，头痛目眩，舌苔滑，脉沉弦等。常用的药有芫花、甘遂、大戟、牵牛子等，代表方剂有十枣汤、舟车丸等。

2.13　十枣汤

　　出自《伤寒论》。由芫花、甘遂、大戟各等分，大枣 10 枚组成。前 3 味药共为末，大枣煎汤，调服药末 1.5～3 克，日 1次，清晨空腹服。方中甘遂味苦性寒，善行经隧水湿，大戟味苦性寒，善泄脏腑水湿，芫花味辛性温，善消胸胁伏饮痰癖，大枣益气护胃，能缓和诸药的峻烈及毒性，使下不伤正。共奏攻逐水饮之功。主治水饮壅盛于里之证。症见咳唾胸胁引痛，心下痞硬，干呕短气，头痛目眩，或胸背掣痛不得息，脉沉弦；或一身悉肿，尤以腰以下为重，腹胀喘满，二便不利。现常用于渗出性胸膜炎、结核性腹膜炎、肝硬化腹水、慢性肾炎等病具有上述症状者。本方为攻逐水饮的峻剂，服用一般宜从小剂量（1.5 克）开始。服药后泻下不止者，可服冷稀粥或冷开水以止之；体虚及孕妇慎用。临床应用十枣汤治疗渗出性胸膜炎 51 例,以芫花、甘遂、大戟各等分为末,每服 3 克,大枣 10～15 枚煎汤,早晨空腹送下,隔日 1 次,以 4～6 剂为度,结果胸水在 11 天内改善者达 96%,20 天内完全消失者达 88.2%,积液平均消失时间为 16.2 天,少数积液吸收后遗留胸痛现象。运用十枣丸治疗肝硬化腹水 5 例,以十枣丸 1.5～6 克,早晨空腹服,大剂 12 克,日分 2 次服,均用大枣汤送下,腹水有不同程度的消退。

2.14 舟车丸

出自《景岳全书》。由牵牛子 120 克,甘遂(面裹煨)、芫花、大戟(俱醋炒)各 30 克,大黄 60 克,青皮、陈皮、木香、槟榔各 15 克,轻粉 3 克组成。研末为丸,每服 3～6 克,日 1 次,清晨空腹温开水送下。方中芫花、甘遂、大戟攻逐胸胁脘腹经隧之水,均为主药。大黄、牵牛子荡涤胃肠,泻水泄热,青皮舒肝而破结气,陈皮理肺脾而畅膈气,槟榔下气利水而破坚,木香疏利三焦而导滞,使气畅水行而肿胀消,轻粉逐水通便,协助诸药分消下泄。共奏峻下逐水,行气破结之功。主治水热内壅,气机阻滞之证。症见水肿水胀,口渴,气粗,腹坚,大小便秘,脉沉数有力。现常用于肝硬化腹水具有上述症状者。本方攻逐之力甚强,正虚及孕妇忌用,方中轻粉、芫花、甘遂、大戟等毒性剧烈,须注意用量,不宜久服,以防中毒。临床应用舟车丸治疗虫积经闭 1 例,症见婚后 3 年未育,2 年前曾患浮肿,继则腹胀闭经,腹胀善饥,便溏,尿少,喜食盐粒,时吐涎沫,四肢沉重,周身乏力,唇白内见丘疹,诊为虫积经闭,药用舟车丸峻剂逐水,第 1 天早晨空腹服用舟车丸 1.5 克,2 小时后呕恶,腹绞痛,3 小时后排出大量水及虫体,腹消大半,隔日晨再服舟车丸 1.5 克,服后反应如前,腹臌消失。

2.15 疏凿饮子

出自《济生方》。由泽泻 12 克，赤小豆 15 克，商陆 6 克，羌活 9 克，大腹皮 15 克，椒目 9 克，木通 12 克，秦艽 9 克，槟榔 9 克，茯苓皮 30 克，生姜皮 4.5 克组成。水煎分 2 次服（原作散剂）。方中商陆味苦辛性平，泻下逐水，通利二便，为主药。槟榔、大腹皮行气导水，茯苓皮、泽泻、木通、椒目、赤小豆利水去湿，使在里之水从二便排出。羌活、秦艽、生姜皮善走皮肤，疏风发表，使在表之水从肌肤而泄。共奏泻下逐水，疏风发表之功。主治表里水湿壅盛之证。症见遍身水肿，喘呼口渴，二便不利。现常用于急性肾炎、肾病综合征等病具有上述症状者。

2.16 攻补兼施剂

是以泻下和补益的药物为主组成的方剂。适用于里实积结而正气内虚证。症见大便秘结，神倦少气，口干咽燥等。常用泻下药大黄、芒硝配伍补益药人参、当归、生地等，代表方剂有新加黄龙汤、增液承气汤等。

2.17 新加黄龙汤

出自《温病条辨》。由生地 15 克，生甘草 6 克，人参（另煎）4.5 克，生大黄 9 克，芒硝 3 克，玄参 15 克，麦冬 15 克，当归 4.5 克，海参 2 条，姜汁 6 匙组成。水煎分 3 次服。方中大黄、芒硝泻热通便，软坚润燥，为主药。玄参、生地、麦冬、海参滋阴增液，人参、甘草、当归补气养血。共奏滋阴益气，泻结泄热之功。主治热结里实，气阴不足之证。症见大便秘结，腹中胀满而硬，神疲少气，口干咽燥，唇裂舌焦，苔焦黄或焦黑燥裂。现常用于肿瘤病患者便秘、结核病患者便秘等病具有上述症状者。

2.18　增液承气汤

出自《温病条辨》。由玄参 30 克，麦冬 25 克，细生地 25 克，大黄 9 克，芒硝 5 克组成。水煎分 2 次服。方中大黄味苦性寒，泄热通便，为主药。生地、麦冬滋阴增液，润肠通便，芒硝软坚化燥。共奏滋阴增液，通便泄热之功。主治热结阴亏的便秘证。症见大便燥结，舌绛苔少，脉细而数。现常用于痔疮患者便秘、肝脓疡病患者便秘、肿瘤病患者便秘等病具有上述症状者。临床应用增液承气汤加减治疗散发性病毒性脑炎 1 例，症见神志不清，谵妄躁动，失语，口向左边㖞斜，手足抽搐频频，便秘 6 日未解，小便短赤自遗，舌红苔黄而干，脉弦滑，服 10 余剂而显效。运用增液承气汤加味治疗流行性出血热少尿期 75 例，基本方由生地、玄参、麦冬、水牛角各 30 克，赤芍、丹皮各 15 克，大黄（开水泡）30 克，芒硝（冲服）30 克，不能口服者可鼻饲或保留灌肠。肠麻痹加枳实、厚朴各 12 克，渴甚加花粉 15 克，呕吐加竹茹 12 克，呃逆加柿蒂 9 克，逆传心包，神昏谵语加安宫牛黄丸，75 例治愈 73 例，死亡 2 例。

第3章 和解剂

3.1 和解剂

由解表药与清里药配伍，祛邪药与扶正药共用，疏肝药与健脾药同使，辛热药与苦寒药并调，滋补药与温凉药相合等不同形式组成。具有和解、解郁、疏畅、调和等作用，以治疗少阳病、肝脾不和、肠胃不和等病证的方剂，统称和解剂。和解剂可分和解少阳、调和肝脾、调和肠胃3类，分别适用于少阳病、肝脾不和、肠胃不和的病证。

凡邪不在半表半里，或虚实各有所急，均不宜用和解剂。若误用和解剂后，轻者贻误病情，迁延难愈；甚则引邪入里，或变生他证。

3.2 和解少阳剂

是以和解少阳的药物为主组成的方剂。适用于邪在少阳胆经之证。症见口苦，咽干，目眩，往来寒热，胸胁苦满，心烦喜呕，默默不欲饮食，脉弦。常用柴胡或青蒿配黄芩等，代表方剂有小柴胡汤、蒿芩清胆汤等。

3.3 小柴胡汤

出自《伤寒论》。由柴胡12克，黄芩9克，人参6克，半夏9克，炙甘草5克，生姜9克，大枣4枚组成。水煎分2次服。方中柴胡味苦辛性微寒，轻清升散，疏邪透表，为主药。黄芩苦寒，善清少阳之邪热，半夏和胃降逆，散结消痞，人参、甘草、生姜、大枣益胃气，生津液，和营卫。共奏和解少阳之功。主治邪犯少阳，邪正相争之证。症见口苦，咽干，目眩，往来寒热，胸胁苦满，默默不欲饮食，心烦喜呕，舌苔薄白，脉弦。现常用于慢性胆囊炎、慢性肝炎、慢性盆腔炎、渗出性胸膜炎、妇人经期感冒发热等病具有上述症状者。临床应用小柴胡汤加减治疗高热 86 例，其中呼吸系统感染 36 例，胆道感染 20 例，泌尿系感染 9 例，产后感染 4 例，败血症 2 例，肝炎 3 例，乙脑 2 例，伤寒 2 例，腮腺炎 5 例，菌痢 3 例。病程 1～30 天，平均 15 天，退热天数 1～5 天，平均 3 天。运用小柴胡汤加味治疗斜视 1 例，症见斜视 1 年余，两眼瞳子斜向左侧 50°～60°，侧面视人，视力减退，舌淡红苔薄白，脉弦细。证属风热入于少阳，药用柴胡 18 克，黄芩、半夏各 12 克，党参、甘草各 9 克，菊花 30 克，黄芪 20 克，当归、山萸肉各 12 克，白芍 15 克，生姜 5 克，大枣 5 枚，连服 1 个月而愈。

3.4 蒿芩清胆汤

出自《重订通俗伤寒论》。由青蒿 6 克，淡竹茹 9 克，仙半夏 5 克，赤茯苓 9 克，黄芩 6 克，生枳壳 5 克，广陈皮 5 克，碧玉散（滑石、甘草、青黛）9 克组成。水煎分 2 次服。方中青蒿味苦辛性寒，清透少阳邪热，黄芩味苦性寒，清泄胆腑邪热，均为主药。竹茹、半夏清化痰热，陈皮、枳壳宽胸畅膈，和胃降逆，赤茯苓、碧玉散清热利湿。共奏清胆利湿，和胃化痰之功。主治少阳湿热痰浊之证。症见寒热如疟，寒轻热重，口苦膈闷，吐酸苦水或呕黄涎而粘，甚则干呕呃逆，胸胁胀痛，舌红苔白腻，脉数而右滑左弦。现常用于急性胆囊炎、急性胃炎、急性肝炎、慢性胰腺炎等病具有上述症状者。临床应用蒿芩清胆汤治疗钩端螺旋体病 13 例，症见发热，头痛，全身酸痛，腓肠肌痛，眼结膜充血，淋巴结肿痛，结果 2 例服 1 剂热退，11 例服 2～4 剂体温正常，其余症状在 2～6 剂消失。运用蒿芩清胆汤加味治疗胆囊炎 48 例，基本方由青蒿 10 克，黄芩 15 克，枳壳、竹茹各 9 克，半夏 10 克，陈皮 6 克，茯苓 15 克，滑石 30 克，生甘草 5 克，青黛（布包）0.2 克，柴胡 10 克，大黄 6 克，龙胆草、车前子各 10 克，绵茵陈 20 克组成，经治疗，显效者 40 例，好转者 6 例，无效者 2 例。

3.5 柴胡达原饮

出自《重订通俗伤寒论》。由柴胡 5 克，生枳壳 5 克，川朴 5 克，青皮 5 克，炙草 2 克，黄芩 5 克，苦桔梗 3 克，草果 2 克，槟榔 6 克，荷叶梗 12 克组成。水煎分 2 次服。方中柴胡味苦辛性微寒，透发外邪，黄芩清泄郁热，均为主药。枳壳、桔梗一升一降，开发上焦之气，厚朴、草果辛烈辟秽，燥湿化痰，宣畅中焦之气，青皮、槟榔下气破结，清痰化积，疏利下焦之气，荷梗善通气宽胸，炙甘草益气和中，调和诸药。共奏宣湿化痰，透达膜原之功。主治痰湿阻于膜原之证。症见胸膈痞满，心烦懊侬，头眩口腻，咳痰不爽，间日发疟，舌苔厚如积粉，扪之糙涩，脉弦而滑。现常用于疟疾、胆系感染等病具有上述症状者。

3.6 调和肝脾剂

是以调和肝脾的药物为主组成的方剂。适用于肝气郁结。横犯脾胃，或脾虚不运，影响肝失疏泄之证。症见胸闷胁痛，脘腹胀痛。不思饮食，大便泄泻，甚则寒热往来。常用的药有柴胡、白芍、白术、甘草等，代表方剂有四逆散、逍遥散、痛泻要方等。

3.7 四逆散

出自《伤寒论》。由炙甘草 6 克，枳实 6 克，柴胡 6 克，芍药 9 克组成。水煎分 2 次（原作散剂）。方中柴胡味苦辛性微寒，疏肝解郁，清热透邪，为主药。枳实下气破结，芍药益阴养血，与柴胡相合而疏肝理脾，甘草益气和中，调和诸药，与白芍配伍而缓急止痛。共奏透邪解郁，疏肝理脾之功。主治阳气内郁之热厥证，或肝脾不和之证。症见手足厥冷，或胸腹疼痛，或泄利下重，脉弦。现常用于慢性肝炎、慢性胆囊炎、胃及十二指肠溃疡、肋间神经痛等病具有上述症状者。临床应用四逆散加青皮治疗乳痈 15 例，全部获愈，其中 1 天愈者 4 例，2 天愈者 10 例，3 天愈者 1 例。运用四逆散加味治疗胃粘膜异型增生 30 例，证属肝气郁结、胃失和降者，基本方由柴胡 10 克，枳实 10 克，赤、白芍各 10 克，炙甘草 5 克，制半夏 10 克，陈皮 6 克组成，经服用 3～6 个月后胃镜复查，其中显效者 25 例，有效者 3 例，无效者 2 例，总有效率为 93.3%。

3.8 柴胡疏肝散

出自《景岳全书》。由柴胡 9 克，陈皮 9 克，川芎 6 克，香附 10 克，枳壳 9 克，芍药 10 克，甘草 4.5 克组成。水煎分 2 次服（原作散剂）。方中柴胡味苦辛性微寒，疏肝解郁，为主药。芍药、川芎和血柔肝止痛，陈皮行气健胃，香附、枳壳疏肝理气，甘草调和诸药，与芍药配伍而缓急止痛。共奏疏肝行气，和血止痛之功。主治肝郁气滞之证。症见胁肋疼痛，胸脘胀闷，寒热往来，舌苔白，脉弦。现常用于慢性胃炎、慢性肝炎、肋间神经痛等病具有上述症状者。临床应用柴胡疏肝汤加减治疗抽动秽语综合征 1 例，证属肝气郁结，气机不畅，症见 10 日前因情志不遂而致精神抑郁，次日出现阵发性干呕，且喉内发出声响，伴噘嘴，双腿弯曲，逐渐加重且发作频繁，约 10 分钟发作 1 次，睡眠时消失，面色红赤，纳呆便干，舌质红，苔黄腻，脉弦滑。药用柴胡 10 克，枳壳 10 克，香附 15 克，川芎 15 克，郁金 15 克，白芍 15 克，芦荟 15 克，旋复花 25 克，代赭石 20 克，龙、牡各 15 克，甘草 15 克，服 10 剂而愈。运用柴胡疏肝汤加减治疗胸胁内伤 80 例，基本方由柴胡、赤芍、白芍、香附、川芎各 9 克，枳壳、陈皮、甘草各 6 克组成，伤气型可加厚朴、木香，伤血型可加丹参、红花、橘络，伤在胸部可加桔梗、薤白，伤在剑突下可加丁香、肉桂，疼痛甚者可加乳香、没药，胸闷咳嗽重者可加厚朴、杏仁，大便不通者可加瓜蒌仁、生大黄，经治疗80例痊愈。

3.9　逍遥散

出自《太平惠民和剂局方》。由柴胡9克，当归9克，白芍9克，白术9克，茯苓9克，炙甘草4.5克，烧生姜6克，薄荷3克组成。水煎分2次服（原作散剂）。方中柴胡味苦辛性微寒，疏肝解郁，为主药。当归、白芍养血补肝，白术、茯苓健脾益气，薄荷助柴胡散肝解郁，生姜温胃和中，炙甘草益气补中，与白芍配伍而缓肝之急。共奏疏肝解郁、健脾养血之功。主治肝郁血虚，脾失健运之证。症见两胁疼痛，寒热往来，头痛目眩，口燥咽干，神疲食少，或月经不调，乳房作胀，舌淡红，脉弦而虚。现常用于慢性肝炎、月经不调、慢性胃炎等病具有上述症状者。临床应用逍遥散加味治疗无黄疸型肝炎253例，症见胁肋胀痛，肝脾肿大，乏力肢软，食欲不振，大便不调，心跳气短，失眠多梦，腰背酸痛，常发寒热，结果肝功完全恢复者36例，好转139例，总有效率68.9%。运用逍遥散加减治疗带下病160例，基本方由柴胡、当归、白芍、白术、茯苓、银花、贯众组成。治疗结果：白带者71例，治愈48例，显效17例，好转6例；黄带者89例，治愈60例，显效20例，好转9例。服药以4～8剂者占多数，本方对输卵管炎引起的带下病疗效较好，但病程较长者约服10～20剂才能获愈，对人工流产（刮宫）引起的带下，一般服3～5剂后见效。

3.10　痛泻要方

引自《景岳全书》。由白术12克，白芍9克，陈皮6克，防风9克组成。水煎分2次服（原作散剂）。方中白术味苦甘性温，健脾燥湿，白芍味苦酸性微寒，柔肝止痛，两药均为主药。

陈皮和中化湿，防风散肝舒脾。共奏补脾疏肝之功。主治肝郁脾虚之证。症见肠鸣腹痛，大便泄泻，泻后仍腹痛，舌苔薄白，脉弦而缓。现常用于过敏性结肠炎、急性肠炎等病具有上述症状者。临床应用痛泻要方加减治疗急性肠炎60例，患者均为成年人，发病时间1~2天，最长不超过4天，均有肠鸣、腹疼、泻频等临床表现，其中大便成水样的39例，稀粥样便17例，脓血样便4例，兼有里急后重者5例，发热者8例，全部患者均经大便镜检确诊。结果多数服1~2剂而愈，无副作用，90%治愈和98%有效。运用痛泻要方合四神丸治疗肠道易激综合征187例，基本方由柴胡15克，白芍20克，防风15克，肉蔻20克，故纸20克，五味子15克，白术15克，陈皮15克组成。7天为1疗程，每疗程后停药3天，患者年龄15~78岁，病程3个月~26年，10年以内者114例，治疗1个疗程者54例，2个疗程者87例，3个疗程者36例，4个疗程者10例，结果治愈者128例，占68.4%，好转者41例，占21.9%，无效者18例，占9.7%，有效的169例，腹泻、腹痛的消失时间平均为6.8天，随诊满于1年者95例，82例未见症状复发，占86%，在症状复发的13例中，再次治疗11例，有效者9例。

3.11 调和肠胃剂

是以调和肠胃的药物为主组成的方剂。适用于邪犯肠胃，寒热互结，症见心下痞满，恶心呕吐，脘腹胀痛，肠鸣下利。常用的药有干姜、黄芩、黄连、半夏等，代表方剂有半夏泻心汤等。

3.12 半夏泻心汤

出自《伤寒论》。由半夏9克，黄芩6克，干姜6克，人参6克，炙甘草6克，黄连3克，大枣4枚组成。水煎分2次服。方中半夏味辛性温，辛开散结，降逆止呕，为主药。干姜辛温祛寒，黄芩、黄连泄热，人参、大枣补益中气，甘草补脾胃而调诸药。共奏和胃降逆，开结除痞之功。主治寒热互结于胃肠之证。症见心下痞满不痛，或干呕，或呕吐，肠鸣下利，舌苔薄黄而腻，脉弦数。现常用于慢性胃炎、胃及十二指肠溃疡、胃神经官能症、慢性肠炎等病具有上述症状者。临床应用半夏泻心汤加减治疗贲门痉挛41例，证属寒热互结，痰瘀交阻于胃。基本方由法半夏、黄芩、甘草、党参、旋复花各10克，黄连、干姜各5克，代赭石、大枣各30克组成。服药最少5剂，最多30剂，平均为10～20剂，29例愈，8例显效，4例无效。运用半夏泻心汤治疗胃及十二指肠溃疡出血48例，病程2～6年，呕血者以炮姜炭易干姜，加小蓟根10克，大便隐血试验阳性者用干姜加阿胶10克，脘腹疼痛者加延胡索10克，结果服药3剂止血者31例，服5剂止血者15例，服10剂止血者2例。

第4章 清热剂

4.1 清热剂

由清热药为主组成。具有清热、泻火、凉血、解毒、滋阴透热等作用，以治疗里热的方剂，统称清热剂。温、热、火3者，有温盛为热、热极似火之别，它们在程度上有异，但在属性上则是一致的。由温、热、火所致的里热证，均可选用清热剂。里热证有在气分、血分、脏腑等之不同，因而清热剂可分为清气分热，清营凉血，清热解毒，气血两清，清脏腑热，清虚热6类。分别适用于气分热盛，营血分热，火毒热盛，气血两燔，脏腑火热，阴虚发热的里热证。

清热剂一般在表证已解，里热正盛，或里热虽盛尚未结实的情况下使用。邪热在表，当先解表。里热成实，则宜攻下，表未解，里已热，宜表里双解。热在气而治血，则将引邪深入。热在血而治气，则血热难平。在运用时尚须注意辨别热证的虚实，分清在脏、在腑；辨别热证真假，苦寒、滋阴药久服每易败胃或内伤中阳，必要时可配用醒胃、和胃之品，在寒凉药中，加用温热药，此属反佐法，但温热药的用量宜轻。

4.2 清气分热剂

是以清气分热的药物为主组成的方剂。适用于热在气分，热盛津伤，或气阴两伤之证。症见壮热烦渴，大汗，恶热，脉洪大；或身热多汗，心胸烦闷，口干舌红等。常用的药有石膏、知母、竹叶、栀子，因热易耗气伤津，又宜配益气生津药人参、麦冬等，代表方剂有白虎汤、竹叶石膏汤等。

4.3 白虎汤

出自《伤寒论》。由石膏 30 克，知母 9 克，炙甘草 3 克，粳米 9 克组成。水煎分 2 次服。方中石膏味辛甘性大寒，清泻肺胃而除烦热，为主药。知母清泄肺胃之热，质润以滋其燥，甘草、粳米益胃护津，使大寒之剂无损伤脾胃之虑。共奏清热生津之功。主治阳明气分热盛之证。症见壮热面赤，烦渴引饮，汗出恶热，脉洪大有力，或滑数。现常用于各种急慢性热性传染病、中暑、糖尿病、急性眼结膜炎等病具有上述症状者。临床应用白虎汤加减治疗流行性出血热 40 例，轻型 16 例，中型 11 例，重例 10 例，危重型 3 例。证属温邪化燥伤津，阴液枯涸，症见高热，易发生神昏谵语，斑疹，吐衄，动风惊厥等，基本方由生石膏 30～300 克，知母 12 克，甘草 10 克，粳米 10 克组成，发热期加双花、连翘、板蓝根，低血压期加人参、麦冬、五味子、丹参，少尿期去粳米，加玄参、生地、寸冬、大黄、芒硝，多尿期加生地、山药、麦冬、五味子、菟丝子、党参，恢复期改用竹叶石膏汤加减治疗。40 例全部治愈，最短 6 天，最长 15 天。运用白虎汤加减配合验方治疗糖尿病 21 例，基本方用生石膏 30～120 克，知母 15 克，元参 30 克，生山药 30 克，石斛 15 克，寸冬 15 克，花粉 15 克，芦根 30 克，甘草 3～6 克组成，一般服上方 3～6 剂后，口渴和饮水量可明显减轻或恢复正常，继用验方治疗，验方药用芡实、白扁豆、益智仁、薏苡仁各 30 克，公鸡 1 只（去尽毛及内脏，洗净）将上 4 味药填于公鸡体腔内，用针线缝好体腔切口，砂锅煮之，以公鸡肉熟为度，依患者食量吃肉喝汤，药滓亦可食之，不计量，日 1 剂或 2 日 1 剂，用 3～5 剂后，可改为每周或 10 天 1 剂，以巩固疗效。

4.4 竹叶石膏汤

出自《伤寒论》。由竹叶 15 克，石膏 30 克，半夏 9 克，麦门冬 15 克，人参 5 克，甘草 3 克，粳米 15 克组成。水煎分 3 次服。方中竹叶味甘淡性寒，石膏味辛甘性大寒，两药清热除烦，均为主药。人参益气，麦冬养阴生津，半夏降逆止呕，甘草、粳米和中养胃。共奏清热生津，益气和胃之功。主治热病后期余热未清之证。症见身热多汗，心胸烦闷，气逆欲呕，口干喜饮，或虚烦不寐，舌红少苔，脉虚数。现常用于流行性感冒、小儿夏季热等病具有上述症状者。临床应用竹叶石膏汤治疗金黄色葡萄球菌败血症余热不退 1 例，证属热病后期，邪退而余热未尽，曾用西药抗菌素和中药黄连解毒汤治疗，但热度长期不退，体温常波动在 38～39℃ 之间。经竹叶石膏汤加味治疗而愈。运用竹叶石膏汤治疗妊娠口疮、喘咳、头痛各 1 例，经治疗均获愈。

4.5 栀子豉汤

出自《伤寒论》。由栀子 9 克，淡豆豉 9 克组成。水煎分 2 次服。方中栀子味苦性寒，以清除邪热，为主药。豆豉除烦，并助栀子清热。共奏清热除烦之功。主治外感热病气分轻证，或余热未清之证。症见身热胸满，心中懊侬，虚烦不眠，甚则反复颠倒，舌红苔微黄，脉数。现常用于神经衰弱、慢性胆囊炎、冠心病等病具有上述症状者。

4.6 清营凉血剂

是以清营凉血的药物为主组成的方剂。适用于热在营分，或在血分之证。症见身热烦扰，口渴或不渴，神昏谵语，吐衄发斑，舌降脉数。常用的药有生地黄、玄参、丹皮、赤芍、犀角等；代表方剂有清营汤、犀角地黄汤等。

4.7　清营汤

出自《温病条辨》。由犀角 2 克，生地黄 15 克，元参 9 克，竹叶心 3 克，麦冬 9 克，丹参 6 克，黄连 5 克，银花 9 克，连翘 6 克组成。水煎分 3 次服。方中犀角味咸性寒，生地味甘苦性寒，两药清营凉血，均为主药。元参、麦冬养阴清热，银花、连翘、黄连、竹叶清热解毒以透邪热，丹参活血以消瘀热。共奏清营透热，养阴活血之功。主治邪热初入营分之证。症见身热夜甚，神烦少寐，时有谵语，目常喜开或喜闭，口渴或不渴，或斑疹隐隐，舌绛而干，脉数。现常用于流行性脑脊髓膜炎、乙型脑炎、斑疹伤寒、猩红热等病具有上述症状者。临床应用清营汤加减治疗皮肤粘膜淋巴结综合征 5 例，急性期药用水牛角、生地、赤芍、丹参、银花、连翘、元参、芦根、麦冬、甘草各 10 克。恢复期用本方加红花、川芎各 10 克，退热时间为 11～16 天，平均 13.5 天，皮疹消退时间 5～7 天，平均 6 天。近期治愈 4 例，好转 1 例，随访 4 例，未见心血管并发症。运用清营汤加减治疗 12 年顽固性盗汗症 1 例，曾经中西医久治无效，每年入冬即盗汗，出汗前有烘热感，后形寒畏冷，口舌干燥，乏力，面足浮肿，脉细数，证属营阴不足，邪热内伏，以清营养阴为法，药用犀角、生地、元参、丹皮、麦冬、白薇，经治疗盗汗渐止，追踪 1 年未见复发。

4.8　犀角地黄汤

出自《备急千金要方》。由犀角 1.5～3 克，生地黄 30 克，芍药 12 克，牡丹皮 9 克组成。水煎分 3 次服。方中犀角味咸性寒，清心、凉血、解毒，为主药。生地凉血止血，养阴清热，芍药、丹皮既能凉血，又能散瘀。共奏清热解毒，凉血散瘀之功。主治热入血分之证。症见吐血、衄血、便血、善忘如狂，漱水不欲咽，胸中烦痛，自觉腹满，大便色黑易解，或昏狂谵语，斑色紫黑，舌绛有刺。现常用于急性白血病、急性黄色肝萎缩、血小板减少性紫癜、流行性脑脊髓膜炎、乙型脑炎、斑疹伤寒、肝昏迷、尿毒症等病具有上述症状者。临床应用犀角地黄汤治疗原发性血小板减少性紫癜11例，均有出血症状，其中皮下出血11例，口腔粘膜出血9例，鼻血7例，便血6例，尿血、呕血、眼结膜下出血者各2例，因大量失血而致昏迷者2例，血小板60,000／mm³ 以下者5例，其余均在 60,000～80,000 之间，11例均有发热，口干畏饮，烦躁不安，面赤，尿黄，出血，舌红苔薄不润，脉滑数等内热积盛之象，经用犀角地黄汤为主治疗，结果6例痊愈，4例显效，1例无效死亡。运用犀角地黄汤治疗急性再生障碍性贫血1例，药用本方加大黄、黄芩、板蓝根、连翘、石膏、知母、葛根、金银花、甘草、服2剂后体温由40.7℃降至36.5℃，便通斑消，咽痛减轻，精神转佳，血红蛋白9.4克，红细胞由 280 万／mm³ 升至 348 万／mm³，白细胞1,600／mm³ 升至 2,800／mm³，淋巴细胞由94%降至44%，后改用清气分湿热与益气养阴之剂而获效。

4.9　清热解毒剂

　　是以清热解毒的药物为主组成的方剂。适用于瘟疫、温毒或疮疡疔毒等热深毒重之证。症见烦躁狂乱、吐衄发狂，或头面红肿，或口糜咽痛等。常用的药有黄连、黄芩、黄柏、栀子、石膏、连翘、板蓝根、升麻、玄参、蒲公英、紫花地丁等；代表方剂有黄连解毒汤、普济消毒饮、仙方活命饮等。

4.10　黄连解毒汤

　　出自《外台秘要》。由黄连9克，黄芩、黄柏各6克，栀子9克组成。水煎分2次服。方中黄连味苦性寒，泻心火，兼泻中焦之火，为主药。黄芩泻上焦之火，黄柏泻下焦之火，栀子通泻三焦之火，导火下行。共奏泻火解毒。主治三焦热盛而津液未伤之证。症见大热烦扰，口燥咽干，错语不眠，或吐血发斑，以及外科痈肿疔毒、舌红苔黄、脉数有力。现常用于蜂窝组织炎等急性化脓性感染、败血症、脓毒血症、痢疾、肺炎、血液病等病具有上述症状者。临床应用黄连解毒汤加减治疗乙型脑炎 56 例，其中重型及暴发型 31 例，轻型及中型 25 例，基本方由黄连 9 克、黄芩 15 克、黄柏 15 克、栀子 9 克、板蓝根 15 克、金银花 15 克组成，高热不退加知母，呕吐加竹茹、代赭石，抽搐不止加止痉散，谵语、昏迷加牛黄丸、紫雪丹，结果痊愈 51 例，进步 1 例，死亡 4 例。运用黄连解毒汤治疗流行性脑脊髓膜炎 12 例，基本方由黄连、黄柏、栀子各等分，兼挟新感者加银花、连翘，头痛者加生石决、杭白芍、刺蒺藜、天麻，便秘者合承气汤，壮热烦渴者加石膏、竹叶、麦冬，痰涎壅盛者合涤痰汤，谵语者加紫雪丹、牛黄丸，神志昏迷者加石菖蒲、远志、竹沥，衄血或见斑疹者加丹皮、生地，结果 12 例全部治愈，其中服 3 剂愈者 4 例，服 4 剂愈者 2 例，服 5 剂愈者 5 例，服 6 剂愈者 1 例，均无后遗症。

4.11　凉膈散

出自《太平惠民和剂局方》由川大黄、朴硝、炙甘草各 600 克，山栀子仁、薄荷、黄芩各 300 克，连翘 1200 克组成。共为粗末，每 6 克加竹叶 3 克、蜂蜜少许，水煎，去滓。日 3 次，饭后服（亦可作汤剂煎服，用量按原方比例酌减）。方中连翘味苦微寒，清热解毒，为主药。黄芩清心胸郁热，山栀通泻三焦之火，引火下行，薄荷、竹叶清疏肺胃心胸之热，芒硝、大黄荡涤胸膈邪热，导热下行，白蜜、甘草既能缓和芒硝、大黄峻泻之功，又可助芒硝、大黄以推导之力。共奏泻火通便，清上泄下之功。主治上中二焦邪郁生热之证。症见身热口渴，面赤唇焦，胸膈烦热，口舌生疮，或咽痛吐衄，便秘溲赤，或大便不畅，舌红苔黄，脉滑数。现常用于麻疹、肺炎、纵膈肿瘤、肺脓肿等病具有上述症状者。临床应用凉膈散加减治疗小儿急性扁桃体炎 32 例，证属肺胃积热，复感风邪，基本方由焦山栀、银花、连翘、淡竹叶、土牛膝、玄参各 6~9 克，生石膏（先煎）20~30 克，生川军（后下）、生甘草各 3~5 克，大青叶 9~15 克，黄芩 4.5~6 克组成。32 例中，年龄最小 16 个月，最大 12 岁，大多用抗菌素无效，除 2 例原有呕吐而中断治疗外，其余均治愈。运用凉膈散加味治疗大叶性肺炎、支气管扩张、高血压脑溢血、纵膈肿瘤各 1 例，均获显效。

4.12 普济消毒饮

出自《东垣试效方》。由黄芩（酒炒）、黄连（酒炒）各 9 克，陈皮、甘草、玄参、柴胡、桔梗各 6 克，连翘、板蓝根、马勃、牛蒡子、薄荷各 3 克，僵蚕、升麻各 2 克组成。水煎分 3 次服（原作散剂）。方中黄连、黄芩味苦性寒，酒炒善清降头面热毒，均为主药。牛蒡子、连翘、薄荷、僵蚕疏散上焦风热；玄参、马勃、板蓝根、桔梗、甘草清解咽喉头面热毒；陈皮理气而疏通壅滞；升麻、柴胡疏散风热，并协诸药上达头面。共奏疏风散邪，清热解毒之功。主治头面热毒之证。症见恶寒发热，头面红肿焮痛，目不能开，咽喉不利，舌燥口渴，舌红苔黄，脉数有力。现常用于流行性腮腺炎、急性颌下淋巴结炎、急性扁桃体炎等病具有上述症状者。临床应用普济消毒饮治疗急性扁桃体炎 69 例，症见发热，咽痛，汗出，便干或便秘，食欲减退，尿黄而少，舌红、苔白厚或黄厚，脉浮数等症，69 例全部咽充血，扁桃体 I 度者 9 例，II 度者 60 例，有脓点者 53 例，结果治愈 65 例，好转 3 例，无效 1 例，总有效率 98.6%。运用普济消毒饮加减治疗流行性腮腺炎 100 例，基本方由银花、连翘、牛蒡子、山栀子、板蓝根、马勃、蒲公英、桔梗组成，发热头痛甚者加桑叶、菊花、薄荷，便秘者加元明粉、元参，高烧者加紫雪丹、或口中含化六神丸（每次 3~5 粒，每天 2~3 次）。患者 2

天愈者 31 例，4 天愈者 46 例，6 天愈者 18 例，8～10 天愈者 5 例。

普济消毒饮煎剂，对甲型和乙型链球菌、肺炎双球菌、金黄色葡萄球菌、白色葡萄球菌均有较好的制菌作用，对其它细菌亦有不同程度的制菌作用。

4.13 气血两清剂

是以清气凉血的药物为主组成的方剂。适用于疫毒或热毒充斥内外，气分、血分均受干扰之证。症见大热烦渴，吐衄，发斑，神昏谵语等。常用清气药石膏、知母配伍凉血药犀角、地黄等，代表方剂有清瘟败毒饮等。

4.14 清瘟败毒饮

出自《疫疹一得》。由生石膏 30 克，生地 12 克，犀角 6 克，黄连 6 克，黄芩 6 克，栀子 10 克，牡丹皮 6 克，玄参 10 克，连翘 15 克，赤芍 6 克，知母 6 克，桔梗 9 克，竹叶 6 克，甘草 6 克组成。水煎分 3 次服（先煎石膏数 10 沸，后下诸药，犀角磨汁和服）。方中石膏味辛性寒，清热泻火，犀角味咸性寒，生地味甘苦性寒，两药凉血养阴，均为主药。知母养阴泻火，山栀、黄连、黄芩、连翘、玄参清热解毒，丹皮、赤芍凉血活血；桔梗、竹叶载药上行；甘草清热解毒，调和诸药。共奏清热解毒，凉血泻火之功。主治热毒充斥，气血两燔之证。症见大热渴饮，头痛如劈，谵语神糊，视物昏瞀，或发斑疹，或吐血衄血，四肢或抽搐，或厥逆，舌绛唇焦，脉沉数，或沉细而数，或浮大而数。现常用于流行性脑脊髓膜炎、重症流感、流行性出血热、败血症等病具有上述症状者。临床应用清瘟败毒饮加减治疗温毒严重麻疹 23 例，证属气血两燔，症见高热，有汗或汗泄不畅，口渴喜饮，舌质绛红，舌苔黄燥，基本方由生石膏 24 克，鲜生地 9 克，净连翘 9 克，焦山栀 9 克，黄芩 4.5 克，粉丹皮 9

克，川黄连 1.5 克，京赤芍 9 克，黑玄参 6 克，金银花 9 克，鲜芦根 30 克组成。若喘咳鼻煽，面苍唇干者，去赤芍、玄参，加麻黄、杏仁、猴枣散。声音嘶哑，咽部红肿，饮水作呛者，加山豆根、挂金灯。泻利频作，黄粘热臭者，加葛根、黄芩改黄连（炒用），口臭牙疳者，加服板蓝根，其中 15 例麻疹合并肺炎，经治疗，23 例患者均获显效。

运用加减清瘟败毒饮治疗四联球菌脑炎 1 例，患儿 6 岁，于 1 个半月前突然呕吐发烧，继之腹痛，头痛，头向左歪，两上肢弯曲，左肩低垂，手指无力，掌握失灵，两下肢痿软，行走跌仆。经住院治疗，症情缓解后出院不久，病情复发，仍见头向左歪，左肩低垂，上午轻烧，下午热盛汗出，患儿疲乏欲睡，颜面苍黄，舌红无苔，脉数。经以本方为主治疗，不久即获痊愈，随访患儿健康如常。

4.15 清脏腑热剂

是以清脏腑热的药物为主组成的方剂。适用于热邪偏盛于某一脏腑所产生的火热之证。根据邪热偏盛于某一脏腑的不同，药物治疗上也有区别，如心经热盛用黄连、栀子、连子心、木通等清心泻火，肝胆实火用龙胆草、夏枯草、青黛等清肝泻火，肺中有热用黄芩、桑白皮、石膏等清肺泄热，热在脾胃，一用防风与石膏、山栀以升散脾胃积热，一用黄连与升麻、生地等以清胃凉血，胃热阴虚用石膏与熟地、麦冬等清胃滋阴，热在肠腑用白头翁、黄连、黄柏等清肠解毒。代表方剂：清心经热有导赤散，清肝胆实火有龙胆泻肝汤，清肺热有泻白散，清脾胃热有泻黄散、清胃散，清胃养阴有玉女煎，清肠腑湿热有白头翁汤、芍药汤等。

4.16 导赤散

出自《小儿药证直诀》。由生地黄9克，木通6克，生甘草梢6克，竹叶9克组成。水煎分2次服（原作散剂）。方中生地味甘苦性寒，凉血滋阴，为主药。木通上清心经之热，下清小肠而利水通淋；生甘草梢清热解毒，调和诸药；竹叶清心除烦。共奏清心养阴，利水通淋之功。主治心经与小肠有热之证。症见心胸烦热，口渴面赤，意欲饮冷，口舌生疮，或小溲赤涩刺痛，舌红，脉数。现常用于急性泌尿系感染、口腔炎、泌尿系结石等病具有上述症状者。临床应用导赤散加减治疗淋证15例，其中砂淋5例，气淋7例，血淋3例，症见小便短涩，痛引脐中，甚则腰胀或痛，苔白腻或薄黄，脉弦数或细数等，砂淋加海金砂、萹蓄、金钱草，血淋加白茅根、生侧柏、小蓟，气淋加厚朴、香附，结果治愈9例，好转6例。运用导赤散加味治疗小儿手足口病50例，患者分3型论治，湿热型26例，本方加板蓝根、重楼、黄芩。热重于湿型15例，加石膏、知母、栀子、连翘、板蓝根、大青叶、重楼、僵蚕。湿重于热型9例，加茯苓、泽泻、苍术、黄柏、板蓝根、重楼、滑石，去生地，结果3剂治愈34例，6剂治愈12例。服药后无效和复发4例，总有效率92%。

4.17 龙胆泻肝汤

出自《医方集解》。由龙胆草（酒炒）6克，黄芩（炒）6克，栀子（酒炒）9克，泽泻12克，木通9克，车前子9克，当归（酒洗）3克，生地黄（酒炒）9克，柴胡6克，生甘草6克组成。水煎分2次服。方中龙胆草味苦性寒，上泻肝胆实火，下清下焦湿热，为主药。黄芩、栀子苦寒泻火，泽泻、木通、车前子清热利湿，使湿热从水道排除，肝经有热易耗伤阴血，加用苦寒燥湿更耗其阴，故用生地、当归滋阴养血，柴胡疏畅肝胆，甘草调中和药。共奏泻肝胆实火，清下焦湿热之功。主治肝胆实火，或肝经湿热下注之证。症见头痛目赤，胁痛口苦，耳聋，耳肿；或阴肿，阴痒，小便淋浊，妇女湿热带下。现常用于急性结膜炎、急性中耳炎、高血压、急性黄疸型肝炎、急性胆囊炎、带状疱疹、急性肾盂炎、膀胱炎、尿道炎、急性盆腔炎、急性前列腺炎等病具有上述症状者。本方药物多为苦寒之性，脾胃虚寒者不宜服用。临床应用龙胆泻肝汤加减治疗急性黄疸性肝炎172例，证属肝胆湿热型，症见食欲不振，尿黄，巩膜及皮肤中度黄染，肝肿大，肝功能损坏，基本方由龙胆泻肝汤去泽泻、车前子、栀子，加土茵陈、红枣组成，连服30~40剂，平均28天治愈。运用龙胆泻肝汤加减治疗急进型高血压1例，症见眩晕头痛，口干口苦，心悸多梦，烦躁易怒，小便黄赤，舌红苔黄腻，脉弦滑，血压200／148mmHg，尿蛋白+++，肾功NPN60mg，视神经乳头水肿。用本方去当归，生地黄，加夏枯草、生龙牡、僵蚕、石菖蒲，4剂症状消失，血压120／86mmHg，2月后痊愈。

4.18　左金丸

出自《丹溪心法》。由黄连9克，吴茱萸1.5克组成。水煎分2次服（原作丸剂）。方中黄连味苦性寒，清热泻火，为主药。吴茱萸辛热，制黄连之寒，又能入肝降逆，使肝胃和调。共奏清肝泻火，降逆止呕之功。主治肝郁化火，肝火犯胃之证。症见胁肋胀痛，嘈杂吞酸，呕吐口苦，脘痞嗳气，舌红苔黄、脉弦数。现常用于急性胃炎、胃及十二指肠溃疡、无黄疸型传染性肝炎等病具有上述症状者。临床应用左金丸加味治疗溃疡病24例，基本方由黄芩12克（代黄连），吴茱萸1.5克组成。若证属肝胃不和者，以本方合四逆散。证属脾胃湿热者，以本方合平胃散。证属脾虚而湿邪郁滞者，以本方合六君子汤等。经治疗，胃脘疼痛及纳差等主要症状均有不同程度的改善。

4.19 泻白散

出自《小儿药证直诀》。由地骨皮 12 克，桑白皮 12 克，炙甘草 3 克，粳米 6 克组成。水煎分 2 次服（原作散剂）。方中桑白皮味甘性寒，泻肺而清郁热，为主药。地骨皮泻肺中伏火，兼退虚热；炙甘草、粳米养胃和中以扶肺气。共奏泻肺清热，止咳平喘之功。主治肺有伏火郁热之证。症见咳嗽、甚则气急欲喘，皮肤蒸热，日晡尤甚，舌红苔黄，脉细数。现常用于急性支气管炎、支气管哮喘、肺气肿合并感染、小儿肺炎等病具有上述症状者。临床应用泻白散加味治疗百日咳 63 例，63 例均属痉咳期，痉咳连声不已，有回拗声，咳吐稠痰而稍止为主要症状，证属肺火内伏者 23 例，本方加百部、马兜铃、杏仁、贝母、黄芩、瓜蒌皮、枇杷叶等以清肺火，伴见咳血、衄血者，加侧柏叶、丹皮、藕节等以凉血止血。属表有风热者 28 例，本方加薄荷、牛蒡子、竹叶、杏仁、连翘、百部等。属风寒外束者 12 例，本方加麻黄、杏仁、前胡、枇杷叶、竹茹、防风等。63 例服药最少者 4 剂，最多者 8 剂，均获痊愈。

4.20 清胃散

出自《兰室秘藏》。由生地黄 12 克，当归身 6 克，牡丹皮 9 克，黄连 4.5 克，升麻 6 克组成。水煎分 2 次服（原作散剂）。方中黄连味苦性寒，清胃中积热，为主药。生地凉血滋阴，丹皮凉血清热；当归养血和血；升麻散火解毒。共奏清胃凉血之功。主治胃有积热，胃火上攻之证。症见牙痛牵引头痛，面颊发热，其齿恶热喜冷，或牙龈溃烂，或牙宣出血，或唇舌颊腮肿痛，或口气热臭，口舌干燥，舌红苔黄，脉滑大而数。现常用于三叉神经痛、口腔炎、牙周炎、慢性胃炎等病具有上述症状者。临床应用清胃散加减治疗牙痛，基本方由清胃散加石膏、知母、银花、连翘组成，治疗牙髓炎、牙周炎等证属胃火的患者 60 余例，均获满意效果。运用加味清胃散治疗复发性口疮 56 例，方由黄连 9 克，生地 45 克，当归 12 克，丹皮 16 克，升麻 12 克，双花 12 克，公英 16 克，连翘 16 克，淡竹叶 12 克，甘草 6 克组成。经治疗，显效 31 例，有效 18 例，无效 7 例，总有效率 87.5%。

4.21　泻黄散

出自《小儿药证直诀》。由藿香 12 克，山栀仁 6 克，石膏 15 克，甘草 6 克，防风 9 克组成。水煎分 2 次服（原作散剂）。方中石膏味辛甘性大寒、栀子味苦性寒，两药清泻脾胃积热，均为主药。防风疏散脾中伏火；藿香芳香醒脾，并助防风升散脾胃伏火；甘草泻火和中，调和诸药。共奏泻脾胃伏火之功。主治脾胃伏火。症见口疮口臭，烦渴易饥，口燥唇干，舌红，脉数。现常用于口腔炎、牙周炎等病具有上述症状者。

4.22　玉女煎

出自《景岳全书》。由石膏 18 克，熟地 15 克，麦冬 6 克，知母、牛膝各 4.5 克组成。水煎分 2 次服。方中石膏味辛甘性大寒，清胃中余热，为主药；熟地滋阴；知母质润，助石膏以清胃热；麦冬养阴，助熟地以滋胃阴；牛膝导热引血下行，以降上炎之火，而止上溢之血。共奏清胃滋阴之功。主治胃热阴虚之证。症见头痛牙痛，齿松牙衄，烦热口渴，舌干红，苔黄而干。现常用于急性口腔炎、舌炎、糖尿病、神经性牙痛等病具有上述症状者。临床应用玉女煎加味治疗牙痛 15 例，证属胃火牙痛，症见牙痛，甚则牵引头痛，或牙龈红肿，或腮颊红肿发热，伴有夜睡不安，不能咀嚼东西，口干欲饮，大便不爽，舌质红，苔或薄黄，脉浮弦滑或兼数。其原因多为蛀齿，以本方加防风、竹叶、淮山药治疗，一般服 2～7 剂即痛止而愈。运用玉女煎加减治疗赖特氏病 1 例，于菌痢后出现发烧，关节肿痛，运动受限，伴尿道炎，眼球结膜充血，口腔溃疡及生殖器糜烂，曾用抗菌素、抗风湿药及激素等治疗无明显效果，改用本方加减，药用生地 30 克，知母 9 克，石膏 30 克，牛膝 9 克，秦艽 15 克，忍冬藤、银花各 15 克，赤芍 12 克，丹皮 12 克，防风 12 克，木瓜 12 克，茯苓 9 克，陈皮 9 克，桑叶 30 克，寻骨风 30 克，经治疗 1 个月，恢复正常，出院半年后随访，情况良好。

4.23 芍药汤

出自《医学六书》。由芍药 15 克，当归、黄连各 9 克，槟榔、木香、甘草各 5 克，大黄 9 克，黄芩 9 克，官桂 3 克组成。水煎分 2 次服（原作散剂）。方中白芍味苦酸性微寒，调和营血，治痢止痛，为主药；黄连、黄芩、大黄清热解毒；当归、肉桂和营行血，木香、槟榔导滞调气；甘草清热解毒，调和诸药，与白芍配伍而缓急止痛。共奏调和气血。清热解毒之功。主治湿热蓄积肠中，气滞失调之证。症见腹痛便脓血，赤白相兼，里急后重，肛门灼热，小便短赤，舌苔黄腻，脉滑数。现常用于细菌性痢疾、阿米巴痢疾、过敏性肠炎、急性肠炎等病具有上述症状者。临床应用芍药合剂（芍药汤去大黄）治疗杆菌性痢疾 46 例，均见发病急、发热、腹痛、泻下脓血粘液、里急后重、不思饮食等症，镜检粪便内均有脓细胞及红细胞。经治疗，1 日内退热者 18 例，2 日内退热者 1 例，其余病例在入院初体温即正常，排便次数在服药 3 日内即恢复正常者 19 例，4 日内恢复正常者 6 例，1 周内恢复正常者 11 例，1 周后恢复正常者 10 例，腹痛及里急后重大都 5 日内消失，46 例均治愈。运用芍药汤加味治疗小儿杆菌痢疾 18 例，入院前都有发热，体温在 37～39℃之间，症见呕吐，腹泻，腹痛，里急后重，抽风昏迷等，大便镜检有红细胞及粘液，血象白细胞增高，基本方由白芍 9 克，黄芩 4.5 克，黄连 4.5 克，槟榔 4.5 克，木香 3 克，当归 3 克，枳壳 4.5 克，陈皮 4.5 克，银花 6 克，焦楂 3 克组成。水煎分 6 次，每日服 3 次，18 例全部治愈。治愈平均住院时间 4.44 天。与用合霉素组 20 例对照，本方的治疗效果优于合霉素。

4.24　白头翁汤

　　出自《伤寒论》。由白头翁 15 克，黄柏 12 克，黄连 6 克，秦皮 12 克组成。水煎分 2 次服。方中白头翁味苦性寒，清血分热毒，为主药。黄连、黄柏、秦皮清热解毒，燥湿治痢。共奏清热解毒，凉血治痢之功。主治热毒赤痢。症见腹痛，里急后重，肛门灼热，泻下脓血，赤多白少，渴欲饮水，舌红苔黄，脉弦数。现常用于急性细菌性痢疾、阿米巴性痢疾、溃疡性结肠炎、滴虫性肠炎、大叶性肺炎、支气管肺炎等病具有上述症状者。临床应用白头翁加大黄汤治疗急性菌痢 48 例。基本方由白头翁 8 克，黄连 6 克，黄柏 10 克，秦皮 12 克，炒大黄 10 克组成。初起有表证者加荆芥、防风、葛根。热重于湿者加马齿苋、苦参、地榆炭。湿重于热者加苍术、藿香、厚朴。腹痛、里急后重甚者加槟榔、木香、焦楂。经治疗，均获痊愈，其中 3 天愈者 29 例，5 天愈者 11 例，7 天愈者 8 例。运用白头翁汤治疗肺炎 67 例，男 48 例，女 19 例，年龄最大 56 岁，最小 3 岁，体温最高 41.4℃，最低 38.2℃，大叶性肺炎 41 例，支气管肺炎 26 例。证属大肠腑热而邪热壅肺。基本方由白头翁 16 克，黄连、黄柏各 6 克，秦皮 9 克组成，16 岁以下减量。风热闭肺者，加杏仁、麻黄、鱼腥草、僵蚕、大青叶、生石膏、葶苈子。痰热壅肿者，加黄芩、生石膏、生甘草、葶苈子、丹参、白花蛇舌草。热烁营阳，加生地、玄参、北条参、丹参、麦冬、花粉。气血两燔，加生地、玄参、麦冬、南沙参。神昏谵语加紫雪丹。经治疗，56 例患者获愈，11 例无效，56 例治愈的患者中，体温恢复正常的时间 3 日者 8 例，5～6 日者 37 例，8～14 日者 11 例。

4.25　清虚热剂

是以清虚热的药物为主组成的方剂。适用于热病后期，邪热未尽，阴液已伤，热留阴分，或肝肾亏损，或久热不退的虚热证。症见暮热早凉，骨蒸潮热，舌红少苔、脉数或细数。常用的药有青蒿、鳖甲、地骨皮、知母等，代表方剂有青蒿鳖甲汤，秦艽鳖甲散、清骨散等。

4.26　青蒿鳖甲汤

出自《温病条辨》。由青蒿 6 克，鳖甲 15 克，细生地 12 克，知母 6 克，丹皮 9 克组成。水煎分 2 次服。方中鳖甲味咸性寒，滋阴退虚热，青蒿味苦辛性寒，清热透络，引邪外出，两药养阴透热，均为主药。生地、知母益阴清热，助鳖甲以退虚热，丹皮凉血透热，助青蒿以透泄伏热。共奏养阴透热之功。主治温病后期，阴虚邪伏之证。症见夜热早凉，热退无汗，舌红苔少，脉来细数。现常用于慢性肾盂肾炎、肾结核、小儿夏季热等病具有上述症状者。临床应用青蒿鳖甲汤加味治疗妇科手术后低热 100 例，因子宫肌瘤、子宫内膜异位症、子宫体癌、功能性子宫出血等施行子宫全切除术者 82 例，子宫次全切除者 7 例，因卵巢囊肿、宫外孕、输卵管卵巢积水等施行附件切除术者 11 例，11 例术后均经各种抗生素治疗体温持续在 37.3～38℃ 左右不退，检查无感染阳性体征。基本方由生地 15 克，炙鳖甲 12 克，青蒿、知母、丹皮、白微、银柴胡、白芍各 10 克，生甘草 5 克组成。术后 5～10 天开始服用本方者 81 例，11～15 天者 19 例，单服本方者 82 例，加用抗菌素者 18 例（大部分系应用本方的初期），显效 70 例服 1～3 剂体温恢复正常，有效 28 例服 4～5 剂体温恢复正常，其余无效。运用青蒿鳖甲汤治疗泡疹性结膜炎 19 例，证属肺经燥热，基本方由本方去丹皮、生地，加柴胡、钩藤、陈皮、白术组成。少则数剂，多则 10 余剂即告痊愈，治愈率100%。

4.27 秦艽鳖甲散

出自《卫生宝鉴》由地骨皮12克，柴胡9克，鳖甲15克，秦艽12克，知母9克，当归9克，青蒿6克，乌梅3克组成。水煎分2次服（原作散剂）。方中鳖甲味咸性寒，滋阴清热，秦艽味苦辛性微寒，清热除蒸，均为主药。知母、青蒿、地骨皮清内热以治骨蒸；当归补血和血；柴胡驱风邪以从外解；乌梅敛阴止汗。共奏滋阴养血，清热除蒸之功。主治风劳之证，症见骨蒸盗汗，肌肉消瘦，唇红颊赤，午后潮热，咳嗽困倦，舌红少苔，脉微数。现常用于肺结核、骨结核等病具有上述症状者。

4.28 清骨散

出自《证治准绳》。由银柴胡10克，胡黄连、秦艽、鳖甲（醋炙）、地骨皮、青蒿、知母各6克，甘草4克组成。水煎分2次服（原作散剂）。方中银柴胡味甘性微寒，善清虚劳骨蒸之热，为主药。知母、胡黄连、地骨皮善消虚热而退有汗骨蒸，青蒿、秦艽可治无汗骨蒸；鳖甲滋阴潜阳，以治虚热；甘草调和诸药。共奏清虚热，退骨蒸之功。主治虚劳骨蒸，或低热日久不退。现常用于结核病、血液病等病具有上述症状者。临床应用清骨散加减治疗创伤发热21例，基本方由银柴胡、地骨皮各18克，黄连、知母各9克，秦艽15克，青蒿（后下）、甘草各6克，白薇30克组成。凡有外伤史，局部有血肿、瘀斑，热型为午后至傍晚体温升高，翌晨热退，自觉发烧，无表证，精神状态尚好，初时白细胞反应性升高，数天后恢复正常，舌质红苔薄白或薄黄，脉细数等均可应用本方治疗。共治21例，20例服1～2剂即退热，1例无效。

4.29 当归六黄汤

出自《兰室秘藏》。由当归 9 克，生地黄 9 克，熟地黄 9 克，黄芩 9 克，黄柏 9 克，黄连 6 克，黄芪 18 克组成。水煎分 2 次服（原作散剂）。方中当归、生地、熟地育阴养血以清内热，均为主药。黄连、黄芩、黄柏泻火除烦、清热坚阴；黄芪益气固表而止汗。共奏滋阴泻火，固表止汗之功。主治阴虚火旺，发热盗汗之证。症见面赤，心烦，口干唇燥，便结溲黄，舌红，脉数。现常用于结核病、风湿病、血液病等病具有上述症状者。临床应用当归六黄汤治疗盗汗、月经过多、复发性口疮及慢性尿路感染各 1 例，证属气火关系失调，经治疗均获愈。运用当归六黄汤加莲子心、麦门冬、麻黄根治疗持续高烧 1 例。症见 10 日前持续发烧，每晚高达 39～40℃ 之间，将近天明，满身盗汗出，始回降至 38.5℃ 左右，口干，舌疮，烦躁不安，舌质红，苔薄黄而干燥少泽，尖端鲜红，脉滑数，服本方 5 剂，盗汗全止，夜热降。

第5章 祛暑剂

5.1 祛暑剂

由祛暑药为主组成。具有祛除暑邪的作用，以治疗暑病的方剂，统称祛暑剂。暑为夏季的主气，属温热或火热之范畴，暑热易伤气，所以暑病一般发热较高，并见口渴、心烦、汗多等津气两伤之证；因夏季气候较潮湿，暑病每多挟湿；夏暑炎热，人们多喜纳凉饮冷，不避风露，又易兼表寒。根据上述暑病的不同特点，祛暑剂可分为祛暑解表、祛暑清热、祛暑利湿和祛暑益气四类。

暑病挟湿较为常见，使用祛暑剂时，每多配伍祛湿之品，但须注意主次轻重，如暑重湿轻，则湿易从热化，祛湿之品不宜过于温燥，以免燥灼津液。如湿重暑轻，则暑为湿遏，祛暑又不宜过用甘寒，以免阴柔碍湿。

5.2 祛暑清热剂

是以祛暑清热的药物为主组成的方剂。适用于夏季感受暑热之证。症见身热心烦，汗多口渴等。常用的药有西瓜翠衣、银花、扁豆花、荷叶等，代表方剂有清络饮等。

5.3 清络饮

出自《温病条辨》。由鲜荷叶边6克，鲜银花9克，丝瓜皮6克，西瓜翠衣6克，鲜扁豆花6克，鲜竹叶心6克组成。水煎分2次服。方中鲜银花味甘性寒，与芳香清散的鲜扁豆花相伍，两药祛暑清热，均为主药。西瓜翠衣清热解暑，丝瓜络清肺透络；鲜荷叶边祛暑清热而舒散；鲜竹叶心清心利水。共奏清解暑邪之功。主治暑热伤肺，邪在气分之证。症见身热口渴不甚，但头目不清，昏眩微胀，舌淡红苔薄白等。现常用于中暑等病具有上述症状者。

5.4 祛暑解表剂

是以祛暑解表的药物为主组成的方剂。适用于暑气内伏，兼外感风寒之证。症见恶寒发热，无汗头痛，心烦口渴等。常用的药有香薷、银花等，代表方剂有新加香薷饮等。

5.5 新加香薷饮

出自《温病条辨》。由香薷 6 克，银花 9 克，鲜扁豆花 9 克，厚朴 6 克，连翘 9 克组成。水煎分 2 次服。方中香薷味辛性微温，发汗解表，祛暑化湿，为主药。鲜扁豆花、银花、连翘清上焦暑热，以除热解渴，厚朴化湿除满。共奏祛暑解表，清热化湿之功。主治暑温初起，复感外寒之证。症见发热头痛，恶寒无汗，口渴面赤，胸闷不舒，舌苔白腻，脉浮而数者。现常用于夏季暑湿感冒等病具有上述症状者。本方治暑夹寒邪之证，以汗不出为使用要点。若纯属暑温为病，发热而有汗者，虽有恶寒，也不宜使用。

5.6 祛暑利湿剂

是以祛暑利湿的药物为主组成的方剂。适用于感冒挟湿之证。症见身热烦渴，胸脘痞闷，小便不利等。常用的药有滑石、茯苓、泽泻等，代表方剂有六一散、桂苓甘露散等。

5.7 六一散

出自《伤寒直格》。由滑石 180 克，甘草 30 克组成。为细末，每服 9~18 克，用纯棉纱布包煎，去滓，日 2 次。方中滑石味甘淡性寒，善清热利小便，为主药。甘草清热和中，与滑石配用，甘寒生津，使小便利而津液不伤。共奏祛暑利湿之功。主治感受暑湿之证。症见身热烦渴，小便不利，或泄泻。现常用于轻度中暑、膀胱炎、泌尿系结石等病具有上述症状者。临床应用加味六一散治疗砂淋1例，症见腰部酸痛，时而排尿不畅，小便混浊而赤，淋沥刺痛，苔白腻，脉弦。药用飞滑石30克，甘草6克，鸡内金18克，琥珀12克，共研细末，分成9包，每次1包，日3次。用金钱草60克，车前草60克，煎汤送服，服药2天后小便通畅，第3天中午尿出结石2块，5天后先后排出11块结石，腰痛腹胀消失，小便自利。继用金钱草，车前草各30克，煎服，连服1周而愈。

5.8　桂苓甘露饮

出自《宣明论方》。由茯苓30克，甘草6克，白术12克，泽泻15克，官桂3克，石膏30克，寒水石30克，滑石30克，猪苓15克组成。共研为末，每服9克，温汤调服。生姜汤调服尤良，日2次。方中滑石味甘淡性寒，清热利湿，为主药。石膏、寒水石清解暑热；官桂助下焦气化，猪苓、茯苓、泽泻利湿，白术健脾；甘草调和诸药，与滑石相配，增强清热利湿。共奏祛暑清热，化气利湿之功。主治中暑受湿之证。症见发热头痛，烦渴引饮，小便不利，以及霍乱吐下等。现常用于中暑、夏季胃肠型感冒等病具有上述症状者。

5.9　清暑益气剂

是以清暑益气的药物为主组成的方剂。适用于暑热伤气，津液受灼之证。症见身热烦渴，倦怠少气，汗多，脉虚等。常用的药有西洋参、西瓜翠衣、石斛、知母等，代表方剂有王氏清暑汤等。

5.10　清暑益气汤

　　出自《温热经纬》。由西洋参 5 克，石斛 15 克，麦冬 9 克，黄连 3 克，竹叶 6 克，荷梗 15 克，知母 6 克，甘草 3 克，粳米 15 克，西瓜翠衣 30 克组成。水煎分 2 次服。方中西洋参味甘微苦性凉，益气生津，养阴清热，西瓜翠衣味甘性寒，清热解暑，两药均为主药。荷梗助西瓜翠衣清热解暑，石斛、麦冬助西洋参养阴清热；知母、竹叶清热除烦；甘草、粳米益气养胃。共奏清暑益气，养阴生津之功。主治中暑受热，气津两伤之证。症见身热汗多，心烦口渴，小便短赤，体倦少气，精神不振，脉虚数等。现常用于中暑等病具有上述症状者。

第6章 温里剂

6.1 温里剂

　　由温热药为主组成。具有温里助阳，散寒通脉等作用，以治疗阴寒在里的方剂，统称温里剂。寒邪致病，有在表在里之分，表寒证当用辛温解表剂治疗，而里寒证当用温里剂治疗，两者不可混淆。里寒证的成因，有因素体阳虚，寒从中生者；有因外寒直中脏腑者；有因表寒证治疗不当，寒邪乘虚入里者；有因服寒药太过，损伤阳气者。根据里寒证的轻重之别，以及所伤部位的不同，本剂又分温中祛寒，回阳救逆、温经散寒3类。

　　本类方剂多由辛温燥热之品组成，运用时应辨清寒热的真假，对真热假寒证不能使用；若病人素体有阴虚、失血之证，不可过剂，以免重伤其阴，寒去热生，或辛热之品劫阴动血；根据四时寒热的变化，应注意药量大小的调谐；素体阳气虚弱，经温里剂治疗，里寒去而阳气仍虚，可另谋温补之剂；温里剂治里寒证，须中病即止。

6.2 温中祛寒剂

　　是以温中祛寒的药物为主组成的方剂。适用于中焦虚寒之证。症见脘腹胀痛，肢体倦怠，手足不温，或吞酸吐涎，恶心呕吐，或腹痛下利，不问饮食，口淡不渴，舌苔白滑，脉沉细或沉迟等。常用的药有干姜、吴茱萸、蜀椒、生姜等，代表方剂有理中丸、吴茱萸汤、小建中汤、大建中汤等。

6.3 理中丸

出自《伤寒论》。由人参 6 克，干姜 5 克，甘草（炙）6 克，白术 9 克组成。共研末，蜜和为丸，如鸡子黄大，服时研碎，温服，日 3 次（亦作汤剂，按原方比例酌定用量）。方中干姜味辛性热，温中焦脾胃而祛里寒，为主药。人参大补元气，助运化而和升降，白术健脾燥湿；炙甘草益气和中。共奏温中祛寒，补气健脾之功。主治中焦虚寒之证。症见自利不渴，呕吐腹痛，不欲饮食，舌淡苔白，脉沉迟等。现常用于胃及十二指肠溃疡、慢性胃炎、慢性结肠炎、局限性回肠炎、细菌性痢疾等病具有上述症状者。临床应用理中汤治疗严重腹胀 1 例，始因发烧，肚腹撑胀，呕吐，阵发性腹痛而住院，现症见 10 余天水米未进，体温降至 35℃，频呕，腹部撑胀，3 天未大便，发烧，药用理中汤加桂枝、大黄、芒硝、石膏、知母，以大米、荷叶为引，服药 1 剂症减，继服上方加减 3 剂症大减。运用理中汤加味治疗慢性口腔溃疡 1 例，患者 3 年来口腔经常溃疡、灼痛、口中时有臭味，牙龈出血，手足心热，近两月病情有所加重，就诊时口腔溃烂灼痛，饮食尚可，倦怠无力，口干不欲饮，尿清，舌淡苔薄白，脉细缓。药用附子 9 克，党参 15 克，炮姜 6 克，白术 9 克，熟地 15 克，甘草 4.5 克。服用 4 剂后口腔溃疡减其大半，食热物未见明显灼痛，再进 3 剂，溃疡痊愈。

6.4 吴茱萸汤

出自《伤寒论》。由吴茱萸 3 克，人参 6 克，大枣 4 枚，生姜 18 克组成、水煎分 3 次服。方中吴茱萸味辛苦性热，温胃散寒，开郁化滞，下气降浊，为主药。人参大补元气，兼能益阴；生姜温胃散寒，大枣益气滋脾，姜、枣相合，尚能调和营卫。共奏温中补虚，降逆止呕之功。主治胃中虚寒，食谷欲呕，胸膈满闷，或胃脘痛，吞酸嘈杂；厥阴头痛，呕吐涎沫；少阴吐利。现常用于慢性胃炎、神经性头痛、妊娠呕吐、胃肠神经官能证、美尼尔氏综合征、药物过敏性呕吐等病具有上述症状者，临床应用吴茱萸汤加味治疗溃疡病34例。证属虚寒，症见胃痛日久，时时发作，痛处喜按，饥饿痛甚，得食痛缓，喜热畏凉，食欲不振，恶心欲呕或吐清水，口不干，舌淡苔白滑，脉缓。经治疗，显效25例，进步8例，无效1例，疼痛消失短者3天，长者25天。运用吴茱萸汤加味治疗慢性胆囊炎3例，均因前医过用苦寒而损伤中阳，导致寒邪干胃，胃气上逆，呕味涎沫，经用吴茱萸汤加味治疗，而获显效。

6.5 小建中汤

出自《伤寒论》。由芍药（酒炒）18克，桂枝9克，炙甘草6克，生姜10克，大枣4枚，饴糖30克组成。前5味水煎2次，取汁，兑入饴糖，分2次温服。方中饴糖味甘性温，益脾气而养脾阴，温补中焦，兼缓肝急，润肺之燥，为主药。桂枝温阳气，芍药益阴血；炙甘草甘温益气，既助饴糖、桂枝益气温中，又合芍药酸甘化阴而益肝滋脾；生姜温胃，大枣补脾，姜、枣又调和营卫。共奏温中补虚，和里缓急之功。主治虚劳里急之证。症见腹中时痛，温按则痛减，舌淡苔白，脉弦细而缓；或心中悸动，虚烦不宁，面色无华；或四肢酸楚，手足烦热，咽干口燥。现常用于胃及十二指肠球溃疡、神经衰弱、再生障碍性贫血、血小板减少性紫癜等病具有上述症状者。临床应用小建中汤治疗遗精1例，症见遗精2年余，1～2日即发生1次，其面色晦暗，食少身倦，头晕心悸，耳鸣，腰酸多梦，舌光无苔，脉细弱。药用桂枝15克，饴糖60克，芍药30克，炙草9克，生姜3片，大枣3枚，牡蛎24克，龙骨24克。患者服3剂遗精止，梦少睡宁，余症均减。运用小建中汤加味治疗蛔虫型腹痛3例，基本方由桂枝6克，白芍6克，炙草6克，大枣4枚，生姜3片，乌梅6克，饴糖30克组成，3例服2～3剂后均愈。

6.6 大建中汤

出自《金匮要略》。由蜀椒 3 克，干姜 4.5 克，人参 6 克，饴糖 30 克组成。前 3 味水煎 2 次，取汁，兑入饴糖 30 克，分 2 次温服。方中蜀椒味辛性热，温脾胃，助命火，散寒除湿，下气散结，为主药。干姜温中散寒，助蜀椒建中阳，散逆气，止痛平呕；人参、饴糖甘温补中而益脾胃。共奏温中补虚，降逆止痛之功。主治中阳衰弱，阴寒内盛之证。症见心胸中大寒痛，呕不能食，腹中寒上冲皮起，见有头足，上下痛而不可触近，舌苔白滑，脉细紧，其则肢厥脉伏，或腹中渡渡有声。现常用于慢性胃炎、溃疡病、慢性胰腺炎、慢性胆囊炎、胆道蛔虫、肠结核等病具有上述症状者。临床应用加味大建中汤治疗胆道蛔虫症 45 例。基本方由干姜、川椒、乌梅、苦楝皮、槟榔、党参各 9 克，饴糖 60 克，黄连、炙甘草各 4.5 克，小儿均减半。经治疗，其中 39 例治愈，4 例进步。运用大建中汤治疗心胸中大寒痛呕不能饮食 6 例，证属中阳不足，阴寒上乘，病程长者 3 年余，短者 2 天，若腹胀满加厚朴、砂仁，寒甚或头痛目眩加吴茱萸，恶寒重加炮附子，哎吐加半夏、生姜，脾虚加白术，白虚加当归，口干加白芍，手足倦或麻痹加桂枝尖。经治疗，均获满意疗效。

6.7 回阳救逆剂

是以回阳救逆的药物为主组成的方剂。适用于阳气衰微，内外俱寒，其至阴盛格阳或戴阳等证。症见四肢厥逆，恶寒蜷卧，呕吐腹痛，下利清谷，精神萎靡，脉沉细或沉微等。常用的药有附子、干姜、肉桂等，代表方剂有四逆汤、回阳救急汤等。

6.8 四逆汤

出自《伤寒论》。由附子（生）5~10 克，干姜 6~9 克，甘草（炙）6 克组成。先煎生附子 1 小时，再加余药同煎，取汁，分2次温服。方中生附子味辛甘性大热，有毒，善补先天命门真火，通行十二经，生用尤能迅速通达内外以温阳逐寒，为主药。干姜温中阳而除里寒，助附子伸发阳气；炙甘草既能解毒，又能缓干姜、生附子辛烈之性。共奏回阳救逆之功。主治少阴病，症见四肢厥逆，恶寒蜷卧，呕吐不渴，腹痛下利，神衰欲寐，舌苔白滑，脉象微细，以及太阳病误汗亡阳之证。现常用于慢性结肠炎、肺心病、肺炎、脱水症等病具有上述症状者。本方是温燥偏重之剂，如见面红、烦躁属"真寒假热"者，服用本方时，以凉服为宜，否则可能反增上燥，而致鼻衄。临床应用针刺配合四逆汤加味中西医结合抢救雷电击伤心跳骤停1例，患者男性，38岁，被雷电击伤，神志昏迷，面色苍白，唇绀，四肢厥冷，呼吸极微，心音听不到，经胸外心脏按摩，针刺人中、合谷、涌泉等穴，并肌肉注射尼可刹米0.375mg，静脉注射50%葡萄糖50ml等治疗，半小时后，心脏可听到间歇微弱的心音，心律不齐，心率28次／分，即予四逆汤加党参、黄芪1剂，重用附子25克，1小时后四肢转温，心率50次／分，自诉心前疼痛，再予原方加红花、当归1剂，药后病情继续好转，再将附子量减半，继服2剂而愈。运用四逆汤加黄连治疗小儿泄泻70例。症见大便溏薄、微热、肢冷、脉微弱、苔薄白。基本方由制附子15克，干姜、甘草各9克，加水350毫升，煎至150毫升，再加黄连9克，微火煎至80毫升，过滤加糖适量，煮沸备用。5个月以下患儿每次3~5ml，6~10个月患儿每次5~8ml，1~1.5岁每次8~10ml，每4小时服1次。结果治愈58例，有效8例，无效4例，治疗时间平均4日。

6.9 回阳救急汤

出自《伤寒六书》。由熟附子9克，干姜5克，肉桂3克，人参6克，白术（炒）9克，茯苓9克，陈皮6克，甘草（炙）5克，五味子3克，半夏（制）9克，生姜3片，麝香0.1克组成。水煎，临服入麝香，分 2 次服。方中附子味辛甘性大热，温里回阳，祛寒破阴，为主药。干姜温中散寒，肉桂温壮元阳；人参、白术、茯苓、甘草、陈皮、半夏补益脾胃，燥湿化痰；麝香通达十二经血脉，五味子酸收，使发中有收，与人参相合，益气生脉。共奏回阳救急，益气生脉之功。主治寒邪直中三阴，真阳衰微之证。症见恶寒蜷卧，四肢厥冷，吐泻腹痛，口不渴，神衰欲寐，或身寒战粟，或指甲口唇青紫，或吐涎沫，舌淡苔白，脉沉微，甚或无脉等。现常用于慢性结肠炎、慢性腹泻、沙门氏菌属感染、中毒性痢疾等病具有上述症状者。本方温燥，中病以手足温和即止，不宜多服。

6.10　黑锡丹

出自《太平惠民和剂局方》。由金铃子（蒸）、胡芦巴（酒浸，炒）、木香、附子（炮）、肉豆蔻（面裹煨）、破故纸（酒浸，炒）、沉香、茴香（炒）、阳起石（酒煮，焙干，研）各30克，肉桂15克，黑锡（即铅，去滓净秤）、硫黄各60克组成。共为细末，酒糊丸，成人每服5克，小儿每服2～3克，盐开水送下，急救可用至9克。方中黑锡味甘性寒，镇摄浮阳，降逆平喘，硫黄味酸性热，温补命火，暖肾消寒，两药均为主药。附子、肉桂温肾助阳，引火归原，阳起石、破故纸、胡芦巴温命门，除冷气；茴香、沉香、肉豆蔻温中调气，降逆除痰，兼能暖肾；川楝子苦寒，监制诸药以防温燥太过，又能利气疏肝。共奏温壮下元，镇纳浮阳之功。主治肾阳衰弱，肾不纳气之证。症见胸中痰壅，上气喘促，四肢厥逆，冷汗不止，舌淡苔白，脉沉微等，以及奔豚气上冲胸，胁腹胀满，或寒疝腹痛，肠鸣滑泄，或男子阳痿精冷，女子血海虚寒，带下清稀等。现常用于哮喘、阳痿等病具有上述症状者。本方为温降镇摄救急之剂，非久病缓治之方，不宜多服久服，否则有铅中毒的危险。临床应用黑锡丹治疗哮喘 1 例，患者哮喘已数年，1 日 1 发至 10 余发不等，病时呼吸喘促，胸腹气紧，提不升，咽不降，气若不续，汗大出，吐泡沫痰，口渴喜热食，苔白薄，日夜发作 5～6 次，伛偻扶坐，不能平卧，服黑锡丹 1 日 3 次，每次 30 粒，第 3 日哮喘减至 1 日 1 发或间日发，第 10 日，哮喘完全停止，续服 10 日，症状完全消失。

6.11　温经散寒剂

是以温经散寒和养血通脉的药物为主组成的方剂。适用于阳气不足，阴血亦弱，复有外寒伤于经络，血脉不利之证。常用温经散寒药桂枝、细辛配伍养血通脉药当归、芍药等，代表方剂有当归四逆汤等。

6.12　当归四逆汤

出自《伤寒论》。由当归 12 克，桂枝 9 克，芍药 9 克，细辛 1.5 克，甘草（炙）5 克，通草 3 克，大枣 8 枚组成。水煎分 3 次服。方中当归味辛甘性温，活血养血，为主药。桂枝温通经脉，白芍养血和营；细辛通血脉，散寒邪；大枣、炙甘草补脾气而调诸药，通草通经脉。共奏温经散寒，养血通脉之功。主治血虚受寒。症见手足厥冷，舌淡苔白，脉沉细或脉细欲绝者。现常用于血栓闭塞性脉管炎、周围静脉炎、多发性神经炎、冻疮等病具有上述症状者。临床应用当归四逆汤加减治疗血栓闭塞性脉管炎 10 例，病程分别为 2 月～3 年。基本方由当归、桂枝、赤芍、通草、川椒、大枣、丹参、益母草、王不留行、川郁金、蒲公英、银花、玄参、附子、鹿角胶、鸡血藤、党参、黄芪、川牛膝组成。经治疗，有 9 例痊愈。运用加味当归四逆汤治疗早期雷诺氏病 2 例，证属阳气虚弱不能温养四末，寒邪外袭，血脉凝涩，1 例用原方加艾叶、红花，服 30 余剂而愈，1 例服 18 剂而愈，随访均未复发。

第7章　表里双解剂

7.1　表里双解剂

由解表药配合泻下药或清热药、温里药等为主组成。具有表里同治的作用，以治疗表里同病的方剂，统称表里双解剂。对于表证未除，里证又急者，如仅用表散，则在里之邪不得去；仅治其里，则在外之邪亦不得其解。针对这种情况，宜使用表里双解剂以表里同治，使病邪得以分消。表里双解剂，根据表里同病的性质不同，有解表攻里、解表清里、解表温里3种分类。至于解表补里法，是治疗表邪未解而有正气不足之证，已在解表剂中介绍，本章不再重复。

使用表里双解剂，应当注意须具备既有表证，又有里证者，方可应用，否则即不相宜。辨别表证与里证的寒、热、虚、实，针对病情选择适当的方剂。分清表证与里证的轻重主次，而后权衡表药与里药的比例，方无太过或不及之弊。

7.2　解表攻里剂

是以解表和泻下的药物为主组成的方剂。适用于既有表寒或表热的症状，又有里实之证。常用解表药麻黄、桂枝、荆芥、防风、柴胡、薄荷配伍泻下药大黄、芒硝等，代表方剂有大柴胡汤、防风通圣散等。

7.3　大柴胡汤

出自《金匮要略》。由柴胡15克，黄芩9克，芍药9克，半夏9克，枳实（炙）9克，大黄6克，生姜15克，大枣5枚组成。水煎分二次服。方中柴胡味苦辛性微寒，透表泄热，为主药。黄芩配柴胡和解清热，以除少阳之邪；大黄、枳实泻阳明热结；芍药缓急止痛，与大黄相配可治腹中实痛，与枳实相伍可治气血不和；半夏降逆止呕，配伍生姜重用，以治呕逆不止；大枣、生姜同用，能调和营卫而和诸药。共奏和解少阳，内泻热结之功。主治少阳、阳明合病。症见往来寒热，胸胁苦满，呕不止，郁郁微烦，心下满痛或心下痞鞕，大便不解或协热下利，舌苔黄，脉弦有力。现常用于急性单纯性肠梗阻、急性胰腺炎、急性胆囊炎、胆道结石等病具有上述症状者。临床应用大柴胡汤加川楝子、延胡索、甘草治疗急性胆囊炎 40 例。均有胸胁疼痛，肝区触压痛，多伴有疼痛放射至右肩背，畏寒发热，恶心呕吐，腹肌紧张，巩膜黄染等症，其中约有半数的患者，尚有咽干口苦，在右季肋下可触及肿大的胆囊或炎症粘连包块。经治疗，35 例痊愈，5 例好转，3 例复发。运用大柴胡汤加延胡索、木香治疗急性胰腺炎 22 例。症见上腹剧烈疼痛及局部疼痛，恶心呕吐，大部分有不同程度的体温升高，舌苔黄厚或黄干，脉弦滑。其中 18 例白细胞计数升高，尿淀粉酶 128 单位者 2 例，其余均在 256 单位以上，在测定血清淀粉酶的 19 例中，有 8 例在 128 单位以上，经配合输液或用阿托品、杜冷丁治疗全部治愈。

7.4　防风通圣散

出自《宣明论方》。由防风、荆芥、连翘、麻黄、薄荷、川芎、当归、白芍（炒）、白术、山栀、大黄（酒蒸）、芒硝（后下）各 15 克，石膏、黄芩、桔梗各 30 克，甘草 60 克，滑石 90 克组成。以上诸药共为粗末，每次 9 克，加生姜 3 片，水煎服，日 2 次（亦作丸剂）。方中防风味辛甘性微温，疏风解表，为主药。与荆芥、麻黄、薄荷配伍增强疏风解表之力，使风邪从汗而解；大黄、芒硝泄热通便，配伍石膏、黄芩、连翘、桔梗清解肺胃之热；山栀、滑石清利湿热，使里热从二便而解；当归、川芎、白芍养血活血，白术健脾燥湿，甘草和中缓急，生姜和胃降逆。共奏疏风解表，泻热通便之功。主治风热壅盛，表里俱实之证。症见憎寒壮热，头目昏眩，目赤睛痛，口苦口干，咽喉不利，胸膈痞闷，咳呕喘满，涕唾稠粘，大便秘结，小便赤涩等。现常用于荨麻疹、神经性头痛、牛皮癣、过敏性紫癜等病具有上述症状者。临床应用防风通圣散加陈皮、半夏治疗顽固性头痛 1 例。症见头痛，以右侧头部及左侧颞部为重，血压高，约 1 个月前发生轻度左面神经瘫痪和轻度言语障碍，大便每周 1 次，脉弦有力，无舌苔，腹部略膨胀，心窝部稍有抵抗，血压 170／90mmHg。经服 3 剂后，不但治好了头痛，而且语言障碍亦得到显著地改善。

7.5　解表清里剂

是以解表和清热的药物为主组成的方剂。适用于既有表寒或表热的症状，又有里热之证。常用解表药麻黄、淡豆豉、葛根配伍清热药黄芩、黄连、黄柏等，代表方剂有葛根黄芩黄连汤、石膏汤等。

7.6　葛根黄芩黄连汤

出自《伤寒论》。由葛根 15 克，甘草（炙）6 克，黄芩 9 克，黄连 9 克组成。水煎分 2 次服。方中葛根味甘辛性凉，既能解表清热，又能升发脾胃清阳之气以治下利，为主药。黄芩、黄连清胃肠之热，燥胃肠之湿；甘草缓中和药。共奏解表清热之功。主治外感表证未解，热邪入里之证。症见身热，下利臭秽，肛门有灼热感，胸脘烦热，口干作渴，喘而汗出，苔黄脉数。现常用于细菌性痢疾、肠伤寒、急性肠炎、小儿泄泻等病具有上述症状者。临床应用葛根黄芩黄连汤治疗急性细菌性痢疾 40 例。最多服药 12 剂，最少服药 2 剂即愈。退热最快的为 4 小时，腹痛消失平均为 4.51 天，里急后重消失平均为 3.47 天，食欲恢复正常平均为 2.5 天，解便次数正常，大便镜检阴性，平均为 4

天，急性症状消失平均为 3.44 天。临床症状完全消失的 39 例。运用加味葛根芩连汤治疗小儿麻痹症 129 例。基本方由葛根、黄芩、黄连、甘草、生石膏、银花、白芍、全蝎、蜈蚣组成。经治疗，结果在患肢呈深度完全麻痹，失去自主运动功能的重型患者 52 例中，痊愈 17 例，好转 35 例。在尚能自主活动，但不能走路，不能站立的中型患者 67 例中，痊愈 33 例。好转 34 例。能自主活动，能站立行走，但肢体软弱无力的轻型患者 10 例，全部治愈。一般中型及轻型病例，多在 1 个月左右痊愈，最快的 1 例仅 1 周而愈。

7.7　石膏汤

出自《外台秘要》。由石膏 30 克，黄连、黄柏、黄芩各 6 克，香豉 9 克，栀子 9 克，麻黄 9 克组成。水煎分 3 次服。方中石膏味辛甘性大寒，清热除烦，为主药。麻黄、豆豉发汗解表，使在表之邪从外而解；黄连、黄芩、黄柏、栀子泻火解毒，使三焦之火从里而泄。共奏清热解毒，发汗解表。主治伤寒里热已炽，表证未解之证。症见壮热无汗，身体沉重拘急，鼻干口渴，烦躁不眠，神昏谵语，或发斑，脉滑数。现常用于败血症、胆囊炎、盆腔炎、胰腺炎、阑尾炎等病具有上述症状者。

7.8　解表温里剂

是以解表和温里的药物为主组成的方剂。适用于外有表证而里有寒象之证。常用解表药麻黄。白芷配伍温里祛寒药干姜、肉桂等，代表方剂有五积散等。

7.9　五积散

出自《太平惠民和剂局方》。由白芷、川芎、炙甘草、茯苓、当归、肉桂、芍药、半夏各 90 克，陈皮、枳壳（炒）、麻黄各 180 克，苍术 720 克，干姜（煨）120 克，桔梗 360 克，厚朴

120 克，生姜 3 片组成。除生姜外，余药均研为粗末（肉桂、枳壳另研），慢火炒令色转，摊冷，次入肉桂、枳壳末，令匀。每次 9 克，入生姜，水煎去渣温服，日 2 次（亦作汤剂，用量按原方比例酌定）。方中麻黄、白芷发汗解表，干姜、肉桂温里祛寒，四药均为主药。苍术、厚朴燥湿健脾，陈皮、半夏、茯苓理气化痰；当归、川芎、芍药活血止痛；桔梗、枳壳理气化滞；甘草和中健脾，调和诸药。共奏发表温里，顺气化痰，活血消积之功。主治外感风寒，内伤生冷之症。症见身热无汗，头痛身疼，项背拘急，胸满恶食，呕吐腹痛，以及妇女气血不和，心腹疼痛，月经不调等。现常用于习惯性感冒、胃肠神经官能症、月经不调、慢性胃肠炎、慢性肝炎等病具有上述症状者。

第8章 补益剂

8.1 补益剂

以补益药为主组成。具有滋养补益人体气血阴阳作用，治疗各种虚证的方剂，统称补益剂。人体虚损不足诸证，归纳起来有气虚、血虚、阴虚、阳虚、气血两虚等。因此，补益剂可分为补气、补血、补阴、补阳以及气血双补五类。

气血阴阳之间的关系十分密切，不可分割，所以常根据气血相生，气为血帅，血为气母等理论，在补血剂中配补气药，如气虚兼血虚者亦可配补血药。由于阴阳互根，相互为用，生理上相互联系，病理上相互影响，因此，补阴剂中可配补阳药，补阳剂中可配补阴药，以达到阴中求阳，阳中求阴之目的。若脾胃功能不足者，应配以健脾益胃药。

补益剂宜文火久煎，空腹或饭前服为佳。应用时应辨清虚证之真假。如外邪未尽，当先祛邪，不能过早补益；如必须补益者，也应扶正祛邪并用。

8.2 补气剂

是以补气的药物为主组成的方剂，适用于脾肺气虚证。症见肢体倦怠乏力，呼吸短气，声低懒言，面色萎白，食欲不振，舌淡苔白，脉浮或虚大。或者虚热自汗，或脱肛、子宫脱垂等。常用药有人参、黄芪、白术、炙甘草等。代表方剂有四君子汤、参苓白术散、补中益气汤等。

8.3　四君子汤

出自《太平惠民和剂局方》。由人参 10 克，白术、茯苓各 9 克，炙甘草 6 克组成。水煎分 2 次服。方中人参甘温大补元气，健脾胃，为主药。白术健脾燥湿，茯苓渗湿健脾，与白术相配促其运化；炙甘草补气和中；调和诸药。共奏益气健脾之功。主治脾胃气虚证。症见面色㿠白，语声低微，四肢无力，食少或便溏，舌质淡，脉细缓。现常用于治疗慢性胃炎、胃及十二指肠溃疡等病具有上述症状者。临床应用四君子汤治疗胃手术后 154 例，以代替或减少补液等术后处理，效果令人满意。处方为党参 9 克，白术 6 克，茯苓 6 克，甘草 3 克，首乌 6 克，白芍 6 克，水煎服，一般于术后 16~24 小时开始服 1 剂，以后于术后 48 小时、72 小时各服 1 剂，全程共服 3 剂。

四君子汤对小白鼠肝脏的糖元及核糖核酸的影响。实验表明，给药组（占 40%）肝糖元明显增加，并有糖元颗粒聚集成较大团块，以中心区为多。用一定剂量的四君子汤对家兔离体小肠运动呈抑制性影响，主要与其抗乙酰胆硷作用有关，表现在使肠管运动的紧张性下降，而不抑制收缩力。四君子汤尚有明显的抗组织胺作用；脾虚患者服用四君子汤后胃肠功能紊乱的症状有所好转，可能与其抗乙酰胆硷及抗组织胺作用有关，同时有一定程度的抗肾上腺素作用。

8.4　六君子汤

出自《妇人良方》。由人参 10 克，白术、茯苓各 9 克，炙甘草 6 克，陈皮 9 克，半夏 9 克组成。水煎分 2 次服。方中四君子汤益气健脾，陈皮理气和胃，燥湿化痰。半夏燥湿化痰，降逆止呕。共奏健脾止呕之功。主治脾胃气虚挟痰湿证。症见不思饮食，恶心呕吐，胸脘痞闷，大便不实，或咳嗽痰多稀白等。现常用于妊娠呕吐、慢性胃炎、胃及十二指肠溃疡具有上述症状者。

临床用六君子汤加减治疗妊娠恶阻症 52 例，服药后 24～96 小时之内呕吐均完全停止（其中 4 例停后有复发），饮食情况迅速好转。服药 1～5 剂后痊愈者 42 例（占 80.77%），进步者 9 例（占 17.3%），1 例无效（占 1.93%）。

8.5 香砂六君子汤

出自《医方集解》。由人参 10 克，白术，茯苓各 9 克，炙甘草 6 克，陈皮 9 克，半夏 9 克，木香 6 克，砂仁 6 克组成。水煎分 2 次服。方中四君子汤益气健脾；半夏燥湿化痰，降逆止呕；陈皮、木香、砂仁理气和胃止痛。共奏健脾和胃，理气止痛之功。主治脾胃虚弱，寒湿内停证。症见胸脘痞闷，呕恶食少，泄泻，或胃寒作痛等。现常用于慢性胃炎、溃疡病以及妊娠呕吐等病具有上述症状者。

8.6 参苓白术散

出自《太平惠民和剂局方》。由莲子肉 500 克，薏苡仁 500 克，缩砂仁 500 克，桔梗 500 克，白扁豆 750 克，茯苓、白术、人参、山药、炙甘草各 1000 克组成。共为细末，每服 6 克，枣汤调下（亦可作汤剂，用量按原方比例酌减）。方中人参、山药、莲子肉益气健脾，和胃止泻，为主药。白术、茯苓、苡仁、扁豆渗湿健脾；砂仁和胃醒脾，理气宽胸；桔梗宣肺利气，载药上行；炙甘草益气和中，调和诸药。共奏健脾益气，和胃渗湿之功。主治脾胃气虚挟湿证。症见食少便溏，或吐泻，四肢乏力，形体消瘦，胸脘闷胀，面色萎黄，苔白腻，脉虚缓者。现常用于慢性胃肠炎、贫血、肺结核、慢性肾炎及其他慢性消耗性疾病中具有上述症状者。临床应用参苓白术散加减治疗脾虚腹泻 18 例。症见身体瘦弱，精神萎靡，面色苍白，或萎黄，脘腹胀满，腹痛喜按，便溏不息，或完谷不化，纳差，舌淡苔薄白，脉细缓，指纹隐淡。以本方随证加减治疗，结果 13 例痊愈，进步 4

例，无效 1 例。

8.7 补中益气汤

出自《脾胃论》。由黄芪 15 克，炙甘草 6 克，人参 6 克，当归 9 克，橘皮 6 克，柴胡、升麻各 3 克，白术 10 克组成。水煎分 2 次服。亦可按原方比例作丸剂，每次 10～15 克，日 2～3 次。方中黄芪补气固表，升阳举陷，为主药。当归与黄芪配伍益气生血；陈皮理气和胃，使本方补而不滞；升麻、柴胡助黄芪升阳和胃。共奏补中益气，升阳举陷之功。主治脾胃气虚证。症见身热有汗，头痛恶寒，渴喜热饮，少气懒言，或饮食无味，四肢乏力，舌质淡苔白，脉虚软无力，及脱肛、子宫下垂、胃下垂、久泻久痢等证属中气虚弱者。现常用于胃下垂、脱肛、子宫下垂、久泻久痢、以及易感冒等病具有上述症状者。因本方为甘温之品，故阴虚内热者忌用。临床用本方治疗子宫脱垂 23 例，每日 1 剂，2 星期为 1 疗程。服药期间每日早晚作胸膝卧式及提肛肌收缩运动，每次 10～20 分钟，治疗期间忌重体力劳动以及暴怒。结果除 2 例未完成 1 疗程外，其余 21 例中治愈率者占 76.2%，进步者占 6.5%，无效者占 14.3%。又用本方治疗 3 例眼睑下垂、眼睁不大、眼上睑不能上举，眼睛发干发酸，有时感觉疼痛等症，均服药半月而获效。

8.8 生脉散

出自《内外伤辨惑论》。由人参 10 克，麦冬 15 克，五味子 6 克组成。水煎分 2 次服。方中人参补肺益气生津，为主药。麦冬养阴清热生津；五味子敛肺止渴生津。三药合用，一补、一清、一敛，共奏益气生津，敛阴止汗之功。主治热伤气津，或久咳肺虚之证。症见汗多体倦，气短口渴，脉虚数。或咳嗽痰少，气短自汗，口舌干燥，脉虚数等。现常用于热病后期，肺结核、慢性支气管炎、心力衰竭，以及急性传染病恢复期等病具有上述症状者。临床应用生脉、四逆注射液治疗 17 例急性心肌梗塞并发心源性休克者疗效满意。结果死亡 1 例，其余 16 例血压全部恢复正常，17 例中合并急性左心衰竭 4 例，室性心动过速与室上性心动过速各 1 例，Ⅱ度房室传导阻滞 1 例。

8.9　人参蛤蚧散

出自《卫生宝鉴》。由蛤蚧 1 对，杏仁 150 克，炙甘草 150 克，人参 60 克，茯苓 60 克，贝母 60 克，桑白皮 60 克，知母 60 克组成。制为散剂，早晚空腹时各服 1 次，每次 6 克，开水送下。方中蛤蚧补肾纳气定喘，为主药。人参大补元气，益肺脾；茯苓益脾渗湿；桑皮、杏仁降气平喘；贝母清热润肺化痰；知母清肺滋肾纳气；炙甘草补气和胃，调和诸药。共奏益气清肺，止咳定喘之功。主治肺虚久咳证。症见咳嗽气喘，痰稠色黄，或咳吐脓血，胸中烦热，身体羸瘦，脉浮虚等。现常用于肺结核，慢性气管炎等病具有上述症状者。

8.10　补血剂

是以补血的药物为主组成的方剂。适用于血虚证。症见头晕眼花，面色萎黄，爪甲苍白，心悸失眠，或月经量少色淡，脉细数无力等。常用的药有当归、熟地、阿胶、何首乌等，代表方剂有四物汤、归脾汤等。

8.11　四物汤

出自《太平惠民和剂局方》。由当归 10 克，熟地 15 克，白芍 10 克，川芎 6 克组成。水煎分 2 次服。方中熟地滋阴养血填精，为主药。当归补血和血调经，白芍养血敛阴，川芎活血行滞，使全方补而不滞。共奏补血调经之功。主治血虚血滞证。症见惊惕头晕，目眩耳鸣，唇爪无华，月经量少，或经闭不行，脐腹作痛，舌质淡，脉弦细或细涩。现常用于贫血、月经不调等病具有上述症状者。方中熟地、芍药均为阴柔之品，易于滞气伤阳，如平素脾胃阳虚，食少便溏者，不宜使用。临床应用四物汤治疗神经性头痛 44 例，效果良好。其表现为头部憋胀疼痛或刺痛，并伴有眩晕、失眠、心悸、腰酸、脉细弱等症。以本方为主加减治疗，近期控制（6 个月未复发）23 例，显效 13 例，好转 7 例，无效 1 例。运用四物汤加减纠正胎位异常 100 例，取得一定疗效，在复查 87 例中，有 73 例胎位转正，9 例未转正。处方：当归 6 克，白芍 9 克，川芎 1.5 克，白术 9 克，茯苓 9 克，每日 1 剂，连服 3 剂，出血者忌服。

8.12 当归补血汤

出自《内外伤辨惑论》。由黄芪 30 克，当归 6 克组成。水煎分 2 次服。方中重用黄芪大补脾肺之气，以资生血之源。当归补血和营，两药合用则阳生阴长，气旺血生。共奏补气生血之功。主治血虚发热证。症见肌热面赤，烦渴欲饮，脉洪大而虚，以及月经期、产后血虚发热头痛；或疮疡溃后，久不愈合等。现常用于各种贫血、过敏性紫癜、功能性子宫出血、白细胞减少、神经衰弱等病具有上述症状者。

8.13 归脾汤

出自《济生方》。由白术 9 克，茯神 10 克，黄芪 12 克，龙眼肉 10 克，酸枣仁 10 克，人参 12 克，木香 5 克，甘草 5 克，当归 10 克，远志 10 克，生姜 6 克，大枣 3 枚组成。水煎分 2 次服。方中黄芪、人参补气健脾，为主药。当归、龙眼肉养血和营，与主药相配伍益气养血；白术、木香以健脾理气，使补而不滞；茯神、远志、枣仁养心安神；甘草、生姜、大枣和胃健脾。共奏益气补血，健脾养心之功。主治心脾两虚，或脾不统血之证。症见心悸怔忡，健忘失眠，多梦易惊，虚热，体倦食少，面色萎黄，舌质淡苔薄白，脉细弱。或便血，妇女崩漏，月经超前，量多色淡等。现常用于神经衰弱、心脏病、功能性子宫出血、血小板减少性紫癜、再生障碍性贫血、胃及十二指肠溃疡出血等病具有上述症状者。临床应用归脾汤治疗神经衰弱720例，痊愈者占2.2%，近愈者占46.4%，好转者占28%。运用归脾汤加减治疗脑外伤后遗综合症88例，治疗前皆诊断为脑震荡、脑挫伤等闭合性颅损伤。治疗结果：痊愈41例（45.5%），显效30例（34%），好转17例（20.5%）。

8.14 炙甘草汤

出自《伤寒论》。由炙甘草12克，人参6克，生地黄30克，桂枝9克，阿胶6克，麦冬10克，麻仁10克，生姜10克，大枣5枚组成。水煎分2次服。方中重用炙甘草甘温益气，缓急养心，为主药。人参、大枣益气补脾养心，生地、麦冬、麻仁、阿胶滋养阴血；桂枝、生姜温阳通脉，使气血流通。共奏益气养血，滋阴复脉之功。主治气血虚弱证。症见脉结代，心悸心慌，或大便干结，舌质淡红少苔，以及干咳无痰，或痰中带血等。现常用于冠心病、病毒性心肌炎、风湿性心脏病，神经衰弱等病具有上述症状者。本方性偏湿，故阴虚内热者忌用。临床用炙甘草汤治疗心律不齐28例，其中男性12例，女性16例，年龄最大56岁，最小4岁。病程最短3个月，最长2年。治疗效果，显效23例，有效4例，无效1例。处方：党参9克，桂枝9克，阿胶9克，生姜9克，生地15克，麦冬9克，麻仁12克，大枣10枚。水煎服，每日1剂。心烦不眠盗汗者，加酸枣仁，心悸加磁砂、龙骨、牡蛎。运用炙甘草汤去麻仁、生姜，加五味子、鸡血藤、龟板、冰糖治疗心绞痛150例，观察效果：显效48例，改善90例，无效12例。

8.15　气血双补剂

是以补气和补血的药物为主组成的方剂。适用于气血俱虚证。症见面色无华，头晕目眩，心悸气短，舌淡，脉虚细无力。常用补气药人参、黄芪、甘草配伍补血药当归、白芍、首乌、阿胶、龙眼肉等，代表方剂有八珍汤、泰山磐石散等。

8.16　八珍汤

出自《正体类要》。由当归 10 克，川芎 6 克，白芍 10 克，熟地 15 克，人参 6 克，白术 10 克，茯苓 10 克，炙甘草 6 克，生姜 6 克，大枣 3 枚组成。水煎分 2 次服。方中熟地、人参益气养血，为主药。白术、茯苓健脾祛湿；当归、白芍养血和营；川芎和血行气；炙甘草益气和中；生姜、大枣调和脾胃。共奏补益气血之功。主治气血两虚证。症见面色苍白或萎黄，头晕目眩，四肢倦怠，气短懒言。心悸怔忡，食欲不振，舌质淡苔薄白，脉细弱或虚大无力。现常用于病后虚弱及各种慢性病、妇人月经不调、胎产崩漏、痈疮及久不收口等病具有上述症状者。临床用加味八珍汤治疗习惯性流产 38 例。流产的次数，最少为 2 胎，最多 5 胎。处方：当归、熟地、白芍、川芎、党参、茯苓、白术、甘草、砂仁、紫苏、生姜、大枣。如气虚加黄芪，血虚加阿胶，虚火盛而呕者，加黄芩、竹茹，虚火引起咽干口燥者，去熟地加生地、玉竹。

8.17　泰山磐石汤

出自《景岳全书》。由人参 5 克，黄芪 10 克，当归 10 克，川断 10 克，黄芩 6 克，白术 10 克，川芎 3 克，芍药 6 克，熟地 10 克，砂仁 3 克，炙甘草 6 克，糯米 5 克组成。水煎分 3 次，空腹服。方中人参、黄芪、白术、炙甘草补脾益气；当归、熟地、芍药、续断补益肝肾，养血和血；黄芩清热，与白术配伍健脾清热以安胎；砂仁理气和中安胎；川芎行气和血；糯米养脾胃而固胎元。共奏益气健脾，养血安胎之功。主治气血两虚，胎元不固之证。症见胎动不安，或屡有堕胎，面色淡白，倦怠无力，不思饮食，舌质淡，苔薄白，脉滑无力。现常用于先兆流产、习惯性流产等病具有上述症状者。

8.18　补阴剂

是以补阴的药物为主组成的方剂，适用于阴虚证。症见肢体羸瘦，面容憔悴，口燥咽干，腰腿酸软，头晕眼花，大便干燥。或骨蒸盗汗，呛咳无痰，颧红、舌红少苔，脉细数。常用的药有地黄、麦冬、天冬、龟板、知母等，或配鹿胶，菟丝子等补阳药，以阳中求阴，代表方剂有六味地黄丸、左归丸等。

8.19　六味地黄丸

出自《小儿药证直诀》。由熟地黄 24 克，山茱萸 12 克，山药 12 克，泽泻 9 克，茯苓 9 克，丹皮 9 克组成，研细末，炼蜜为丸，每丸重 15 克。成人每次 1 丸，日 3 次。亦可水煎服，用量按原方比例酌减。方中熟地滋肾填精，为主药。山茱萸温补肝肾而涩精；山药滋肾益脾；三药合用，三阴并补；泽泻清泻肾火，并防熟地之滋腻；丹皮清泻肝火，并制山茱萸之温；茯苓淡渗脾湿，以助山药益脾。共奏滋补肝肾之功。主治阴虚证。症见腰膝酸软，头晕目眩，耳鸣耳聋，盗汗遗精，或骨蒸潮热，手足心热，舌红少苔，脉细数。现常用于肺结核、肾结核、慢性肾盂肾炎、高血压病，以及更年期综合证等慢性疾病具有上述症状者。临床应用六味地黄丸治疗中心视网膜、脉络膜病变 5 例，结合临床辨证加减，结果 4 例治愈，1 例好转。

8.20 左归丸

出自《景岳全书》。由熟地 240 克，山药 120 克，枸杞 120 克，山茱萸 120 克，川牛膝 90 克，菟丝子 120 克，鹿胶 120 克，龟胶 120 克组成。制为蜜丸，每丸重 15 克，早晚空腹各服 1 丸。方中熟地滋肾填精，为主药。山茱萸、枸杞子、菟丝子补益肝肾；山药补益脾肾；龟板胶、鹿角胶峻补精血，其中鹿角胶偏于补阳，有阳中求阴之义；牛膝强壮筋骨。共奏滋补肾阴之功。主治真阴不足之证。症见头目眩晕，腰酸腿软，自汗盗汗，口燥咽干。舌红少苔，脉细或数等。现常用于慢性肾炎、肾结核以及更年期综合证等病具有上述症状者。本方组成是以阴柔滋阴为主，久服易滞脾碍胃，在运用时，宜加入陈皮、砂仁等理气醒脾胃药。

8.21 一贯煎

出自《柳州医话》。由北沙参、麦冬、当归各 10 克，生地黄 30 克，枸杞子 12 克，川楝子 5 克组成。水煎分 2 次服。方中重用生地为主药，滋阴养血以补肝肾。沙参、麦冬、当归、枸杞子益阴而柔肝。更配少量川楝子疏泄肝气，虽性味苦寒，但配入大量滋阴养血药中，则无伤阴之害。诸药合用，共奏滋养肝肾，疏肝理气之功。主治肝肾阴虚，肝气不舒证。症见胸脘胁痛，吞酸吐苦，咽干口燥，舌红少津，脉细弱或虚弦等。现常用于慢性肝炎、溃疡病、神经官能症、高血压、肋膜炎、肋间神经痛、慢性睾丸炎等病具有上述症状者。本方滋腻之药较多，对于兼有停痰积饮者，不宜使用。

8.22 大补阴丸

出自《丹溪心法》。由黄柏、知母各 120 克，熟地黄、龟板各 180 克组成。共碾为末,猪脊髓适量蒸熟，捣如泥状，炼蜜，混合拌匀和药粉为丸，每丸约重 15 克。每日早晚各服 1 丸，淡盐开水送服，或水煎服。方中以熟地、龟板滋补真阴，潜阳制火，猪脊髓、蜂蜜俱为血肉甘润之品，用以填精补阳，以生津液，黄柏苦寒泻相火以坚真阴，知母苦寒，上以清润肺热，下以滋润肾阴。诸药合用，共奏滋阴降火之效。主治肝肾阴虚，虚火上炎之证，症见骨蒸潮热，盗汗遗精，咳嗽咳血，心烦易怒，足膝疼热或痿软，舌红少苔，尺脉数而有力等。现常用于甲状腺机能亢进、肾结核、糖尿病等病具有上述症状者。本方黄柏、知母两药苦寒，对于脾胃虚弱，食少便溏者应慎用。临床应用加味大补阴丸治疗肺结核大咯血 10 例，该病例均经中西医结合治疗后，肺结核大咯血不止，证属肺肾阴虚，虚火上炎，灼伤肺络所致。用本方加味：生地 12 克，熟地 12 克，焦山枝 6 克，知母 9 克，龟板 30 克，麦冬 15 克，牛膝 9 克，枇杷叶 9 克，侧柏叶 30 克、旱莲草 30 克，治疗效果：10 例中 9 例血止，1 例无效，一般服 1～2 剂则显效，再服即止。

8.23 石斛夜光丸

出自《原机启微》。由天门冬、人参、茯苓各 60 克、熟地黄、生地黄、麦门冬各 30 克、菟丝子、甘菊花、草决明、杏仁、干山药、枸杞、牛膝、五味子各 23 克，蒺藜、石斛、肉苁蓉、川芎、炙甘草、枳壳、青葙子、防风、川黄连、乌犀角、羚羊角各 15 克组成。共碾细末，筛净，炼蜜和丸，每丸重 10 克，早晚各服 1 丸，淡盐汤送下。方中以二冬、二地、五味子、石斛生津养血，菟丝子、枸杞、牛膝、肉苁蓉滋阴补肾；人参、茯苓、甘草、山药益脾补肺；枳壳、川芎、菊花、杏仁、防风、草决明、蒺藜、青葙子疏风清热；黄连、犀角、羚羊角平肝泻心凉血。诸药合用，共具平肝熄风，滋阴明目之功。主治肝肾不足，阴虚火旺之目疾。症见瞳神散大，视物昏花，羞明流泪，头晕目眩，以及内障等。现常用于青光眼、白内障等病具有上述症状者。

8.24　补肺阿胶汤

出自《小儿药证直诀》。由阿胶 45 克，牛蒡子 7.5 克，炙甘草 7.5 克，马兜铃 15 克，炒杏仁 6 克，炒糯米 30 克组成。共为末，每服 3～6 克，水煎后温服（亦作汤剂，阿胶另加开水炖化，共分 3 次服）。方中阿胶味甘性平，滋阴补肺，养血止血，为主药。牛蒡子疏风热，利咽膈；马兜铃清肺热，化痰止咳；杏仁润肺止咳；糯米、甘草滋养脾阴，且能甘润补肺。共奏养阴补肺，镇咳止血之功。主治肺虚热盛之证。症见咳嗽气喘，咽喉干燥，咯痰不多或痰中带血，脉浮细数，舌红少苔。现常用于肺结核、支气管扩张并咯血等病具有上述症状者。

8.25　龟鹿二仙胶

出自《医方考》。由鹿角 5000 克，龟板 2500 克，枸杞子 1500 克，人参 500 克组成。先将鹿角锯截，刮净，水浸，用火熬龟、鹿成胶，再将人参、枸杞熬膏和入，每晨取 3 克，清酒调化，淡盐开水送服。方中鹿角通督脉而补阳，龟板通任脉而补阴；人参大补元气，枸杞滋补肾阴。共奏填补精髓，益气壮阳之功。主治肾中阴阳两虚，任、督精血不足之证。症见全身瘦弱，遗精阳萎，两目昏花，腰膝酸软。现常用于各种贫血、阳萎等病具有上述症状者。

8.26　七宝美髯丹

出自《医方集解》。由何首乌 300 克，白茯苓 150 克，怀牛膝 150 克，当归 150 克，枸杞、菟丝子、破故纸各 120 克（黑芝麻拌炒）组成。共碾细，炼蜜丸，每丸重 10 克，早晚各服 1 丸，淡盐开水送服。方中何首乌味甘苦涩性微温，润补肝肾，坚筋骨而固精，为主药。枸杞、菟丝、芝麻补肝肾，固精止遗；牛膝补肝肾，坚筋骨，强腰膝；当归补血养肝，共奏滋肾水，益肝血之功。主治肝肾不足之证。症见须发早白，齿牙动摇，梦遗滑精，腰膝酸软等。现常用于须发早白、神经衰弱等病具有上述症状者。

8.27 二至丸

出自《医方集解》。由女贞子、旱莲草各适量组成。女贞子适量，蒸熟阴干，碾细筛净，将旱莲草适量水煮 3 次，取汁煎熬，浓缩成流浸膏，加适量蜂蜜拌匀，将女贞子粉末拌入和为丸。每丸约重 15 克，早晚各服 1 丸，开水送下。方中女贞子味甘苦性凉，滋肾养肝，旱莲草味甘酸性寒，养阴益精，凉血止血。共奏补肾养肝之功。主治肝肾阴虚之证。症见口苦咽干，头昏眼花，失眠多梦，腰楚酸软，下肢痿软，遗精，早年发白等。现常用于神经衰弱症、须发早白等病具有上述症状者。

8.28 补阳剂

是以补阳的药物为主组成的方剂，适用于肾阳虚之证。症见腰膝酸痛，四肢不温，酸软无力，少腹拘急冷痛，小便不利，或小便频数，阳萎早泄，肢体羸瘦，消渴，脉沉细或尺脉沉伏等。常用的药有附子、肉桂、杜仲、巴戟天、补骨脂等，代表方剂有肾气丸、右归丸等。

8.29 肾气丸

出自《金匮要略》。由干地黄 240 克，山药 120 克，山茱萸 120 克，泽泻 90 克，茯苓 90 克，牡丹皮 90 克，桂枝 30 克，附子（炮）30 克组成。方中干地黄滋补肾阴，山茱萸、山药滋补肝脾，且滋补肾阴，桂枝、附子温补肾阳，泽泻、茯苓利水渗湿，丹皮清泻肝火。共奏温补肾阳之功。主治肾阳不足之证，症见腰痛脚软，下半身常有冷感，少腹拘急，小便不利，或小便反多，舌质淡而胖，苔薄白不燥，尺脉沉细。以及脚气、痰饮、消渴、转胞等证。现常用于冠心病、妊娠中毒症、慢性肾炎、前列腺炎、红斑性狼疮、阿迪森氏病、粘液性水肿、慢性气管炎等病具有上述症状者。临床应用薛氏加减肾气丸治疗慢性肾炎6例，基本方由熟地12克、山药、山萸、泽泻、丹皮、肉桂、车前子、淮牛膝各3克、茯苓9克、附子1.5克组成。结果浮肿逐渐减退或减轻，尿量增多，尿蛋白消失或减少，肾功能改善，食欲增加，体力增强，血压降低。治疗过程中未发现有副作用，获满意疗效。运用肾气丸治疗老年性白内障284例，不合并糖尿病、肾炎等疾患，亦无显著的眼底和前眼部病变。接受治疗最短者1个半月，最长者9年半。结果568只患眼的总有效率81.4%，本方对改善和阻止老年性白内障的进一步发展有显著的疗效。

8.30　右归丸

出自《景岳全书》。由大怀熟地240克、山药（炒）120克，山茱萸（微炒）90克，枸杞（微炒）120克，鹿角胶（炒）120克，菟丝子（制）120克，杜仲（炒）120克，当归90克，肉桂60～120克，附子（制）60～180克组成。共为细末，配做蜜丸，每丸重15克。早晚各服1丸，开水送下（亦做汤剂，用量按原方比例酌情增减）。方中肉桂、附子、鹿角胶温补肾阳，填精补髓，熟地、山茱萸、山药、菟丝子、枸杞、杜仲滋阴益肾，养肝补脾，当归补血养肝。共奏温补肾阳，填精补血之功。主治肾阳不足，命门火衰之证。症见久病气衰神疲，畏寒肢冷，或阳萎遗精，阳萎无子，或大便不实，甚则实谷不化，或小便自遗，或腰膝软弱，下肢浮肿等。现常用于冠心病、妊娠中毒症、慢性肾炎、原发性高血压、前列腺炎、红斑性狼疮、阿迪森氏病、粘液性水肿、慢性支气管炎、希汉氏病等病具有上述症状者。临床应用右归丸加减治疗遗传性小脑型共济失调1例，症属肾气虚弱。症见步履蹒跚，左右摇摆，头昏耳鸣，记忆衰退，形寒肢冷，腰膝无力，舌淡苔薄，脉细尺部无力。药用淡附片6克，肉桂 4 克，鹿角霜、杜仲、山药、怀牛膝、全当归各 9 克，菟丝子、龟板、枸杞、熟地、制首乌各 12 克。服 20 剂症状减轻。再加生地 12 克，服 50 剂后病情显著好转。

第9章 安神剂

9.1 安神剂

由重镇安神或滋养安神药为主组成。具有安神作用，以治疗神志不安疾患的方剂，统称安神剂。神志不安的病因很多，就本剂所治之症而言，一为外受惊恐，或肝郁化火，内扰心神，表现为惊恐、喜怒、烦躁不宁等，一般多属实证，须应用重镇安神治法，以达到镇心安神，清热除烦的目的；二为忧思过度，心肝血虚，心神失养或心阴不足，虚火内扰，表现为惊悸、健忘、虚烦不寐，一般多属虚证，须应用滋养安神治法，以达滋阴降火，养血安神的目的。安神剂，根据所治证候虚实的不同，大致可分为重镇安神和滋养安神两类，此外，因热、因痰而致者，分别在清热剂、祛痰剂介绍，在此不作重复。

安神剂中的重镇安神类多由金石组成，不宜久服，以免有碍脾胃运化。素体脾胃不健，宜加用补脾和胃药。

9.2 重镇安神剂

是以重镇安神的药物为主组成的方剂。适用于心肝之阳偏亢之证。症见烦乱，目眩，失眠，惊悸，怔忡等。常用的药有朱砂、磁石、龙齿、珍珠母等，代表方剂有朱砂安神丸、珍珠母丸、磁朱丸等。

9.3 朱砂安神丸

出自《医学发明》。由朱砂 15 克，黄连 18 克，灸甘草 16 克，生地黄 8 克，当归 8 克组成。共为细末，制丸，每次 6～9 克，睡前开水送下。（亦作汤剂，用量按原方比例酌情增减，朱砂研细末水飞，以药汤送服）。方中朱砂味甘性寒，重镇安神，黄连味苦性寒，清热除烦，两药均为主药。当归养血，生地滋阴；甘草调和诸药。共奏镇心安神，泻火养阴之功。主治心火偏亢，阴血不足之证。症见心烦神乱，失眠，多梦，怔忡，惊悸，胸中懊侬，舌红，脉细数。现常用于神经衰弱、心肌炎、精神抑郁症等病具有上述症状者。本方朱砂有毒，不宜多服或久服。临床应用朱砂安神丸合磁朱丸治疗夜游症 1 例，证属火热内扰神魂，症见每于睡梦中惊起，启门而出，跌仆于田野荒丘，依然沉睡。诊时见患者神态如常，自觉心烦耳鸣，夜卧而出并不知觉，唯多梦易惊，舌红苔黄，脉弦数。药用生地 60 克，黄连 18 克，当归 30 克，甘草 15 克，煅磁石 30 克，建曲 18 克，以上六味研末和蜜为丸，外以朱砂 9 克，水飞为丸衣，丸如黄豆大，早晚各服 1 次，每服 30 克，服完 2 料丸剂而病愈。

9.4　珍珠母丸

出自《普济本事方》。由珍珠母 22.5 克，当归、熟地各 45 克，人参、酸枣仁、柏子仁各 30 克，犀角、茯神、沉香、龙齿各 15 克组成。共为细末，炼蜜为丸，如梧子大，辰砂为衣，每服 40～50 丸，金银花、薄荷汤冲下，日午，夜卧服。方中珍珠母味咸性寒，平肝潜阳，为主药。龙齿镇心安神；枣仁、柏子仁、茯神安神定志，宁心入寐；人参、当归、熟地养血滋阴，益气生血；犀角凉肝镇惊，沉香摄纳浮阳，辰砂镇惊安神；金银花、薄荷清热凉肝。共奏滋阴养血，镇心安神之功。主治阴血不足，肝阳偏亢之证。症见神志不宁，少寐，时而惊悸，头目眩晕，脉细弦。现常用于神经衰弱、精神分裂症等病具有上述症状者。

9.5　磁朱丸

　　出自《备急千金要方》，由磁石 60 克，朱砂 30 克，神曲 120 克组成。共为细末，炼蜜为丸，如梧子大，每服 6 克，日 2 次，开水送服。方中磁石味咸性寒，益阴潜阳，重镇安神；朱砂味甘性寒，安神定志；神曲健脾助运，以防石药伤胃，与蜂蜜补中和胃。共奏重镇安神，潜阳明目之功。主治心肾不交之证。症见心悸失眠，耳鸣耳聋，视物昏花等。现常用于神经衰弱、癫痫等病具有上述症状者。临床应用磁朱丸治疗幻听 7 例。7 例患者，或为精神分裂症以幻听为突出症状，或系精神分裂症经过治疗后基本症状消失而残留幻听者。用磁朱丸治疗，每次 6～10 克，每日 1～2 次，一般以 1 个月为 1 疗程。治疗后，显效 3 例，好转 3 例，无效 1 例。7 例中有心肾不交症状的 6 例，有较好疗效，其中 1 例没有心肾不交症状，则无效。运用磁朱丸治疗瞳孔散大 2 例，其中 1 例有合并症，用磁朱丸为主先后服药 20 余剂获愈，另 1 例无合并症，经门诊治疗，共服药 6 剂，计服磁朱丸 43 克，即告痊愈。

9.6　滋养安神剂

　　是以滋养安神的药物为主组成的方剂。适用于阴血不足，虚阳偏亢之证。症见虚烦少寐，心悸盗汗，梦遗健忘，舌红苔少。常用的药有生地、麦冬、酸枣仁、柏子仁等，代表方剂有酸枣仁汤、天王补心丹、甘麦大枣汤等。

9.7　酸枣仁汤

　　出自《金匮要略》。由酸枣仁（炒）15～18 克，甘草 3 克，知母 8～10 克，茯苓 10 克，川芎 3～5 克组成。先煎酸枣仁，再入余药水煎分 3 次服。方中酸枣仁味甘酸性平，养肝血而安心神，为主药。川芎调养肝血，茯苓宁心安神，知母清润泄火；甘草清热和药。共奏养血安神，清热除烦之功。主治虚劳虚烦不得眠之证。症见心悸盗汗，头目眩晕，咽干口燥，脉细弦。现常用于神经衰弱等病具有上述症状者。临床应用中药复方酸枣汤治疗神经衰弱 209 例，其中包括惊悸不寐、失眠、健忘等症。产生的原因大多是肾阴亏损，阴虚火旺，心肾不交，肝血不足，魂无所归。经治疗，有效率达 90%。

复方酸枣仁汤对大脑确有催眠和镇静作用，能抑制其过度亢进和兴奋的神经细胞，让长期处在紧张或紊乱状态下的皮质细胞，有充分休息和调节的机会，从而促进使兴奋和抑制恢复平衡各器官的功能自然恢复正常。

9.8　天王补心丹

出自《摄生秘剖》。由生地黄（酒洗）120 克，人参、丹参（微炒）、元参（微炒）、白茯苓、五味子（烘）、远志（炒）、桔梗各 15 克，当归身（酒洗）、天门冬、麦门冬、柏子仁（炒）、酸枣仁各 60 克，朱砂 12 克组成。共研为末，炼蜜为小丸，朱砂为衣。每服 9 克，温开水送下（亦作汤剂，用量按原方比例酌减）。方中生地味甘苦性寒，滋阴养血，为主药。玄参、天冬、麦冬甘寒滋润以清虚火，丹参、当归养血安神；人参、茯苓益气宁心，酸枣仁、五味子收敛心气而安心神；柏子仁、远志、朱砂养心安神；桔梗载药上行。共奏滋阴养血，补心安神之功。主治阴亏血少，心肾阴虚之证。症见虚烦少寐，心悸神疲，梦遗健忘，大便干结，口舌生疮，舌红少苔，脉细而数。现常用于神经衰弱、更年期综合症、心肌炎等病具有上述症状者。临床应用加味天王补心丹治疗精神病 62 例。经吐、下法治疗之后，可应用于恢复期，如虚弱患者，可先以此方调补，再予吐下，然后以此方善后。62 例均获治愈，有的再次发作，复用此法施治亦获效。运用天王补心丹加味治疗慢性结膜炎 1 例，病者患急性结膜炎未彻底治疗，并在灯光下坚持工作，20 余天来，目红干涩畏光，视物不清，并见午后心烦，夜多恶梦，经用西药及中医清心、凉肝、活血、滋肾阴等法治疗未见效。以天王补心丹为主方随症加减，服 10 剂后，诸症悉除，续服丸剂善后。

补心丹加味（人参 15 克，麦冬、五味子各 30 克，玄参、炮附子、远志、公丁香、甘草各 15 克，丹参、茯神、枣仁、天冬、柏子仁、红花、当归各 30 克，生地 120 克，蒲黄 18 克，按常法水煎成 100%浓度。）对由异丙肾上腺素所致的健康雄小鼠实验性心肌梗塞具有满意的拮抗作用，该方不仅能防止上述药物所致的缺血性心电图改变和心肌病理学损害，而且对缺血心肌的生化代谢也有良好影响，如通过对心肌琥珀酸脱氢酶、三磷酸腺甘酶活化的作用，进而改善细胞线粒体呼吸和电子传递系统促使线粒体能量转换，并使心肌兴奋——收缩耦联机制正常化，同时该方还能改善动物的非特异性防御功能和应激状态。

9.9　甘麦大枣汤

出自《金匮要略》。由甘草 9 克，小麦 9～15 克，大枣 5～7 枚组成。水煎分 3 次服。方中甘草味甘性平，和中养心。甘缓急迫，为主药。小麦养心安神；大枣补益脾气，缓肝急并治心虚，共奏养心安神；和中缓急之功。主治心虚、肝郁而致的脏躁证。症见精神恍惚，常非伤欲哭，不能自主，睡眠不安，甚则言行失常，呵欠频作，舌红苔少。现常用于神经衰弱、癔病、轻症精神分裂症等病具有上述症状者。临床应用甘麦大枣汤加龙骨、牡蛎治疗精神分裂症 79 例，均病程较长，虽经长期反复使用多种抗精神病药治疗无效或疗效较差，基本方由灸甘草 10 克，淮小麦、龙骨、牡蛎各 30 克，大枣 5 枚组成。若精神运动性兴奋明显者，加磁石、制大黄。幻觉明显者，加磁朱丸、六味地黄丸。妄想明显者，加石菖蒲、陈胆星、萱草。失眠明显者，加酸枣仁、合欢皮、夜交藤。治疗结果，痊愈 5 例，显效 23 例，好转 34 例，无效 17 例。运用甘麦大枣汤加味治疗小儿遗尿证 28

例，基本方由炙甘草 20～25 克，淮小麦 18 克，炙桑螵蛸 9 克，炒益智仁 9 克，菟丝子 9 克，大枣 8 枚组成。经治疗，显效 13 例，有效 15 例。

第10章　开窍剂

10.1　开窍剂

　　由芳香开窍药为主组成。具有开窍醒神的作用，以治疗神昏窍闭之证的方剂，统称开窍剂。神昏窍闭之证，多由邪气壅盛，蒙蔽心窍所致，其证候有热闭与寒闭的不同。热闭由温邪热毒内陷心包所致，治宜清热开窍；寒闭由寒湿痰浊之邪蒙蔽心窍所致，治宜温通开窍。故本类方剂可分为凉开与温开两类。

　　开窍剂，无论凉开还是温开，只适用于邪盛气实的闭证，如症见口噤，两手握固，脉象有力，可用开窍剂；对于汗出肢冷，气微遗尿，口开目合的脱证，即使神志昏迷，也不宜使用。对阳明腑实证而见神昏谵语者，治宜寒下，不宜用开窍剂；若阳明腑实而兼有邪陷心包之证，应根据病情的轻重缓急，以掌握应用开窍与寒下的先后主次，或两者并用。开窍剂中的芳香开窍药物，善于辛散走窜，宜制丸、散剂或注射剂，不宜作汤剂，否则药性挥发，影响疗效。开窍剂久服易耗伤元气，临床多用于急救，中病即止，不可久服。

10.2　凉开剂

　　是以芳香开窍和清热解毒药物为主组成的方剂。适用于温邪热毒内陷心包的热闭之证。症见高热，神昏谵语，甚或痉厥。其他如中风、痰厥及感触秽浊之气，卒然昏倒，不省人事；证有热象者，亦可选用。常用芳香开窍药麝香、冰片、郁金配伍清热解毒药牛黄、犀角、黄连、石膏等，代表方剂有安宫牛黄丸、紫雪丹、至宝丹、回春丹等。

10.3 安宫牛黄丸

出自《温病条辨》。由牛黄、郁金、犀角、黄芩、黄连、雄黄、山栀子、朱砂各 30 克，梅片、麝香各 7.5 克，珍珠 15 克，金箔（适量）组成。共为极细末，炼蜜为丸，每丸 3 克，金箔为衣，蜡护，每服 1 丸，大人病重体实者，日再服，甚至日 3 服；小儿服半丸，不知，再服半丸。方中牛黄味苦甘性凉，清心解毒，豁痰开窍，麝香味辛性温，开窍醒神，均为主药。犀角清心凉血解毒；黄连、黄芩、山栀清热泻火解毒，助牛黄以清心包之火；冰片、郁金芳香辟秽，通窍开闭，以加强麝香开窍醒神；朱砂、珍珠镇心安神，以除烦躁不安；雄黄助牛黄以豁痰解毒；蜂蜜和胃调中，金箔重镇安神。共奏清热开窍，豁痰解毒之功。主治温热病，热邪内陷心包，痰热壅闭心窍，以及中风昏迷、小儿惊厥属热闭之证。症见高热烦躁，神昏谵语等。现常用于乙型脑炎、肝性昏迷、急性脑出血昏迷、流行性脑脊髓膜炎、中毒性痢疾、尿毒症、中毒性肝炎等病具有上述症状者。临床应用针灸配合安宫牛黄丸治疗急性脑出血昏迷 16 例。采用轻而短的手法针刺人中等穴的同时，内服安宫牛黄丸，用鼻饲法灌服，每日 1～4 丸，随证增减，经治疗，9 例生命获得挽救，其中 3 例完全恢复健康。

10.4 紫雪丹

出自《外台秘要》。由石膏、寒水石、滑石、磁石各 1500 克，犀角、羚羊角各 150 克，青木香、沉香各 150 克，玄参、升麻各 500 克，甘草（炙）240 克，丁香 30 克，朴硝 5000 克，硝石 96 克，麝香 1.5 克，朱砂 90 克，黄金 3000 克组成。将石膏、寒水石、滑石、磁石砸成小块，加入黄金水煎煮 2 次，去渣；入玄参、木香、沉香、升麻、甘草、丁香等煎煮 3 次，合并煎液滤过，滤液浓缩成膏。朴硝、硝石粉碎入膏中，搅匀，干燥，粉碎成细粉。犀角、羚羊角锉研成细粉，朱砂水飞或粉碎成级细粉，将麝香研细，与朴硝等粉末及上述犀角、羚羊角、朱砂粉末配研，过筛，混匀而成。口服，一次 1.5～3 克，日 2 次，小儿酌减。方中石膏、寒水石、滑石甘寒清热，羚羊角清肝熄风以解痉厥，犀角清心以解热毒，麝香芳香开窍，以上各药，均为主要部分。玄参、升麻、甘草清热解毒，玄参养阴生津；朱砂、磁石；黄金重镇安神；青木香、丁香、沉香行气宣通；朴硝、硝石泄热散结。共奏清热开窍，镇痉安神之功。主治温热病，热邪内陷心包，以及小儿热盛惊厥之证。症见高热烦躁，神昏谵语，痉厥，口渴唇焦，尿赤便闭等。现常用于乙型脑炎、流行性脑脊髓膜炎、猩红热、小儿麻疹、小儿高烧惊厥、肝性昏迷等病具有上述症状者。

10.5 至宝丹

出自《太平惠民和剂局方》。由生乌犀屑（研）、生玳瑁屑（研）、琥珀（研）、朱砂（研，飞）、雄黄（研，飞）各 30 克，龙脑（研）、麝香各 7.5 克，牛黄（研）15 克，安息香 45 克（为末，以无灰酒搅澄飞过，滤去沙土，约得净数 30 克，慢火熬成膏）、金箔（半入药、半为衣）、银箔（研）各 50 片组成。研末为丸，每丸重 3 克，每服 1 丸，服前研碎，开水送服，小儿半丸（原方用人参汤化服）。主治中暑、中风、小儿惊厥和温病痰热内闭之证。症见神昏谵语，身热烦躁，痰盛气粗，舌红苔黄垢腻，脉滑数等。现常用于脑血管意外、肝性昏迷、乙型脑炎、癫痫等病具有上述症状者。本方原用人参汤化服，对于病情复杂正气虚弱者，借助人参益气扶正，与辛香开窍药配合，对苏醒神志，扶正祛邪，功效较著，但以脉虚者为宜。

10.6 小儿回春丹

出自《敬修堂药说》。由川贝母、陈皮、木香、白豆蔻、枳壳、法半夏、沉香、天竹黄、僵蚕、全蝎、檀香各 37.5 克，牛黄、麝香各 12 各，胆南星 60 克，钩藤 240 克，大黄 60 克，天麻 37.5 克，甘草 26 克，朱砂适量组成。共研为细末，制为小丸，每丸重 0.09 克。口服，周岁以下，每次 1 丸，1～2 岁，每次 2 丸，日 2～3 次。方中牛黄清热解毒，豁痰开窍，息风定惊，麝香芳香开窍，川贝母、天竹黄、胆南星、法半夏清热化痰，钩藤、天麻、全蝎、僵蚕息风镇痉，朱砂重镇安神；大黄清热泻火，去积导滞，使痰热从肠腑而解；枳壳、木香、陈皮、沉香、白豆蔻、檀香调理气机，使气畅痰消，痰热不致内生；甘草调和诸药。共奏开窍定惊，清热化痰之功。主治小儿急惊，痰热蒙蔽之证。症见发热烦躁，神昏惊厥，或反胃呕吐，夜啼吐乳，痰嗽哮喘，腹痛泄泻等。现常用于小儿高烧惊厥等病具有上述症状者。本方对脾肾虚寒所致之慢惊风不宜应用。

10.7 温开剂

是以芳香开窍和辛温行气的药物为主组成的方剂。适用于中风、中寒、痰厥的寒闭之证。症见突然昏倒，牙关紧闭，神昏不语，苔白脉迟等。常用芳香开窍药苏合香、麝香、冰片配伍辛温行气药沉香、丁香等，代表方剂有苏合香丸、紫金锭等。

10.8 苏合香丸

出自《太平惠民和剂局方》。由白术、青木香、乌犀屑、香附子（炒，去毛）、朱砂（研，水飞）、诃子（煨，去皮）、白檀香、安息香（别为末，用无灰酒 1 升熬膏）、沉香、麝香（研）、丁香、荜茇各 60 克，龙脑（研）、苏合香油（入安息香膏内）各 30 克、乳香（别研）30 克组成。为细末，用安息香膏并炼白蜜和剂，制丸，每丸重3克。每服1丸，温开水送下，日1或2次，小儿用量酌减。方中苏合香、麝香、冰片、安息香等芳香开窍，均为主药。青木香、白檀香、沉香、乳香、丁香、香附行气解郁，散寒化浊，并能解除脏腑气血之郁滞；荜茇散寒开郁；犀角解毒，朱砂镇心安神；白术补气健脾，燥湿化浊；煨诃子收涩敛气，与诸香药配伍，可防止辛香太过。共奏芳香开窍，行气止痛之功。主治中风、中气或感受时行瘴疬之气等证。症见突然昏倒，牙关紧闭，不省人事，苔白，脉迟，或中寒气闭，心腹猝痛，甚则昏厥，或痰壅气阻，突然昏倒等。现常用于癔病、冠心病心绞痛、食物中毒、癫痫等病具有上述症状者。本方香窜走泄，有损胎气，孕妇慎用。临床应用苏合香丸配合西药治疗急性心肌梗塞5例，症状表现以心前区剧痛为重点，过去多用吗啡类药物止痛，有容易成瘾及抑制呼吸的副作用，应用苏合香丸后，4例明显好转，其中1例急性后壁心肌梗塞自觉服药后半小时顿觉心胸开朗感，并无副作用。运用苏合香丸救治木薯中毒2例，症见发冷，头晕，胸闷，呕吐，重者肢冷，手足微抽，面青唇绀，鼻扇，气促，呈半昏迷状态，脉伏，经以温开水磨苏合香丸1枚灌服，2例均治愈。

10.9　通关散

出自《丹溪心法附余》。由猪牙皂、细辛各等分组成。研极细末，和匀，吹少许入鼻中取嚏。方中皂角味辛性温，祛痰开窍，细辛味辛性温，宣散开窍。共奏通关开窍之功。主治中恶客忤或痰厥所致的闭证。症见口噤气塞，人事不省，牙关紧闭，痰涎壅盛。现常用于癫痫、脑血管意外、颅脑外伤等病具有上述症状者。本方为外用的临时急救方法，苏醒后应按病情辨证治疗。

10.10　紫金锭

出自《片玉心书》。由山慈姑 90 克，红大戟 45 克，千金子霜 30 克，五倍子 90 克，麝香 9 克，雄黄 30 克，朱砂 30 克组成。共研为末，糯米糊作锭子。口服，一次 0.6～1.5 克，日 2 次；外用醋磨，调敷患处。方中麝香芳香开窍，行气止痛；山慈姑清热消肿；雄黄辟秽解毒；千金子霜、红大戟逐痰消肿，朱砂重镇安神；五倍子涩肠止泻。共奏内服开窍化痰，辟秽解毒，并有缓下降逆作用；外敷有消肿散结之功。主治感受秽恶痰浊之证。症见脘腹胀闷疼痛，呕吐泄泻；外敷疗疔疮疖肿。现常用于食物中毒、疔疮疖肿等病具有上述症状者。方中千金子霜、红大戟等俱有毒，小儿用量宜减；麝香芳香走窜，孕妇宜慎用。

第 11 章　固涩剂

11.1　固涩剂

由固涩药物为主组成。具有收敛固涩的作用，以治疗气血精津滑脱散失之证的方剂，统称固涩剂。气血精津的滑脱散失，因病因及病位的不同，其表现有自汗盗汗、肺虚久咳、遗精滑泄、小便失禁、久泻久痢和崩漏带下等不同。因此，本类方剂根据其不同作用，分为固表止汗，敛肺止咳，涩肠固脱，涩精止遗和固崩止带 5 类。

固涩剂收涩作用较强，凡实邪所致的自汗盗汗，久咳不已，遗精滑泄，小便失禁，泻痢日久，崩漏带下等，均非本法所宜。

11.2　固表止汗剂

是以固表止汗的药物为主组成的方剂。适用于卫外不固，或阴虚有热之自汗、盗汗症。常用的药有黄芪、牡蛎、麻黄根、浮小麦等，代表方剂有牡蛎散、玉屏风散等。

11.3　玉屏风散

出自《丹溪心法》。由防风 30 克，黄芪 30 克，白术 60 克组成。共研细末，每服 6～9 克，日服 2 次（亦可水煎服，用量按原方比例酌减）。方中黄芪益气固表，白术健脾益气，两者相伍，使气旺表实，则汗不外泄，邪不内侵。防风辛温而散，有疏风散邪之功，与黄芪相合，固表不留邪，祛邪不伤正。共奏益气固表止汗之功。主治表虚自汗证。症见恶风，面色㿠白，舌淡苔薄白，脉浮虚等。现常用于慢性鼻炎、过敏性鼻炎、呼吸道感染等病具有上述症状者。临床用玉屏风散治疗 32 例常患感冒、气管炎、肺炎等疾病的体弱儿童，每月服玉屏风散15天，经3个半月观察治疗，一直未发病者11例，感冒仅发一次者13例，感冒2次者7例，因未按时服药而无效者1例。对16例手术后恶风自汗者使用玉屏风散，平均服药5剂，均获痊愈。

11.4 牡蛎散

出自《太平惠民和剂局方》。由黄芪、麻黄根、牡蛎各30克组成。共为粗末，每服9克，用小麦30克水煎冲服，日2次。（亦可按原方比例酌减用量，如小麦30克，水煎服）方中牡蛎益阴潜阳，除烦敛汗，为主药。黄芪益气固表；麻黄根专于止汗；小麦益心气，养心阴，止汗泄。共奏固表敛汗之功。主治阳浮自汗证。症见身常汗出，夜卧尤甚，久而不止，心悸惊惕，舌淡苔白，脉细弱。现常用于植物神经功能失调所致自汗盗汗，及肺结核之盗汗等病具有上述症状者。临床用牡蛎散治疗28例患者，其中盗汗15例，自汗6例，自汗兼盗汗者7例。治疗结果，痊愈20例，基本痊愈5例，减轻1例，无效2例，服药2～5剂者18剂，6～10剂者5例，10剂以上者5例。

11.5 敛肺止咳剂

是以敛肺止咳的药物为主组成的方剂。适用于久咳肺虚，气阴耗伤，喘促自汗，脉虚数等。常用的药有五味子、罂粟、壳、乌梅、人参、阿胶等，代表方剂有九仙散。

11.6 九仙散

出自《医学正传》。由人参、款冬花、桔梗、桑白皮、五味子、阿胶、贝母各2克，乌梅、罂粟壳各6克组成。共为细末，作1剂，加生姜1片，大枣1枚，水煎分2次服。方中罂粟壳敛肺止咳，人参补气益肺，并为主药。阿胶养阴益肺；五味子、乌梅敛肺止咳；款冬花、贝母止咳化痰，降气平喘；桑白皮清肺止咳；桔梗止咳化痰。共奏敛肺止咳，益气养阴之功。主治肺虚气弱证，症见久咳不已，咳甚则气喘自汗，舌淡苔白，脉虚数等。现常用于慢性支气管炎、支气管哮喘、胸膜炎及肺炎恢复期等病具有上述症状者。但因本方敛肺止咳之力颇强，故凡久咳不已，而内多痰涎，或外有表邪者，切勿使用，以免留邪为患。

11.7 涩肠固脱剂

是以涩肠固脱的药物为主组成的方剂。适用于脾肾虚寒所致之泻痢日久，滑脱不禁等证。常用的药有赤石脂、肉豆蔻、诃子、五味子、补骨脂、肉桂、人参、白术等。代表方剂有真人养脏汤、四神丸、桃花汤等。

11.8 真人养脏汤

出自《太平惠民和剂局方》。由人参、甘草各 6 克，当归、木香各 9 克，白术、肉豆蔻、诃子各 12 克，白芍 15 克，罂粟壳 20 克，肉桂 3 克组成。水煎分 2 次服。方中罂粟壳涩肠止泻，肉桂温肾暖脾，共为主药。肉豆蔻、诃子温脾肾，止泻痢；人参、白术益气健脾；当归、白芍养血和营，木香调气止痛；甘草调和诸药，缓急止痛。共奏涩肠固脱，温补脾肾之功。主治脾肾虚寒证。症见久泻久痢，大便滑脱不禁，腹痛喜暖喜按，或下痢赤白，日夜无度，倦怠食少，舌淡苔白，脉沉迟等。现常用于慢性肠炎、慢性细菌性痢疾、肠结核等病具有上述症状者。临床用真人养脏汤化裁治疗小儿虚寒性泄泻 13 例，均获痊愈。其中食积者加神曲、山楂，滑脱者加石榴皮、柿蒂，小便不利者加车前子、木通、茯苓。

11.9 四神丸

出自《证治准绳》。由肉豆蔻、五味子各 60 克，补骨脂 120 克，吴茱萸 30 克组成。共为细末，用生姜 24 克，大枣 100 枚，煮熟取枣肉，和末为丸。每服 6～9 克，日 2 次 (亦可水煎服，用量按原方比例酌减)。方中补骨脂温补肾阳，为主药。肉豆蔻暖脾止泻，行气消食；吴茱萸和生姜温中祛寒；五味子收敛止泻，大枣补脾养胃。共奏温补脾肾，涩肠止泻之功。主治脾肾虚寒证。症见五更泻泄，不思饮食，腹痛腰酸肢冷，神疲乏力，舌淡苔薄白，脉沉迟无力等。现常用于慢性结肠炎、过敏性结肠炎、肠结核等病具有上述症状者。临床用四神丸治疗五更泻 20 例，结果痊愈 16 例，显效 4 例，全部有效。治疗过敏性结肠炎 1 例，病史长达 9 年，腹痛泄泻，日 3～5 次。服四神丸 20 天后，大便成形，每日排便 1～2 次，再服 10 天，诸证消失。停药观察 1 个月，疗效巩固。

四神丸对肠管的自发活动有明显抑制作用，并能对抗乙酰胆碱引起的肠痉挛，还可对抗氯化钡引起的肠痉挛。

11.10　桃花汤

出自《伤寒论》。由赤石脂 30 克，粳米 30 克，干姜 9 克组成。水煎分 2 次服。方中赤石脂体重性温，涩肠固脱为主药。干姜温中祛寒；粳米养胃和中。共奏温中涩肠之功。主治脾胃虚寒证。症见久痢不愈，大便脓血，色暗不鲜，小便不利，腹痛喜暖喜按，舌淡苔白，脉微细等。现常用于慢性阿米巴痢疾、慢性菌痢、慢性肠炎等病具有上述症状者。临床用本方加禹余粮、炒地榆、山药、秦皮、龙骨、牡蛎，治疗慢性阿米巴痢疾 4 例，其病程为半年至 2 年不等，服药 3～5 剂即见效，继用健脾和胃法调理 1 周后痊愈。

11.11　涩精止遗剂

是以补肾涩精及固肾止遗的药物为主组成的方剂。适用于肾虚失藏，精关不固之遗尿滑精，或肾虚不摄，膀胱失约之遗尿尿频等症。常用的药有沙菀、蒺藜、莲须、芡实、桑螵蛸、益智仁等，代表方剂有金锁固精丸、桑螵蛸散、缩泉丸等。

11.12　金锁固精丸

出自《医方集解》。由沙菀、蒺藜、芡实、莲须各60克，龙骨、牡蛎各30克组成。以莲子肉粉糊为丸。再服9克，淡盐汤或开水送服，日3次（亦可按原方用量比例酌减，加入适量莲子肉，水煎服）。方中沙菀、蒺藜补肾涩精，为主药。莲子清心宁神；龙骨、牡蛎、莲须、芡实涩精止遗。共奏补肾涩精之功。主治肾虚精亏证。症见遗精滑泄，神疲乏力，四肢酸软，腰痛耳鸣，舌淡苔白，脉细弱等。现常用于植物神经功能紊乱、重症肌无力等病具有上述症状者。临床应用金锁固精丸治疗重症肌无力患者1例，症见右眼上睑完全下垂，四肢无力，蜷卧不起，咀嚼困难，喘息短气，遗精滑泄，腰膝冷痛，服金锁固精丸12克，日服3次，2周后病情明显好转，数月痊愈，随访6年未见复发。

11.13　桑螵蛸散

出自《本草衍义》。由桑螵蛸、远志、菖蒲、龙骨、人参、茯神、当归、龟板各30克组成。共为细末，睡前人参汤调下6克（亦可水煎服，用量按原方比例酌减）。方中桑螵蛸补肾益精，固脬止遗，为主药。龙骨、龟板滋肾固涩；人参、当归、茯苓益气养血；菖蒲、远志安神定志，交通心肾。共奏调补心肾，涩精止遗之功。主治心肾两虚证。症见小便频数，或色如米泔，遗尿滑精，心神恍惚，健忘食少，舌淡苔白，脉细弱等。现常用于尿崩症、糖尿病、神经衰弱、神经性尿频等病具有上述症状者。临床用桑螵蛸散加减治疗子宫脱垂并有小便频数，及子宫口渗液较多者，疗效显著。如某患者子宫脱垂8年，伴头昏气短、神疲乏力，小便频数，宫口时流黄水，舌淡苔白，脉虚弱。服桑螵蛸散加黄芪、柴胡、升麻，4剂后子宫明显回缩，继服3剂而愈。

11.14 缩泉丸

出自《妇人良方》。由乌药、益智仁各等分组成。共为细末，酒煎山药末糊为丸。每服6克，日服2次（亦可水煎服。用量按原方比例酌定）。方中益智仁温肾纳气，暖脾摄精，固涩缩尿，为主药。乌药温肾散寒；山药健脾补肾。共奏温肾祛寒，缩尿止遗之功。主治下焦虚寒证。症见小便频数，小儿遗尿，舌淡苔白，脉沉迟等。现常用于神经性尿频、尿崩症、骨髓炎等病具有上述症状者。但因本方药简力薄，若证情较甚者，仍需酌加温补固涩之品，以提高疗效。临床用缩泉丸加牡蛎、枸杞、熟地、炙附子、桃仁、甘草治疗30多年顽固性便秘1例，症见大便秘结，夏轻冬重，腰酸尿频，肛门疼痛，舌暗少苔，脉沉细而迟。服药20剂，诸症消失而愈。

11.15 固崩止带剂

是以固崩止带的药物组成的方剂。适用于妇人血崩及带下等症。常用的药有椿根皮、黑荆芥、赤石脂等，代表方剂有固经丸、完带汤等。

11.16 固经丸

出自《医学入门》。由黄芩、白芍、龟板各30克，椿根皮21克，黄柏9克，香附7.5克组成。共为细末，酒糊为丸，每服9克，日服2次（亦可水煎服，用量按原方比例酌定）。方中龟板滋阴降火而益肾；白芍敛阴益血以柔肝；黄芩、黄柏清热泻火以止血；椿根皮固经止带，燥湿清热；香附调气解郁而和血。共奏滋阴清热；止血固经之功。主治阴虚内热证。症见经行不止，崩中漏下，血色深红，或夹紫黑闷块，心胸烦热，腹痛溲赤，舌红，脉弦数等。现常用于生殖系统炎症所致月经不调、功能性子宫出血等病具有上述症状者。

11.17　震灵丹

出自《太平惠民和剂局方》。由禹余粮、紫石英、赤石脂、丁头代赭石各 200 克，乳香、五灵脂、没药各 100 克，朱砂 50 克组成。共研细末，另取糯米粉 200 克炒熟，与药粉和匀，水泛为丸，朱砂包衣。每服 6 克，日服 2 次。方中赤石脂、禹余粮、紫石英、赭石暖宫固下，养血止崩；乳香、没药、五灵脂活血化瘀，理气止痛；糯米粉补肺健脾，益气温中。共奏止血化瘀之功。主治冲任虚寒，瘀阻胞宫证。症见崩漏下血，色紫红或紫黑，夹有血块，小腹疼痛拒按，舌紫黯，脉沉细而弦等。现常用于功能性子宫出血、产后出血过多等病具有上述症状者。本方配伍是收敛化瘀并用，对真元虚衰而无瘀滞者，不宜使用。

11.18　完带汤

出自《傅青主女科》。由白术、出药各 30 克，车前子、苍术各 9 克，白芍 15 克，人参 6 克，陈皮、黑芥穗各 1.5 克，柴胡 1.8 克，甘草 3 克组成。水煎分 2 次服。方中白术、苍术、人参、山药、甘草益气健脾，燥湿固下；白芍、陈皮、柴胡柔肝升阳；车前子导湿下行；黑芥穗祛风胜湿以止带。共奏补中健脾，化湿止带之功。主治脾虚肝郁，湿浊下注证。症见带下色白或淡黄，清稀无臭，面色㿠白，倦怠便溏，舌淡苔白，脉缓或濡弱。现常用于生殖系统慢性炎症所致白带增多等病具有上述症状者。临床用完带汤加女贞子 9 克，治疗白带增多症 100 例，均获良效，随访病例无一复发。运用完带汤加合欢皮、女贞子、当归、黄柏、黑大豆，除可治疗带下症外，并能兼治闭经及月经不调。

第12章 理气剂

12.1 理气剂

由理气药物为主组成。具有行气或降气的作用，以治疗气滞、气逆病证的方剂，统称理气剂。气乃一身之主，升降出入，周行全身，温养内外。一旦致病因素作用于机体，往往使气之升降失常，导致气机郁结或气逆不降等病证。气机郁结者，当行气以解郁散结为治；气逆上冲者，则须降气以降逆平冲为治。因此，本类方剂根据其不同作用，分为行气与降气两类。

理气药多属芳香辛燥之品，易伤津耗气，应用当适可而止，勿使过剂。年老体弱、孕妇或素有崩漏吐衄者，更应慎用。

12.2 行气剂

是以行气通滞和疏肝解郁的药物为主组成的方剂。适用于气机郁滞之脘腹胀满，嗳气吞酸，或胸胁胀痛，疝气痛，月经不调，痛经等证。常用的药物有陈皮、厚朴、木香、枳实、川楝子、乌药、香附、小茴香、橘核等，代表方剂有越鞠丸、金铃子散、半夏厚朴汤、枳实薤白桂枝汤、橘核丸、天台乌药散、暖肝煎、厚朴温中汤等。

12.3 越鞠丸

出自《丹溪心法》。由苍术、香附、川芎、神曲、栀子各等分组成。共为细末，水泛为丸。每服6~9克，日2次（亦可水煎服，用量按原方比例酌定）。方中香附行气解郁，以治气郁，为主药。川芎活血祛瘀，以治血郁；栀子清热泻火，以治火郁；苍术燥湿运脾，以治湿郁；神曲消食导滞，以治食郁。共奏行气解郁之功。主治气郁证。症见胸膈痞闷，脘腹胀满，嗳腐吞酸，恶心呕吐，饮食不消等。现常用于慢性胃炎、胃神经官能症、胃及十二指肠溃疡、肝炎、胆囊炎、肋间神经痛等病具有上述症状者。临床用越鞠丸加减治疗胃扭转1例，症见脘腹胀满不适，隐痛，恶心，食少便溏，服药10剂，诸证消失，钡透胃已复正。用越鞠丸化裁治疗4例气滞型精神病患者，均获痊愈出院。

12.4 金铃子散

出自《素问病机气宜保命集》。由金铃子、延胡索各30克组成。共为细末，每服9克，日2次（亦可水煎服，用量按原方比例酌定）。方中金铃子疏肝气，泄肝，为主药。延胡索行气活血，共奏行气疏肝，活血止痛之功。主治肝郁化热证。症见心腹胁肋诸痛，时发时止，口苦，舌红苔黄，脉弦数等。现常用于胃及十二指肠溃疡、慢性胃炎、病毒性肝炎等病具有上述症状者。临床应用金铃子散加减治疗胃痛患者15例，无论火郁，酒肉腻滞，肝气犯胃等，均1剂痛止，2剂痊愈。

12.5 半夏厚朴汤

出自《金匮要略》。由半夏、茯苓各12克，厚朴、生姜各9克，苏叶6克组成。水煎分2次服。方中半夏化痰散结，降逆和胃，为主药。厚朴下气除满；茯苓甘淡渗湿；生姜辛温散结，和胃止呕；苏叶芳香行气，理肺舒肝，共奏行气散结，降逆化痰之功。主治梅核气。症见咽中如有物梗阻，吐之不出，咽之不下，胸胁满闷，苔白润，脉弦缓等。现常用于瘿病、胃神经官能症、食道痉挛、慢性咽炎等病具上述症状者。临床用半夏厚朴汤治疗梅核膈19例，病程由半日至半年不等。均获满意疗效。运用半夏厚朴汤加减治疗慢性咽炎2例，其病程长达2年，均服药20余剂痊愈。

12.6 枳实薤白桂枝汤

出自《金匮要略》。由枳实、厚朴、瓜蒌各 12 克，薤白 9 克，桂枝 6 克组成。水煎分 2 次服。方中枳实下气破结，消痞除满；薤白辛温通阳，宽胸散结；桂枝通阳散寒，降逆平冲；瓜蒌涤痰散结；厚朴下气除满。共奏通阴散结，祛痰下气之功。主治胸痹。症见胸闷而痛，甚或胸痛彻背，喘息咳唾，短气，舌苔白腻，脉沉弦或紧等。现常用于冠心病、心绞痛、肋间神经痛、肋软骨炎等病具有上述症状者。临床应用枳实薤白桂枝汤合瓜蒌薤白白酒汤、瓜蒌薤白半夏汤加减，治疗非化脓性肋软骨炎，多数患者服药后短期内症状减轻或消失，极少复发。

12.7 橘核丸

出自《济生方》。由橘核、海藻、昆布、海带、川楝子、桃仁各 30 克，厚朴、木通、枳实、延胡索、桂心、木香各 15 克组成。共为细末，酒糊为丸。每服 9 克，日 2 次（亦可水煎服，用量按原方比例酌定）。方中橘核行气治疝，为主药。木香、川楝子行气止痛；桃仁、延胡索活血散结；桂心温肝肾而散寒；枳实、厚朴破气行滞；木通利血脉而除湿；海藻、昆布、海带软坚散结。共奏行气止痛，软坚散结之功。主治寒湿疝气。症见睾丸肿胀偏坠，或坚硬如石，或痛引脐腹，舌淡苔白，脉沉弦等。现常用于睾丸鞘膜积液、睾丸炎，附睾炎等病具有上述症状者，临床应用橘核丸加减治疗睾丸水肿，疗效显著。一般服药 6 剂，肿势消退，平均服药 20～28 剂，诸证痊愈。

12.8 天台乌药散

出自《医学发明》。由天台乌药、川楝子各 12 克，高良姜、槟榔各 9 克，木香、小茴香、青皮各 6 克，巴豆 70 粒组成。巴豆与川楝子同炒黑，去巴豆，水煎，冲入适量黄酒服，日 2 次。

方中乌药行气疏肝，散寒止痛，为主药。木香、小茴香、青皮、高良姜行气散结，祛寒除湿；槟榔直达下焦，行气化滞而破坚；川楝子与巴豆同炒，既减川楝子之寒性，又可增强其行气破结之力。共奏行气疏肝；散寒止痛之功。主治寒疝气滞证。症见小肠疝气，少腹痛引睾丸，舌淡苔白，脉沉迟或弦等。现常用于腹外疝、痛经、睾丸疾患等具有上述症状者。临床用天台乌药散加减治疗寒凝气滞，肝郁横逆之疝气、腹痛、胃痛、虫痛、痛经等，均获满意效果。

12.9 暖肝煎

出自《景岳全书》。由当归6～9克，肉桂3～6克，枸杞9克，小茴香、乌药、茯苓各6克，沉香3克，生姜3片组成。水煎分2次服。方中当归、枸杞温补肝肾，肉桂、小茴香温肾散寒；乌药、沉香理气止痛；茯苓渗湿健脾；生姜散寒和胃。共奏暖肝温肾，行气止痛之功。主治肝肾阴寒证。症见小腹疼痛，疝气，舌淡苔白，脉沉弦等。现常用于腹外疝、腹痛、不育症等病具有上述症状者。临床应用暖肝煎加减治疗5年不育患者1例，症见少腹隐痛，睾丸阴冷潮湿，遇寒则收缩牵引。查精子数3000万／ml，异常精子50%，2小时内有活动力精子30%，服药10剂后症状改善，1月后精子数5000万／ml，异常精子20%，有活动力者超过60%，诸证悉除，其妻怀孕。运用暖肝煎加减治疗缩阳症1例，症见阴茎抽痛缩入，外观阴茎消失，少腹疼痛，牵引阴囊，服药3剂症减，15剂痊愈。

12.10 厚朴温中汤

出自《内外伤辨惑论》。由厚朴、陈皮各30克，茯苓、草蔻仁、木香、甘草各15克，干姜2克组成。按原方比例酌定用量，加生姜3片，水煎分2次服。方中厚朴行气消胀，燥湿除满，为主药。草蔻仁温中散寒，燥湿除痰；陈皮、木香行气宽中；干姜、生姜温脾胃，散寒邪；茯苓、甘草渗湿健脾和中。共奏温中行气，燥湿除满之功。主治寒湿伤脾证。症见脘腹胀满或疼痛，不思饮食，四肢倦怠，舌淡苔白腻，脉沉迟等。现常用于急、慢性肠炎、胃炎、胃及十二指肠溃疡等病具有上述症状者。

12.11　降气剂

是以降气的药物为主组成的方剂。适用于肺胃气逆之证。症见咳喘、呕吐、噫气、呕逆等。常用的药有苏子、杏仁、沉香、旋复花、代赭石、陈皮、丁香、柿蒂等。代表方剂有苏子降气汤、定喘汤、旋复代赭汤、橘皮竹茹汤、丁香柿蒂散等。

12.12　苏子降气汤

出自《太平惠民和剂局方》。由苏子、半夏各9克，当归、厚朴、前胡、炙甘草各6克，肉桂3克组成。用时加生姜2片、大枣1枚、苏叶2克，水煎分2次服。方中苏子降气祛痰，止咳平喘，为主药。半夏、厚朴、前胡止咳平喘；肉桂温肾纳气；当归养血补肝，又治咳逆上气；略加生姜、苏叶散寒宣肺，甘草、大枣和中调药。共奏降气平喘，祛痰止咳之功。主治上实下虚，痰涎壅盛之证。症见喘咳短气，胸膈满闷，或腰痛脚弱，或肢体浮肿，舌淡苔白滑，脉沉等。现常用于支气管哮喘、慢性支气管炎、肺气肿、肺心病等具有上述症状者。临床用苏子降气汤加沉香、白果、杏仁、五味子治疗支气管哮喘10例，结果显效5例，有效5例。运用苏子降气汤去肉桂、生姜、当归，加葶苈子、黄芩、生大黄治疗支气管扩张，服药3剂，咯血止，咳嗽减，继用枇杷膏巩固而愈。

12.13　定喘汤

出自《摄生众妙方》。由白果、麻黄、款冬花、杏仁、桑白皮、半夏各9克，苏子、黄芩各6克，甘草3克组成。水煎分2

次服。方中麻黄宣肺散邪平喘，白果敛肺定喘祛痰，共为主药。苏子、杏仁、半夏、款冬花降气平喘，止咳祛痰；桑白皮、黄芩清泄肺热，止咳平喘；甘草调和诸药。共奏宣降肺气，祛痰平喘之功。主治风寒外来，痰热内蕴证。症见痰多气急，痰稠色黄，哮喘咳嗽，舌淡苔黄腻，脉滑数等。现常用于慢性支气管炎、支气管哮喘等病具有上述症状者。临床应用定喘汤加减治疗婴幼儿急性毛细支气管炎 30 例，均获痊愈，其中 3 天内哮鸣音消失，喘憋减轻者 28 例，平均住院日数为 4 天，较单用西药组平均住院 7 天为短。运用本方治疗慢性喘息性支气管炎 100 例，总有效率达 97%，显效占 83%。

12.14　四磨汤

出自《济生方》。由人参、沉香各 3 克，槟榔、天台乌药各 9 克组成。水煎分 2 次服。方中乌药行气疏肝以解郁；沉香顺气降逆以平喘，槟榔行气化滞以除满；人参益气扶正。共奏行气降逆；宽胸散结之功。主治肝气郁结证。症见胸膈烦闷，上气喘急，心下痞满，不思饮食，舌淡苔白，脉沉弦等。现常用于肝炎、胆囊炎、肩周炎、乳腺炎等病具有上述症状者。临床应用四磨汤去人参、槟榔，加青皮、赤芍、公英、沙参、白花蛇草治疗乳汁郁积性乳腺炎 1 例，症见乳房胀痛，有鸡卵状硬块，伴干咳胸痛，烦燥易怒，口苦厌食，脉弦滑。服药 6 剂而愈。

12.15　旋复代赭汤

出自《伤寒论》。由旋复花、代赭石、半夏各 9 克，人参、炙甘草各 6 克，生姜 10 克，大枣 12 枚组成。水煎分 2 次服。方中旋复花下气消痰，降逆止噫，为主药。代赭石重镇降逆；人参益气补虚，炙甘草温益中气；大枣养胃补脾；生姜温胃化痰，散寒止呕；半夏祛痰散结，降逆和胃。共奏降逆化痰，益气和胃之功。主治胃气虚弱，痰浊内阻证。症见心下痞硬，噫气不除，舌苔白滑，脉弦而虚等。现常用于胃肠神经官能症、胃扩张、幽门不完全性梗阻、溃疡病等病具有上述症状者。临床应用旋复代赭汤治疗眩晕呕吐患者 50 例，其中胃炎、胃溃疡 6 例，神经官能症 11 例，高血压、美尼尔氏症、癔病、脑膜炎后遗症各 1 例，结果 34 例症状消失，14 例减轻，2 例无效。

12.16　橘皮竹茹汤

出自《金匮要略》。由橘皮、竹茹各 12 克，人参 3 克，生姜 9 克，甘草 6 克，大枣 5 枚组成。水煎分 2 次服。方中橘皮理气和胃，降逆止呕，竹茹清胃止呕，共为主药。人参补气扶正；生姜和胃止呕，甘草、大枣益气和胃，调和诸药。共奏降逆止呕，益气清热之功。主治胃虚有热，气逆不降之证。症见呃逆或干呕，舌红苔薄黄，脉虚数等。现常用于妊娠呕吐、幽门不完全性梗阻、手术后呃逆等病具有上述症状者。临床以橘皮竹茹汤加减治疗顽固性呃逆 10 余年患者，症见呃逆频作，嗳气恶心，时吐涎沫，睡眠不安，饮食难进，便秘溲赤。服药 6 剂而愈，随访 4 个月无复发。

12.17　丁香柿蒂汤

出自《证因脉治》，由丁香、生姜各 6 克，柿蒂 9 克，人参 3 克组成。水煎分 2 次服。方中丁香温胃散寒，下气止呃；柿蒂降逆止呃；人参益气补虚，生姜温胃降逆。共奏温中益气，降逆止呃之功。主治胃气虚寒证。症见呃逆不已，胸痞脉迟等。现常用于治疗膈肌痉挛、神经性呃逆等病具有上述症状者。临床用丁香柿蒂散治疗顽固性呃逆 2 例，均获痊愈。运用丁香柿蒂散合旋复代赭汤、瓜篓薤白汤化裁，治疗贲门痉挛 1 例，服药 1 月而愈。

第 13 章　理血剂

13.1　理血剂

凡以理血药物为主组成，具有活血调血或止血作用，以治疗血瘀或出血证的方剂，统称理血剂。生理状态下，血液周流不息地循行于脉管之中，灌溉五脏六腑，濡养四肢百骸。一旦某种原因，造成血行不畅或离经妄行，均可造成血瘀为患或出血之证。因此，根据本类方剂的不同作用，分为活血祛瘀和止血两类。

13.2　活血祛瘀剂

是以活血祛瘀药物为主组成的方剂。适用于蓄血及瘀血证。如瘀积肿痛，外伤瘀肿，，瘀阻经脉之半身不遂，瘀血内停之胸腹诸痛，以及经闭、痛经、产后恶露不行等。常用的药有川芎、桃仁、红花、丹参等。代表方剂有桃核承气汤、血府逐瘀汤、复元活血汤等。

活血祛瘀剂能促进血行，性多破泄，易于动血、坠胎，故月经过多者及孕妇均当慎用。

13.3　桃核承气汤

出自《伤寒论》。由桃仁、大黄各 12 克，桂枝、芒硝、甘草各 6 克组成。水煎分 2 次服。方中桃仁破血祛瘀，大黄下瘀泄热，共为主药。桂枝通行血脉，助桃仁破血祛瘀；芒硝泻热软坚，助大黄下瘀泄热；甘草益气和中，调和药性。共奏破血下瘀之功。主治下焦蓄血证。症见少腹急结，小便自利，谵语烦渴，至夜发热，继则其人如狂，舌黯，脉沉实或涩等。现常用于盆腔炎、附件炎、肠梗阻等病具有上述症状者。临床应用桃核承气汤治疗急性坏死性肠炎 22 例，结果治愈 19 例，死亡 2 例，转外科 1 例。运用桃核承气汤加黄芩、黄连、木香、马齿苋治疗暴发型痢疾 26 例，痊愈 22 例，死亡 2 例，无效 2 例。

13.4　血府逐瘀汤

　　出自《医林改错》。由桃仁 12 克，红花、当归、生地、牛膝各 9 克，赤芍、枳壳各 6 克，川芎、桔梗各 5 克，柴胡、甘草各 3 克组成。水煎分 2 次服。方中桃仁、红花、赤芍、川芎、当归活血祛瘀；牛膝祛瘀通脉，引血下行；柴胡疏肝解郁；桔梗、枳壳开胸行气，生地凉血清热，养血润燥，甘草调和诸药。共奏活血祛瘀，行气止痛之功。主治气滞血瘀证。症见头痛日久不愈，痛如针刺，固定不移，或烦燥易怒，入暮潮热，或呃逆日久，心悸怔忡，舌黯红，脉涩或弦紧等。现常用于冠心病、高血压、神经官能症、脑震荡后遗症等病具有上述症状者。临床应用血府逐瘀汤加蒿本治疗高血压病 31 例。症见头痛、头晕、眼睑充血等。一般服药 2～5 剂症状消除，随访 2～3 次，无 1 例复发。运用血府逐瘀汤治疗急性弥漫性血管内凝血 22 例，其中 19 例有出血现象，16 例休克。结果治愈 16 例，好转 1 例，无效 4 例，死亡 1 例。

13.5　复元活血汤

　　出自《医林改错》。由大黄 30 克，柴胡 15 克，瓜蒌根、当归、桃仁各 9 克，红花、穿山甲、甘草各 6 克组成。水煎分 2 次服。方中重用大黄荡涤留瘀败血，柴胡疏肝调气，共为君药。当归、桃仁、红花活血祛瘀，消肿止痛；穿山甲破瘀通络；瓜蒌根消瘀散结，清热润燥；甘草缓急止痛，调和诸药。共奏活血祛瘀，疏肝通络之功。主治外伤瘀血证。症见跌打损伤，瘀血留于胁下，痛不可忍，舌黯脉弦涩等。现常用于肋间神经痛、肋软骨炎、软组织损伤等病具有上述症状者。临床应用复元活血汤治疗肋软骨炎 9 例。发病时间在 1～6 周内，一般服药 1～2 剂，肿痛明显减轻，5～7 剂，基本痊愈。运用复元活血汤治疗跌打损伤数百例，均获良好效果。

13.6　七厘散

出自《良方集腋》。由血竭 30 克，麝香、冰片各 0.4 克，乳香、没药、红花各 5 克，朱砂 4 克，儿茶 7.5 克组成。共研细末，每服 0.22～0.15 克，黄酒或温水送服，日 2 次。外用适量，以酒调敷伤处。方中血竭、红花活血祛瘀；乳香、没药祛瘀行气，消肿止痛；麝香、冰片行气活血，走窜经络；朱砂镇心安神；儿茶清热止血。共奏活血散瘀，止痛止血之功。主治跌打损伤，筋断骨折之瘀血肿痛，或刀伤出血等。现常用于烧伤、烫伤、带状疱疹以及冠心病、心肌炎等病具有上述症状者。临床应用七厘散加减治疗带状疱疹 11 例。一般药 1～2 剂疼痛停止，2～3 剂斑丘疹开始消退，4～6 剂水疱变干、结痂，疗程平均 4.6 天，全部治愈。运用七厘散加减治疗冠心病 100 例，其中心绞痛 76 例，陈旧性心梗伴心绞痛 13 例，陈旧性心梗 3 例，隐型冠心痛 8 例，结果显效 14 例，改善 49 例，无效 24 例，加重 3 例。

13.7　补阳还五汤

出自《医林改错》。由黄芪 120 克，当归、赤芍各 6 克，地龙、川芎、红花、桃仁各 3 克组成。水煎分 2 次服。方中重用黄芪大补元气，使气旺以促血行，为主药。当归、川芎、赤芍、桃仁、红花、地龙活血通络。共奏补气活血通络之功。主治中风后遗症，症见半身不遂，口眼歪斜，语言塞涩，口角流涎，下肢痿废，小便频数或遗尿不禁，苔白脉缓等。现常用于脑血管意外后遗症、小儿麻痹后遗症等病具有上述症状者。临床应用补阳还五汤治疗偏瘫 12 例，7～18 天痊愈者 5 人；24～90 天痊愈者 7 人，效果满意。运用补阳还五汤治疗坐骨神经痛 100 例，结果痊愈 89 例，显效 7 例，好转 2 例。

13.8　失笑散

出自《太平惠民和剂局方》。由五灵脂、蒲黄各等分组成。共研细末，每服 6 克，用黄酒或醋冲服，日 2 次（亦可水煎服，用量按原方比例酌定）。方中五灵脂、蒲黄相须为用，通利血脉，祛瘀止痛。用醋或黄酒冲服，取其活血脉，行药力，加强活血止痛作用。共奏活血祛瘀，散结止痛之功。主治瘀血证。症见心腹剧痛，或产后恶露不绝，或月经不调，少腹急痛，舌黯，脉涩等。现常用于心绞痛、宫外孕等病具有上述症状者。临床应用失笑散合胶艾四物汤为主，治疗宫外孕 18 例，其中陈旧性 16 例，亚急性 2 例，服药 10～20 剂，均获痊愈。运用失笑散加减治疗冠心病 46 例，服药 1 个月为 1 疗程，结果在有心绞痛的 44 例中，显效 12 例，改善 27 例，无效 5 例，无 1 例加重。

13.9　丹参饮

出自《时方歌括》。由丹参 30 克，檀香、砂仁各 5 克组成。水煎分 2 次服。方中重用丹参活血祛瘀，为主药。檀香、砂仁、行气宽中止痛。共奏活血祛瘀；行气止痛之功。主治血瘀气滞证。症见心胃诸痛，舌黯，脉弦涩等。现常用于慢性胃炎、溃疡病、慢性胰腺炎等病具有上述症状者。临床应用丹参饮加延胡索、苏叶、白术、厚朴等，不仅对胃痛有效，对上腹部疼痛性疾病，如肝炎、胆囊炎、胰腺炎等效果均佳。

13.10　温经汤

出自《金匮要略》。由吴茱萸、当归、阿胶、麦冬各 9 克，芍药、川芎、人参、桂枝、丹皮、半夏、生姜、甘草各 6 克组成。水煎分 2 次服。方中吴茱萸、桂枝温经散寒，兼通血脉；当归、川芎活血祛瘀，养血调经；阿胶、芍药、麦冬养血益阴；丹皮祛瘀通经,并退虚热;人参、甘草、生姜、半夏益气和胃,以资化源。共奏温经散寒,祛瘀养血之功。主治冲任虚寒,瘀血阻滞证。症见月经不调,漏下不止,傍晚发热,手心烦热,少腹里急或久不受孕,舌黯,脉沉细或涩等。现常用于功能性子宫出血、慢性盆腔炎等病具有上述症状者。临床应用温经汤加减治疗卵巢囊肿1例,症见月经衍期,量少色暗,右下腹痛,右穹窿有一肿块,服药10剂,症状减轻,继进数剂,诸症消失而愈。

13.11　生化汤

出自《傅青主女科》。由当归25克,川芎9克,桃仁6克,干姜2克,甘草2克组成。水煎分2次服,或酌加黄酒同煎。方中重用当归补血活血,祛瘀生新,为主药。川芎活血行气;桃仁活血祛瘀;干姜入血散寒,温经止痛;黄酒温散以助药力,甘草调和诸药。共奏活血化瘀,温经止痛之功。主治产后血虚受寒证。症见恶露不行,小腹冷痛,舌淡或有瘀斑,脉沉迟或涩等。现常用于子宫内膜炎、胎盘残留、子宫肥大等病具有上述症状者。临床应用温经汤加丹皮、熟地、红花、艾叶、煨姜、治疗小产后胎盘残留22例,服药2~6剂,其残留胎盘自动流出,22例均获痊愈。运用温经汤加芥穗、益母草治疗子宫肥大症15例,其病程多为3~19年,子宫最小者7.5×6cm,最大者12×10cm,服本方30日为1疗程,结果痊愈7例,有效4例,无效4例。

13.12　活络效灵丹

出自《医学衷中参西录》。由当归、丹参、生明乳香、生明没药各15克组成。水煎分2次服。方中当归活血养血;丹参活血祛瘀,乳香、没药活血祛瘀,行气止痛。共奏活血祛瘀,通络止痛之功。主治气血凝滞证。症见心腹疼痛,腿痛臂痛,跌打瘀肿,内外疮疡,癥瘕积聚,舌黯,脉弦涩等。现常用于心绞痛、宫外孕、脑血栓形成、坐骨神经痛等病具有上述症状者。临床应用活络效灵丹合红藤煎加减治疗阑尾脓肿1例，症见右下腹肿块，逐渐增大，压痛明显，神疲乏力，胃纳不佳等。服药12剂，诸证消失而愈。

13.13 桂枝茯苓丸

出自《金匮要略》。由桂枝、茯苓、丹皮、桃仁、芍药各9克组成。炼蜜为丸，每服3～5克，日2次（亦可水煎服，用量按原方比例酌定）。方中桂枝温通血脉，茯苓渗利下行而益心脾之气，既有助于行瘀，又有利于安胎，共为主药。丹皮、芍药、桃仁化瘀清热，白蜜缓和诸药。共奏活血化瘀，缓消癥块之功。主治胞宫血瘀证。症见妊娠胎动不安，漏下不止，腹痛拒按，舌黯，脉涩等。现常用于治疗月经不调、痛经、前列腺肥大、精神分裂症等病具有上述症状者。临床用桂枝茯苓丸加红花、大黄、牛膝、益母草、泽兰治疗前列腺肥大5例，除1例无效，其余4例服药10剂后，症状消失，小便通利。

13.14 大黄䗪虫丸

出自《金匮要略》。由大黄、干地黄各300克，黄芩、桃仁、杏仁、水蛭、虻虫、蛴螬各60克，䗪虫、干漆各30克，芍药120克，甘草90克组成。共为细末，炼蜜为丸。每服3克，日2次（亦可水煎服，用量按原方比例酌减）。方中大黄逐瘀攻下，凉血清热，䗪虫攻下积血，共为主药。桃仁、干漆、蛴螬、水蛭、虻虫活血通络，攻逐瘀血；黄芩助大黄以清瘀热；杏仁助桃仁以润燥结，且破血降气；生地、芍药养血滋阴；甘草和中补虚，调和诸药。共奏祛瘀生新之功。主治五劳虚极之证。症见形体羸瘦、腹满不能饮食，肌肤甲错，两目黯黑，舌黯，脉沉细而涩等。现常用于跌打损伤、瘀肿疼痛、肝硬化等病具有上述症状者。临床应用大黄䗪虫丸治疗痹症1例，症见环跳穴处剧痛，状如针刺，有灼热感，入夜尤甚，举步艰难，服药 3 丸，夜间痛减，继服 20 余丸而愈。。

13.15 止血剂

是以止血药物为主组成的方剂。适用于血液离经妄行而致的吐血、衄血、咳血、便血、崩漏等各种出血证。常用的药有侧柏叶、小蓟、槐花、灶心土、艾叶等，代表方剂有十灰散、四生丸、小蓟饮子、槐花散、黄土汤、胶艾汤等。

13.16 十灰散

出自《十药神书》。由大蓟、小蓟、荷叶、侧柏叶、茅根、茜草根、牡丹皮、棕榈皮、山栀、大黄各等分组成。各药烧存性，为末。藕汁或萝卜汁磨京墨适量，调服 9 克，日 2 次（亦可水煎服，用量按原方比例酌定）。方中大蓟、小蓟、荷叶、茜草根、侧柏叶、白茅根凉血止血；棕榈皮收涩止血；栀子清热泻火；大黄导热下行；丹皮凉血祛瘀，使血止而不留瘀。本方烧炭存性，以加强收涩止血作用。用藕汁或萝卜汁京墨调服，意在增强清热凉血止血之功。共奏凉血止血之功。主治血热妄行之证。症见呕血、吐血、咯血、咳血、舌红脉数等。现常用于肺结核、支气管扩散、胃溃疡等病具有上述症状者。临床应用十灰散治疗肺结核咯血 27 例，显效 20 例，有效 2 例，无效 5 例。一般服药 4～6 天即能止血，平均止血时间为 5 天。

13.17 四生丸

出自《妇人良方》。由生荷叶、生艾叶各 9 克，生柏叶 12 克，生地黄 15 克组成。水煎分 2 次服。方中侧柏叶凉血止血，为主药。生地清热凉血，养阴生津；荷叶、艾叶止血散瘀，使血止而不留瘀。共奏凉血止血之功。主治血热失血证。症见吐血、衄血、血色鲜红、口干咽燥、舌红或绛、脉弦数等。现常用于肺结核、支气管扩张之咯血及胃溃疡吐血等病具有上述症状者。

13.18 咳血方

出自《丹溪心法》。由青黛、诃子各 6 克，瓜蒌仁、海石、山栀子各 9 克组成。水煎分 2 次服。方中青黛、栀子清肝泻火凉血，共为主药。瓜蒌仁、海石清热降火，润燥化痰；诃子敛肺止咳。共奏清火化痰，敛肺止咳之功。主治肝火犯肺证。症见咳嗽痰稠带血，咯吐不爽，或心烦易怒，胸胁刺痛，颊赤便秘，舌红苔黄，脉弦数。现常用于支气管扩张、肺结核咯血等病具有上述症状者。

13.19 槐花散

出自《本事方》。由槐花、柏叶各 12 克，荆芥穗、枳壳各 6 克组成。水煎分 2 次服。方中槐花专清大肠湿热，凉血止血，为主药。柏叶助槐花凉血止血，芥穗疏风止血，枳壳下气宽肠。共奏清肠止血，疏风下气之功。主治肠风脏毒证。症见便前出血，或便后出血，或粪中带血，以及痔疮出血，色红或晦暗，舌红苔白或薄黄，脉数等。现常用于痔疮、阿米巴痢疾、溃疡病等疾病具有上述症状者。

13.20 小蓟饮子

出自《济生方》。由生地 30 克，小蓟、滑石各 15 克，木通、蒲黄、藕节、淡竹叶、山栀子各 9 克，当归、炙草各 6 克组成。水煎分 2 次服。方中小蓟凉血止血，为主药。藕节、蒲黄凉血止血，并能消瘀；滑石清热利水通淋；木通、竹叶、栀子清泄心、肺、三焦之热；生地养阴清热，凉血止血，当归养血和血；甘草调和诸药。共奏凉血止血，利水通淋之功。主治下焦瘀热证。症见血淋，尿中带血，小便频数，赤涩热痛，舌红，脉数等。现常用于泌尿系感染、泌尿系结石等病具有上述症状者。临床应用小蓟饮子加减治疗急性肾炎 2 例，症见头面浮肿，小便不利，尿少黄赤，心烦口渴，舌尖红少苔，脉浮数，服药 9～20 剂，均痊愈。

13.21　黄土汤

出自《金匮要略》。由灶心土 30 克，干地黄、白术、附子、阿胶、黄芩、甘草各 9 克组成。先将灶心土煎取汤，再煎余药，分 2 次服。方中灶心土温中止血，为主药。白术、附子温脾阳而补中气；生地、阿胶滋阴养血；更配苦寒之黄芩与甘寒滋润之生地，共同制约白术、附子过于温燥之性；甘草调和诸药。共奏温阳健脾，养血止血之功。主治脾阳不足、中焦虚寒证。症见大便下血，或吐血、衄血，及妇人崩漏，血色暗淡，四肢不温，面色萎黄，舌淡苔白，脉沉细无力等。现常用于慢性胃肠道出血、功能性子宫出血等病具有上述症状者。临床应用黄土汤加丹皮治疗上消化逆出血 23 例，用红砖 120 克代灶心土，先捣碎水浸泡，取澄清液煎药，结果痊愈 22 例，无效 1 例。

13.22　胶艾汤

出自《金匮要略》。由阿胶、艾叶、当归各 9 克，川芎、甘草各 6 克，芍药、干地黄各 12 克组成。水煎去渣，或加酒适量，入阿胶化，分 2 次服。方中阿胶补血止血，艾叶温经止血，共为主药。熟地、当归、芍药、川芎补血调经，活血调血；甘草调和诸药；入清酒助药力运行。共奏补血止血，调经安胎之功。主治冲任虚损证。症见崩中漏下，月经过多，淋漓不止，或半产后下血不绝，或妊娠下血，腹中疼痛，舌淡，脉沉细等。现常用于先兆流产、产后子宫复旧不全等病具有上述症状者。临床用本方加减治疗先兆流产 41 例，痊愈 36 例，好转 5 例。

第 14 章　治风剂

14.1　治风剂

凡是运用辛散祛风或熄风止痉的药物为主组成，具有疏散外风或平熄内风的作用，治疗风病的方剂，统称治风剂。风病的范围甚广，病情变化亦很复杂，概言之，可分内风、外风两大类。外风是指风邪侵入人体，留于肌表、经络、筋肉、骨节等所致；内风是指内脏病变所致的风病。在治疗上，外风宜疏散，内风宜平熄。因此，根据本类方剂的功能特点，分为疏散外风和平熄内风两类。

运用治风剂，首先必须辨别风病的属内、属外，分别其寒热虚实。若属外风，则宜疏散，不宜平熄；属于内风，则宜平熄，切忌辛散。若风邪夹寒，夹热，夹湿，夹痰，则应与祛寒，清热，化湿，化痰等法合参。

14.2　疏散外风剂

是以辛散祛风药物为主组成的方剂。适用于外风所致的头痛、眩晕、风疹、湿疹等病。常用的药有防风、川芎、白芷、荆芥、白附子等。代表方剂有大秦艽汤、消风散、川芎茶调散、牵正散、小活络丹等。

14.3　大秦艽汤

出自《素问病机气宜保命集》。由秦艽 90 克，甘草、川芎、当归、白芍、石膏、独活各 60 克，羌活、防风、黄芩、白芷、白术、生地、熟地、茯苓各 30 克，细辛 15 克组成。为散，每次 30 克，水煎去渣服，日 2 次（亦可水煎服，用量按原方比例酌减）。方中秦艽祛风通络，为主药。羌活、独活、防风、白芷、细辛祛风散邪；当归、白芍、熟地养血柔筋；川芎活血通络；黄芩、石膏、生地凉血清热；甘草调和诸药。共奏祛风清热，养血活血之功。主治风邪初中经络证。症见口眼㖞斜，舌强不能言，手足不能运动，苔白脉浮等。现常用于面神经麻痹、破伤风等病具有上述症状者。本方风药较多，辛燥太过，有耗伤阴血之弊，临床宜斟酌加减。

14.4 消风散

出自《外科正宗》。由当归、生地、防风、蝉蜕、知母、苦参、胡麻、荆芥、苍术、牛蒡子、石膏各3克，木通、甘草各1.5克组成。水煎分2次服。方中荆芥、防风、牛蒡子、蝉蜕疏风透表，为主药。苍术散风除湿；苦参清热燥湿；木通渗利湿热；石膏、知母清热泻火；当归、生地、胡麻养血活血，滋阴润燥；甘草清热解毒，调和诸药。共奏疏风养血，清热除湿之功。主治风疹、湿疹。症见皮肤出疹色红，或遍身云片斑点，瘙痒，破后渗出津水，苔白或黄，脉浮数有力等。现常用于过敏性皮炎、稻田性皮炎、神经性皮炎、药物性皮炎等病具有上述症状者。临床应用消风散化裁治疗变应性亚败血症1例，患者罹病3年，中西药物均不能控制其发作，用本方加黄藤、丹皮、土茯苓、僵蚕、贝母，服药70天，症状消失，唯指关节仍呈梭状改变。运用消风散治疗湿疹44例，平均服药20剂，结果近期治愈38例，基本治愈6例。

14.5 川芎茶调散

出自《太平惠民和剂局方》。由川芎、荆芥各120克，白芷、羌活、甘草各60克，细辛、防风各45克，薄荷240克组成。共为细末，每服6克，日2次，清茶调下（亦可水煎服，用量按原方比例酌减）。方中川芎、白芷、羌活疏风止痛，为主药。细辛散寒止痛，重用薄荷清利头目，搜风散热；荆芥、防风辛散上行，以疏上部风邪；甘草调和诸药，用清茶调下，取茶叶苦寒之性，既可上清头目，又能制约风药过于温燥升散，使升中有降。共奏疏风止痛之功。主治头风证。症见偏正头痛，或巅顶作痛，恶寒发热，目眩鼻塞，舌苔薄白，脉浮等。现常用于慢性鼻炎、鼻窦炎、神经性头痛等病具有上述症状者。临床应用川芎茶调散治疗偏头痛 126 例，主要表现为左右颞颥部疼痛，交替发作，经久不已，伴呕吐、嗜睡、烦燥疲乏，便秘等症。总有效率达 83.3%。

14.6 牵正散

出自《杨氏家藏方》。由白附子、僵蚕、全蝎各等分组成。共为细末，每服 3 克，日 2 次（亦可水煎服，用量按原方比例酌情增减）。方中白附子祛风化痰，并长于治头面之风，僵蚕、全蝎祛风止痉，三药合用，力专效著。共奏祛风化痰止痉之功。主治中风面瘫、口眼㖞斜，甚或面部肌肉抽动，苔白脉浮滑等。现常用于面神经麻痹、三叉神经痛等病具有上述症状者。临床应用牵正散为主加减，和姜汁为糊，外敷患处，治疗倍耳氏面瘫 33例，结果痊愈 29 例，好转 2 例，无效 2 例。运用 50%复方牵正散注射液（白附子、僵蚕、全蝎、当归、蜈蚣）取患侧地仓、颊车、阳白等穴，轮流作穴位注射。共治疗面神经麻痹 418 例，疗程 7～42 天，治愈率为 90%。

14.7 玉真散

出自《外科正宗》。由南星、防风、白芷、天麻、羌活、白附子各等分组成。共为细末，每服 3 克，用热酒或童便调服。外用适量，敷患处（亦可水煎服，用量按原方比例酌定）。方中天南星、白附子祛风化痰，解痉止痛；羌活、防风、白芷疏散经络中之风邪，驱邪外出，天麻熄风解痉，热酒与童便有通经络，行气血之功。共奏祛风化痰、解痉止痛之功。主治破伤风。症见牙关紧闭，口撮唇紧，身体强直，角弓反张，苔白脉弦紧等。现常用于破伤风、百日咳、狂犬病等病具有上述症状者。临床应用玉真散治疗破伤风3例，外敷并内服，每日3次，每次9克，平均4.8天治愈。用酒调玉真散外敷，治疗扭挫外伤所致腱鞘炎，一般3～5天肿痛消失，功能恢复。

14.8　小活络丹

出自《太平惠民和剂局方》。由川乌、草乌、地龙、天南星、乳香、没药各66克组成。共为细末，炼蜜为丸，每服3克，陈酒或温开水送服，日2次。方中川乌、草乌祛风除湿，温通经络，为主药。天南星燥湿化痰，除经络中之痰湿；乳香、没药行气活血；地龙通经活络；加陈酒以助药势。共奏祛风除湿，化痰通络，活血止痛之功。主治风寒湿邪留滞经络之痹证。症见肢体筋脉挛痛，关节屈伸不利，疼痛游走不定，以及中风日久不愈，手足不仁，经络中有湿痰死血，腰腿沉重，或腿臂间作痛，苔白脉沉弦等。现常用于脑卒中后遗症、风湿性关节炎、类风湿性关节炎等病具有上述症状者。

14.9　平熄内风剂

是以平肝熄风或补养熄风的药物为主组成的方剂。适用于内风证。常用的药有羚羊角、钩藤、石决明、天麻、菊花、牡蛎、地黄、白芍、阿胶、鸡子黄、肉苁蓉等，代表方剂有羚角钩藤汤、镇肝熄风汤、大定风珠、地黄饮子等。

14.10　羚角钩藤汤

出自《通俗伤寒论》。由羚角片4.5克，桑叶6克，京川贝12克，鲜生地、竹茹各15克，双钩藤、滁菊花、茯神木、生白芍各9克，生甘草2.4克组成。水煎分2次服。方中羚羊角、钩藤凉肝熄风，清热解痉，为主药。合桑叶、菊花以加强熄风之效；白芍、生地养阴增液以柔肝舒筋；贝母、竹茹清热化痰；茯神木平肝、宁心安神；生甘草调和诸药。共奏凉肝熄风，增液舒筋之功。主治肝经热盛，热极动风证。症见高热不退，烦闷躁扰，手足抽搐，发为痉厥，甚则神昏，舌绛而干，脉弦而数等。现常用于流行性乙型脑炎、原发性高血压等病具有上述症状者。临床应用羚角钩藤汤治疗流行性乙型脑炎 8 例，均获痊愈，无后遗症。运用羚角钩藤汤加石决明或珍珠母治疗抽搐症 1 例，症见肢体抽搐，牙关紧闭，颈项强直，角弓反张等。患者服药后，效果满意。

14.11　镇肝熄风汤

出自《医学衷中参西录》。由怀牛膝、生赭石各 30 克，生龙骨、生牡蛎、生龟板、生杭芍、玄参、天冬各 15 克，川楝子、生麦芽、茵陈各 6 克，甘草 4.5 克组成。水煎分 2 次服。方中重用怀牛膝引血下行，补益肝肾。代赭石、龙骨、牡蛎降逆潜阳，镇肝熄风；龟板、玄参、天冬、白芍滋养阴液，以制阳亢；茵陈、川楝子、生麦芽助主药清泄肝阳之有余，条达肝气之郁滞；甘草调和诸药。共奏镇肝熄风，滋阴之功。主治肝肾阴亏，肝阳上亢证。症见头目眩晕，目胀耳鸣，脑部热痛，心中烦热，肢体渐觉不利，口角渐形歪斜，甚或眩晕颠仆，昏不知人，移时苏醒，或醒后不能复原，舌红，脉弦长有力等。现常用于高血压病、嗜铬细胞瘤、脑血管意外等病具有上述症状者。临床应用镇肝熄风汤治疗高血压病 66 例。其中Ⅱ期高血压病 50 例，治疗后显效 30 例，改善 19 例，无效 1 例，Ⅲ期高血压病 16 例，治疗后显效 6 例，改善 9 例，基本无效 1 例，总有效率 93.7%。

14.12　天麻钩藤饮

出自《杂病证治新义》。由天麻、山栀、黄芩、杜仲、益母草、桑寄生、夜交藤、朱茯神各9克，钩藤、川牛膝各12克，石决明18克组成。水煎分2次服。方中天麻、钩藤、石决明平肝熄风，为主药。山栀、黄芩清热泻火；益母草活血利水；牛膝引血下行；桑寄生、杜仲补益肝肾；夜交藤、朱伏神安神定志。共奏平肝熄风，清热活血，补益肝肾之功。主治肝阳偏亢，肝风上扰证。症见头痛、眩晕、失眠等。现常用于破伤风、高血压病、脑血管意外等病具有上述症状者。临床应用天麻钩藤饮治疗破伤风2例。症见头痛、项强、四肢抽搐，角弓反张，牙关紧闭，不省人事，服药7~15剂均痊愈。

14.13　阿胶鸡子黄汤

出自《通俗伤寒论》。由陈阿胶、双钩藤各6克，生白芍、络石藤各9克，石决明15克，大生地、生牡蛎、茯神木、各12克，清炙草1.8克，鸡子黄2枚组成。水煎分2次服。方中阿胶、鸡子黄滋阴血，熄风阳。生地、芍药、甘草酸甘化阴，柔肝熄风；钩藤、石决明、牡蛎镇肝潜阳；茯神木平肝安神，络石藤舒筋通络。共奏滋阴养血，柔肝熄风之功。主治阴虚动风证。症见筋脉拘急，手足瘈疭，类似风动，或头目眩晕，舌绛苔少，脉细数等。现常用于治疗神经衰弱、老年性震颤、高血压病等病具有上述症状者。

14.14　大定风珠

出自《温病条辨》。由生白芍、干地黄、麦冬各18克，生龟板、生牡蛎、炙甘草、鳖甲各12克，阿胶9克，麻仁、五味子各6克，鸡子黄2枚组成。水煎去渣，再入鸡子黄搅匀，分2次服。方中鸡子黄、阿胶滋阴养液以熄内风，为主药。地黄、麦冬、白芍滋阴柔肝；龟板、鳖甲滋阴潜阳；麻仁养阴润燥；牡蛎平肝潜阳；五味子、炙甘草酸甘化阴。共奏滋阴熄风之功。主治温病邪热久羁，热灼真阴，或因误用汗、下重伤阴液之动风证。症见神倦瘛疭，舌绛少苔，脉气虚弱等。现常用于流行性乙型脑炎、伤寒等病具有上述症状者。临床应用大定风珠治疗流行性乙型脑炎 39 例，症见神倦瘛疭，脉气虚弱，服药后痊愈 36 例，死亡 3 例。

14.15　地黄饮子

出自《黄帝素问宣明论方》。由熟干地黄、巴戟天、山茱萸、石斛、肉苁蓉、附子、五味子、官桂、白茯苓、麦冬、菖蒲、远志各等分组成。加生姜、大枣、薄荷适量，水煎服，用量按原方比例酌定。方中熟地黄、山茱萸滋补肾阴，肉苁蓉、巴戟天温壮肾阳，共为主药。附子、肉桂协上药以温养真元，摄纳浮阳；麦冬、石斛、五味子滋阴敛液，使阴阳相配；菖蒲、远志、茯苓交通心肾，开窍化痰；生姜、大枣、薄荷为引，以调和营卫。共奏滋肾阴，补肾阳，开窍化痰之功。主治瘖痱证。症见舌强不能言，足废不能用，口干不欲饮，苔浮腻，脉沉细弱等。现常用于脊髓空洞症、脑血管意外后遗症、高血压病等病具有上述症状者。临床应用地黄饮子加减治疗脊髓空洞症 5 例，其表现为肌肤麻木、肌肉萎缩，时而瞤动，步履艰难，语言不清等。服本方 1 月余，症状体征均有一定改善，近期疗效满意。运用地黄饮子加减治疗全身性瘙痒 180 例，结果痊愈 103 例，显效 42 例，无效 35 例，总有效率为 80.5%。

第 15 章 治燥剂

15.1 治燥剂

　　凡用苦辛温润或甘凉滋润的药物为主组成，具有轻宣燥邪或滋养润燥的作用，以治疗燥证的方剂，统称治燥剂。燥证有外燥和内燥之分。外燥是外感燥邪所致，随着气候的差异，其发病又有凉燥与温燥之不同。内燥是脏腑精亏液耗所致，从发病部位来说，有上燥、中燥、下燥之别。治疗方法，外燥宜轻宣，内燥宜滋润，凉燥宜温宣，温燥宜清宣。因此，本类方剂根据其功能特点，分为轻宣润燥和滋阴润燥两类。

　　治燥剂多为滋腻之品，易于助湿碍气，故素体多湿者忌用；脾虚便溏以及气滞、痰盛者亦应慎用。

15.2 轻宣润燥剂

　　是以轻宣温润药或清宣润肺药为主组成的方剂，适用于外感凉燥或温燥之证。常用的药有苏叶、桔梗、前胡、杏仁、桑叶、沙参、麦冬等，代表方剂有杏苏散、桑杏汤、清燥救肺汤等。

15.3 杏苏散

　　出自《温病条辨》。由苏叶、半夏、茯苓、前胡、苦桔梗、枳壳、甘草、生姜、橘皮、杏仁各 6 克，大枣 2 枚组成。水煎分 2 次服。方中苏叶、前胡解表散邪；杏仁、桔梗宣肺利气；半夏、茯苓祛湿化痰；枳壳、橘皮理气宽胸；生姜、大枣、甘草调和营卫。共奏轻宣凉燥，宣肺化痰之功。主治外感凉燥证。症见头微痛，恶寒无汗，咳嗽痰稀，鼻塞嗌干，苔白脉弦等。现常用于慢性支气管炎、支气管扩张、肺气肿等病具有上述症状者。

15.4 桑杏汤

出自《温病条辨》。由桑叶、象贝母、香豉、栀皮、梨皮各3克，杏仁4.5克，沙参6克组成。水煎分2次服。方中桑叶、香豉宣肺散邪；杏仁宣肺利气；沙参、贝母、梨皮润肺止咳；栀子清泄胸膈之热。共奏清宣润燥之功。主治外感温燥，邪在肺卫证。症见身不甚热，，干咳无痰，咽干口渴，舌红苔薄白，脉浮数等。现常用于上呼吸道感染、麻疹、百日咳等病具有上述症状者。临床应用桑杏汤治疗百日咳72例，其中69例服药3剂，诸症消失，33例服药5~10剂痊愈。

15.5 清燥救肺汤

出自《医门法律》。由冬桑叶9克，石膏7.5克，人参、杏仁各2克，甘草、胡麻仁、枇杷叶各3克，真阿胶2.4克，麦冬3.6克组成。水煎分2次服。方中桑叶清宣肺燥，为主药。石膏清肺经之热；麦冬润肺金之燥；杏仁、枇杷叶利肺气；阿胶、胡麻仁润肺养阴；人参、甘草益气和中。共奏清燥润肺之功。主治温燥伤肺证。症见头痛身热，干咳无痰，气逆而喘，咽喉干燥、鼻燥、心烦口渴，舌干无苔，脉虚大而数等。现常用于呼吸道感染、肺炎、肺结核等病具有上述症状者。临床应用清燥救肺汤加减治疗偏瘫1例，症见头痛咳嗽，咽干口燥，实然呕吐，继则语言不出，肢体偏瘫。服本方3剂，诸证悉除。运用清燥救肺汤治疗失音85例，结果痊愈84例，无效1例，治愈患者中服药1~3剂者45例，4~6剂者33例，7剂以上者6例。

15.6 滋阴润燥剂

是以滋阴润燥的药物为主组成的方剂。适用于脏腑津液不足之内燥证。常用的药有沙参、麦冬、生地、玄参等，代表方剂有养阴清肺汤、麦门冬汤、增液汤等。

15.7 养阴清肺汤

出自《重楼玉钥》。由大生地 6 克，麦冬、玄参各 5 克，生甘草、薄荷各 2 克，贝母、丹皮、炒白芍各 3 克组成。水煎分 2 次服。方中生地养肾阴；麦冬养肺阴；玄参清火解毒；丹皮凉血消肿；贝母润肺化痰；白芍敛阴泄热；薄荷散邪利咽；甘草和药解毒。共奏养阴清肺之功。主治白喉。症见喉间起白如腐，不易拨去，咽喉肿痛，鼻干唇燥，或咳或不咳，呼吸有声，似喘非喘，舌红，脉数等。现常用于扁桃体炎、咽喉炎、鼻咽癌等病具有上述症状者。临床应用养阴清肺汤加减治疗白喉 213 例，服药后多数于第 2 天退热，白膜消退最快者 2 天，最迟者 12 天，平均 5.5 天，杆菌培养转阴最快者 2 天，最迟者 12 天，平均 6.4 天。213 例中，痊愈 192 例，死亡 21 例。运用养阴清肺汤治疗急性扁桃体炎 100 例，有效率 85%。

15.8 百合固金汤

出自《医方集解》。由生地黄 6 克，熟地黄 9 克，麦冬 5 克，百合、白芍、当归、贝母、生甘草、玄参、桔梗各 3 克组成。水煎分 2 次服。方中熟地滋阴补肾，生地凉血止血，共为主药。麦冬、百合、贝母润肺养阴，化痰止咳；玄参滋阴凉血，清退虚火，当归养血润燥；白芍养血益阴；桔梗宣肺止咳；甘草调和诸药。共奏养阴润肺，化痰止咳之功。主治肺肾阴虚证。症见咳痰带血，咽喉燥痛，手足心热，骨蒸盗汗，舌红少苔，脉细数等。现常用于肺结核、气管炎、支气管扩张等病具有上述症状者。临床应用百合固金汤治疗自发性气胸 11 例，轻者单用本方，重者配合抽气减压，并适当用抗生素，其气胸消失最快者为 2 天，最慢者 20 天，平均 11 天。运用百合固金汤治疗慢性肝炎 1 例，症见少腹作胀，嗳气频作，肝功异常，服用本方后，症状消失，肝功逐渐恢复正常，随访 1 年，未再发作。

15.9   麦门冬汤

出自《金匮要略》。由麦门冬 60 克，半夏 9 克，人参、粳米各 6 克，甘草 4 克，大枣 3 枚组成。水煎分 2 次服。方中重用麦冬，滋养肺胃之阴，且清虚火，为主药。半夏下气降逆，和胃化痰；人参、粳米、甘草、大枣补中和胃，益气生津。共奏滋养肺胃，和中降逆之功。主治肺胃阴虚证。症见咳逆上气，咯痰不爽，或咳吐涎沫，口干咽燥，手足心热，气逆呕吐，舌红少苔，脉虚数等。现常用于肺结核、慢性支气管炎、胸膜炎、胃溃疡、胃粘膜脱垂等病具有上述症状者。临床应用麦门冬汤治疗溃疡病 19 例，服药后症状明显好转，止痛效果显著，治疗 45～120 天后，经 X 线复查 8 例，其中 4 例龛影或变形消失，另 4 例较前好转。

15.10   琼玉膏

引自《洪氏集验方》。由人参 750 克，生地黄 8000 克，白茯苓 1500 克，白蜜 5000 克组成。以生地黄汁（无鲜生地时，将干生地熬取汁）入蜂蜜与人参、茯苓细末，和匀，放瓷罐内封存，再服 6～9 克，日 2 次。方中生地黄滋阴壮水，为主药。白蜜养肺润燥；人参、茯苓补脾益气；茯苓又能利湿化痰。共奏滋阴润肺，益气补脾气功。主治肺阴亏损证。症见虚劳干咳，咽燥咯血，肌肉消瘦，气短乏力，舌红少苔，脉细数等。现常用于肺结核、支气管扩张、肺炎、胸膜炎等病具有上述症状者。

15.11   玉液汤

出自《医学衷中参西录》。由生山药 30 克，生黄芪、知母各 15 克，五味子、天花粉各 9 克，生鸡内金 6 克，葛根 4.5 克组成。水煎分 2 次服。方中山药补脾固肾以止便数，润肺生津止口渴，黄芪升阳益气，助脾气上升，复其散精达肺之职，共为主药。知母、天花粉滋阴润燥止渴；鸡内金助脾之运化，消谷生津，葛根升阳布津，以溉五脏；五味子敛阴生津，固肾涩精。共奏益气生津，润燥止渴之功。主治消渴病之气不布津，肾虚胃燥证。症见口渴引饮，小便频数量多，或小便混浊，困倦气短，舌红少苔，脉虚细无力等。现常用于糖尿病、尿崩症等病具有上述症状者。

15.12 增液汤

出自《温病条辨》。由玄参 30 克，麦冬、细生地各 24 克组成。水煎分 2 次服。方中重用玄参养阴生津，润燥清热，为主药。麦冬滋液润燥，生地养阴清热。共奏滋阴清热，润燥通便之功。主治阳明温病，津液不足，大便秘结，或下后 2、3 日，下证复现之证。症见大便秘结，口渴、舌红而干，脉沉无力等。现常用于肠结核、痔疮、结肠过敏、慢性胰腺炎等病具有上述症状者。临床应用增液汤化裁治疗放疗所致口腔反应 120 例，症见口干，温而引饮，牙龈红肿，口腔粘膜潮红或白斑，甚则溃烂，疼痛难忍，治疗后痊愈 41 例，显效 65 例，好转 13 例，无效 1 例。

第16章 祛湿剂

16.1 祛湿剂

  由祛湿药为主组成。具有化湿利水，通淋泄浊的作用，以治疗水湿病证的方剂，统称祛湿剂。湿邪为病，有外湿、内湿之分。外湿者，每因久处湿地，或淋雨涉水，感受湿邪所致。症见恶寒发热，头胀身重，周身疼痛，面目浮肿；内湿者，每因姿食生冷，酒酪过度，脾阳失运水湿所致，症见胸脘痞闷，呕恶泄利，黄疸，淋浊，足胕浮肿等。肌表与脏腑由于经络的沟通，表湿可以内传脏腑，里湿亦可外溢肌肤，故外湿与内湿，亦可相兼并存。湿邪为病，常有风、寒、暑、热相兼，人体有虚实强弱之别，所犯部位有上下表里之分，病情有寒化、热化之异。因此，祛湿之法亦较为复杂。大抵湿邪在上在外者，可表散微汗以解之；在内在下者，可芳香苦燥以化之，或甘淡渗利以除之。从寒化者，宜温阳化湿；从热化者，宜清热祛湿。体虚湿盛者，又当祛湿扶正兼顾。祛湿剂可分为燥湿和胃、清热祛湿、利水渗湿、温化不湿、祛风胜湿五类。

  湿邪其性重着粘腻，易于阻碍气机，故祛湿剂中，常配伍理气药；祛湿剂多由辛香温燥或甘淡渗利之药组成，易于耗伤阴津，故对素体阴虚津亏者宜慎用。

16.2 燥湿和胃剂

  是以燥湿和胃的药物为主组成的方剂。适用于湿浊阻滞，脾胃不和之证。症见脘腹痞满，嗳气吞酸，呕吐泄泻，食少体倦等。常用的药有苍术、陈皮、藿香、白豆蔻等，代表方剂有平胃散、藿香正气散等。

16.3　平胃散

出自《太平惠民和剂局方》。由苍术 15 克，厚朴、陈皮各 9 克，甘草（炒）4 克，生姜 2 片，干枣 2 枚组成。水煎分 2 次服（原作散剂）。方中苍术味辛苦性温，善除湿运脾，为主药。厚朴行气化湿，消胀除满；陈皮理气化滞；甘草和中，调和诸药，生姜、大枣调和脾胃。共奏燥湿运脾，行气和胃之功。主治湿滞脾胃之证。症见脘腹胀满，不畏饮食，口淡无味，呕吐恶心，嗳气吞酸，肢体沉重，怠惰嗜卧，常多自利，舌苔白腻而厚，脉缓。现常用于慢性胃炎、胃肠神经官能症、急性胃炎、小儿消化不良、胃及十二指肠溃疡等病具有上述症状者。临床应用平胃散加味治疗胃肠神经官能症 1 例，症见呃逆频繁发作 5 月余，面色苍黄少华，纳呆腹胀，乏力，舌白腻，脉濡缓。西药治疗未效，遂改服中药。药用苍术 9 克，厚朴 9 克，陈皮 6 克，甘草 3 克，法半夏 12 克，绵茵陈 15 克，云茯苓 12 克，丁香 4.5 克。服 5 剂后腹胀消，呃逆渐止，续用健脾法而痊愈。运用平胃散加味引产 4 例。症见脘腹胀闷，饮食少进，倦怠口淡，大便溏薄，苔白腻厚，基本方由厚朴、陈皮各 12 克，苍术 9 克，甘草 6 克，玄明粉（冲）12 克，枳实 12 克组成，经治疗 4 例均取得肯定疗效。

16.4　藿香正气散

出自《太平惠民和剂局方》。由大腹皮、白芷、紫苏、茯苓各 6 克，半夏曲、白术、陈皮、厚朴、苦桔梗各 9 克，藿香 12 克，甘草（炙）4.5 克，生姜 3 克，大枣 1 枚组成。水煎分 2 次服（原作散剂）。方中藿香味辛性微温，既能辛散风寒，又能芳香化浊，且兼升清降浊而治霍乱，为主药。苏叶、白芷辛香发散，芳化湿浊；半夏、陈皮燥湿和胃，降逆止呕；白术、茯苓健脾运湿，和中止泻；厚朴、腹皮行气化湿，畅中除满；桔梗宣肺利膈，既利于解表，又益于化湿；生姜、大枣、甘草调和脾胃。

共奏解表化湿，理气和中之功。主治外感风寒，内伤湿滞之证。症见霍乱吐泻，发热恶寒，头痛，胸膈满闷，脘腹疼痛，舌苔白腻等。现常用于急性胃肠炎、食物中毒、胃肠型感冒等病具有上述症状者。临床应用藿香正气散加减治疗急性肠炎30例。症见轻度全身不适，脐周微痛，腹胀，食欲不振，肠鸣泄泻，每日达4～8次，呈粥样或水样，浅黄色或有泡沫。经治疗，一般在第2天即见效或痊愈。运用藿香正气散治疗胃肠型过敏性紫癜1例，症见腹痛，黑色稀便，全身皮肤出现出血点，以四肢为著，经服本方1剂后，恶心、呕吐、腹痛明显好转，能进饮食，5剂后症状大减，服10剂痊愈。

16.5 清热祛湿剂

是以清热祛湿的药物为主组成的方剂。适用于湿热外感，或湿热内盛，湿热下注之证。症见黄疸，午后身热，胸闷，腹胀，或脚膝肿痛等。常用的药有茵陈蒿、薏苡仁、山栀、滑石等，代表方剂有茵陈蒿汤、三仁汤、八正散等。

16.6 茵陈蒿汤

出自《伤寒论》。由茵陈30克，栀子15克，大黄9克组成。水煎分3次服。方中茵陈蒿味苦性微寒，善清利湿热，退黄疸，为主药。栀子通利三焦，导湿热下行，引湿热自小便出；大黄泻热逐瘀，通利大便。共奏清热、利湿、退黄之功。主治湿热黄疸之证。症见一身面目俱黄，黄色鲜明，腹微满，口中渴，小便不利，舌苔黄腻，脉沉数。现常用于急性黄疸型传染性肝炎、急性胆囊炎、胆石症、钩端螺旋体等病具有上述症状者。临床应用茵陈蒿汤加减治疗小儿黄疸型急性传染性肝炎115例。症见疸色鲜明，寒热纳呆，乏力尿黄，肝大，肝功损害，基本方由茵陈15克，山栀9克，黄柏4.5克，大黄3克，龙胆草4.5克，鸡骨草30克，赤芍9克，桃仁6克，川楝子9克，木通6克组成。

结果退黄时间最快者 2 天，最慢者 22 天，痊愈需 30 天左右。运用茵陈蒿汤加减治疗胆汁性肝硬化 1 例，症见眼球及全身黄疸，上腹不适，食后腹胀，纳呆，伴恶心呕吐，尿少色如浓茶，神倦，恶寒，头昏晕，面色苍黄憔悴，舌苔薄白，脉细软。先用本方合四君子汤加麦芽，又用苍术、砂仁、陈皮或山药、鸡内金等配合治疗，服 65 剂而愈。

16.7 三仁汤

出自《温病条辨》。由杏仁 15 克，飞滑石 18 克，白通草 6 克，白蔻仁 6 克，竹叶 6 克，厚朴 6 克，生薏苡仁 18 克，半夏 10 克组成。水煎分 3 次服。方中杏仁味苦性微温，开达肺气以利上焦，白蔻仁味辛性温，芳香化湿，利气以理中焦，苡仁味甘淡性微寒，淡渗利湿，疏泄下焦，三药宣通化浊，均为主药。半夏、厚朴行气散满，除湿消痞；滑石、通草、竹叶渗利湿热。共奏宣畅气机，清利湿热之功。主治湿温初起的湿重热轻之证。症见头痛恶寒，身重疼痛，面色淡黄，胸闷不饥，午后身热，舌白不渴，脉弦细而濡。现常用于肠伤寒、胃肠炎、肾盂肾炎、支气管肺炎、术后肠粘连等病具有上述症状者。临床应用三仁汤加减治疗肾盂肾炎 15 例，均有不同程度的尿蛋白、脓细胞，中段尿培养均阳性。基本方由三仁汤加连翘、茯苓组成，热重加柴胡、黄芩，尿道痛加车前子、琥珀、黄柏，腰痛甚加木瓜、杜仲，尿中细菌难消失加马齿苋、金钱草、连翘、苦参。结果 12 例痊愈，3 例好转。

16.8 甘露消毒丹

引自《温热经纬》。由飞滑石 450 克，绵茵陈 330 克，淡黄芩 300 克，石菖蒲 180 克，川贝母、木通各 150 克，藿香、射干、连翘、薄荷、白豆蔻各 120 克组成。共为细末，每服 9 克，开水调服，日 2 次（或以神曲糊丸，每丸 9 克；亦可按原方用量比例酌减，水煎服）。方中藿香味辛性微温，茵陈味苦性微寒，两药清热利湿，芳香化浊，宣通气机，均为主药。滑石清热利湿并解暑，木通清热利湿，引湿热从小便而出；黄芩清热燥湿，连翘清热解毒；贝母、射干清咽散结；石菖蒲、白蔻仁、薄荷芳香化浊，行气悦脾。共奏利湿化浊；清热解毒之功。主治湿温时疫，邪在气分之证。症见发热困倦，胸闷腹胀，肢酸咽肿，身黄，颐肿口渴，小便短赤，吐泻，淋浊，舌苔淡白或厚腻或干黄。现常用于肠伤寒、黄疸型传染性肝炎、胆囊炎、急性胃肠炎等病具有上述症状者。临床应用甘露消毒丹治疗小儿急性传染性肝炎 26 例。症见纳呆，尿黄，发热，，倦怠，恶心呕吐，咳嗽，舌红，苔薄白或白黄，脉弦滑。以甘露消毒丹原方生药粗末煎服，结果黄疸指数 13～20 单位者 9 例，均在 2 周内降至正常，谷丙转氨酶高者 24 例，在 3 周内降至正常，食欲均在 1～5 日内恢复，20 例在治疗后肝仍可触及 1.5～2cm。运用甘露消毒丹加减治疗 8 年低热 1 例，8 年前患急性胃肠炎后遗留低热，持续不退，迭经治疗未效，经检查除 X 线钡餐透视提示十二指肠溃疡外，其余均无异常发现。症见形体消瘦，面色萎黄，倦怠无力，四肢酸痛，少气懒言，胸腹满闷，嗜睡，诊时亦睡意频见，胃纳时呆时可，大便不畅，小便黄浊，舌质淡红苔黄厚腻，脉弦濡，体温 37.8℃。辨证为湿温病在气分，秽浊湿热蔓延内外，用甘露消毒丹去薄荷加苏叶水煎服，服 2 剂后病情好转，续服 8 剂而病愈。

16.9　连朴饮

出自《霍乱论》。由制厚朴 6 克，黄连（姜汁炒）、石菖蒲、制半夏各 3 克，香豉（炒）、焦山栀各 9 克，芦根 60 克组成。水煎分 2 次服。方中厚朴味苦辛性温，行气化湿，黄连味苦性寒，清热燥湿，均为主药。山栀、豆豉清宣胸脘之郁热，菖蒲芳香化湿而悦脾，半夏燥湿降逆而和胃；芦根清热化湿，和胃止呕。共奏清热化湿，理气和中之功。主治湿热蕴伏，胃失和降，脾失升清之证。症见霍乱吐利，胸脘痞闷，小便短赤，舌苔黄腻。现常用于肠伤寒、急性胃肠炎等病具有上述症状者。

16.10 蚕矢汤

出自《霍乱论》。由晚蚕砂 15 克，生苡仁、大豆黄卷各 12 克，陈木瓜 9 克，川连（姜汁炒）9 克，制半夏、黄芩（酒炒）、通草各 3 克，焦山栀 5 克，陈吴萸（泡淡）1 克组成。水煎分 2 次服。方中蚕砂味辛甘性微温，和胃化湿，治霍乱转筋，为主药。木瓜化湿和中，舒筋活络，与蚕砂相伍，善治霍乱转筋；大豆黄卷，化湿而升清，薏苡仁利湿而降浊，兼能舒筋；黄芩、黄连、焦栀清解热邪，兼可燥湿；半夏降逆止呕，通草渗湿利浊，疏通经络；少用吴茱萸，既可助半夏降逆，又协黄连降火止呕。共奏清利湿热，升清降浊之功。主治湿热内蕴，扰于脾胃的霍乱吐泻转筋之证。症见霍乱吐泻，腹痛转筋，口渴烦躁，舌苔黄厚而干，脉濡数。现常用于肠伤寒、急性胃肠炎等病具有上述症状者。

16.11 八正散

出自《太平惠民和剂局方》。由车前子 15 克，瞿麦 10 克，萹蓄 12 克，滑石 18 克，山栀子仁 9 克，炙甘草 4.5 克，木通 6 克，大黄（面裹煨）9 克，灯蕊草 3 克组成。水煎分 3 次服（原作散剂）。方中瞿麦、木通味苦性寒，两药泻热利湿，利尿通淋，均为主药。萹蓄、山栀、滑石、车前子、灯蕊草皆清热利湿，导邪从小便而出；大黄泄热降火；甘草和药缓急。共奏清热泻火，利水通淋之功。主治湿热下注，发为热淋、石淋之证。症见小便浑赤，溺时涩痛，淋漓不畅，甚或癃闭不通，小腹急满，口燥咽干，舌苔黄腻，脉滑数。现常用于膀胱炎、尿道炎、急性前列腺炎、泌尿系结石、肾盂肾炎等病具有上述症状者。临床应用八正散治疗泌尿道感染 28 例，其中急性肾盂肾炎 19 例，慢性肾盂肾炎急性发作 7 例，肾炎并泌尿道感染 1 例，前列腺肥大并感染 1 例，除 1 例慢性肾盂肾炎急性发作无效外，其余全部治愈，治愈率为 96.4%。运用八散加减治疗产后及术后尿潴留 32 例。证属肾虚、气虚、挟有气滞。基本方由萹蓄、瞿麦、滑石各 15 克，木能 3 克，车前子 9 克，甘草梢 6 克，元明粉（分冲）9 ～15 克组成。有发热合并泌尿系感染者，酌加栀子、黄连、蒲公英、紫地丁、败酱草。阴虚加生地、麦冬、沙参。结果服药 4 小时即能自动排尿者 15 例，服药 4～8 小时内排尿，仍不通畅，须 2～5 剂始愈者 17 例。

16.12　二妙散

出自《丹溪心法》。由黄柏（炒）、苍术（米泔浸炒）各 15 克组成。水煎分服（原作散剂）。方中黄柏味苦性寒，善于清热，苍术味苦性温，善于燥湿。共奏清热燥湿之功。主治湿热下注之证。症见下肢痿软无力，或足膝红肿热痛，或带下，或下部湿疮，小便短黄，舌苔黄腻。现常用于小儿麻痹后遗症、多发性神经炎、下肢静脉曲张、闭塞性脉管炎、坐骨神经痛、风湿性关节炎等病具有上述症状者。临床应用二妙丸加味治疗痹、痿证各 1 例，痿证例证属湿热所致，症见发热 3 天后，两手持物无力，双脚不能行走。药用苍术 30 克，黄柏 20 克，牛膝 15 克，续断 15 克，鸡血藤 25 克，银花 25 克，板蓝根 25 克，蒲公英 50 克，连翘 15 克，大青叶 15 克，石斛 25 克，滑石 20 克，甘草 7.5 克。服 4 剂后，可站立行走数步，续以上方治疗半个月而愈。痹证例证属湿热所致，症见腹痛，服用蓖麻片后，全身起疙瘩，瘙痒，下肢肿，关节疼痛，步行艰难，药用苍术 15 克，生地 15 克，赤芍 15 克，防风 15 克，白藓皮 15 克，地肤子 15 克，地骨皮 15 克，防己 10 克，秦艽 15 克，忍冬藤 25 克，鸡血藤 25 克，夜交藤 25 克，以上方加减治疗半月而愈。运用二妙散煎剂治疗传染性肝炎 40 例，36 例临床主要症状消失，转氨酶降到 40 单位以下，4 例降到 80 单位以下，主要症状消失或减轻。

16.13　利水渗湿剂

是以利水渗湿的药物为主组成的方剂。适用于水湿壅盛所致的癃闭、淋浊、水肿、泄泻等证。症见小便不利，水肿身重，大便稀或水样便，或眩晕，或呕恶等。常用的药有茯苓、泽泻、猪苓等，代表方剂有五苓散、五皮散等。

16.14　五苓散

出自《伤寒论》。由猪苓 9 克，泽泻 15 克，白术 9 克，茯苓 9 克，桂枝 6 克组成。为末，每服 3～6 克，日 3 次（亦作汤剂）。方中泽泻味甘淡性寒，利水渗湿，为主药。茯苓、猪苓利水蠲饮；白术健脾化湿；桂枝既解表散寒，又温化膀胱而利小便。共奏利水渗湿、温阳化气之功。主治外有风寒，内聚水湿及痰饮之证。症见头痛发热，烦渴欲饮，水入即吐，小便不利，舌苔白，脉浮；或水肿，泄泻，小便不利，呕吐；或脐下动悸，吐涎沫而头眩，短气而咳等。现常用于急性肾炎、传染性肝炎、美尼尔氏综合征、脑积水等病具有上述症状者。临床应用五苓散治疗急性肾炎 40 例。40 例均为较重病例，有明显的水肿、高血压、血尿及肾功能减退，部分病例伴有腹水和肾性心力衰竭，以 1 日总药量重症者 9 克，中等者 6 克，轻症者 3 克，7 日为 1 疗程，并配合保温（尤其肾区保温），减盐饮食及安静休息，40 例全部有效，平均住院日数为 164 天。运用五苓散治疗传染性肝炎 3 例，证属湿热黄疸，症见右胁下胀闷不舒、食欲不振、腹胀、肝大、黄疸、小便黄赤、经本方治疗、均获痊愈。

五苓散对健康人、正常小鼠和家兔均无利尿作用，在代谢障碍时，却具有显著利尿的作用，并能促进局限性水肿的吸收。在抗菌素所引起口渴、呕吐、尿量减少时，机体的抵抗力显著减弱，通过给于五苓散可改善全身状况，恢复机体对细菌的抵抗力，加上抗菌素的抗菌作用，能使体温下降，症状改善。

16.15 猪苓汤

出自《伤寒论》。由猪苓、茯苓、泽泻、阿胶（烊化）、滑石各 9 克组成。水煎分 2 次服。猪苓味甘淡性寒，渗湿利水而泄热，为主药。茯苓、泽泻渗利小便，滑石清热通淋；阿胶滋阴润燥。共奏利水清热养阴之功。主治水热互结，邪热伤阴之证。症见小便不利，发热，口渴欲饮，或心烦不寐，或兼有咳嗽，呕恶，下利，或小便涩痛，点滴难出，小腹满痛等。现常用于泌尿系感染、肾炎等病具有上述症状者。临床应用猪苓汤治疗急性膀胱炎 107 例。基本方由猪苓 10 克，茯苓 18 克，滑石 15 克，阿胶（烊化）6 克组成。尿短淋沥加车前子，尿时涩痛加石苇、乌药，尿血加白茅根、茜草炭，肾附素亏加元参，腰痛加桑寄生、怀牛膝，107 例均服药 1～6 剂而痊愈。运用猪苓汤治疗流行性出血热休克期 13 例，基本方由猪苓 30 克，泽泻 30 克，茯苓 15 克，阿胶 30 克（隔水烊化约 30 毫升，加糖另服），有腹泻者加滑石 10 克，13 例患者中，11 例在休克期前阶段给药后，9 例中止进入休克期后阶段，2 例进入休克期后阶段，另 2 例先经西药治疗，因治疗棘手，在进入休克期后阶段改用猪苓汤治疗，结果 13 例无 1 例死亡。服药 1 剂者 9 例，2 剂者 4 例，第 2 剂药均在给服首剂后 12 小时服用，而在用西药治疗的对照组的同期患者，有 3 例死亡。

16.16 防己黄芪汤

出自《金匮要略》。由防己 12 克，黄芪 15 克，甘草（炒）6 克，白术 9 克，生姜 3 克，大枣 1 枚组成。水煎分 2 次服。方中防己味苦辛微寒，祛风行水，黄芪味甘性微热，益气固表，行水消肿，两药均为主药。白术补气健脾，助脾运化；甘草培土和中，调和诸药；姜、枣调和营卫。共奏益气祛风、健脾利水之功。主治风水、风湿的表虚之证。症见汗出恶风，身重，小便不利，舌淡苔白，脉浮。现常用于慢性肾炎、心脏病水肿、肝硬化腹水、风湿性关节炎等病具有上述症状者。临床应用加减防己黄芪汤治疗晚期血吸虫病腹水 34 例。基本方由防己 9 克，黄芪 12克，白术 9 克，猪苓 9 克，茯苓 12 克，泽泻 9 克，车前子 12克，杜赤豆 30 克，川椒目 3 克，生姜皮 1.5 克组成，本方对血象及肝功能的改善似无作用，而对于症状改善，黄疸消退有一定效果。结果有效 27 例，无效 5 例，恶化 2 例。运用防己黄芪汤合天仙藤散加减治疗妊娠肿胀 7 例，7 例患者均系第 1 胎，年龄在 22～30 岁之间，妊娠月份分别为 6～9 个月，病程为 4～7天。若兼有肝阳上亢、头痛、眩晕、血压偏高者，可酌加钩藤、菊花、石决明、黄芩等。结果 4 例服药 3 天肿消，2 例服药 4 天肿消，1 例肿胀减退。

16.17 五皮散

出自《华氏中藏经》。由生姜皮、桑白皮、陈橘皮、大腹皮、茯苓皮各 9 克组成。共为粗末，9 克水煎去渣温服，日 2 次（亦作汤剂）。方中茯苓皮味甘淡性平，利水渗湿，兼补脾助运化，为主药。生姜皮辛散水饮，桑白皮肃降肺气，以通调水道；大腹皮行水气，消胀满；陈橘皮和胃气，化湿浊。共奏利湿消肿，理气健脾之功。主治脾虚湿盛，泛滥肌肤之证。症见一身悉肿，肢体沉重，心腹胀满，上气喘急，小便不利，苔白腻，脉沉缓。现常用于肾性浮肿、心性浮肿、妊娠浮肿、血管神经性水肿等病具有上述症状者。临床应用大剂量五皮散加减治疗慢性肾炎26 例，基本方由茯苓皮、大腹皮、桑白皮各 60 克，地骨皮 30克，姜皮、猪苓各 15 克组成。血压高加杜仲，恶心、呕吐、咳嗽、气短加陈皮、半夏，胃脘不适加白术。症状好转，检查尿仍有改变时加肉桂、当归、党参、熟地，原方茯苓皮、大腹皮、地骨皮、桑白皮各减去半量，结果痊愈 5 例，有效 16 例，好转 4 例，无效 1 例。运用五皮散加玉米须治疗妊娠水肿 43 例，基本方由桑白皮 15 克，茯苓皮 9 克，大腹皮 12 克，陈皮 9 克，生姜皮 6 克，玉米须（干）30 克或鲜品 60 克组成。肿甚加猪苓 9 克，泽泻 9 克，恶阻加竹茹 9 克，白术 12 克，代赭石 15 克，咳嗽加杏仁 6 克，百合 9 克，喘加苏子 12 克。经治疗，均获得满意的效果。

16.18　温化水湿剂

是以温化水湿的药物为主组成的方剂。适用于湿从寒化和阳不化水的痰饮、水肿、痹证及寒湿脚气等证。症见目眩心悸，肢体浮肿，肢体沉重疼痛，手足不温，大便稀溏，苔白滑，脉沉等。常用的药有桂枝、附子、白术等，代表方剂有苓桂术甘汤、真武汤等。

16.19　苓桂术甘汤

出自《金匮要略》。由茯苓 12 克，桂枝 9 克，白术 6 克，甘草（炙）6 克组成。水煎分 3 次服。方中茯苓味甘淡性平，健脾渗湿，祛痰化饮，为主药。桂枝温阳化水，平冲降逆；白术健脾燥湿；甘草益气和中。共奏温化痰饮，健脾利湿之功。主治中阳不足的痰饮证。症见胸胁支满，目眩心悸，或短气而咳，舌苔白滑，脉弦滑。现常用于慢性支气管炎、支气管哮喘、慢性肾炎等病具有上述症状者。临床应用苓桂术甘汤治疗心包积液 1 例，证属脾虚湿盛、湿邪上犯，症见发热已半月余，咳嗽，胸闷且痛，气喘，水肿，脉沉细无力。药用本方加黄芪、防己、丹参等，共服 10 余剂而愈。运用苓桂术甘汤治疗咳而遗尿症 1 例，症见产后咳嗽月余，咳嗽时小便滴滴而出，夜间咳嗽尤甚，小便也淋漓尤多，就诊时已病 16 个月，纳食正常，痰咯不多而色白，舌苔薄白，脉弦细。药用茯苓 15 克，桂枝 6 克，白术 9 克，甘草 3 克，服 3 剂症大减，6 剂咳止，遗尿亦愈。

16.20　真武汤

出自《伤寒论》，，由茯苓 9 克，芍药 9 克，白术 6 克，生姜 9 克，附子（炮）9 克组成。水煎分 2 次服。方中附子味辛甘性大热，温肾暖土，扶阳散寒，为主药。茯苓健脾渗湿，以利水邪；生姜既助附子温阳祛寒，又配茯苓以温散水气；白术健脾燥湿；白芍利小便，缓急止腹痛。共奏温阳利水之功。主治脾肾阳虚，水气内停之证。症见小便不利，四肢沉重疼痛，腹痛下利，肢体浮肿，口不渴，苔白，脉沉；或发热而汗出不解，心下悸，头眩，身瞤动，振振欲擗地等。现常用于慢性结肠炎、慢性肾炎、心性浮肿、醛固酮增多症、甲状腺功能低下、肠结核、美尼尔氏综合症等病具有上述症状者。临床应用真武汤加减治疗充血性心力衰竭 15 例，其中心功能 IV 级者 7 例，III 级者 7 例，II 级者 1 例，首次心力衰竭者 3 例，反复发作 2～3 次者 9 例，4 次以上者 3 例。治疗是在用抗感染、祛风湿的同时，给予真武汤加活血化瘀药。基本方由附子 9～18 克，茯苓 15～30 克，白术、白芍、桃仁、琥珀各 9 克，生姜 9～15 克，红花 6～9 克组成。治疗后心力衰竭基本纠正 1 例，显效 6 例，有效 5 例，无效 3 例。运用真武汤治疗内耳眩晕症 41 例。证属肾阳虚，膀胱气化无权，水气上冲，清阳不升所致，症见眩晕、耳鸣、重听、部分病人有心悸、肉瞤等。基本方由附子 8 克，白术 10 克，茯苓 12 克，生姜 10 克，白芍 6 克，细辛 3 克，桂枝 5 克，五味子 6 克，川芎 8 克组成。结果治愈 35 例，好转 6 例。

真武汤具有强心利尿、促进胃肠吸收、排除体内残余物质的作用。

16.21　实脾散

出自《重订严氏济生方》。由厚朴（姜制）、白术、木瓜、木香、草果仁、大腹子、附子（炮）、白茯苓、干姜（炮）各6克，甘草（炙）3克，生姜3克，大枣1枚组成。水煎分2次服（原作散剂）。方中附子味辛甘性大热，温脾肾，助气化，散寒湿，干姜味辛性热，温脾阳，助运化，散寒水，两药均为主药。茯苓、白术健脾燥湿，淡渗利水；木瓜芳香醒脾，化湿利水；厚朴、木香、大腹子、草果下气导滞，化湿行水；甘草、生姜、大枣调和诸药，益脾和中。共奏温阳健脾，行气利水之功。主治阳虚水肿之证。症见下肢肿甚，手足不温，口中不渴，胸腹胀满，大便溏薄，舌苔厚腻，脉沉迟。现常用于慢性肾炎、肝硬化腹水、心性浮肿等病具有上述症状者。临床应用实脾饮加减治疗重证肝硬化腹水1例，证属气郁脾肾两虚，症见腹部胀满，食欲不振，嗳气吞酸，四肢倦怠，步行艰难。药用本方加党参12克，木通9克，泽泻9克，郁金9克，陈皮4.5克，服5剂症状缓解，继服本方加四君、归脾丸40余剂而痊愈。

16.22　萆薢分清饮

出自《丹溪心法》。由益智、川萆薢、石菖蒲、乌药各10克组成。水煎分2次服。方中萆薢味苦性寒，利湿化浊，为主药。益智温肾阳，缩小便，止遗浊；乌药温肾寒，暖膀胱，止尿频；石菖蒲化浊除湿，去膀胱虚寒。共奏温肾利湿，分清化浊之功。主治下焦虚寒，湿浊下注之证。症见小便白浊，频频无度，白如米泔，凝如膏糊。现常用于乳糜尿、慢性前列腺炎、慢性膀胱炎等病具有上述症状者。临床应用萆薢分清饮加减治疗痉中痒痛1例，证属湿热下注膀胱尿道，兼见阴伤。症见1位8岁男性患儿，阴茎中段奇痒疼痛6年余，舌质淡红，苔薄微黄，脉细数。药用萆薢12克，苡仁12克，木瓜4.5克，生地12克，竹叶6

克，赤芍6克，当归6克，玄参9克，银花12克，苦参9克，六一散12克，服5剂痒痛大减，连服20剂获愈。运用萆薢治疗肾结核并血尿2例，均见腰痛、尿频、尿中带血。先服萆薢分清饮，药后尿即转清，此后乃逐一减去辅佐药，仅用萆薢1味，每日9克，水煎服，分别服半年和2年，症状改善，血尿停止，未发生任何副作用。

16.23　祛风胜湿剂

是以祛风胜湿的药物为主组成的方剂。适用于外感风湿的痹证及寒湿脚气等证。症见头痛，身痛，腰膝顽麻，肢体困重，或足胫肿重无力等。常用的药有独活、独活、防风、秦艽等，代表方剂有羌活胜湿汤、独活寄生汤等。

16.24　羌活胜湿汤

出自《内外伤辨惑论》。由羌活、独活各6克，藁本、防风、甘草（炙）、川芎各3克、蔓荆子2克组成。水煎分2次服。方中羌活味辛苦性温，善祛上部风湿，独活味辛苦性微温，善祛下部风湿，两药能散周身风湿，舒利关节而通痹，为主药。防风、藁本、蔓荆子祛风湿，止头痛；川芎活血祛风止痛；甘草调和诸药。共奏祛风胜湿之功。主治风湿在表之证。症见肩背痛不可回顾，头痛身重，或腰脊疼痛，难以转侧，苔白，脉浮。现常用于感冒、风湿性关节炎、神经性头痛等病具有上述症状者。

16.25　独活寄生汤

出自《备急千金要方》。由独活9克，寄生18克，杜仲9克，牛膝9克，细辛3克，秦艽9克，茯苓12克，肉桂心1.5克，防风9克，川芎6克，人参10克，甘草6克，当归12克，芍药9克，干地黄15克组成。水煎分3次服。方中独活味辛苦性微温，善祛下焦与筋骨间之风寒湿邪，为主药。细辛散寒止痛，防风祛风胜湿，秦艽除风湿而舒筋；寄生、杜仲、牛膝祛风湿兼补肝肾；当归、川芎、地黄、白芍养血又兼活血；人参、茯苓补气健脾；桂心温通血脉；甘草调和诸药。共奏祛风湿，止痹痛，益肝肾，补气血之功。主治风寒湿痹着日久，肝肾不足，气血两虚之证。症见腰膝疼痛，肢节屈伸不利，或麻木不仁，畏寒喜温，心悸气短，舌淡苔白，脉象细弱。现常用于慢性关节炎、风湿性坐骨神经痛等病具有上述症状者。临床应用独活寄生汤加味治疗坐骨神经痛 19 例，基本方由独活 15 克，桑寄生 20 克，秦艽 15 克，细辛 5 克，川芎 15 克、防风 15 克，狗脊 25 克、菟丝子 25 克，续断 40 克，黄芪 25 克，稀莶草 20 克，当归 15 克，红花 10 克，党参 25 克，牛膝 15 克，甘草 10 克组成。因外伤引起，痛甚者加炙乳没，腿沉重加生苡仁，麻木加木瓜、黑木耳，寒重加桂枝。19 例患者均疗效满意。运用独活寄生汤加减治疗颞颌关节功能紊乱综合征 40 例，基本方由熟地、牛膝、杜仲、桑寄生、当归、白芍、川芎、党参、茯苓、甘草、羌活、独活、细辛、桂心、秦艽、防风组成。经过服药 3～30 剂，痊愈 38 例，显效 2 例。

16.26 鸡鸣散

出自《证治准绳》。由槟榔 15 克，陈皮、木瓜各 9 克，吴萸、紫苏叶各 3 克，桔梗、生姜和皮各 5 克组成。水煎凌晨空腹冷服。方中槟榔味辛苦性温，行气逐湿，为主药。木瓜舒筋活络，并能化湿；陈皮健脾燥湿，理气行滞；紫苏叶、桔梗宣通气机，外散表邪，内开郁结；吴茱萸、生姜温化寒湿，降逆止呕。共奏行气降浊，宣化寒湿之功。主治寒湿脚气。症见足胫肿重无力，麻木冷痛，恶寒发热，或挛急上冲，甚至胸闷泛恶等。现常用于脚气病、丝虫病等病具有上述症状者。临床应用鸡鸣散治疗湿脚气 12 例，服药 1 剂而愈者 4 例，2 剂而愈者 5 例，3 剂而愈者 3 例。运用鸡鸣散治疗丝虫病 52 例，证多属寒湿凝滞经脉，基本方由槟榔 60 克，木瓜 30 克，干姜 30 克，陈皮 30 克，桔梗 30 克，苏叶 30 克，吴萸 30 克，茯苓 30 克，羌活 30 克组成。共为细末，分为 50 包，每天 13 时 30 分开始服药，每隔 1 小时服 1 次，每次 1 包，每天服 5 次，10 天为 1 疗程，结果脚肿全消者 34 例，半消者 11 例，好转者 7 例。

第 17 章　祛痰剂

17.1　祛痰剂

由祛痰药为主组成，具有消除痰饮作用，以治疗各种痰病的方剂，统称祛痰剂。凡咳嗽喘促、眩晕呕吐、癫狂惊痫及痰核瘰疬等病证属痰浊为患者，均可选用祛痰剂。根据痰的性质和治法的不同，祛痰剂又可分为燥湿化痰、清热化痰、润燥化痰、温化寒痰和治风化痰五类，分别适用于湿痰、热痰、燥痰、寒痰和风痰所致的疾病。

祛痰剂多为行消之品，不宜久用，应中病即止。有咯血倾向者，不宜用温燥的祛痰剂，以防引起大量咯血。外感咳嗽初起有表证者，宜先用宣肺解表剂，不宜早用清润化痰之品。

17.2　燥湿化痰剂

是以燥湿化痰的药物为主组成的方剂，适用于湿痰证。症见咳嗽痰多易咯，胸脘痞闷，恶心呕吐，眩晕心悸，舌苔白滑或白腻，脉缓或弦滑等。常用药物有陈皮、半夏、橘红等，代表方剂有二陈汤、温胆汤、茯苓丸等。

17.3　二陈汤

出自《太平惠民和剂局方》。由半夏 9 克，橘红 9 克，茯苓 6 克，炙甘草 3 克，生姜 3 克，乌梅 1 个组成。水煎分 2 次服。方中半夏燥湿化痰，和胃止呕，为主药。橘红理气燥湿化痰；茯苓健脾渗湿；生姜降逆化痰，并助半夏、橘红行气消痰；乌梅收敛肺气，使祛痰而不伤肺气；炙甘草调和诸药。共奏燥湿化痰，理气和中之效。主治湿痰证。症见咳嗽痰多，色白易咯，胸膈痞闷，恶心呕吐，肢体困倦，或头眩心悸，舌苔白腻，脉滑等。现常用于慢性支气管炎及肺气肿、消化性溃疡、美尼尔氏病、妊娠恶阻、小儿流涎等病具有上述症状者。临床应用二陈汤合平胃散加减治疗慢性支气管炎 55 例，其中合并肺气肿者 33 例，全部病例均有效，咳喘症状一般在 1 周内改善，而且时间肺活量和膈肌运动功能也有一定改善。把二陈汤改用散剂治疗重度单纯性甲状腺肿 7 例，一般疗程为 15 天，结果痊愈 5 例，改善 2 例。

17.4　温胆汤

出自《三因极一病证方论》。由半夏 6 克，竹茹 6 克，枳实 6 克，陈皮 9 克，炙甘草 3 克，茯苓 5 克，生姜 3 克，大枣 1 枚组成。水煎分 2 次服。方中半夏降逆和胃，燥湿化痰，为主药。竹茹清热化痰，止呕除烦；枳实行气消痰；陈皮理气燥湿化痰；茯苓健脾渗湿以助消痰；生姜、大枣、炙甘草益脾和胃，调和诸药。共奏理气化痰，清胆和胃之效。主治胆胃不和，痰热内扰之证。症见虚烦不眠，或呕吐呃逆，眩晕胸闷，惊悸不宁，舌苔黄腻，脉滑数或弦数等。现常用于消化性溃疡、美尼尔氏病、高血压病、脑动脉硬化、神经官能症、更年期综合征、冠状动脉硬化性心脏病等病具有上述症状者。临床应用加味温胆汤治疗美尼尔氏病 62 例，椎——基底动脉供血不足 6 例，均取得较好疗效。

17.5　茯苓丸

出自《指迷方》。由半夏 60 克，茯苓 30 克，炒枳壳 15 克，风化朴硝 7.5 克组成。诸药共研为细末，加姜汁适量，煮糊为丸，每服 6 克，姜汤或温开水送下，日 2 次。方中半夏燥湿化痰，为主药；茯苓健脾渗湿以助消痰；枳实理气宽中；朴硝软坚润下；姜汁可减轻半夏的毒性，又可化痰。共奏燥湿行气涤痰之功。主治痰湿内停之证。症见两臂酸痛或四肢浮肿，或咳嗽痰多，胸脘满闷、舌苔白腻、脉弦滑等。现常用于周围神经炎、甲状腺功能减退、慢性支气管炎、肺气肿等病具有上述症状者。

17.6 清热化痰剂

　　是以清热和化痰的药物为主组成的方剂，适用于热痰证。症见咳嗽痰黄，粘稠难咯，舌红苔黄腻，脉滑数等。常用药物有黄芩、黄连、栝蒌、胆南星、半夏等，代表方剂有清气化痰丸、小陷胸汤等。

17.7 清气化痰丸

　　引自《医方考》。由栝蒌仁、陈皮、黄芩、杏仁、枳实、茯苓各30克，胆南星、制半夏各45克组成。诸药共研细末，以姜汁适量为丸，每服6克，温开水送下，日2次（亦可水煎服，用量按原方比例酌减）。方中胆南星清热化痰；栝蒌仁助胆南星清肺热而化热痰；枳实、陈皮理气消痰散结；茯苓健脾渗湿；杏仁宣肺止咳；半夏燥湿化痰。共奏清热化痰、理气止咳之效。主治痰热蕴肺之证。症见咳嗽痰黄，粘稠难咯，胸膈痞满，舌红苔黄腻，脉滑数等。现常用于肺炎、急性支气管炎、慢性支气管炎急性发作、支气管扩张并感染等病具有上述症状者。

17.8 小陷胸汤

　　出自《伤寒论》。由黄连6克，半夏12克，栝蒌30克组成。水煎分2次服。方中栝蒌清热化痰，宽胸散结，为主药。黄连清热泻火；半夏降逆和胃化痰。共奏清热化痰，宽胸散结之功。主治痰热互结之证。症见胸脘痞闷，按之则痛，或咳嗽，咯痰黄稠，舌苔黄腻，脉滑数或浮数等。现常用于胸膜炎、肋间神经痛、支气管炎、肺炎、急慢性胃炎、胆囊炎等病具有上述症状者。临床应用小陷胸汤合桂枝加桂汤治疗血管神经性头痛有近期疗效，一般3～5剂后头痛症状即明显减轻。

17.9　滚痰丸

引自《丹溪心法附余》。由大黄（酒蒸）、黄芩（酒洗）各240克，煅礞石30克，沉香15克组成。诸药共为细末，水泛为丸，每服6～9克，日2次，温开水送下。方中煅礞石下气平喘，逐痰定惊；大黄通便泻热；黄芩清上焦之热；沉香调理气机。共奏泻火逐痰之功。主治实热顽痰之证。症见癫狂惊悸，狂躁不安，或怔忡昏迷，或咳喘痰稠，或胸脘痞闷，眩晕耳鸣，大便秘结，舌红、苔黄厚而腻，脉滑数有力等。现常用于躁狂抑郁性精神病、癫痫、慢性支气管炎、支气管哮喘等病具有上述症状者。本方药力峻猛，只用于实热顽痰，久积不去而身体壮实者，体虚及孕妇患者慎用。临床应用滚痰丸合桂枝加桂汤加减治疗脑外伤后综合征30例，其中22例症状基本消失，6例明显好转，1例好转。

17.10　润燥化痰剂

是以润肺化痰的药物为主组成的方剂，适用于燥痰证。症见痰稠而粘，咯之不爽，咽喉干燥，或有呛咳，声音嘶哑等。常用的药有贝母、栝蒌等，代表方剂有贝母栝蒌散等。

17.11　贝母栝蒌散

出自《医学心悟》。由贝母5克，栝蒌3克，天花粉、茯苓、橘红、桔梗各2.5克组成。水煎分2次服。方中贝母清热润肺，化痰止咳；栝蒌清热涤痰而润燥；天花粉清热化痰，生津润燥；茯苓健脾利湿；橘红理气化痰；桔梗宣肺降逆，祛痰止咳。共奏润肺清热，化痰止咳之功。主治肺燥有痰之证。症见咳嗽喘促，咯痰不爽，咽喉干燥而痛，舌红少苔而干等。现常用于慢性支气管炎、支气管哮喘、支气管扩张、肺结核、矽肺等病具有上述症状者。

17.12 温化寒痰剂

是以辛温和化痰的药物为主组成的方剂，适用于寒痰证。症见咳嗽喘促，咯痰清稀色白，胸膈痞闷，舌苔白滑或白腻等。常用的药有干姜、细辛、五味子、苏子等，代表方剂有苓甘五味姜辛汤、三子养亲汤等。

17.13 苓甘五味姜辛汤

出自《金匮要略》。由茯苓12克，甘草6克，干姜9克，细辛6克，五味子6克组成。水煎分2次服。方中干姜辛热，既温肺散寒以化痰饮，又温运脾阳以祛湿；细辛温肺散寒，助干姜温化痰饮；茯苓健脾利湿以消痰；五味子敛肺止咳；甘草和胃，调和诸药。共奏温化痰饮之功。主治寒饮内停之证。症见咳嗽痰多，清稀色白，胸满喘促，舌苔白滑，脉弦滑等。现常用于慢性支气管炎、肺气肿、支气管哮喘、支气管扩张等病具有上述症状者。

17.14 三子养亲汤

出自《韩氏医通》。由白芥子6克，苏子9克，莱菔子9克组成。将3药捣碎，用白色纱布包裹，煎汤频服。方中白芥子温肺利气，宽胸消痰；苏子降气化痰，止咳平喘；莱菔子消食导滞，行气祛痰。共奏化痰消食，止咳平喘之功。主治痰壅气滞的咳喘证。症见咳嗽喘促，痰多色白，胸闷食少，舌苔白腻，脉滑等。现常用于慢性支气管炎、支气管哮喘、支气管扩张、肺气肿、肺源性心脏病等病具有上述症状者。本方对年老体弱者，不宜单方久服，如需久服，应配用调补脾肺或健脾益肾之品。临床应用三子养亲汤合桂附理中汤（痰饮丸）分别治疗慢性支气管炎195例和97例，总有效率分别达到88%和85.6%，大部分病例治疗后体质增强，感冒次数减少，提示有增强机体抵抗力的作用。

17.15　冷哮丸

出自《张氏医通》。由麻黄、生川乌、细辛、花椒、白矾、炙皂角、半夏曲、胆南星、杏仁、生甘草各 30 克，紫菀、冬花各 60 克组成。上药共研细末，加姜汁适量调糊为丸，每服 6 克，温开水送下，日 2 次（亦可水煎服，用量按原方比例酌减）。方中麻黄、川乌、细辛温肺化痰，宣肺平喘；川椒温中除湿；白矾、皂角消痰除满；半夏曲、胆南星化痰降逆；杏仁、紫菀、冬花化痰止咳平喘；甘草调和诸药。共奏温肺化痰之效。主治风寒喘咳。症见喘促气急，不得平卧，咳嗽咯痰，遇冷即发，胸膈满闷，舌苔白滑，脉浮滑或弦滑等。现常用于支气管哮喘、喘息型支气管炎、慢性支气管炎、肺气肿等病具有上述症状者。本方主要用于咳喘发作时的治疗，一旦病情控制，即应换用或配用调补脾肺的方剂，以增强机体抵抗力，减少咳喘的复发。

17.16　治风化痰剂

是以宣散风邪或平肝息风药与化痰药配伍组成的方剂，适用于风痰证。因风痰证由外感风邪或内风挟痰所致，故治风化痰剂又分疏风化痰和息风化痰两法。

疏风化痰法，适用于风邪犯肺的咳喘证。症见恶风发热，咳嗽咯痰，舌苔薄白等。常用的药有荆芥、紫菀、桔梗、百部、陈皮等，代表方剂有止嗽散等。

息风化痰法，适用于内风挟痰之证。症见眩晕头痛，或发癫痫，甚则昏厥，不省人事等。常用的药有天麻、半夏、茯苓等，代表方剂有半夏白术天麻汤、定痫丸等。

17.17　止嗽散

出自《医学心悟》。由桔梗、紫菀、荆芥、百部、白前各1000克，炙甘草375克，陈皮500克组成。诸药共研细末，每次6克，日2～3次，温开水送下（亦可水煎服，用量按原方比例酌减）。方中紫菀、百部、白前止咳化痰；桔梗、陈皮宣降肺气，祛痰止咳；荆芥疏散风邪以解表；甘草调和诸药；荆芥、桔梗、甘草相配，又有清利咽喉而止痛的作用。共奏疏风宣肺，化痰止咳之功。主治风邪犯肺之咳喘证。症见咳嗽，咽痒，咯痰，或微有恶寒发热，舌苔薄白，脉浮等。现常用于急性支气管炎、慢性支气管炎、百日咳、流行性感冒等病具有上述症状者。临床应用止嗽散加减治疗百日咳28例，水煎少量频服，日1剂，结果治愈19例，好转6例，无效3例（其中1例合并肺炎）。治愈者一般服药5～7天。运用本方加减水煎服，治疗外感咳嗽280例（包括上呼吸道感染，急性支气管炎及肺炎等），其中238例发病均在15天以内，结果治愈273例，占97%，平均服药3剂略强，7例疗效不满意，全部病例均无不良反应。

17.18　半夏白术天麻汤

出自《医学心悟》。由制半夏9克，天麻、茯苓、橘红各6克，白术15克，甘草4克，生姜1片，大枣2枚组成。水煎分2次服。方中制半夏燥湿化痰，降逆止呕；天麻平肝息风，善止眩晕，两药合用，是治疗风痰眩晕头痛的常用配伍；白术、茯苓健脾渗湿，以治生痰之源；橘红理气化痰；生姜、大枣调理脾胃。共奏燥湿化痰，平肝息风之功。主治风痰内扰之证。症见眩晕头痛，胸闷恶心呕吐，舌苔白腻，脉弦滑等。现常用于高血压病、美尼尔氏病、脑震荡后遗症、脑动脉硬化、前庭神经炎等病具有上述症状者。临床应用半夏白术天麻汤加减治疗美尼尔氏病28例，均取得控制发作，症状改善或消失的满意疗效。运用本方加减治疗结核性脑膜炎 7 例，结果表明，本方具有降低脑压，止呕、止痉等作用，全部病例均获满意疗效，随访观察 5 年，患者健康状况良好。因结核性脑膜炎病程长，故不过早停药，症状消失后，仍需继续服药，以巩固疗效。

17.19　定痫丸

出自《医学心悟》。由天麻、川贝母、半夏、茯苓、茯神各 30 克，胆南星、石菖蒲、全蝎、甘草、僵蚕、琥珀、灯心草各 15 克，陈皮、远志各 22 克，丹参、麦冬各 60 克，朱砂 9 克组成。诸药共为细末，再用甘草 120 克熬膏，加竹沥 100 毫升，姜汁 50 毫升，和匀调药为小丸，每服 6 克，日 2 次，温开水送下（亦可水煎服，用量按原方比例酌减）。方中竹沥清热化痰，镇惊醒神，配姜汁化痰开窍；胆南星清热化痰，镇静定痫；半夏、陈皮、川贝母、茯苓、麦冬祛痰降逆，兼防阴伤；丹参、石菖蒲化瘀开窍；全蝎、僵蚕息风定痉；天麻平肝息风以消风痰；朱砂、琥珀、远志、灯心草、茯神镇惊安神，以助解痉定痫；甘草益气扶正，调和诸药。共奏豁痰开窍，息风定痫之功。主治痰热内扰的癫痫、癫狂证。症见意识突然丧失而跌倒，肌肉强直，抽搐，口吐白沫或喉中痰鸣，不久苏醒，或狂躁不安，舌红苔黄腻或白腻，脉弦滑或滑数等。现常用于癫痫、精神分裂症、躁狂忧郁症等病具有上述症状者。临床应用本方治疗癫痫 21 例，总有效率为 85.7%。运用定痫丸合风引汤加减治疗癫痫 31 例，其中 9 例随访 2 年未复发，11 例基本控制，5 例好转，其余无效。总有效率为 80.6%。

第18章 消导化积剂

18.1 消导化积剂

由消导药为主组成的具有消食导滞，化积消癥作用的方剂，统称消导化积剂。本章主要讨论消食导滞和消痞化积剂两类，分别用于宿食积滞和癥瘕痞块证。

消导剂与泻下剂均有消除有形实邪的作用，但在临床应用中，两者有所区别。消导剂作用较缓和，用于饮食积滞和逐渐形成的脘腹痞块而病情较缓或病程较长者。泻下剂作用较峻猛，用于里实积聚和便秘等证而病情较急或病程较短者。

消导化积剂虽较泻下剂作用缓和，但毕竟是克伐之剂，故对于纯虚无实之证，应予禁用。治疗期间，应禁食生冷油腻及难消化食品。

18.2 消食导滞剂

是以消食导滞的药物为主组成的方剂，适用于食积证。症见脘腹痞闷，厌食嗳腐，恶心呕吐，或腹痛泄泻等。常用的药有山楂、神曲、莱菔子、枳实等，代表方剂有保和丸、枳实导滞丸等。

若脾胃虚弱，饮食不消，或食积日久，损伤脾胃者，除消导药外，尚须配伍益气健脾之品，如人参（或党参）、白术、茯苓等组成补消兼施之剂，代表方剂有健脾丸、枳术丸等。

18.3 保和丸

出自《丹溪心法》。由山楂180克，神曲60克，半夏、茯苓各90克，陈皮、连翘、莱菔子各30克组成。共研细末，水泛为丸，每服 6～9 克，日 2 次，温开水送下（亦可水煎服，用量按原方比例酌减）。方中山楂消食化滞，尤善消肉食油腻之积，为主药。神曲消食健脾，善消酒食陈腐之积；莱菔子消食下气，善消谷面之积；半夏、陈皮行气化滞，和胃止呕；茯苓健脾利湿，和胃止泻；因食积易于化热，故又佐以连翘清热散结。共奏消食和胃之功。主治各种食积证。症见脘腹痞满、胀痛、嗳腐吞酸，厌食、恶心呕吐，或大便泄泻，舌苔厚腻，脉滑等。现常用于消化不良、急性或慢性胃肠炎、慢性胃炎、慢性胰腺炎等病具有上述症状者。临床应用本方加减治疗婴幼儿消化不良属食积证者69 例，结果痊愈 61 例，进步 5 例，无效 3 例。运用保和丸加减治疗急性胆道感染 20 例，其中单纯性胆囊炎 7 例，胆石症伴胆囊炎 9 例，胆管炎 4 例，结果显效（症状体征消失，化验正常）14 例，好转（症状消失，化验正常，仍有轻度体征）5 例，无效1 例。

18.4　枳实导滞丸

出自《内外伤辨惑论》。由大黄 30 克，枳实（麸炒）、炒神曲各 15 克，茯苓、黄芩、黄连、白术各 9 克，泽泻 6 克组成。共研细末，水泛小丸，每服 6～9 克，温开水送下，日 2 次（亦可水煎服，用量按原方比例酌减）。方中大黄攻积泻热，使积滞邪热从大便而出；枳实助大黄行气消积，除脘腹之胀满；佐以黄芩、黄连清热燥湿止痢；茯苓、泽泻利水渗湿，亦可止泻；白术健脾燥湿；神曲消食和胃。共奏消导化积，清热祛湿之功。主治湿热食积，内阻肠胃之证。症见脘腹胀痛，下痢泄泻，或大便秘结，小便短黄，舌苔黄腻，脉滑数等。现常用于急性消化不良、胃肠炎、细菌性痢疾、急性或慢性胆囊炎等病具有上述症状者。本方是消食导滞之剂，若腹泻、痢疾而无积滞者不宜使用。

18.5　木香槟榔丸

引自《丹溪心法》，由木香、槟榔、青皮、陈皮、莪术、黄连、黄柏各 30 克，大黄 15 克，制香附、牵牛子各 60 克组成。诸药共研细末，水泛小丸，每服 3～6 克，温开水送下，日 2 次。方中木香、槟榔行气化滞，消脘腹痞满，且能除里急后重，为主药。牵牛子、大黄泻热通便导滞；青皮、陈皮行气化积；香附、莪术疏肝解郁，调理气血；枳壳行气导滞，健胃消食；黄连、黄柏清热燥湿止痢。共奏行气导滞，攻积泻热之功。主治积滞内停，湿热内蕴之证。症见脘腹痞满胀痛，大便脓血，里急后重，或大便秘结，舌苔黄腻，脉沉实等。现常用于急性胃肠炎、细菌性痢疾、溃疡性结肠炎等病具有上述症状者。临床上，凡便秘、腹泻、痢疾患者只要内有积滞而无外感表证，正气未虚者，均可根据中医辨证使用本方。体弱正虚者则应慎用。

18.6　枳术丸

引自《脾胃论》。由炒枳实 30 克，白术 60 克组成。共研细末，水泛为丸，每服 6～9 克，温开水送下，日 2 次（亦可水煎服，用量按原方比例酌减）。方中白术健脾祛湿以助脾之运化；枳实行气导滞，消痞除满；白术用量重于枳实 1 倍，是以益气健脾为主。共奏健脾消痞之功。主治脾虚气滞，饮食停积之证。症见脘腹痞满或胀痛，食欲不振，或腹中肠鸣，舌淡苔白滑，脉虚等。现常用于胃下垂、慢性胃炎、胃神经官能症、消化不良等病具有上述症状者。临床应用枳术丸合升陷汤加减，治疗胃下垂、子宫脱垂及脱肛，均取得较好疗效。

18.7　健脾丸

出自《证治准绳》。由白术（麸炒）75 克，木香、黄连、甘草各 22 克，茯苓 60 克，人参 45 克，炒神曲、陈皮、砂仁、炒麦芽、山楂、山药、煨肉豆蔻各 30 克组成。共研细末，水泛小丸，每服 6~9 克，温开水送下，日 2 次（亦可水煎服，用量按原方比例酌减）。方中人参、白术、茯苓、甘草补气健脾；山楂、神曲、麦芽消食化滞；木香、砂仁、陈皮理气和胃；山药、肉豆蔻健脾止泻；黄连清热燥湿。共奏健脾消食之功。主治脾胃虚弱，饮食内停之证。症见食少难消，脘腹痞闷，大便溏薄，苔腻微黄，脉象虚弱等。现常用于消化不良、慢性胃肠炎、胃神经官能症、结肠过敏、肠结核等病具有上述症状者。临床应用健脾丸配合附子理中丸治疗五更泄（一种慢性腹泻，以黎明时腹痛肠鸣，随即腹泻，泻后则舒为特征，多伴有畏寒怕冷，腰膝酸软等症，属肾虚泄泻）24 例，治疗方法：健脾丸（蜜丸，每丸重 3 克）每日 3 次，每次 1 丸，饭后服，同时服用附子理中丸每日 2 次，每次 1 丸。结果治愈 22 例，效果不显而停药者 2 例，治愈时间最短者 8 天，最长 1 个月。

18.8　消痞化积剂

是以化积消食，行气活血，软坚散结的药物为主组成的方剂。适用于腹部的癥积痞块之证。症见两胁下扪及肿块（肝、脾肿大），或脘腹痞硬，胀满疼痛，食欲不振，身体消瘦等。常用的药有枳实、厚朴、半夏、鳖甲、芍药、丹皮、桃仁等，代表方剂有枳实消痞丸、鳖甲煎丸等。

18.9　枳实消痞丸

出自《兰室秘藏》。由干姜 3 克，炙甘草、炒麦芽、茯苓、白术各 6 克，半夏曲、人参各 9 克，厚朴 12 克，枳实、黄连各 15 克组成。诸药共研细末，水泛为丸，每服 6~9 克，日 3 次，温开水送下（亦可水煎服，用量酌情增减）。方中枳实行气消痞除满，为主药。厚朴行气消胀；黄连清热燥湿，半夏曲消食和胃散结，干姜辛散温中祛寒，三药配伍，辛开苦降，调理气机，共助枳实、厚朴行气消痞；人参、白术、茯苓、甘草益气健脾；麦芽消食和胃。共奏消痞除满，健脾和胃之功。主治脾虚气滞、寒热互结之证。症见脘腹痞满，不欲饮食，倦怠乏力或腹中胀痛，便秘或腹泻，舌淡苔腻，脉弦等。现常用于消化不良、慢性胃炎、慢性肠炎、慢性胰腺炎、慢性胆囊炎等病具有上述症状者。

18.10　鳖甲煎丸

出自《金匮要略》。由鳖甲90克，射干、黄芩、鼠妇（又称地虱炒）、干姜、大黄、桂枝、石韦、厚朴、瞿麦、紫葳、阿胶各22.5克，柴胡、蜣螂（炒）各45克，芍药、丹皮、䗪虫（炒）各37克，炙蜂巢30克，赤硝90克，桃仁15克，人参、半夏、葶苈子各7.5克组成。取草木灰1.5公斤，黄酒5公斤，浸灰内过滤取汁，煎鳖甲成胶状；其余22味药共研细末，将鳖甲胶放入药粉，炼蜜和匀为小丸，每次3克，每日3次，温开水送下。方中鳖甲软坚消癥；黄酒活血通经；赤硝、大黄、䗪虫、蜣螂、鼠妇活血逐瘀消癥；柴胡、黄芩、白芍调理肝气；厚朴、射干、葶苈子、半夏理气舒郁祛痰浊；干姜、桂枝温中散结；人参、阿胶补气养血，扶助正气；桃仁、丹皮、紫葳、蜂巢活血化瘀；瞿麦、石韦利水祛湿。共奏消癥化积之功。主治各种癥瘕积聚之证。症见胁下或腹中积块，腹痛，消瘦，饮食减少，时有寒热发作，或女子闭经，舌质紫黯，或有瘀斑，脉涩等。现常用于疟疾、慢性肝炎、肝硬化、血吸虫病等病具有上述症状者。临床应用鳖甲煎丸治疗251例晚期血吸虫病肝脾肿大，治疗后，肝脾均有不同程度软化和缩小，有效率为100%，疗效巩固率为80%。

第19章 驱虫剂

19.1 驱虫剂

由驱虫药为主组成，具有驱虫、止痛、消积的作用，以治疗人体寄生虫病的方剂，统称驱虫剂。人体内的寄生虫种类很多，常见的有蛔虫、蛲虫、钩虫、绦虫等消化道的寄生虫，其成因多为饮食不洁，误食沾染虫卵的食物而引起。症见脐腹作痛，时发时止，痛而能食，面色萎黄，或青或白，或生虫斑，或嘈杂呕吐清水，舌苔剥落，脉乍大乍小。迁延日久，可见肌肉消瘦，肚大青筋外露，成为疳积。此外，唇内有红白点，是蛔虫的见症；肛门作痒，是蛲虫的独有特点；便下白色节片，是绦虫的特征；嗜食异物、面色萎黄、虚肿，则为钩虫的表现。本类方剂能驱虫、消积，对治疗上述虫证均可酌情选用。运用驱虫剂，首先要辨别虫的种类，以选择针对性强的方药，还应根据人体正气的虚实和兼证的寒热，适当与清热药、温里药、消导药、补益药相配伍。常用的药有乌梅、苦楝根皮、使君子、榧子、槟榔等，代表方剂有乌梅丸等。

驱虫剂宜空腹服用，有的还应忌食油腻。为助虫体排除，宜配合泻下药物，驱虫后，可适当调理脾胃。驱虫药多系攻伐之品，对年老、体弱、孕妇宜慎用。注意用量，过大则易伤正或中毒，不及则达不到驱虫的目的。

19.2 乌梅丸

出自《伤寒论》。由乌梅 480 克，细辛 180 克，干姜 300 克，黄连 480 克，当归 120 克，附子（炮）180 克，蜀椒（炒）120 克，桂枝 180 克，人参 180 克，黄柏 180 克组成。用 50%醋浸乌梅一宿，去核打烂，和余药打匀，晒干，研末，加蜜制丸如梧桐子大，每服9克，日1~3次，空腹温开水送下（现亦作汤剂，用量按原方比例酌减）。方中乌梅味酸性平，制蛔而安其扰动，使蛔静而痛止，为方中主药。蜀椒、细辛味辛能驱蛔，性温可温脏祛寒；桂枝、附子、干姜加强温脏祛寒；人参、当归补气养血；黄连、黄柏味苦可下蛔，性寒能清上热，又能缓和方中诸药之过于温热，以防伤阴之弊。共奏温脏安蛔之功。主治蛔厥证，以及寒热错杂而正气虚弱的久痢、久泻之证。症见心烦呕吐，时发时止，食入吐蛔，手足厥冷，腹痛，或久痢、久泻。现常用于胆道蛔虫症、慢性痢疾、慢性肠炎等病具有上述症状者。临床应用乌梅丸治疗胆道蛔虫症225例，其中包括偏寒型、寒热错杂型、偏热型。偏寒型用乌梅15~30克，槟榔、川楝子各15克，花椒、桂枝、熟附子各6克，细辛、干姜各3克。寒热错杂型用上方加黄柏9克，黄连6克。偏热型用寒热错杂方去桂枝、干姜、附子、细辛。治愈率97.6%，有效率100%。

19.3　肥儿丸

出自《太平惠民和剂局方》。由神曲（炒）300克，黄连（去须）300克，肉豆蔻（面裹煨）150克，使君子（去皮）150克，麦芽（炒）150克，槟榔120克，木香60克组成。共为细末，猪胆汁为丸，如粟米大，3岁小儿每服3克，日2次，年龄小者酌减，大者酌增。方中使君子味甘性温，槟榔味辛苦性温，两药杀虫消积，均为主药。神曲、麦芽健脾和中，消积食；黄连泻郁热，肉豆蔻健胃止泻，木香理中气而止腹痛，猪胆汁泻肝胃之热。共奏杀虫消积，健脾清热之功。主治虫积腹痛，消化不良之证。症见面黄体瘦，纳呆，肚腹胀满，脐周时痛，发热口臭，大便稀溏。现常用于小儿蛔虫症、小儿慢性消化不良、小儿营养不良等病具有上述症状者。

19.4　化虫丸

出自《太平惠民和剂局方》。由胡粉（即铅粉）1500克，鹤虱1500克，槟榔1500克，苦楝根1500克，白矾370克组成。共为细末，水泛为丸，如麻子大，1岁儿服5丸，空腹时米汤送服。方中鹤虱苦辛平，有小毒，驱杀蛔虫；苦楝根皮苦寒有毒，既可驱杀蛔虫，又可缓解腹痛；槟榔驱蛔，行气缓泻而排出虫体；枯矾解毒伏虫；铅粉有毒，性能化虫。共奏驱杀肠中诸虫之功。主治肠中诸虫。症见发作时腹中疼痛，往来上下，其痛甚剧，呕吐清水，或吐蛔虫。本方药性强烈且具毒性，使用时当适可而止，服后应调补脾胃。若虫未尽，可间隔1周再服。

第 20 章　涌吐剂

20.1　涌吐剂

由涌吐药为主组成，具有涌吐痰涎、宿食、毒物等作用，以治疗痰厥、食积、误食毒物的方剂，统称涌吐剂。本剂可使停蓄在咽喉、胸膈、胃脘的痰涎、宿食、毒物从口中吐出。常用于中风、癫狂、喉痹之痰涎壅盛，宿食停留胃脘，毒物尚留胃中，以及干霍乱吐泻不得等，属于病情急迫而又急需吐出之证。常用的药有瓜蒂、皂角等，代表方剂有瓜蒂散、救急稀涎散等。

涌吐剂作用迅猛，易伤胃气，应中病即止，年老体弱、孕妇产后均宜慎用。若服后呕吐不止者，可服用姜汁少许，或服用冷粥、冷开水等以止之。若吐仍不止，则应根据所服吐剂的不同而进行解救，如服瓜蒂散而吐不止者，可服麝香 0.03～0.06 克，或丁香 0.3～0.6 克解之；若吐后气逆不止，宜予和胃降逆之剂以止之；若药后不吐者，则应助其涌吐，常以翎毛或手指探喉，亦可多饮开水，以助其吐。服药得吐后，须避风，以防止吐后体虚而患外感。需注意调理脾胃，宜用稀粥调养，切勿骤进油腻及不易消化之食物，以免重伤胃气。

20.2　瓜蒂散

出自《伤寒论》。由瓜蒂（熬黄）4 克，赤小豆 4 克，豆豉 9 克组成。将前 2 味药研细末和匀，每服 1～3 克，用豆豉 9 克煎汤送服。方中瓜蒂味苦性寒，善吐痰涎宿食，为主药。赤小豆味酸，能祛湿除烦满，与瓜蒂相伍，具有酸苦涌泄之性；豆豉煎汤调服，宣解胸中之邪气，与赤小豆配伍，可和胃气而使吐不伤正。共奏涌吐痰涎宿食之功。主治痰涎宿食壅滞胸脘之证。症见胸中痞硬，懊𢙐不宁，气上冲咽喉不得息，寸脉微浮。现常用于误食毒物、宿食等病具有上述症状者。本方瓜蒂苦寒有毒，体虚患者，须禁用；若宿食已离胃入肠，或痰涎不在胸膈，均须禁用。

20.3　救急稀涎散

出自《圣济总录》。由猪牙皂角15克，白矾30克组成。共为细末，每服2～3克，温水调下。方中皂角味辛咸性温，辛能开窍，咸能软坚，可涤除浊腻之痰，为主药。白矾酸苦涌泄，能化顽痰，并有开闭催吐之效。共奏开关涌吐之功。主治中风闭证。症见喉中痰声漉漉，气闭不通，胸中烦闷，两目昏花，或倒仆不省，或口角似歪，脉滑实有力。现常用于脑血栓、慢性咽炎等病具有上述症状者。本方是催吐之剂，当痰稀涎出，咽喉疏通后，宜随证改用他药继调之。

第 21 章　痈疡剂

21.1　痈疡剂

由消除痈疡药为主组成。具有解毒消肿、托里排脓、生肌敛疮的作用，以治疗体表痈、疽、疔、疮、丹毒、流注、瘰、瘤、瘰疬等，以及内在脏腑的痈疽等病证。体表痈疡辨证，须将体表局部症状和全身情况结合在一起辨证，以此分为阴阳虚实，及其善恶顺逆、肿形高起、范围局限、根脚收缩、皮肤红赤、灼热等属于阳证；外形平塌、坚硬或棉软、范围松散、皮色不变等属于阴证。痈疡发于内在脏腑，如肺痈、肠痈等，在辨证上须分寒热虚实、已成脓或未成脓。体表痈疡的治法有内治法和外治法两类，方剂学所要介绍的，主要是用于前者的方剂。内治法有消、托、补3法之分，消法用于痈疡尚未成脓的初期，根据证候的不同，消法包括解表、通里、清热、温通、祛痰、行气、活血行瘀等；托法用于痈疡中期，可使内毒移深就浅，促其易溃、易敛，托法有内托和补托之分，前者是消散透脓为主，兼以扶正，后者是扶正与透脓两顾，补法用于痈疡后期，气血双虚而见脓液清稀、疮口久溃不敛等症，通过补益使气血充实，促其溃处生肌收敛，对未溃者可托毒外透，使其速溃早敛。痈疡发于内在脏腑的治法，是以清热解毒、逐瘀排脓、散结消肿为主，清热解毒、逐瘀排脓的方药，可使毒解瘀化，肿结自消，脓排腐祛，可使溃处易于修复。常用的药有双花、连翘、穿山甲、皂刺、乳香、没药、黄芪、薏苡仁等，代表方剂有仙方活命饮、五味消毒饮、四妙勇安汤、大黄牡丹汤、阳和汤等。

临床运用痈疡剂，须根据病情变化，随证加减使用；痈疡已成，固执内消一法，则易损伤气血，以至难溃、难敛。毒盛使用托，应注意解毒，防止余毒留恋。化脓迟缓，须注意攻透，力求毒随脓泄，防止内陷。体表痈疡火毒炽盛时，禁用温补。痈疡余毒未尽时，不宜用纯补。

21.2　仙方活命饮

出自《校注妇人良方》。由白芷、贝母、防风、赤芍、生归尾、甘草节、皂角刺（炒）、穿山甲（炙）、天花粉、乳香、没药各3克，金银花、陈皮各9克组成。水煎分2次服（或水酒各半煎服）。方中金银花味甘性寒，清热解毒，为主药。防风、白芷疏散外邪，使热毒从外透解；归尾、赤芍、乳香、没药活血散瘀，以消肿止痛；贝母、花粉清热散结；山甲、皂刺通行经络，透脓溃坚；陈皮理气，甘草解毒、和中。共奏清热解毒，消肿溃坚，活血止痛之功。主治痈疡肿毒初起，热毒壅聚，气滞血瘀之证。症见痈疡红肿焮痛，或身热微恶寒，苔薄白或黄，脉数有力。现常用于蜂窝织炎、乳腺炎、化脓性扁桃体炎等病具有上述症状者。临床应用仙方活命饮治疗阑尾脓肿30例，基本方由金银花、连翘、花粉、贝母、皂刺、生地、丹皮、赤芍、归尾、甘草、蒲公英、乳香、没药组成。经治疗，27例痊愈，3例中转手术，成功率为90%，无1例死亡。平均住院时间14日，随访7例未见复发。运用仙方活命饮加减治疗重症有头疽129例，热毒型加用清热解毒之药，正虚型合八珍汤，阴虚型合六味地黄汤，单纯中药治疗者82例，短期（7天左右）加用抗菌素治疗者47例，疗程15～20天14例，21～30天20例，31～40天17例，41～50天29例，51～60天21例，60天以上者28例，结果痊愈127例，占98.5%，死亡2例，占1.5%，其中1例死于败血症，1例因年老体虚并发紫癜性肾炎，死于肾功能衰竭，129例病例入院前多数经过抗菌素治疗无效。

仙方活命饮在试管内对乙型链球菌有高度抑制作用，对葡萄球菌抑制作用也很强，但对大肠杆菌及绿脓杆菌无效。

21.3　五味消毒饮

出自《医宗金鉴》。由银花 20 克，野菊花、蒲公英、紫花地丁、紫背天葵子各 15 克组成。水煎分 2 次服。方中金银花味甘性寒，清热解毒，为主药。地丁、天葵、蒲公英、野菊花均有清热解毒之功，并能凉血散结以消肿痛。共奏清热解毒，消散疔疮之功。主治火毒结聚的痈疮疔肿。症见初起局部红肿热痛，或发热恶寒，或疮形如粟，坚硬根深，状如铁钉，舌红苔黄，脉数。现常用于蜂窝织炎、乳腺炎、化脓性扁桃体炎、淋巴结炎、腮腺炎等病具有上述症状者。临床应用五味消毒饮治疗颜面疔 20 例，症见局部焮赤肿痛，中央有粟米状的脓头，麻痒疼痛，伴有恶寒发热，心烦口渴，恶心呕吐，食少便秘，舌苔白腻或黄腻，脉沉实或弦有力。以本方为主，酌情配合外用药外敷，均取得较满意的效果。运用五味消毒饮加减治疗慢性骨髓炎 7 例，症见局部肿胀疼痛，溃后流脓久不收口，以致形成瘘管，长期不愈，或反复破溃，基本方由银花、蒲公英、紫花地丁、牛膝、白芷、甲珠、蜈蚣、全虫组成，酌配以外用药。经治疗，均获治愈。

21.4　四妙勇安汤

出自《验方新编》。由金银花、玄参各 90 克，当归 30 克，甘草 15 克组成。水煎分 3 次服。方中金银花味甘性寒，清热解毒，为主药。玄参泻火解毒，当归活血散瘀，甘草解毒缓痛。共奏清热解毒，活血止痛之功。主治热毒炽盛之脱疽。症见患肢红肿灼热，溃烂腐臭，疼痛剧烈，或见发热口渴，舌红脉数。现常用于血栓闭塞性脉管炎、栓塞性大静脉炎等病具有上述症状者。临床应用四妙勇安汤加减治疗血栓闭塞性脉管炎 25 例，发病部位均在下肢。虚塞型加附子、干姜、桂枝、鸡血藤、黄芪。气滞血瘀型加红花、桃仁、泽兰、王不留行。热毒型加蒲公英、地丁、黄芩、黄柏、气血两虚加党参、黄芪、白术、去玄参和金银花。经治疗，痊愈者 10 例，好转者 11 例，未效者 4 例，总有效率达 84%。运用四妙勇安汤加味治疗慢性肝炎 33 例。患者均治疗病程长，远期疗效不佳，HBsAg 持续阳性，其中慢性迁延性者 12 例，慢性活动性者 21 例。基本方由玄参、生黄芪、土茯苓各 30 克，当归、升麻各 15 克，忍冬藤、白茅根各 60 克，甘草 10 克，黄疸加茵陈、苦参，脾大加鸡内金、炮山甲，寒湿困脾加干姜、苍术、白术，瘀血加丹参、川芎，出血明显加仙鹤草、参三七。30 剂为 1 个疗程，均配合用维生素，2 例加辅酶 Q_{10}，结果显效 25 例，有效 6 例，无效 2 例，总有效率 94%。

21.5 犀黄丸

出自《外科全生集》。由犀黄 3 克，麝香 15 克，乳香、没药（各去油）各 100 克，黄米饭 100 克组成。前 4 味共为细末，用黄米饭捣烂为丸，每次 9 克，日 3 次。方中牛黄味苦甘性凉，清热解毒，豁痰散结，为主药。麝香辛窜，既能活血散结，又能通经活络；乳香、没药活血祛瘀，消肿定痛；黄米饭调养胃气。共奏解毒消痈，化痰散结，活血祛瘀之功。主治火郁、痰瘀热毒壅滞而致的乳岩、横痃、瘰疬、痰核、流注、肺痈、小肠痈等证。症见局部有大小不等的肿块，肿块坚如石，形体消瘦，溃后难以收敛，或漫肿疼痛，皮色如常，或发生部位不固定，易走窜等。本方药物多辛香走窜，不宜久服，孕妇忌服。临床应用西黄丸加味治疗颈淋巴结结核 1 例，用抗痨药治疗未效，穿刺后感染溃破，流豆渣样脓液黄水，基本方由西黄丸加昆布、海藻、夏枯草、牡蛎等药组成，外敷五行丹、桃花五宝丹，获得较好疗效，愈后肌肤光泽如常，无疤痕溃留。

21.6 牛蒡解肌汤

出自《疡科心得集》，由牛蒡子 10 克，薄荷 6 克，荆芥 6 克，连翘 10 克，山栀 10 克，丹皮 10 克，石斛 12 克，玄参 10

克，夏枯草 12 克组成。水煎分 2 次服。方中牛蒡子味辛苦性寒，疏散头面风热，为主药。薄荷、荆芥发汗解表；连翘清热解毒，散结消痈；丹皮、山栀、夏枯草泻火凉血，玄参泻火解毒，与石斛相伍，滋阴清热。共奏疏风清热，凉血消肿之功。主治痈肿兼有风热表证。症见外痈焮红肿痛，寒轻热重，汗少口渴，小便黄，或牙痛，苔白或黄，脉脬数。现常用于颈淋巴结炎、牙周炎、流行性感冒等病具有上述症状者。

21.7　海藻玉壶汤

出自《医宗金鉴》。由海藻、昆布、半夏（制）、陈皮、青皮、连翘、贝母、当归、川芎、独活、甘草节各 3 克，海带 1.5 克组成。水煎分 2 次服。方中海藻、昆布、海带味咸性寒，化痰软坚，均为主药。青皮、陈皮疏肝理气，当归、川芎、独活活血而通经脉，促进瘿病消散；贝母、连翘散结消肿；甘草调和诸药。共奏化痰软坚，消散瘿瘤之功。主治肝脾不调、气滞痰凝之证。症见颈部瘿瘤，坚硬如石，推之不移，皮色不变。现常用于颈部癌肿、甲状腺腺瘤、甲状腺肿大等病具有上述症状者。

21.8　透脓散

出自《外科正宗》。由生黄芪 12 克，当归 6 克，穿山甲 3 克，皂角刺 5 克，川芎 9 克组成。水煎分 2 次服（临服入酒 1 杯亦可）。方中生黄芪味甘性微温，益气托毒，为主药。当归、川芎养血活血；山甲、皂刺消散通透，软坚溃脓；用酒少许，增强行血活血。共奏托毒溃脓之功。主治正虚不能托毒之证。症见痈疡肿痛，内已成脓，外不易溃，漫肿无头，或酸胀热痛。现常用于各种化脓性感染具有上述症状者。

21.9 阳和汤

出自《外科全生集》。由熟地 30 克，肉桂（去皮，研粉）3 克，麻黄 2 克，鹿角胶 9 克，白芥子 6 克，姜炭 2 克，生甘草 3 克组成。水煎分 2 次服。方中熟地味甘性微温，补营养血，为主药。鹿角胶填精补髓，强壮筋骨，藉血肉有情之品，助熟地以养血；炮姜、肉桂温中有通，温散寒凝；麻黄开腠理以达表，白芥子祛皮里膜外之痰；生甘草化毒和药。共奏温阳补血，散寒通滞之功。主治阴疽之阳虚寒凝证。症见患处漫肿无头，疼痛无热，皮色不变，口中不渴，舌苔淡白，脉沉细。现常用于骨结核、慢性骨髓炎、类风湿性关节炎、血栓闭寒性脉管炎等病具有上述症状者。临床应用阳和汤合犀黄丸治疗骨结核 60 例，以阳和汤为主方，阳虚者重用肉桂、炮姜、白介子的用量，并配合犀黄丸等内外同治。疗程 5 个月左右，结果 X 线证实骨质完全愈合，临床症状消失者 19 例，骨质的破坏停止，部分吸收好转，临床症状减轻者 8 例，临床症状减轻，但未经 X 线复查者 33 例。运用阳和汤加味治疗坐骨神经炎 30 例，结果病例疗程一般为 10～20天，大都服药 1～2 剂后自觉发热汗出，疼痛即有缓解，服药 5～8 剂后，疼痛明显减轻，病程短而痛剧者疗效高，疗程也短，反之则疗程较长而疗效亦差，服药期间未见不良反应。

21.10 内补黄芪汤

出自《外科发挥》。由黄芪（盐水拌炒）、麦门冬、熟地黄（酒拌）、人参、茯苓各 10 克，甘草（炙）、白芍（炒）、远志（炒）、川芎、肉桂、当归（酒拌）各 5 克，生姜 3 斤，大枣 1 枚组成。水煎分 2 次服。方中黄芪味甘性微温，益气生肌，为主药。人参、茯苓、甘草健脾益气；当归、熟地、白芍、川芎养血补肝；肉桂温助阳气，麦冬滋阴养心，远志宁心安神。共奏补益气血、养阴生肌之功。主治痈疽溃后的气血双虚之证。症见痈疽溃处作痛，倦怠懒言，纳差，寐少，自汗口干，间或发热经久不退，舌淡苔薄，脉细弱。现常用于慢性溃疡、慢性骨髓炎等病具有上述症状者。

21.11　苇茎汤

出自《备急千金要方》。由苇茎 30 克，薏苡仁 30 克，冬瓜子 24 克，桃仁 9 克组成。水煎分 2 次服。方中苇茎味甘性寒，清肺泄热，为主药。冬瓜仁、薏苡仁清化痰热，利湿排脓；桃仁活血祛瘀，润肠通便。共奏清肺化痰，逐瘀排脓之功。主治热毒蕴肺，痰瘀互结之证。症见肺痈咳嗽，微热，甚则咳吐腥臭痰，胸中隐隐作痛，肌肤甲错，舌红苔黄腻，脉滑数。现常用于肺脓疡、大叶性肺炎、支气管扩张、肺气肿等病具有上述症状者。临床应用苇茎汤合桔梗汤加味治疗肺脓疡 12 例，除 1 例因故中断治疗外，全部治愈，治疗时间最短者 6 天，最长者 16 天，平均为 9.5 天。运用苇茎汤加减治疗小儿急性支气管炎 200 例，轻型138 例，重型 62 例，病程 1～2 日，基本方由鲜芦根 30 克，冬瓜子、薏苡仁各 12 克，桃仁、杏仁、前胡、白前各 4.5 克，苏子、莱菔子、玉蝴蝶各 6 克，胆星 3 克组成，每日 1 剂，分 3～4 次温服，年长儿可 1 次顿服，结果治愈 169 例，无效 31 例，治愈率 84.5%。

21.12　大黄牡丹汤

出自《金匮要略》。由大黄 18 克，牡丹皮 9 克，桃仁 12克，冬瓜子 30 克，芒硝 9 克组成。水煎顿服。方中大黄泻肠间瘀热结聚，清热解毒，丹皮味苦辛性寒，清热凉血，均为主药。芒硝软坚散结，助大黄荡涤速下，桃仁性善破血，助牡丹皮、大黄活血散瘀，并能通便，冬瓜仁清湿热，排脓散结消痈。共奏泻热破瘀、散结消肿之功。主治肠痈初起的湿热瘀滞之证。症见右少腹疼痛拒按，甚则局部有痞块，小便自调，时时发热，自汗出，复恶寒，或右足屈而不伸，脉滑数。现常用于急性阑尾炎、子宫附件炎、盆腔炎、输精管结扎术后感染等病具有上述症状者。临床应用大黄牡丹汤加减治疗急性阑尾炎 100 例，其中包括阑尾穿孔合并腹膜炎 9 例，阑尾包块 7 例，18 例加用抗菌素，平均 6.5 天治愈，仅 1 例病情加重转手术治疗。运用大黄牡丹汤加苍术、薏苡仁、甘草，治疗 74 例输精管结扎术后局部感染的患者，症见附睾肿大，精索粗硬，掣引小腹胀痛及腰痛不适，或伴有头晕，食欲不振，小便黄赤，大便干燥，或感染不重，仅有局部疼痛不适，结果均治愈。

大黄牡丹汤加当归、银花、连翘、枳壳、桔梗、甘草对家兔实验，可增强机体全身和局部网状内皮系统的防御能力。

21.13　薏苡附子败酱散

出自《金匮要略》。由薏苡仁 30 克，附子 6 克，败酱草 15 克组成。水煎分 2 次服（原作散剂）。方中薏苡仁味甘淡性微寒，利湿消肿，为主药。败酱草排脓解毒；附子辛温，助苡仁散寒湿，并藉以行郁滞之气。共奏排脓消肿之功。主治肠痈的寒湿瘀血互结之证。症见肠痈已成脓，身无热，肌肤甲错，腹皮急，如肿胀，按之濡软，脉数。现常用于急性阑尾炎合并化脓、阑尾周围脓肿、慢性阑尾炎等病具有上述症状者。临床应用薏苡附子败酱散加味配合抗菌素治疗阑尾脓肿 36 例，基本方由熟附子 1.5 克，薏苡仁 30 克，败酱草 30 克，桃仁、红花、广木香各 9 克组成，日 2 剂，服 4 次，第 4 天起每日改服 1 剂，服 2 次，直至肿块消失为止。服中药期间，肌注青霉素，每日 80 万单位，分 4 次注射，本组除 1 例因复发性腹膜炎行手术引流外，其余 35 例全部脓肿消失，平均住院天数 5 天。

THE ENGLISH–CHINESE ENCYCLOPEDIA OF PRACTICAL TCM
(Booklist)

英汉实用中医药大全

(书目)

VOLUME	TITLE	书名
1	ESSENTIALS OF TRADITIONAL CHIN ESE MEDICINE	中医学基础
2	THE CHINESE MATERIA MEDICA	中药学
3	PHARMACOLOGY OF TRADITION-AL CHINESE MEDICAL FORMULAE	方剂学
4	SIMPLE AND PROVEN PRESCRIPTION	单验方
5	COMMONLY USED CHINESE PATENTMEDICINES	常用中成药
6	THERAPY OF ACUPUNCTURE AND MOXIBUSTION	针灸疗法
7	*TUINA* THERAPY	推拿疗法
8	MEDICAL *QIGONG*	医学气功
9	MAINTAINING YOUR HEALTH	自我保健
10	INTERNAL MEDICINE	内科学

V. G. Gorshkov

Gorškov, Viktor G.

Physical and Biological Bases of Life Stability

Man, Biota, Environment

With 37 Figures

Springer-Verlag

Berlin Heidelberg New York
London Paris Tokyo
Hong Kong Barcelona
Budapest

Professor Dr. Victor G. Gorshkov

St. Petersburg Nuclear Physics Institute
Gatchina, St. Petersburg 188350, Russia

ISBN 3-540-57049-7 Springer-Verlag Berlin Heidelberg New York
ISBN 0-387-57049-7 Springer-Verlag New York Berlin Heidelberg

Library of Congress Cataloging-in-Publication Data. Gorshkov, V. G. (Victor G.), 1935- Physical and biological bases of life stability: man, biota, environment / V. G. Gorshkov. p. cm. Includes bibliographical references and index. ISBN 3-540-57049-7 (Berlin: acid-free paper). – ISBN 0-387-57049-7 (New York: acid-free paper) 1. Environmental policy. 2. Man–Influence on nature. 3. Biotic communities. 4. Ecosystem management. I. Title. GE170.G68 1994 363.7–dc20 94-21157

© Springer-Verlag Berlin Heidelberg 1995
Printed in Germany

The use of general descriptive names, registered names, trademarks, etc. in this publication does not imply, even in the absence of a specific statement, that such names are exempt from the relevant protective laws and regulations and therefore free for general use.

Typesetting: Data conversion by Springer-Verlag
SPIN: 10080719   55/3140 - 5 4 3 2 1 0 - Printed on acid-free paper

Preface

It is well known that the biochemical processes of life on Earth are maintained by the external solar radiation and can be reduced to the synthesis and decomposition of organic matter. Man has added the synthesis and decomposition of various industrial products to these natural processes. On one hand, biological synthesis may only be conducted within the rather narrow margins of parameters of the environment, including temperature, humidity, concentrations of the inorganic substances used by life (such as carbon dioxide, oxygen, etc.) On the other hand, the physical and chemical composition of the environment suffers significant changes during those processes of synthesis and decomposition.

The maximum possible rate of such change due to the activity of living beings can exceed the average geophysical rates of change of the environment due to activity of terrestrial depths and cosmic processes by a factor of ten thousand. In the absence of a rigid correlation between the biological synthesis and decomposition, the environment would be greatly disturbed within a decade and driven into a state unfit for life. A lifeless Earth, however would suffer similar changes only after about a hundred thousand years. Preservation of the existing state of the environment is only possible with strict equality between the rates of biological synthesis and decomposition, that is, when the biochemical cycles of matter are virtually closed.

The environment of living beings is regularly subjected to sudden external perturbations such as volcanic eruptions, the fall of large meteorites, and other major geophysical and cosmic fluctuations. Return to the initial state after such perturbations can only be achieved through the compensation of such changes by the living beings, distorting the biochemical cycles from their closed states. The enormous power of synthesis and destruction developed by the Earth biota is necessary to quickly compensate for the various external perturbations.

Numerous different species of living organisms can exist in the present environment, including various domesticated plants and animals. However, an arbitrary set of living things with adequate life capacity cannot maintain the stability of the environment. It is only a strictly defined set of species, forming rigidly correlated communities, which is capable of keeping the environment in a state fit for life. Each species in the community fulfills its precisely prescribed role in stabilizing the environment. There are no "lazybone" species in the community performing no work, and, moreover, there are no villain species that would disrupt the internal correlation of the community. It is the full set of such natural communities which comprises the Earth biota. Within a time period of several thousand years, only random variations around its stable state could take place and the biota should not have to adapt to any random change in the environment (Sect. 3.9).

The evolutionary transition from one stable state of the biota and its habitat to another takes about a million years; that is the time of species formation.

Thus processes in outer space and in the Earth's core, external with respect to the biosphere, result in a directional change of the environment. Such changes should have brought the terrestrial environment to a state unfit for life, similar to those found on the surface of Mars or Venus, in several million years. Solar radiation by itself does not change the composition of the environment and does not affect the processes in the Earth's core. Using solar radiation as a source of energy, life organizes the processes of transformation of the environment, basing them on the dynamically closed matter cycles, their fluxes exceeding the fluxes of destruction of the environment by the external forces by many orders of magnitude. This is what enables the biota to compensate for practically any adverse changes in the environment by directional change of biochemical cycles from their closed character. This is how life can ensure the stability of an environment fit for its own existence.

It is apparent, however, that there is some threshold level of perturbation of both the natural biota and the environment above which the stability of both is broken. Man's activities during the pre-industrial era did not produce any apparent changes in the natural biota. The biota of non-perturbed natural communities was then capable of compensating for every perturbation of the environment produced by man's activities. There arose no problems of protecting the environment from pollution, and so there was no need for any closed cycle technologies. Such a situation prevailed until the beginning of the industrial era in the last century.

During the present century a significant restructuring of natural biota has occurred, and the rate of pollution of the environment by industrial wastes has drastically increased. As a result the perturbed biota has lost its capacity to compensate for anthropogenic perturbations, and the environment has started to change on a global scale. Any directional change in the existing environment means the loss of its stability and is thus unfavorable for the biota and man.

Escape from the situation thus formed is usually thought to be in a transition to no-waste technologies and to ecologically clean energy sources. However, that is no solution to the task of preserving the environment. Any industrial activity by man is based on energy consumption and involves land use and hence transforming the natural biota. The present-day land biota, perturbed by man, is not only incapable of compensating for anthropogenic perturbations, but perturbs the environment itself at a rate similar in order of magnitude to that generated by the industrial enterprises themselves (Sect. 4.11). Further perturbation of natural biota via ever-increasing industrial activities based on ecologically absolutely clean energy sources may drive the biota into a totally open state. In that case the rate of perturbation of the environment by the perturbed biota will exceed many-fold that due to activities of modern industrial enterprises. The transition to no-waste technologies will not result in any practical changes in the situation. It will only overcome the apparent local pollution. It is not possible to substitute the natural biota by a technosphere operating, similar to the biota, by the reproducible solar energy: information fluxes in the biota exceed the maximum possible information fluxes in the technosphere by 15 orders of magnitude (Sect. 2.8).

The real breakthrough consists in recovering the natural biota to the extent necessary to support stability of the environment on a global scale. That calls for a reduction in the scope of industrial activities and in the overall human energy consumption on the planet by means of negative population growth.

This book aims to clarify the laws by which the natural biota and man function. That way, the admissible threshold of perturbation disrupting the stability of the biosphere may be estimated, as well as the necessary reductions of contemporary anthropogenic perturbations.

The book is structured as follows: The first chapter briefly describes the contents of the monograph, gives the principal quantitative results and stresses the most important conclusions. The subsequent chapters expound in fine detail on, and produce detailed quantitative arguments and evidence for, the individual claims set forth in the first chapter. The author hopes that the reader will have a clear enough understanding of the message after reading that chapter. As for the more detailed information on any particular question it can be found in one of the follow-up chapters.

Acknowledgements. The author expresses his sincere gratitude to Bert Bolin for his helpful critical comments on the CO_2 problem; to Paul Damon for valuable discussions of the radiocarbon data and the action of the Le Chatelier principle in the biosphere; to Viktor Dolnik for many years of discussing the problems of general biology; to Mikhail Filatov for discussions and critical comments on molecular biology; to Valery Gavrilov for discussing the energetics of birds; to Vadim Gorshkov for consulting the author on problems of botany and general ecology; to Motoo Kimura for providing the author with a voluminous set of key studies in the neutral theory; to Alexey Kondrashov for long discussions on the problems of evolution; to Kirill Kondratiev for cooperation and help in joint studies and for discussion of problems of climatology; to Kym Losev for valuable discussion of the water cycle and the principal ecological problems; to James Lovelock for his extended written communication with the author discussing the Gaia hypothesis and the problems of local adaptation; to Mikhail Prokofiev for his critical comments on general scientific questions and for help in translating the manuscript into English; to Valentin Rybchin for affording the author opportunities in teaching and discussing the problems of genetic engineering; to Leonid Rodin for frequent discussions of problems of global ecology, and for introducing the author to classic studies on the subject; to Semyon Sherman for his fruitful cooperation in many problems of ecology; to Galina Stepanova for help in composing the text; to Peter Williams for his constructive critical review of the first ecological study by the author (Gorshkov, 1979); and to Georgy Winberg for his strong support of the author's work, numerous consultations in all the questions of biology, and permission to use unique books from his private library. This work was partly supported by International Science Foundation (grant N R2Y000).

St. Petersburg   *V. Gorshkov*

Table of Contents

1. Ecological Stability

1.1 Introduction

The aim of all ecological studies is to give a scientific answer to the question: just what are the normal conditions of human existence and how may these be secured for both the present and future generations? Man exists in his environment. Therefore ecological studies should first of all provide for conservation of an environment fit for man's existence.

If the result shows that changes in the environment are mainly controlled by erroneous management of business, the ecological problem would turn into a problem of finding out possible ways of organizing these activities such that they do not alter the environment (Schneider, 1989a). The problems of protecting the wilderness areas and of preserving wild species in both the fauna and flora would then only be secondary, related mainly to catering to the aesthetic tastes of man. Preserving the unique gene pools of the wild species in their natural conditions, as well as in reserves, zoos, and gene banks would then become a purely applied interest, having nothing to do with the ecological task of protecting the environment. Reserves, negligibly small in their areal extent, would serve merely as wild nature memorials, fit only for studies by some narrow circle of dedicated experts. It is apparent that many wild species can only survive if at least 30% of habitable land surface is withdrawn from industrial use (Wilson, 1989). However, mankind will certainly never go to those extremes if all the above is true, and the respective species would be doomed to die out without causing any great concern in the general public.

If, on the other hand, it appears that the communities of natural biospheric species completely control and support the existing state of the environment in which man himself exists, then protection of the wilderness areas, preservation of the natural communities of all the wild species and estimating the threshold of admissible perturbations in the natural biota become the central problem and task of ecology. The restructuring of industry towards a lower level of environmental pollution is then reduced to a local task of second priority which is, strictly speaking, not related to ecology itself.

The task of the present study is to demonstrate that it is impossible to preserve a stable environment fit for man's existence within the prevailing tendencies in restructuring the natural biota and the biosphere.

1.2 Biological Regulation of the Environment

Now, what exactly are the environment, the biota, and the biosphere? All the fundamental notions used by natural science are characterized by their measurable properties. Since the knowledge of these properties is enriched as science develops, the definitions of these fundamental notions change too with time. For example, such fundamental definitions as those of mass and energy have passed through some impressive changes during the last hundred years or so (Sect. 2.6). The term *biota* was initially introduced to combine the two notions of fauna and flora. The environment includes substances and bodies from the biota with which the given living organism interacts. Following Vernadsky (1945) the biosphere is understood to be the global biota plus its environment. The biosphere also includes the external environment (such as the upper atmospheric layers, for example), in which one can find no living beings, but which is intimately connected with the immediate environment of the biota. However, all such definitions only indicate the study target. As our knowledge accumulates, these concepts are filled with new content.

The environment is first of all characterized by certain concentrations of chemical substances consumed by living beings. For those organisms busy destroying organic matter (such as bacteria, fungi, and animals) the important concentrations are those of such organic matter and of oxygen in soil, water, and air, while for plants, which synthesize such organic matter, they are the concentrations of inorganic substances: carbon dioxide, certain chemical compounds including nitrogen, phosphorus, and many other elements used in the bodies of living organisms. The question arises then, whether the concentrations of all those compounds (often called nutrients, biogenes, or biogenic elements, Kendeigh, 1974; Ivanoff, 1972, 1975) in the environment are random from the point of view of the biota, or whether the concentrations are established by the biota itself, and maintained by it at an optimal level for life?

In the first case, the biota should function continuously, adapting to the changing environment. However, concentrations of inorganic nutrients may change by about 100 % within time periods of the order of a hundred thousand years due to geochemical processes alone (Budyko et al., 1987; Barnola et al., 1991). Thus, during the lifespan of life in general, which already covers several billions of years, the concentration of practically every nutrient should have changed by several orders of magnitude, reaching values at which no life can exist at all. The Earth's environment should have reached a state similar to that found on the other planets within the solar system (cf. Sect. 2.7).

Naturally, the biota is incapable of altering such natural parameters as the extraterrestrial flux of solar radiation, the rate of Earth's rotation, the magnitude of tides, the terrestrial relief, or the level of volcanic activity. However, adverse changes and random fluctuations in these characteristics may be compensated for by the biota via directional change of concentrations of nutrients in the environment, which it controls, so that the overall reaction is similar to the action of the Le Chatelier principle in physical and chemical stable states (Lotka, 1925; Redfield, 1958; Lovelock, 1972, 1982).

At a prescribed flux of solar radiation the Earth's surface temperature is controlled by the rate of evaporation of moisture from the surface, by the concentrations of certain atmospheric gases producing the greenhouse effect, mainly water vapor and carbon dioxide, and by the albedo – that is, the coefficient of reflectance of solar radiation by the atmosphere and the Earth's surface (Sect. 2.7). The present day average surface temperature is 15 °C (Allen, 1955). A change of that value by 100 °C in either direction would also have resulted in all life perishing. A practically unequivocal conclusion follows: namely that living beings should not use any substances whose concentrations are not subject to biological regulation. Hence, these substances should not be included in the concept of the environment. Moreover, biologically regulated processes and concentrations of substances should define the values of characteristics of the environment such as temperature, the spectral composition of solar radiation reaching the Earth's surface, the regime of evaporation and water precipitation on land.

The measurable natural parameters affecting the biota, supported by the biota at a certain quantitative levels, and liable to directional change by the biota in response to external forces, may be found step by step. In what is to follow we are going to include in the concept of the biosphere only those characteristics that are controlled by the biota. The components of nature bearing traces of former life activity in the geological past (the traces of late biospheres, Vernadsky, 1945), not subject to contemporary biospheric forcing, will be excluded from such concepts. We shall further call "nutrients" only those substances (biospheric components) whose concentrations are controlled by the biota (Redfield, 1958). If we stick to such definitions, no preliminary hypothesising is necessary concerning components of nature with which the biota interacts, and which might be controlled by life (Redfield, 1958; Lovelock, 1972). The presence or the absence of such control can be directly or indirectly found by empirical means.

1.3 Means of Biological Regulation of the Environment

The effect of biota upon the environment can be reduced to the synthesis of organic matter from inorganic components, and to the decomposition of that matter into its inorganic components, and, hence, to a changing ratio between the stores of organic and inorganic substances in the biosphere. The rate of synthesis of the organic matter defines production of, and that of decomposition, destruction of, that matter. Since the organic substances entering living organisms bear a constant ratio to the chemical elements forming them, production and destruction are usually measured by the mass of organic carbon synthesized or destroyed per unit time. On average, synthesizing 1 g of organic carbon in the biota requires the absorption (or release in case of destruction) of 42 kJ of energy (Kendeigh, 1974; Odum, 1983). Production or destruction of 1 tonne (t) of organic carbon per year (1 t C/year) corresponds to energy absorption or release at a power of 1.3 kW. The power of biota should be understood as its production, measured in energy units.

The biota is capable of producing local concentrations of nutrients in the environment differing by 100% or more from the concentrations in the external environment (where no living beings function), when the fluxes of synthesis and destruction of organic matter per unit surface area (called productivity and destructivity) exceed the physical fluxes of nutrient transport. Such a situation is found in soil, where the physical flux of nutrient diffusion is significantly lower than biological productivity. That is why soil is enriched by organic matter and by the inorganic substances necessary for plant life, as compared to lower ground layers where there are no living organisms. Hence, local concentrations of nutrients in soil are biologically regulated.

Concentrations of dissolved carbon dioxide (CO_2) in the depths of oceans are several times larger than at the surface. At the same time the surface concentration of CO_2 is at equilibrium with that in the atmosphere. If life ceased in the ocean, all the concentrations at depths and at the surface would even out. The concentration of CO_2 at the surface and in the atmosphere would then increase severalfold! That could result in catastrophic changes in the scope of the greenhouse effect and in the planetary climate within decades. Hence, the oceanic biota determines the atmospheric concentration of CO_2 and thus regulates the greenhouse effect, keeping the surface temperature at a level acceptable for life in general (Sect. 4.9).

The $N/P/O_2$ concentration ratios in oceanic waters coincide with the ratios of these elements absorbed during synthesis (released during destruction) of the organic matter of living bodies in the ocean. That consideration points to biotic control of these components in the ocean as well (Redfield, 1958).

If the physical fluxes of nutrient transport exceed biological productivity by a factor of several hundred, the concentrations of those nutrients in the environment may only differ from their concentrations in the external environment by several tenths of one per cent due to activities of living beings. However, if the biota acquires any appreciable advantage that way (in other words, if such changes fall within the margin of biotic resolution), these differences will be supported by the biota in that direction. The resulting difference in concentrations will trigger physical fluxes of nutrients from the external environment to internal and back again. Such fluxes will keep on flowing until the concentrations in the external and internal environments even out, that is the concentration of nutrients in both media reaches an optimal value for the biota. Thus biota is also capable of regulating the global concentrations of nutrients in the external environment, so the latter should also be included in the definition of the biosphere.

For example, excessive carbon dioxide in the external environment may be transformed into comparatively inactive or dead organic forms by the biota. Conversely, lack of carbon dioxide in the external environment may be compensated for by the biota by decomposing such organic stores. These stores of organic matter are contained in soil humus, in peat, in the wood of living and dead trees, and in the dissolved organic matter in the ocean (the oceanic humus). More than 95% of all the organic matter of the biosphere is stored in these media. Apparently, the constant concentrations of not only carbon dioxide but also oxygen in both the atmosphere and the ocean are supported by the biota using those stores. So far, neither the value nor the direction of change of stores of organic matter in the biosphere are measurable with the required accuracy on a global scale. They are only known to an order of magnitude. However, these changes may be assessed from other data (Sect. 4.11).

1.4 The Action of the Le Chatelier Principle in the Biosphere

Stores of organic and inorganic carbon in the biosphere coincide in their order of magnitude, see Fig. 1.1. The ratio of these stores to the productivity of global biota yields the time period of biological turnover of the biogenic store in the biosphere, which is of the order of tens of years (Fig. 1.1). Hence, were synthesis of organic matter to take place with no decomposition to accompany it, all the inorganic carbon in the biosphere would be used up and transformed into organic substances in a few decades. Similarly, were only decomposition to take place, all the organic carbon in the biosphere would vanish in decades.

It is found, from measurements of the concentration of carbon dioxide in air bubbles entrapped in ice cores of different ages from Antarctica and Greenland, that the concentration of carbon dioxide in the atmosphere remained constant to within measurement error over the last several thousand years (Oeschger and Stauffer, 1986). It remained within the same order of magnitude over time periods of several hundred thousand years that is for time periods exceeding the turnover time by the factor of 10^4 (Barnola et al., 1991). It follows quite unequivocally from these data that the global annual average fluxes of biological synthesis and destruction of organic matter coincide with each other, to an accuracy of four digits, that is compensate each other to the relative accuracy of 10^{-4} (Fig. 1.1).

Inorganic carbon is released into the atmosphere in the process of degasing (including volcanic activity, filtration from the mantle, etc.) and is stored in sedimentary rocks, leaving the biosphere in the processes of weathering. The biota has no effect on the carbon emission from the Earth's core. The land biota can slightly change the rate of weathering (Schwartzman and Volk, 1989). The difference between emissions and sedimentation yields the net flux of inorganic carbon into the atmosphere. It appears that this flux is positive and is of the same order of magnitude as emissions and depositions. Thus emissions and depositions of inorganic carbon do not compensate each other. The ratio of the present-day store of inorganic carbon in the biosphere to its net geophysical flux corresponds to a timescale of around one hundred thousand years. In other words, that store should have increased about ten thousand fold during a time span of about a billion years. However, that never actually happened. Hence, some compensating process must function, and that process is the storage of organic carbon in sedimentary rocks. Direct studies have demonstrated that the stores of organic carbon, accumulated over approximately one billion years and dispersed through the sedimentary layer about one kilometer thick, exceed the stores of both the organic and inorganic

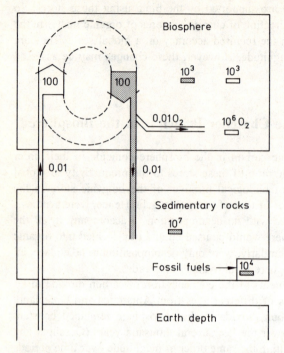

Fig. 1.1. Annual fluxes and stores of carbon in the biosphere. Stores of carbon are given by underlined figures in Gt C. Fluxes of carbon are given by figures at arrows in Gt C/year. Fluxes of carbon going into store as organic matter are shaded and underlined by thick shaded lines, respectively. Clear arrows give the fluxes of inorganic carbon. The stores of inorganic carbon and oxygen (in Gt O_2) in the biosphere are underlined by thick blank lines. The flux of organic carbon going to deposits in sedimented rocks is equal to the difference between its synthesis and destruction in the biosphere. That flux coincides with the net flux of inorganic flux entering the biosphere, to a relative accuracy of about 10^{-4}. Fluxes of synthesis and destruction coincide with each other to about the same level of accuracy. That situation works to hold constant the stores of carbon in its organic and inorganic form in the biosphere during the whole of *Phanerozoi* (6×10^8 years).

carbon used by life in the biosphere by about four orders of magnitude; Fig. 1.1 (Budyko et al., 1987).

It also definitely follows from the above that the net geophysical flux of inorganic carbon into the biosphere and the flux of organic carbon buried into sedimentary rocks (which is equal to the difference between production and destruction) have, on average, coincided to an accuracy of four digits, that is to a relative accuracy of 10^{-4}.

Thus the first four digits in the values of production and destruction coincide over a time period of about ten thousand years. The four digits left in the difference between production and destruction coincide with those giving the net geophysical flux of carbon over hundreds of millions of years. Hence, during geological time periods biota has been controlling up to eight digits in the values of production and destruction, that is, the resolution of biota is extremely high, because the random coincidence of different values to so high an accuracy is extremely improbable (for details see Sect. 4.3).

The amount of oxygen in the atmosphere exceeds that necessary to decompose all the organic carbon in the biosphere by three orders of magnitude. That is so because the oxygen released during synthesis of the organic carbon deposited in sedimentary rocks did not stay in those sedimentary rocks but instead entered the atmosphere in its free form. The process of burial of the organic carbon in sedimentary rocks, going on even now with its flux being equal to only one ten thousandth of biological production by the biosphere, provides for the constancy of concentrations of oxygen and of carbon dioxide in the biosphere.

The organic carbon buried in sedimentary rocks leaves the biological cycle and should thus be excluded from the definition of the biosphere. These stores remain intact for all of the natural biota. Man has started to use fossil fuel, found in the form of concentrated deposits of coal, oil, natural gas, which together contain about one thousandth of the total organic carbon contained in sedimentary rocks (Meadows et al., 1974, 1992; Skinner, 1986).

Thus Fig. 1.1 testifies in favor of the biological regulation of concentrations of various substances in the biosphere. The natural Earth biota is organized so as to be capable of supporting, to the highest level of accuracy, a state of environment fit for life. The question arises, why does the biota develop that enormous power of biological production? Indeed, it seems that it would have been sufficient to have had power four orders of magnitude lower. However, geophysical processes are not constant in their nature. They are subject to large fluctuations such as catastrophic volcanic eruptions, falls of large meteorites, etc. If the biota were slow to reestablish the normal state of environment, many species would be forced to exist in abnormal conditions for quite long periods of time. Such a situation could have resulted in a quick extinction of species and in a loss of capability to compensate for perturbations of the environment by the biota. The enormous power reached by the biota makes it possible for it to repair all the natural perturbations of the environment in the shortest time possible, shorter than a few decades. Such short-lived perturbations of the environment are safe for any living species.

1.5 Violations of the Le Chatelier Principle in the Contemporary Biosphere

The enormous power that the Earth biota develops, however, conceals a potential danger of quick destruction of the environment. If the correlated interaction between the species in the natural communities was disrupted, the environment could be completely perturbed (changed by about 100 %) in just a few decades. If all of the biota was exterminated, the environment would change to the same degree by geophysical factors alone in hundreds of thousand of years. Therefore, breaking up the natural structure of the biota through the transformation of nature by man presents a threat to nature exceeding that of complete extermination of the biota (complete desertification) by a factor of ten thousand.

It is well known by now that global changes of the environment do take place at the present time: the atmospheric concentration of CO_2 is quickly increasing; see Fig. 1.2. That effect strengthens the greenhouse effect and may yet lead to increase in the surface temperature of the planet. For a long time that build-up of carbon dioxide in the atmosphere has been related to combustion of fossil fuel alone (coal, oil, natural gas). It would be reasonable to expect that the biota both on land and in the sea reacts to that increase in accordance with the Le Chatelier principle, absorbing the excess carbon dioxide from the atmosphere.

However, the global analysis of land use practices (Houghton et al., 1983, 1987; Houghton, 1989) indicates that organic carbon is decreasing instead of increasing over large areas of the continental biosphere, the rate of emission of carbon from the continental biota and organic stores in soil into the atmosphere coinciding in its order of magnitude with the rate of emission of fossil carbon during combustion of coal, oil, and natural gas (Watts, 1982; Rotty, 1983). Hence, the biota violates the Le Chatelier principle in lands subject to direct industrial and agricultural use.

The Le Chatelier principle, characterizing the degree of stability of the system, is manifested in that the net rate of absorption of carbon by the biota (at low relative perturbations of the environment) is proportional to the increase in carbon concentration in the environment with respect to the non-perturbed preindustrial state. When the Le Chatelier principle is satisfied the proportionality coefficient in that relation should be positive. The analysis of rate of emission of fossil carbon and of accumulation of carbon in the atmosphere makes it possible to determine the validity of that coefficient with time for continental biota as a whole; see Sect. 4.12. Prior to the beginning of the last century, land biota had been following the Le Chatelier principle, that is it remained weakly perturbed by man. During that time the Earth biota was compensating every impact of man upon the biosphere, and no problem of environmental pollution arose.

From the beginning of the last century land biota ceased absorbing excess carbon from the atmosphere, increasing the environmental pollution precipitated by industrial enterprises from then on, instead of decreasing it. That means that the structure of the global biota appeared to be perturbed on a global scale. Taking into account that all of man's activities transform the biosphere, one may estimate the threshold anthropogenic forcing, at which the Le Chatelier principle ceases to function in the biota, i.e., the threshold beyond which the biota and its environment lose their stability. The area of cultivated land amounted to less than 5% of total land area during the preindustrial era, and man was using no more than 20% of the net primary production from those areas. As a result the overall anthropogenic share of consumption of biospheric net primary production did not exceed 1%. The present day share of anthropogenic consumption of the biospheric net primary production is almost an order of magnitude higher than that value. One may find a detailed account of that estimate below, based on different approaches and on various empirical data (see Sect. 4.12 and Chap. 5).

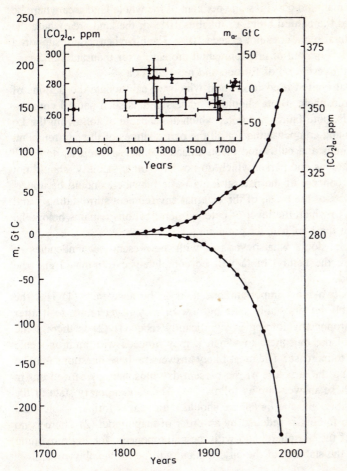

Fig. 1.2. The observed global changes of carbon stores. m_a is the increase of the mass of atmospheric carbon according to measurement data on CO_2 concentration in the atmosphere, $[CO_2]_a$, (after 1958: (Watts, 1982; Gammon et al., 1986; Trivett, 1989)) and in ice cores (prior to 1958: (Friedli et al., 1986; Oeschger and Stauffer, 1986; Leuenberger et al., 1992)); m_f is the depletion of fossil carbon due to combustion of coal, oil, and natural gas (Starke, 1987, 1990; Reviere and Marton-Lefevre, 1992). According to ice-core data the global build up of the atmospheric carbon store had started before combustion of fossil fuel was initiated. That means that global changes in the environment are related to changes of carbon stored in the global biota, and hence to perturbation of the stability of the latter.

It follows quite unequivocally from the data on changes in the global cycle of carbon that, on the one hand the threshold of admissible forcing of the biosphere is much lower than the present-day consumption by man, that is below about 10 %. On the other hand, the biosphere is apparently capable of compensating for any perturbations initiated by mankind provided the share of consumption by mankind does not exceed 1 % of the net primary production by the biosphere. It is then irrelevant whether mankind occupies one per cent of the whole land area where he completely perturbs the natural biota, or inhabits 10 % of the land area where the perturbation of natural biota does not exceed 10 %. The biosphere could support a mankind completely ignorant of environmental protection for thousands of years, while that mankind overran all of Europe and most of Asia.

We now have arrived at a position from which we can update the notions of the biota and the biosphere. Biota should be understood as such natural communities of individuals, both fauna and flora, which are capable of following the Le Chatelier principle and compensating for all the perturbations of the environment. (Domesticated animals and cultivated plants raised by man, as well as domestic patches of land, gardens and parks, which do not have inner stability, should not be included in the concept of the natural biota.) The biosphere should be understood as a stable state of the biota, of the external environment surrounding it and interacting with it, in which the level of external perturbations remains below the action threshold for the Le Chatelier principle.

There may be no doubt whatsoever that with the present-day tendencies of transgressing nature the natural biota will be completely exterminated and the biosphere destroyed.

There are then two most important questions to be answered: (1) Has the biosphere irreversibly left its stable state by now or may it yet return to it after contemporary anthropogenic forcing is significantly reduced? (2) Is there some other stable state of the biosphere to which it may proceed with anthropogenic forcing continuing to increase? The most likely answers to those questions may be obtained by studying the structure of the present-day biosphere as carried out in this monograph. These answers are as follows: (1) The contemporary state of the biosphere is reversible, and the biosphere should return to its former stable state if its anthropogenic forcing is reduced by an order of magnitude; (2) There is no other stable state of the biosphere, and with the anthropogenic forcing remaining at its present level the stability of the environment will be irreversibly ruined.

1.6 Biosphere as a "Free Market"

How does the natural biota function, and how is such a high degree of control over the levels of synthesis and destruction of organic matters in the biosphere maintained? The governing principle determining the functioning of life at any level is competitive interaction between autonomous, mutually uncorrelated individuals. The same principle constitutes the foundation of a free market. It is well known that the accuracy to which prices are determined in a free market is very high. No simulations employing modern mathematical models and computer software can reach this level, so as to be substituted for the action of the market itself. Rejection of the free market approach leads to a loss of such accuracy and to growing non-productive expenditure. The market was not been invented by man. It can prevail because at its foundation lie the actions of living people – the members of the human population. Modern markets are but an adjustment of the basic principles of life to existing human culture and civilization. So what does the free market look like in the biosphere?

Any living being combines extremely complex correlations at molecular, cellular, individual and social levels. The principal feature of life is the fact that, due to this extreme complexity of correlational ties, any given type of correlation in the biota is unstable and decays with time. For a separate individual such a decay means death. The existing types of correlation between living individuals may be maintained only within the population of such individuals. In the course of time the successive offspring of a single individual inevitably accumulate decay changes (deleterious substitutions) in their hereditary program (see Sects. 3.4–6). The relative number of "decay individuals" in the offspring of a normal individual is a quantitative characteristic of a species. The decay individuals are mostly capable of breeding no less actively than the normal ones. To maintain the level of organization in the population all the decay individuals must be either prevented from breeding or eliminated from the population. These functions may be the responsibility of the normal individuals, which, in conditions natural for the given species, have the highest competition capacity. This feature of the normal individuals is most important. The program of elimination of the decay individuals from the population might itself be subject to decay. Identification of decay individuals and their elimination from the population is realized in the process of competitive interaction between all the individuals (Chap. 3).

When the environmental conditions deviate from natural, i.e. the population leaves its ecological niche, the competition capabilities of the normal and decay individuals even out. The criteria by which the normal individuals are distinguished from the decay ones become void. The process of decay is constantly going on, so during such periods the relative number of decay individuals in the population (i.e. the genetic diversity of the population) grows exponentially. The proportion of normal individuals diminishes and they can completely vanish from small populations. However, following a return to normal environmental conditions the maximum competitive capacity of the normal individuals is restored and they expel the decay individuals from the population (Sect. 3.9).

Were the normal individuals to vanish completely from any such population, they would be restored upon return to natural conditions (but not to conditions deviating from the natural). Such would be the end result of inverse mutations and genetic recombination in the course of mating between the decay individuals (see Sects. 3.10,11).

Note also that decay individuals are always present in the population in its stationary state due to the permanent character of decay processes; however under natural conditions their frequency of occurrence is low.

Only the population as a whole, but not the isolated sequential offspring of one individual may enjoy stability. If competitive interaction is neutralized ("switched-off") a decay individual cannot be distinguished from a normal one at all. In this case the population degenerates into several isolated progeny sequences from various individuals. Due to the ongoing process of decay such individuals keep accumulating decay traits and finally the species dies out.

Complex intercorrelated interaction of various individuals in the social structures is maintained via competitive interaction of such structures. For social insects, such as ants, this would be competitive interaction between different anthills in the population of such anthills. In exactly the same way the correlated interaction of individuals from different species in the community may be maintained by way of competitive interaction of different communities (however, they should be identical in their speciation). The simplest type of such a community is lichen, consisting of mutually correlated species of algae and fungus. Such a correlation is maintained through competitive interaction between various individual lichens in the population of lichen of the given species. The correlated formation of social structures like anthills or the communities of different species may be envisaged as the hyperindividual. The internal correlations in hyperindividuals should be maintained by way of their competitive interaction and stabilization selection in the respective hyperpopulation (Chap. 3).

Evidently, stabilization of the existing type of internal correlation of the living individuals based on their competitive interaction and selection in the population is possible only in cases where all the individuals within this population are completely mutually independent and non-correlated with each other. In the opposite case, expulsion of a decay individual from the population becomes impossible in exactly the same way a defective organ cannot be expelled from the body. It also follows from this reasoning that maintaining an inner correlation between the individuals in any population by way of centralized government of that population as a whole is impossible in principle. In other words neither the population nor the hyperpopulation should be considered as superorganisms.

1.7 Biospheric Communities

The most complex type of correlation among living formations, i.e. more complex hyperindividuals, is the correlation between the individuals of different species in the communities. It is particularly this type of correlation which makes possible the operation of the Le Chatelier principle in biota with respect to external perturbations of the environment. Complexity of organization of various individuals in the community and high diversification of the community species composition serves to maintain environmental stability.

To do this, every species executes some strictly prescribed function in stabilizing the environment, operating in a correlated interaction with other species in the community. In conditions where nutrients are artificially fed into and wastes evacuated from the environment, communities fall apart. For instance, urban sparrows have kept their species stability for thousands of years even though they are now out of the natural communities they had once been part of. The introduction of pigeons to those sparrows does not result in the appearance of any new community. The same applies to any and every species of domesticated animal and cultivated plant.

As with separate individuals, each given community has a finite size, occupies a definite space region and decays with time. This decay takes the form of a loss of capacity the community formerly had of maintaining stable local environmental conditions with a high degree of accuracy. This change in the capabilities of the community eventually leads to its expulsion from the environment by the new communities constantly forming. The only organization remaining stable may be the population of communities, i.e. the hyperpopulation.

The size of a separate community is determined by the area in which the synthesis and destruction fluxes of organic matter may, under normal conditions, be balanced by this community to the highest possible accuracy, and where the biotic regulation of the deviations from this balance, forced, as they were, by perturbations of the environment, is at its maximum. Indirect estimates demonstrate that the linear size of any internally correlated community existing in the biosphere does not exceed a few dozen meters (Chap. 5). Quick expulsion of the decayed communities leads to an apparent homogeneity of the hyperpopulation of the communities, occupying a vast surface of the Earth, which is usually called the ecosystem (Odum, 1983).

The correlation of the species in a community may be quite rigid. For example, lichen consists only of the strictly determined species of the algae and the fungus. Certain insect species are capable of feeding off only one single plant species. It is exactly this correlation which provides a wide range of reactions of the community to any possible fluctuations of external conditions. When such correlation breaks, the range of possible reactions narrows in exactly the same way that the range of possible reactions of the separate organs of the body is narrower than the range of such reactions for the body as a whole. The term "adaptation" can characterize neither the interaction between separate organs within the body, nor that between the male and female in bisexual populations, nor the relations between the various casts in the social structures of the insects. All such interactions are but correlations in the sense described above. Similarly, the term adaptation cannot be substituted for the notion of intercorrelation between individuals of different species in a community.

The term adaptation may characterize the interaction of individuals with components of the environment that cannot be regulated by the biota.

The normal genome of an individual contains the information on adaptation to all its natural habitats in which the individuals from that species may find themselves, including possible adaptive morphological changes in the offspring of an individual dependent on the environment. The adaptation to natural environment (the adaptation program) is a necessary but subsidiary part of the information in the normal genome. The principal part is the information concerning action on the environment by the individual (feeding, general behavior, population density, etc.). It is part of an individual belonging to the given species within a given community, and it serves to stabilize the optimal natural environment. It is a stabilization program. Functioning of the whole community is optimized that way, i.e. it is a program for stabilization (but not adaptation) of each separate species. All the normal individuals should produce an optimal, instead of maximum, offspring, which would provide for the best regime of functioning of the whole community.

Numerous species may exist which are unnatural for a given community, but which are well adapted to the given environment, sometimes even better than the species natural to that community, their normal genome being, however, free of a stabilization program. Such "gangster" species destroy the internal correlation in the community, as well as the environment. As a result the community containing such species is supplanted by communities free of such gangster species. Thus selection of the species with necessary stabilization programs is carried out in the biota.

Large animals are present in practically every community of the biosphere. Consequently, communities including such animals are the ones of the highest competitive capacity. The feeding territories of large animals include many separate communities, and a population of a species of large animal sometimes occupies a territory in which all the population of communities, i.e. hyperpopulation dwells. However, the destructive capacity of all large animals (the rate at which they destroy the organic matter) constitutes less than 1 % of the total destructive capacity of the community (see Fig. 1.3 and Chap. 5). Hence, under natural conditions the mammals are a "superfine tuning" of the community. The largest animals have never been the masters of the biosphere as is usually claimed. Violation of this rule always leads to distortion of the communities and to extinction of the large animals. The disappearance of dinosaurs did not perturb the biota to any great extent. It did not affect the capability of the biota to compensate for unfavorable external fluctuations of the environment. Communities keep the destructive capacity of large animals low in the same way as they control the other global characteristics of the environment which equally affect the whole hyperpopulation of the communities. The communities of plants and single-cell beings completely control the number of large animals exactly as they do the concentrations of various substances in the external environment. It may be said that the large locomotive animals jointly present a certain component of the external environment, which, together with concentrations of the biochemically active substances, are kept at certain levels by the hyperpopulation of the communities consisting of plants and microorganisms; see Fig. 1.3.

Extermination of an entire hyperpopulation of communities is irreversible, as is the case with any biological species. (The known examples of such irreversible exterminations of natural communities are the rape of the steppes and the tropical forests.) Following a heavy perturbation of a considerable number of communities comprising a hyperpopulation, the natural communities maintaining closed cycles of matter and a stable environment are restored. Quantitatively, the degree to which the matter cycle is closed may be characterized by the value of its breach, which is equal to the difference between the synthesis and destruction fluxes, divided by the synthesis flux. In the cultivated, constantly perturbed agricultural

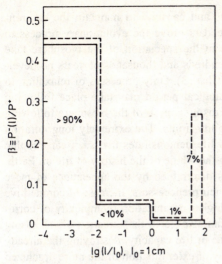

Fig. 1.3. Distribution of the rate of destruction of organic matter with body size of individuals destroying the organic matter (bacteria, fungi, animals) on land. $\beta = P^-(l)/P^+$, $P^-(l)$ is the spectral density of destruction, produced by individuals of body size l, P^+ is the production of land vegetation (net primary production), see Chap. 5. The solid line gives the universal distribution found in all the non-perturbed ecosystems (Sect. 5.6). The area enveloped by the solid curve is equal to unity. Numbers in per cent give the relative input from various parts of the histogram. The dashed line describes the present-day distribution on land, accounting for the anthropogenic perturbation. The area under the anthropogenic peak (7%) corresponds to man's food, plus cattle fodder, plus consumption of wood (Sect. 6.5). The difference between the areas under the dashed and the solid lines characterizes the breach of the biochemical cycle. It is obtained from the measurement data on the global carbon cycle, and is close to the area of the anthropogenic peak (Sect. 4.12).

areas this value is always at a level of several tens per cent. Meanwhile, the moment a perturbation terminates (e.g., after complete wood cutting, fires, or natural disasters) the level of breach quickly lowers, reaching 1% in just a few decades. However, the relaxation to the background breach of hundredths of a per cent takes hundreds of years, following multiple changes of speciation in the plant cover and restoration of the natural age distribution of the vegetation. If a considerable part of the hyperpopulation of the communities is destroyed more often than once in every few hundred years, the background breach is never reached, and the environment begins to disintegrate.

1.8 Evolution Rates

The described mode of stabilization of the biota and the environment also makes possible the evolution of the biological species and of their communities. Only those species which do not decrease the overall competitive capacity of the community can take a firm hold in the biosphere, e.g. they do not lower the average level of closedness of the matter cycles and capacity to maintain the environmental stability by the community. Paleodata prove the evolutionary process to be extremely slow. Noticeable changes in the speciation of the biosphere take several million years. On the scale of hundreds and thousands of years no development can occur in the biosphere (see Chap. 3). Only processes of relaxation to the stable state typical of the given geological period may take place following natural external forcings or processes of disintegration of the biosphere following such perturbations which exceed its stability limits. The extremely long duration of the existence of the biosphere and of life demonstrates that such catastrophic perturbations have never occurred during the whole of the history of life on Earth.

The direction of evolution is always determined by the appearance of more competitive forms and the expulsion of their predecessors. Increase of competitive capacity may not always be caused by higher organization (complexity of correlation) of the living beings. Evolution can also go in the direction of increasing aggressive competitiveness at the expense of life capacity, destroying the already achieved level of organization, i.e. by way of extermination of the more organized but less aggressive individuals by those more aggressive but less organized ones. Such a process could, in principle, lead to complete disorganization, and, finally, to extinction of life. In particular, this might happen if both the separate living beings and the social structures and communities were to physically grow in size without any restriction; such a growth is accompanied by an increase in their respective competitive capacities. The growth in physical size would lead to fewer individuals in the population, and, finally, complete correlation between all parts of the population, thus stopping the competitive interaction and natural selection. Besides, the reduction of the number of independently functioning living beings would block the operation of the well-known statistical law of large numbers – the only means of damping fluctuations known to nature. Thus such a development would lead to an unlimited increase of fluctuations in the processes of synthesis and destruction of organic matter in a community, and to further inability of the community to keep them intercorrelated (Chaps. 4 and 5).

The overall duration of life and the available paleodata show that there existed in nature some acting agents, which stopped (at least prior to the anthropogenic perturbation of the biosphere) the tendency of evolution in the direction of disrupting the foundation of life. Among such agents is the lack of abundance of nutrients in the environment. Abundance corresponds to a situation where the store of nutrients in the environment is much larger than their expenditure (production) in the course of evolution (or progress), that is where the time of evolution is much less than the time of biological cycling of the nutrients, i.e. the residence or turnover time (Chap. 4).

The timescale of the biospheric evolution is determined by the rate of change in speciation of the biosphere, i.e. by the average lifespan of a species. As noted above, this lifespan, according to paleodata, is of the order of a million years. The timescale of the biological cycling of nutrients in the environment is equal to the ratio of the nutrient store and the productivity of the biota, and is of the order of

10 years; Fig. 1.1. Thus it is 10^5 times shorter than the timescale of evolution. As a result, the evolution of natural biota takes place under conditions of strictly limited natural resources, extremely far from those of abundance. Any evolutionary change disrupting the correlation between the synthesis and destruction of the organic matter in a community appears impossible, since a complete local distortion of the environment (due to the extremely high power of the biota to synthesize and destroy organic matter) occurs much faster than such a change. This distortion, should it take place, would lead to an immediate loss in competitive capacity of such a community and to its expulsion.

1.9 Progress

However, following a transition from genetic evolution to scientific-technological progress in free market conditions, the changes speed up. The timescale of the technology overhaul shrinks to several years and becomes considerably less than the timescale of deterioration of the biospheric resources (i.e. the timescale of their imaginary anthropogenic cycling). In such a situation mankind faces a seeming abundance of natural resources. Deterioration of natural resources occurs too slowly and cannot affect technology. Resource-spending technologies appear to be competitively stronger and quickly expel all the resource-conserving technologies, including the natural communities of the biosphere.

The economic progress attains its maximum rate and efficiency of exploitation of natural resources when the maximum number of competing technical units ("technological communities") takes part in solving a given problem. The minimal size of such a technological unit is determined by the correlation radius within a plant (factory) needed to solve this particular task. In the conditions of a seeming abundance of natural resources the market economy inevitably leads to a maximum possible rate of expenditure of such resources and to their deterioration.

Renunciation of competitive interaction and market economy through a transition to its centralized control on a global scale might help to regulate progress and reduce the rate of deterioration of the environment. However, when there remains competitive interaction with the "external environment", which develops on the basis of market economy, the centrally controlled system will lose its competitive capacity and eventually be expelled. Due to lower efficiency in the use of natural resources the centrally controlled system might under those conditions develop local rates of deterioration of these resources that would exceed the overall maximum reached by the market economy. The existence of the centrally governed system might only be possible under conditions of complete isolation when competitive interaction with the external world is stopped. This is equivalent to either the absence or annihilation of the latter.

Parallel to global deterioration of the environment by the progressing market economy there may exist certain localities in which the environment remains in a stationary state or is even apparently improved on the basis of the open cycle of matter. That would mean constant introduction of new amounts of matter needed for consumption into, and removing the wastes from, such a location. This principle is also employed by nature to maintain the life of a separate individual. It is employed by man to keep stationary the state of his personal dwelling, lot, park, or any other cultural complex. However the breach of the local cycle means that the existence of such an artificially stable area is paid for by ever deepening deterioration of the environment for the rest of the biosphere. The garden in bloom, an artificially clean lake or river, kept in such a state on the basis of an open matter cycle, is much more dangerous for the biosphere as a whole than wasted, desertified land.

For resource-spending technologies operating in free market conditions to lose their competitive capacity against the most resource-conserving ones, the cycling time for the environmental resources involved in the technological processes must be considerably less than the timescale of the technology overhaul. Taking the current value of the latter at about 10 years, we conclude that the timescale for complete cycling of all the resources involved should not be more than 1 year. However, for most of the non-renewable resources of energy and materials the timescale of their deterioration is of the order of a hundred years. To reduce the cycling timescale for technological resources it is necessary to either increase the rate of their consumption several hundredfold, or reduce respectively the amount of resources consumed. In other words, either quickly spend all the non-renewable resources or refuse to spend them at all. Only after satisfying these conditions will the economy actually become "ecological". In the opposite case the economic progress related to spontaneous increase in competitive capacity must inevitably lead to complete deterioration of all the resources and to destruction of the environment fit for life.

Note that the natural biota does not use non-renewable resources. Starting to use them is only dangerous if there is evolution or progress. Only if the latter two processes take place is there a possibility of development in the direction of disrupting the environment. In a conservative state, when evolution and progress are absent (when the timescales of these processes are infinitely long) the initially closed matter cycles cannot be disorganized by the existing communities, even if they randomly turn to using the non-renewable resources; in such a case these resources will be automatically restored. Free market mechanisms described in Sects. 1.6 and 1.7 are used by biota only to stabilize an individual's or a hyper-individual's internal organization. A direct free market mechanism could never be used by the biota in the evolution of species (Sects. 3.15, 3.16 and 4.14).

Let us look at the two possibilities mentioned for attaining resource-conserving technologies, while operating in conditions of progress in a free market economy. The first of them − connected with accelerating the rate of consumption of resources many hundredfold (the current civilization is still attuned to this possibility) − is not a real possibility. It could only bring positive results in the case where such an acceleration could happen instantly, i.e. during a time interval short enough for the ongoing progress not to have been able to disrupt the biosphere noticeably, without spoiling the environment and decimating the biota. In reality such an acceleration and a respective increase in consumption must inevitably take too long. During such an inevitable period of the rate of consumption gradually picking-up, the ongoing resource-consuming progress would surely bring the biosphere into a state unfit for life.

1.10 Conservation of the Biosphere

The second possibility connected with a refusal altogether to further spend the non-renewable resources is quite realistic. The present-day consumption of energy by civilization is 90 % based on non-renewable resources. Renunciation of the latter would lead to a tenfold reduction in energy consumption. The human population should then be reduced by the same factor. This would in turn reduce the anthropogenic perturbation of the continental biota by the same factor of ten, which would let the latter return to within the margin of the Le Chatelier principle. Let us stress that consuming energy at its present level even after a transition to the so-called ecologically clean energy resources would still mean destructively perturbing the natural biota and the biosphere (Fig. 1.4). The whole process of reduction should be prolonged so as to let the technological progress in free market conditions restructure itself to the resource-conserving technologies. This could feasibly happen in a few decades to a hundred years, in which the biosphere would not be rendered completely unfit for life: its anthropogenic perturbation would gradually diminish. During such a period a global transition to one-child families (this rate corresponds to a 2 % annual reduction of the population) will reduce the population during the next century exactly by the needed factor of ten.

It should be stressed that the transition from the current population growth (of about 2 % a year) to its reduction at the same rate would not produce any economic problems. The demographic stress the society now suffers raising children would then turn into respective stress from the elders. The level of stress is then determined as the number of children under 15 and elders over 60 years per one person in the 15–60 age bracket. The lowest demographic stress is suffered by the stationary population (neither growing nor shrinking). However, in the contemporary technologically developed society, all children must pass through a costly period of learning and training. On the other hand, the present-day elders maintain their health and working capacity for a long time and can practically always earn their own living. This fact leads to a situation in which the economic stress from a child heavily exceeds that from an elder. In the end the transition from a growing population to its reduction at the same rate would decrease the economic stress upon society severalfold and it could even appear to be less than in the stationary state. In such a situation the economic stress would have to be determined as a ratio of the number of non-working people to the number of those working. Traditionally the fear of depopulation is associated with the loss (inevitable in the past) of competitive capacity by a nation reducing its population as compared to one increasing it. This danger would be eliminated if all nations started to reduce their populations proportionately.

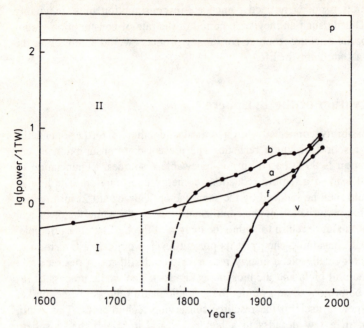

Fig. 1.4. Energy consumption and environmental stability. Horizontal lines are as follows: p is the global power of gross primary production by the whole biosphere; v is the global consumption by all the natural herbivore vertebrates (see Fig. 1.3 and Sect. 5.6). The v-line coincides with the threshold of the ecologically admissible anthropogenic consumption of biospheric production (Sect. 4.12). Curvilinear lines are as follows: f is the power of fossil fuel combusted; a is anthropogenic consumption of biospheric production (man's food, animal fodder, wood consumption; see Sect. 6.5); b is the reduction of organic stores on land. Ranges: I – the ecologically permitted value of anthropogenic consumption. All the anthropogenic perturbations of the biota and the environment are compensated by the natural biota; II – the global consumption of primary production by small invertebrates of the natural biota, who perform the principal work of stabilizing the environment; see Chaps. 3–5. Anthropogenic consumption in that range is ecologically prohibited, since it results in forcing the natural communities out and in violating stability of the biota and the environment.

The program of reducing anthropogenic perturbation and of returning to the margin of the Le Chatelier principle might be successful on one condition: the economic expansion to cultivation and development of new parts of the biosphere, yet unspoiled by civilization, must be stopped totally and immediately on a global scale. Then these parts may become the active sources of restoration of the biosphere. Such a demand calls for the minute inventory of the still intact parts of the biosphere; it should be undertaken without any delay, using all available technological capabilities.

The most productive continental communities are forests and bogs. The highest productivity is demonstrated by the tropical communities. Their productivity exceeds that of the respective communities in temperate zones by a factor of four, see Chap. 5. In accordance with the Le Chatelier principle, when seeking to compensate for the perturbation of the environment, a unit range occupied by virginal tropical forests and bogs would be equivalent to four such ranges of virginal forests and bogs in mid-latitudes. Non-perturbed virginal forests and bogs do not affect their environment. In particular, forests are neither releasers nor absorbers of oxygen. The fact that a forest is a closed system with respect to oxygen means that all the oxygen produced by plants is immediately utilized by other individuals of the forest community. The forest starts to alter its environment only when the latter is perturbed, and its reaction is to compensate for the perturbation.

The secondary forest growing in the wood-cut areas possesses approximately a thousand times worse capacity for compensating environmental perturbations as compared to its virginal predecessor, see Chaps. 4 and 5. In billions of years of evolution nature has mastered the most effective means for reactivating the Le Chatelier principle in the shortest possible time. The damaged forest areas are inhabited by repair species which organize the repair community and quickly reduce the degree of breach of the natural cycles. Then successive substitution (succession) of repair species takes place, during which the degree of breach keeps reducing. Apparently in about 300–500 years this process is finished and the forest returns to its initial unperturbed state (it may only happen if the damaged part is surrounded by non-perturbed areas, i.e. the hyperpopulation of the natural communities still exists), see Chap. 4. If man interferes with the succession process, pursuing his economic profit and tries to grow the most valuable tree species too speedily (e.g., processes the cut areas by herbicides, weeds out the non-valuable species) the process of repairing the cycles slows down.

Periodic felling of mature, economically profitable wood (every 50 years or so) interrupts the restoration of the virginal forests of the closed matter cycles, capable of compensating for environmental perturbations. To return to the natural biosphere it would be necessary to extend the time between such wood-cuts to 300–500 years, i.e. globally reduce the cutting by a factor of six to ten. Since at present more wood is cut everywhere than grows naturally, so that the forested areas globally shrink, the reduction factor should at least reach ten. The same figure was obtained above for the scale of population reduction.

It follows from Fig. 1.4 that large vertebrates may envisage the biosphere as an energy processing engine which stabilizes the environment and provides them with the energy necessary for their existence; however this engine operates at an efficiency level of about 1 %. The remaining 99 % of the power of the biosphere is consumed by small invertebrates and is spent on stabilizing the environment.

As demonstrated in Sect. 1.5, the action of the Le Chatelier principle in continental biota appeared to be disrupted as soon as the share of biotic production consumed by man throughout the continents exceeded 1 %.

The development of civilization, based on and boosted by the free market, under conditions of unlimited energy resources, may be compared to the effect of doping in a sportsman's body. Such a development opens the way to reach good results within a short time period, with the standard of living of all the people becoming very high, but only at the price of destroying the natural biota. Using various waste cleaning and disposal techniques produces an illusion of ecological well-being. However, extermination of the natural biota results in irreversible global changes of the environment.

The so-called highly developed regions (or countries) have only been able to reach their level of prosperity without completely destroying their natural environment because the nature of the developing regions, not yet spoiled by civilization, keep compensating for the devastation wrought upon nature on the global scale. The virgin nature of the developing regions took it upon itself to stabilize the global environment. Without all that biota, 99 % of the gross product of the developed regions would have had to be spent on conserving the environment. In that case there could have been no development of the economy of those regions. The development of the "developed" regions is borrowed.

To stop further destruction of the biosphere, all the developed regions should pay an international tax to those still having some natural biota, not spoiled by civilization, and that tax should exceed the possible income from using the resources of that biota. It is completely inadmissible to use the economic potential of the developed regions to speed up the extraction of resources from the virgin nature of the developing ones.

Trying to raise the standard of living of people in the developing regions to that enjoyed in the regions already developed via the free market economy by extracting the highest economic profit from the exploited natural resources will inevitably result in a global ecological catastrophe. Provided the population of the planet remains at its present level or even grows, the modern standard of living available in the developed regions can only be given to every man on Earth at the cost of the complete destruction of the environment fit for life. Supporting a stable level with the natural biota and environment remaining intact is only possible for a human population that is an order of magnitude smaller than the present one.

If some unused natural resources are still available, the rate of economic growth and the standard of living of the whole population may be increased if a working part of the population (labor force) is imported. That is how North America was conquered. This also explains the present-day demographic policy of the developing countries, particularly in Latin America. However, such a policy results in a quick destruction of natural communities in the biosphere. At the start of the industrial revolution such a development only resulted in local perturbations of the biosphere. But with modern levels of technology such a policy inevitably leads to irreversible global perturbations of the environment, thus significantly lowering the probability of following generations surviving.

The policy pursued in developing the natural resources of Russia also produces significant doubts. In Siberia and the extreme North of Russia the largest areas on the planet still conserved exist, featuring the natural biota only slightly affected by industrial activities. That biota is of enormous value for the whole of mankind, not just for Russia. It is the duty of the developed countries to help Russia preserve that biota, which would be in the best interests of both Russia itself and all the countries of the world. The remaining natural communities of Russia should not be destroyed. That is why the West should help Russia overcome its present-day economic difficulties, to prevent the otherwise inevitable economic development and destruction of a piece of natural biota unique in its scale.

1.11 A Transition to the Noosphere?

An alternative for the further development of civilization is to liquidate competition between groups of people, including countries, and proceed to a globally correlated civilization based on centralized government, i.e. to start constructing the noosphere. In this case any species of untamed living organisms outside their natural communities would present an enormous global danger to the environment: breaking from under control and breeding in natural proportions without any restraint, such species would be capable of destroying the environment much quicker than man does now; remember the enormous power of synthesis and destruction of organic matter that the biota is capable of developing on the scale of the whole biosphere. Note that examples of the destruction of the environment following the introduction of new species into it are numerous and well-known. Therefore, all the remnants of the perturbed continental biota, including wild species unfit for taming must be destroyed. The only biota kept by man would then be represented by a small number of cultivated species. However an incredible multitude of both living organisms and technological objects would then have to be governed and controlled on a global scale within the noosphere under conditions to prevent the recovery of large numbers that would inevitably precipitate growing fluctuations in the processes of synthesis and destruction of biological and technological products. These could finally destroy the environment and bring civilization to its downfall.

With the destruction of natural biota biological regulation of the environment will be lost. The flux of information, extracted from solar energy by the natural biota exceeds the maximum possible information fluxes in the computers of the whole of civilization by 15 orders of magnitude (Sect. 2.8). Thus it appears unrealistic to expect to be able to construct a noospheric system for regulating the environment which would be as efficient as the biotic one. Therefore, even if some completely waste-free technological cycles are organized in place of the natural biota, running on ecologically clean energy sources which do not alter the state of the environment, the latter will be subject to biotically uncontrolled natural fluctuations, which might destroy the environment fit for man in just a short time (Sects. 2.7, 4.12).

Hence the noosphere in the form described above is Utopia. Noosphere is only possible as a stable ecological niche for the existence of civilized man, and with technological progress taking place that niche is only possible if the natural biota is preserved over most of the planet, while the overall energy consumption by the planetary human population is brought down to an ecologically permissible level (Fig. 1.4).

Moreover, even with the construction of a noosphere commanding stable global environment and possessing an efficiency equal to that of the biosphere, no less than 99% of all the energy and manpower (labor) of such a civilization would have to be spent maintaining the stability of the global environment. Since the limit of energy consumption by mankind compatible with climate stability coincides with the power of the biosphere itself (Fig. 1.4 and Sect. 6.6), man in the noosphere would have less power available to satisfy the needs of civilization than he would command in a stationary biosphere, where he would not have to bother stabilizing the global environment.

These are strong grounds for believing that the biosphere (which consists of natural biota developed in the course of evolution, interacting with the environment) presents the only system capable of stabilizing the environment under any external perturbations. Consequently, preservation of the natural communities and the existing species in numbers capable of satisfying the Le Chatelier principle with respect to the global perturbations of the environment must be envisaged as the main condition for further life on this planet. To do that, virginal nature has to be preserved on the larger part of the Earth's surface instead of in tiny reservations, zoos, parks and gene banks.

2. Solar Energy and Ordered Processes in Inanimate Nature

2.1 Decay of Ordered States

We may constantly observe ordered macroscopic processes in nature: wind, generation of clouds, precipitation, the flow of rivers, etc. The ordered motion of molecules of a substance is always envisaged as the opposite of their chaotic (non-correlated) thermal motion. The ordered character of such motion means that a single molecule or a group of molecules appears to be related (correlated) in its motion to that of another such molecule or group of molecules. For example, all the molecules of water in a river have a downstream velocity component. During turbulent flow in whirlpools macroscopic groups of molecules feature identical angular velocities. The phenomenon of wind means that all the molecules of air have a common velocity component.

Molecules taking part in macroscopic motion interact with other molecules of the medium in which such motion occurs. An enormous number of finite states may result from that interaction: during elastic collision a molecule may change the direction in which it moves, while during nonelastic collision it may transmit its energy to a molecule of the medium. All the final states of the two interacting molecules are apparently equally probable. In other words, only an infinitely small fraction of molecules interacting with the medium will retain their velocity component from the initial ordered motion after the interaction, and almost always that component will be transformed and transmitted to molecules of the medium. Hence an ordered correlated motion will decay into disordered chaotic movement of molecules. The energy of that ordered motion dissipates and is transformed into thermal energy. Note that such decay only takes places if a transition is possible from the initial into a large number of final states. A set of objects initially organized into one and the same initial state, will then be transformed into another set with differing final states. Such a transition is envisaged as a transition from order to chaos. The existing order must always be initially organized via some preparatory act.

Since decay and dissipation of energy go on permanently, any ordered process may only be supported if there exists an influx of energy to it from another ordered process. Clouds may only form because water vapor condenses. The latent heat of evaporation released during condensation generates macroscopic motions of the molecules of air, so that cyclones, tornadoes, etc. may form, accompanied, as it were, by strong winds. The energy of wind also gradually dissipates, transforming itself into heat. Evaporation, precipitation, and wind can only exist because the Earth constantly gets energy from the Sun. The solar energy generates all forms of ordered macroscopic processes on Earth. The heat into which the solar radiation transforms (dissipates) is scattered into cosmic space as thermal radiation. As a result the average temperature of the Earth remains approximately constant. The inhomogeneity of heating of the surface of Earth also results in ordered macroscopic fluxes of matter, in both the atmosphere and the ocean. Energy capable of transforming into the energy of ordered macroscopic processes under terrestrial conditions, i.e. at approximately constant temperature and pressure, and of producing work, is called free energy in contrast to thermal energy, which is related to chaotic movement of the molecules, the latter being incapable of producing any work (Sommerfeld, 1952).

Prior to the discovery of the law of energy conservation, it was only free energy capable of producing work which was understood as energy in general. Free energy is not conserved. In the course of work that energy is transformed into other forms of energy, gradually dissipating and transforming into thermal energy. The empirical law of energy conservation means that the amount of energy does not change during such transformations (the so-called first law of thermodynamics). Only scattering and decay of the initial free energy takes place. That decay always goes in the direction of the lower degree of order of that energy. By itself, thermal energy is already incapable of performing any work. That law was also discovered to be empirical (the second law of thermodynamics). However, in many fields of science, such as economics, biology, etc., only free energy is meant when one speaks generally about energy. Following that tradition, in what is to follow we shall omit the word "free" when speaking about any ordered form of energy capable of producing work. In most cases thermal energy is simply called heat.

All the versatile natural processes observed are but various forms of decay of the ordered states of matter and of dissipation of energy they contain. The overall set of states of matter, rich in their energy, combines into the energy resources of the planet Earth. These resources either have the form of kinetic energy of the correlated motion of various material elements (such as the flux of solar radiation, the hydraulic energy of river flow and oceanic waves, the energy of tides, wind energy) or of the accumulated potential energy of correlated bonds between these various material elements (such as gravitational energy, the latent heat of condensation and freezing, chemical and nuclear energy). Other forms of potential energy include the equatorial to polar surface temperature contrasts, the surface to ground water temperature gradients of the oceanic, sea, and lake waters. The nuclear energy, the gravitational energy of displacement of the Earth depths and the energy of tides, have been preserved since the time of formation of the solar system. All other forms of energy resources are generated by the solar radiation.

When decay processes come to their end, all the forms of potential energy first transform into the energy of ordered motion, which then suffers dissipation and is scattered as thermal energy of the chaotic movement of separate molecules. Hence, the final result of such a decay is the minimum of potential energy. However, at low rates of dissipation inverse processes may take place, and the ordered kinetic energy is then transformed into potential energy, which may accumulate. For example, the latent energy of water vapor condensation is accumulated in the atmosphere via evaporation, combustible organic matter accumulates via the absorption of solar radiation by green plants, electric energy is accumulated in either chemical or hydrogravitational installations, etc. Depending on the initial moment of observations either a direct transformation of potential energy to kinetic or an inverse one may be observed in any process of oscillation or in the process of wave propagation. An example of a non-fading sequence of such transition is given by the comets in their highly elliptic orbits. In that case the system does not tend to a minimum of either potential or kinetic energy.

Via the decay of an energy-rich ordered state of matter all the various macroscopic processes may be generated. All the meteorological phenomena taking place in nature, all the activities of living organisms ever to have existed on Earth, and, finally, all the power stations, engines, and machines designed and built by man, are but examples of that diversity. The theoretical laws of these physical and chemical processes, discovered by man, aim to forecast the direction in which the initial state of the system will change. However, every time that initial state itself must be either prepared or independently prescribed.

Decay processes are characterized by the direction and duration of the decay itself. When no decay takes place, the processes may only be characterized by rates at which the measurable variables change: fluxes, speed of movement, oscillation frequencies, etc. The duration of such decay-free processes (including stationary, periodic, or those randomly fluctuating around their stationary values) may be formally obtained mathematically, substituting the changing measurable variable itself by the measurable rate of its change. That may either be the time of cycling (e.g., m/q, where m is the mass of organic matter, and q is the rate of metabolism), or the period of oscillation, or of rotation ($2\pi/\omega$, ω is the angular frequency). Time only acquires a physical meaning when the processes start fading and decaying, i.e., when the envisaged process has a start and a finish. Kinetic energy not subject to decay may be observed in the rotation of the planets and in such experimentally discovered phenomena as superconductivity and superfluidity.

All the phenomena either observed in everyday life or detected in the course of scientific experiments are irreversible processes of decay of the initial state. In the absence of decay processes no observable events develop in time. To measure the decay processes taking place at the surface of the planet, the periods of the diurnal and annual rotation of the Earth are usually used. The accumulated potential energy, not subject to decay (such as that in fossil fuel, for example) does not change until it is used by man. The absolute geochronology of the Earth is only known and available because of the decay of unstable isotopes of chemical elements.

2.2 Solar Energy

Since radiation from the Sun generates practically all the decay processes at the surface of the Earth, we list below the characteristics of the solar radiant energy necessary for our exposition of energy. The spectrum of solar radiation is close to an equilibrium Planck blackbody radiation at an absolute temperature of $T_S \approx$ 6000 K (Newkirk, 1980). The average temperature of the Earth's surface is 15 °C or $T_0 \approx 288$ K (Mitchell, 1989). Due to such a large difference in temperature the solar radiation incident upon the Earth's surface is practically a pure source of free energy, which may be transformed into ordered macroscopic motions at an efficiency close to unity (Sommerfeld, 1952). Following the well-known Carnot principle (Sommerfeld, 1952), which reflects the second law of thermodynamics, that radiation may be transformed into work at a maximum efficiency of $\eta = (T_S - T_0)/T_S = 0.95$ under terrestrial conditions, that is at constant temperature T_0. The maximum efficiency does not depend on the means employed to trap the solar energy, whether it is the kinetic energy of equilibrium radiation of photons contained in a cavity, or the potential energy of chemical bonds synthesized in the course of photochemical reactions, etc. There exist no means to obtain a flux of solar radiation larger than that coming from the Sun's surface (that is, without additional energy expenditure) or of a radiative temperature exceeding the solar temperature itself. Were the situation different, the efficiency of transformation could be raised above the cited maximal value. If additional energy is expended (one might use the solar radiation itself for its source), the solar radiation might be transformed into a flux of radiation of arbitrary temperature; however, on condition that the efficiency of such transformation does not exceed the maximum possible one. A particular case of such a transformation is concentrating the solar energy by the so-called nonimaging optics (Cooke, et al., 1990; Winston, 1991).

The existing average distribution of solar energy among the various macroscopic processes at the Earth's surface along with the present forms and frequencies of all the fluctuations found in it, together form the climate of the planet Earth.

The extraterrestrial power of the solar radiation incident upon the Earth is equal to (cf. Willson, 1984)

$$\pi r_E^2 I_S = 4\pi r_E^2 I = 1.7 \times 10^{17}\,\text{W},$$
$$I_S = 4I = (1367 \pm 3)\,\text{W/m}^2, \qquad\qquad (2.2.1)$$
$$I = 340\,\text{W/m}^2,$$

where I_S is the solar constant, its natural variability not exceeding 0.1 % (Hansen and Lacis, 1990); r_E is the Earth's radius. Due to rotation of the Earth, the solar energy incident upon the Earth's cross section of area πr_E^2 is distributed over the surface of the planet ($4\pi r_E^2$), and energy fluxes within the atmosphere and ocean; I is the average relative flux per unit area of the Earth's surface.

If all the incident energy were totally absorbed, the value of I would be defined by the orbit of the planet. In fact part of that energy is reflected from the planet surface, so that planets become visible among the stars. That reflected fraction of the solar radiant energy is called the planetary albedo A. The albedo of the planet Earth is 30% at present. To 83% of its value that albedo is controlled by reflection in the atmosphere and only to 17% by reflection from the Earth's surface (Schneider, 1989a), see Fig. 2.1 below. The averaged absorbed flux of solar radiation per unit surface area is

$$I_e = I(1 - A) = 240 \, \text{W/m}^2. \tag{2.2.2}$$

The atmosphere absorbs about one-third of the value of I_e. As compared to I the average flux of solar radiation absorbed by the surface of the Earth is decreased by the factor of about two in the result (see Eq. (2.2.1)) (Schneider, 1989a, Fig. 2.1) and amounts to:

$$I_0 \approx 150 \, \text{W/m}^2 \, . \tag{2.2.3}$$

That value includes the complete flux density of free energy which the Earth receives from space.

The absolute temperature of air is proportional to the average energy of motion of its molecules. The absolute temperature of the Sun's surface T_S is proportional to the average energy of the solar photons. Similarly, the absolute temperature of the Earth's surface, T_0, is proportional to the average energy of heat photons.

In its equilibrium state, when the temperature of the Earth's surface does not change, the energy of solar radiation incident upon the Earth coincides with the thermal radiation escaping from the Earth's surface. This means that, on average, each photon of solar radiation decays into $n = T_S/T_0 \approx 20$ photons of terrestrial thermal radiation re-emitted to space. It is because of that decay of solar photons that all the ordered processes we observe occur at the surface of the Earth.

Were the Sun to send the same amount of energy to Earth in the form of thermal radiation (so that the temperature of the Sun would coincide with that of the Earth, $T_S = T_0$) the Earth's temperature would remain the same, but no decay of solar photons would be possible, and, hence, no ordered processes would take place at the surface of the planet. The Earth would then remain warm, as it actually is, but no dynamic processes would occur on it, and no life would exist (certain ordered processes would still be possible due to the rotation of Earth around its axis, and orbit around the Sun, so that the day-to-night, and the summer-to-winter temperature contrasts would be present, but they would in no way compare to those actually observed on Earth now).

Table 2.1 lists the distribution of the solar and other forms of energy available at the Earth's surface among various macroscopic motions.

Geothermal energy, its power being around 30 TW, is generated via the processes of density distribution in the Earth's core and the processes of radioactive decay in these depths. The upper limit of power released in the course of redistribution of masses may be estimated from the dimensional constants as a value of the order of $M_E g r_E / t_E = 3 \times 10^3$ TW, where $M_E = 6 \times 10^{24}$ kg is the mass, $r_E = 6 \times 10^6$ m is the radius, and $t_E = 5 \times 10^9$ years is the age of the Earth, $g = 9.8 \, \text{m/s}^2$ is the acceleration of free fall. Hence, redistribution of density by about 1% of its possible value is capable of explaining the available geothermal

Table 2.1. Energy fluxes at the Earth's surface

Power source sink	Power		References
	TW	Fraction, %	
Solar power distribution:	(1.7×10^5)	(100)	Willson, 1984
Atmospheric and surface absorption	10^5	69	Ramanathan, 1987; Schneider, 1989a
Surface absorption	8×10^4	46	Schneider, 1989a
Evaporation expenditure	4×10^4	24	Schneider, 1989a
Available eddy heat flux	$\sim 1 \times 10^4$	7	Schneider, 1989a
Equator to poles heat fluxes:			Kellogg and Schneider, 1974
atmospheric	$\sim 3 \times 10^3$	2	Peixoto and Oort, 1984
oceanic	2×10^3	1	Chahine, 1992
Land absorption	2×10^4	13	Ramanathan, 1987 Schneider, 1989a
Evaporation power by land (evapotranspiration)	5×10^3	3	Lvovitsh, 1974 Brutsaert, 1982
Plants (transpiration)	3×10^3	2	Brutsaert, 1982
Wind power (dissipation power)	2×10^3	1	Gustavson, 1979 Brutsaert, 1982
Oceanic waves (dissipation power)	1×10^3	0.6	Brutsaert, 1982
Photosynthetic power	10^2	0.06	Whittaker and Likens, 1975
Gravitational power of precipitation	10^2	0.08	Lvovitsh, 1974
River hydraulic power (300 m fall of global runoff)	3	2×10^{-3}	Lvovitsh, 1974 Skinner, 1986
Other renewable powers: geothermal	30	0.02	Berman, 1975 Skinner, 1986 Starr, 1971
Volcanic and geyser	0.3	2×10^{-4}	Starr, 1971
Tidal	1	6×10^{-4}	Hubbert, 1971
Moonlight	0.5	3×10^{-4}	Allen, 1955
Present-day consumption by mankind	10	6×10^{-3}	Starke, 1987, 1990 Skinner, 1986
Human-induced increase of greenhouse effect	10^3	0.6	Dickinson and Cicerone, 1986

energy. That power generates all the ordered processes of production of ores in the lithosphere and changes in the environment at an efficiency not exceeding 10^{-3}. The global power of these ordered processes does not exceed 10 GW, that is, it remains four orders of magnitude below the photosynthetic power of the global biota (Brimhall, 1991).

2.3 The Physical States of Dynamic Equilibrium

If there is no flux of free energy, the molecules of a medium remain in a state of thermal (thermodynamic) equilibrium. At such an equilibrium the number of molecules possessing energy ε is proportional to their Boltzmann exponent $\exp(-\varepsilon/k_B T)$ where $k_B = 1.4 \times 10^{-23}$ J/(K molecule) is the Boltzmann constant, and T is the absolute temperature (T K $= t\,°C + 273.16$ K). In particular, if ε is equal to the kinetic energy of molecules, the Boltzmann distribution transforms into the Maxwell distribution of velocities. These distributions are established in the course of random noncorrelated interaction of molecules among themselves, their transitions into any arbitrary states remaining equally probable. As a result the overwhelming majority of molecules appear to occupy those states that are more numerous. That state of matter is the one with minimal organization.

Instead of the state of an individual molecule, thermodynamics studies the state of a macroscopic group of molecules occupying a volume comparable to that of the human body. The measurement unit for such estimates is the mole, which contains $N_A = 6.02 \times 10^{23}$ molecules (the Avogadro number). This number of molecules is contained in the amount of substance whose mass in grams is numerically equal to its atomic mass, i.e. coincides with the number of protons and neutrons in that molecule (to the accuracy of the binding energy of the nucleus). The number, n_E, of moles of matter having the energy $E = N_A \varepsilon$ is given by the expression

$$n_E = ce^{-E/RT}, \qquad R = k_B N_A = 8.3 \text{ J mole}^{-1}\text{K}^{-1}, \qquad c = \text{const.} \quad (2.3.1)$$

In the absence of external flux of energy, molecules in their chaotic thermal motion may form a group of N molecules which randomly organize by themselves into an ordered macroscopic motion. Such a phenomenon is called fluctuation. However, the relative frequency (probability) of fluctuations occurring in N molecules is proportional to $1/\sqrt{N}$. That proportionality is called the law of large numbers. Considering the general character and importance of that widely known law, we are going to take a numerical example to demonstrate its action in the interest of further exposition.

Consider the velocity of motion of the center of masses of a group of N molecules in a given direction. We denote that velocity as X, and the velocity component of each molecule from that group along the same direction as x_i. Defining the velocity of the center of mass of a group of molecules we have:

$$X = \frac{1}{N}\sum_{i=1}^{N} x_i. \qquad (2.3.2)$$

The average velocity of such molecules and of any group of molecules in a stationary cell filled with gas or liquid is equal to zero: $\bar{X}_i = \bar{x}_i = 0$. Conducting serial measurements of the velocity of a group of molecules one may obtain the average squared velocity for that group:

$$\overline{X^2} = \overline{\left(\frac{1}{N} \sum_{i=1}^{N} x_i \right)^2} = \frac{1}{N^2} \sum_{i=1}^{N} \overline{x_i^2} + \frac{1}{N^2} \sum_{i \neq j} \sum_{j} \overline{x_i x_j}. \qquad (2.3.3)$$

If molecules move in a non-correlated fashion, the second term on the right will be equal to zero. Recalling that the average squared velocities for each molecule are equal to each other, we find for the average velocity of a group of molecules:

$$\sqrt{\overline{X^2}} = \frac{1}{\sqrt{N}} \sqrt{\overline{x^2}}. \qquad (2.3.4)$$

That equation essentially expresses the law of large numbers. The principal assumption needed to retrieve that law was zeroing the second term in (2.3.3). If molecules move in a correlated fashion, so that, for example, N molecules are emitted at equal velocities in one and the same direction, we find the average velocity of the center of gravity of that group of molecules to be equal to the average velocity of each molecule. That may be directly seen from (2.3.3). In that case the second term in (2.3.3) is much larger than the first one, and equals $\bar{x}^2$. Therefore, the second term controls the degree of correlation among the molecules in the group: if its observed value is less than or equal to the first term in its order of magnitude (that is when the law of large numbers is satisfied), molecules may be assumed to move chaotically. The correlation distance in gas appears to be of the order of the size of the molecules themselves, which is much smaller that the average distance between the molecules in that medium (the mean free path).

One may thus derive the law of large numbers for any variable presentable as a sum of its components. In particular, the value of X in (2.3.2) may be envisaged as an average x_i from a set of N independent measurements. Equation (2.3.4) corresponds to the well-known law of decreasing standard deviation at large N.

The dimensionless ratio $r_{ij} = \overline{x_i \cdot x_j} / (\sqrt{\overline{x_i^2}} \cdot \sqrt{\overline{x_j^2}})$ is the simplest correlation characteristic possible; it is the well-known correlation coefficient. However, the correlation coefficient only reflects the presence of a linear correlation between two variables, so that it may adequately describe any nonlinear correlation while these correlating variables show relatively small changes. Generally speaking, if these relative changes are large and the coefficient of correlation is zero, that does not mean a lack of correlation at all. For example, if two variables are related to each other as $x^2 + y^2 = 1$, one may average over the whole circle $\overline{xy} = 0$ and the presence of eddy motions within a large group of molecules will bring the same result, Eq. (2.3.3), as one would find in the case of a totally uncorrelated motion. To find nonlinear relations one must use more sophisticated correlation functions. However, during small relative changes of variables any nonlinear correlations linearize. In our example we obtain $x \equiv x_0 + \Delta x$, $y \equiv y_0 + \Delta y$; and $\Delta x / x_0 \sim \Delta y / y_0 \ll 1$ a dependence $r_{xy} \equiv \overline{\Delta x \Delta y} / (x_0 y_0) = -1$.

Assume that matter consists of internally correlated groups of particles (of domains) which are mutually non-correlated. The r_{ij} is nonzero only inside the group. The average linear size of such a group (the radius of correlation of domains) may be estimated at small relative changes by calculating the sum

$$\frac{\sum_{ij} |r_{ij}| R_{ij}}{N^2}, \qquad R_{ij} = |x_i - x_j|$$

over these N particles, i, and j for which all their r_{ij} differ from zero (within the experimental accuracy), the value R_{ij} giving the distance between the particles i and j. The correlation radius may similarly be prescribed for any measurable characteristic of these particles, defining the value r_{ij}. The internal correlation for various objects may be extremely diverse. It is described by various correlators found by alternative averaging techniques. Both complete lack of, and deficiency of, correlation may always be described (at small relative changes) by the respective value of the correlation coefficient.

The mean squared velocity of the molecules describes the macroscopic characteristics of a substance: its temperature and gas pressure. Temperature and pressure are only meaningful for objects of sufficient macroscopic size. Since the number of molecules in $1\,cm^3$ of a solid body or in $1\,dm^3$ of gas is close to the Avogadro number, that is $N \sim 10^{23}$, fluctuations of external macroscopic characteristics become practically unobservable for compact objects exceeding $0.1\,\mu m$ in size. However with the particle size diminishing below that level, fluctuations of both temperature and pressure become noticeable, and particles start to move randomly in the medium – they display Brownian motion. Temperature and pressure lose any meaning for particles of the size approaching that of molecules. The chemical kinetics and catalytic reactions in a living individual are characterized by the averaged measurable characteristics of large groups of their molecules. For fluctuations of their characteristics to be sufficiently small, the size of such groups should be large enough. We conclude that the minimal size of living individuals should be three to four orders of magnitude larger than the size of an individual molecule.

2.4 The Stability of Physical States

A typical feature of the state of thermal equilibrium, in which all its molecules interact in a non-correlated manner, is that all the characteristics of that state remain unchanged when the volume of that gas or liquid is divided into arbitrary macroscopic parts. Each such part containing a sufficiently large number of molecules will possess characteristics (such as temperature, pressure, etc.) identical to those of the whole volume.

The least ordered state of matter is the most stable one. Stability of a state means that after a short external perturbation the system returns to its initial state and remains in it for an unlimited length of time. For example, if a group of molecules is either decelerated or accelerated, its Maxwell distribution of velocities is eventually recovered in accordance with the average temperature of the medium. Sustaining a state means that the measurable characterizing variables (such as temperature, pressure, average velocity of its center of gravity, etc.) do not change with time. Such a state is called stationary. Clearly, any stationary state actually existing is stable, because certain external perturbations are always present.

One should stress that a stationary state is described by permanent macroscopic measurable variables. Individual molecules incessantly collide with each other in a stationary state of thermal equilibrium, changing their velocities, direction of movement, and internal level of excitation.

If an external perturbation is permanently present, such as the flux of the solar energy falling upon the surface of the Earth, the state of the matter changes and reaches another level, stable with respect to that perturbation. Such a level corresponds to equilibrium between the generation of new and the decay of old ordered macroscopic motions, typical for the given form of matter. On average, that new level features a higher degree of order than in the absence of perturbation. Stationarity and stability of such a state means that after averaging over the lifetime of such ordered motions, we find that its measurable characteristics remain constant with time. The flow of a river may be considered stationary, despite the constant generation and decay of turbulent eddies in any local part of that stream. Stationarity and stability of a flow are characterized by its constant average flow rate, by the constant distribution of angular velocities, by the lifetime of its turbulent eddies, etc. The Earth's climate is characterized by the constant annual mean temperature, pressure, annual mean wind direction and speed, the average number of cyclones and anticyclones, the amplitudes of the diurnal and seasonal oscillations of temperature. Note that during the whole lifespan of life on Earth temperature fluctuations have never reached amplitudes such that oceanic waters would either totally evaporate or freeze.

If the flux of energy is constant, only macroscopic processes of the average degree of order may be sustained for an unlimited length of time, their decay permanently compensated by their generation. Thus in the case of a stable dynamic equilibrium the ratio of the number of decays of ordered states to the number of their spontaneous generations is equal to unity.

Macroscopic processes of a significantly higher than average level of order are only generated as rare fluctuations with limited lifetimes (tornadoes, for example). The more highly a fluctuation is organized, the lower is the probability of its spontaneous generation and the rarer such fluctuations are. Thus rare fluctuations are always unique. Among rare fluctuations the ones of most interest are those whose energy dissipation is the lowest. Although both rarely appearing and quickly dissipating, such fluctuations have sufficiently long lifetimes and that is why they are empirical in the first place (such as thunderballs, for example). Among such fluctuations are those wave processes which slowly fade losing their ordered character (tsunami). However rare fluctuations do not, as a rule, produce any input to the average state and its characteristics.

The average degree of order of macroscopic processes, which are generated by a given flux of external energy, does not change with time, i.e. remains stationary, if an equal amount of waste thermal energy is evacuated from it. The states of a stationary average order are sometimes called non-equilibrium dissipative structures, since they are sustained by an external flow of energy (Nicolis and Prigogine, 1977; Prigogine, 1978). However, recalling that they remain stable only in a constant flow of external energy, we may call them states of dynamic equilibrium. (The state of dynamic equilibrium is vividly illustrated by an example of a bird or a helicopter, hanging motionless in the air (hovering flight (Weis-Fogh, 1972)). All the man-made engines operating in a stable regime are also examples of stationary states of dynamic equilibrium.)

With increasing flux of energy the degree of order of average constantly sustained macroscopic processes and of fluctuations generated increases. Now fluctuations, which had been rare at lower energy levels, may be permanently sustained, and fluctuations which had been extremely rare may become more frequent. If a system sustaining a stationary macroscopic process of low order is introduced to such a flux of energy, that process appears to be unstable in that flow, and within a measurable finite period of time it transforms into a more ordered stable state of dynamic equilibrium, corresponding to the average level of order in the flux of energy fed to it. After averaging over periodic oscillations and frequent fluctuations, the new state of dynamic equilibrium also becomes stable, and, hence, is completely determined by the value and character of the external flux of energy. The decrease of that flux of energy results in an inverse sequence of events, so that the level of order in macroscopic processes falls (Schuster, 1984).

Thus there always exists a certain state of dynamic equilibrium of every observed physical and chemical process occurring at a given flux of external energy. With that external flux changing, the stability of such a state is violated. Below we shall call that stability "physical". Macroscopic processes of order both above and below the average become unstable and are only encountered as rare fluctuations. In other words, rare fluctuations spontaneously occurring within a prescribed flux of energy do not possess physical stability.

It is well known that the level of order of a system can only increase either when external energy is fed into it, or when heat is evacuated from it (e.g., when gas transforms into liquid, or liquid into solid). When external variables reach certain values, the level of correlation between various particles in the system and its degree of internal order both increase stepwise. That process continues via interaction of molecules of the system with each other and via the reduction of the number of stable states of separate molecules when the total energy of the system decreases. Similar sharp changes in the level of correlation between various parts of the system may also happen within the external flux of energy if certain critical values of the measurable parameters of such a flow are reached (Haken, 1982).

All the processes of change of stable order of physical systems, precipitated by changes to their environments beyond certain critical values, e.g., when external energy is fed to the system or its thermal energy is evacuated from it are traditionally called critical phenomena or phase transitions (Haken, 1982). Phase transitions may either result in increase or in decrease of the order of the system, depending on the direction in which its external parameters change (Schuster, 1984).

We shall cite well-known examples of phase transitions which follow the change in the external flux of energy. With the flow rate of fluid increasing it proceeds from laminar to turbulent flow. With temperature lapse rates increasing disordered mixing of liquid rises to an ordered cellular convection (the Bénard cell forms). At low levels of optical pumping a laser emits radiation as an ordinary light bulb, radiating a wide spectrum of random frequencies, but with increasing pumping power all its atoms start to radiate in a correlated coherent manner at a single frequency, and all the other frequencies vanish from its spectrum. Similar phenomena take place during chemical reactions: if an energy-rich flow of monomers is produced, stationary states may be found with equality of polymer generation and decay, or, alternatively, periodic temporal and spatial changes in the concentration or substances (Haken, 1984; Nicolis and Prigogine, 1977). Products of some autocatalytic chemical reactions containing equal number of right- and left-handed molecules (the racemate) can transform to an ordered chirally pure state containing only right- or left-handed molecules through a bifurcational process of spontaneous breaking of the mirror symmetry when the flux of organized external energy introduced to, or flux of thermal energy evacuated from, the system reach the critical values (Morozov, 1978; Goldanskii and Kuz'min, 1989, Avetisov and Goldanskii, 1993).

2.5 Physical Self-Organization

During the last few decades major advances have been made in studying the behavior of physical systems in an external flux of energy, i.e. systems having a state of dynamic equilibrium (Schuster, 1984). It has been demonstrated that phase transitions from one stable state to another, triggered by changes in the characteristics of the external flux of energy, and taking place at critical values of these characteristics, could be described by comparatively simple non-linear equations. Moreover, systems of completely different physical and chemical nature often appeared to be described by similar equations. These finding resulted in combining such physical results into a single branch of science of such physical and chemical systems, which has been named "synergetics" (Haken, 1982, 1984).

Any changes in the values of physical variables are only known to an accuracy prescribed by the available resolution of the experimental instrumentation used. Thus any initial condition may only be described to within the margin of such errors. Forecasts of the development of such systems, following the laws of their behavior, will all contain certain ambiguities (stemming from those initial conditions). After certain systems proceed past their threshold levels in the flux of external energy, that uncertainty begins to grow exponentially with time so that such a system may proceed from any initial to practically any final condition or state. That system will still retain its stability in the sense that all its final states will not deviate too far from its given average (will be "attracted" to a certain fixed value). These values are called "strange attractors" (Schuster, 1984; Eckman and Ruelle, 1985). Attractors are average values of measurable characteristics of common stable systems, such as those oscillating in either a fading or non-fading mode. A system with a strange attractor behaves chaotically, although it is described by simple deterministic classical equations, which do not include any quantum uncertainties (Eckman and Ruelle, 1985).

Such equations with strange attractors are expected to describe phenomena of turbulence in nature. Many researchers hope to similarly describe the phenomenon of stability of life (Nicolis and Prigogine, 1977; Haken, 1984). However, in contrast to phase transitions, life and death are irreversible.

Following the above developments the observed characteristics of phase transitions are often described using biological terminology, on the grounds, first of all, of the seeming analogy between the manifestations of physical-chemical order and the processes of life. E.g., by analogy with the creation of previously nonexisting new genetic information, i.e. self-organization of the living species in the course of evolution, the process of growth of order in physical-chemical systems, taking place when external energy is fed to them, is called self-organization (Nicolis and Prigogine, 1977). Substitution of the unstable physical state by a stable one occurring then, is called selection (Haken, 1982, 1984), while the interaction between the unstable and stable states is called competition. In that sense the notions of selection and competition may apparently be applied to any physical and chemical processes, associated with transitions from some initial to a certain stable final state, proceeding via several unstable intermediate states. One may thus speak about selection among the several competing oscillation maxima (modes) in a laser (Haken, 1982, 1984), as well as about competition and selection among the various competing chemical and physical reactions (Nicolis and Prigogine, 1977), which may, with various probabilities, stem from a given initial state. The two possibilities for a cloud either to dissipate in the sky or to precipitate to the ground are also envisaged as competition and selection among the two alternatives, and similar treatment may be given to the well-known fact that only one river flows out of a lake (Odum, 1983).

Self-organization, competition, and selection among all the chemical and physical processes are related to the stable state of dynamic equilibria. The possible types of competition between the various ordered states and selection among them are then totally determined by the characteristics of the flux of external energy fed to them (Schuster, 1984). It is evident that rate fluctuations which occur spontaneously in small numbers around the state of dynamic equilibrium cannot compete with each other. Selection is manifested as decay and vanishing of all the rare physical fluctuations. It is demonstrated in the next section that there exist clear-cut differences between the content of all the above notions, as applied to animate and inanimate systems. Therefore, we shall indicate below as "physical" the commonly used terms of stability, self-organization, competition, and selection, when applied to physical and/or chemical systems.

2.6 The Measurable Variables:
Dimensions and Mutual Correlations

Natural sciences cover the domain of knowledge that includes information on the quantitative measurable variables of natural objects. That information may be reduced to indicating the variability range for those numerical values, and to the empirically found relations of both fundamental and correlation character between the various measurable variables. The experimentally observed values of measurable variables and the correlations between them are what we call the laws of nature. They are expressed by equalities ($=$). All the numerical values obtained during measurement and all the empirically found correlation relations (i.e. all the equalities) have finite nonvanishing experimental uncertainties.

A combination convenient in one or other respect may always be constructed from several measurable variables, and a certain symbol and meaning may be ascribed to such a combination. It is essentially a definition, a "substitution" of variables, and, in contrast to the laws of nature, it should be presented by an identity ($\equiv$). For example, if some measurable variable $z(t)$ changes at a rate $\dot{z}(t) \equiv dz(t)/dt$ with time, a relative rate of that change may be introduced; we denote it as $k(t)$:

$$\frac{\dot{z}(t)}{z(t)} \equiv k(t) \quad \text{or} \quad \frac{\dot{z}(t)}{z(t - \tau(t))} \equiv K(t), \tag{2.6.1}$$

where the lag function $\tau(t)$ may be prescribed arbitrarily. Expressions of the form (2.6.1) are identities; they only describe the procedure of substitution of variables, so they contain no additional information that was formerly unavailable. They may be written for any variable. Such expressions only turn into equalities if a law of temporal change is known for $k(t)$ or $K(t)$, and $\tau(t)$, independent of $z(t)$.

So later all the identities agree with the newly introduced notations, which are uniquely related to independent variables already introduced, that is to substitution of variables. Equalities are used to relate the variables carrying independent information.

The choice of measurement units depends on considerations of convenience, and, generally speaking, on the observer's wishes. Observed correlation dependencies between arbitrary measurable variables cannot depend on the choice of units for their measurement and description, so they must be invariant with respect to the choice of such units. If this is not so the correlation dependence is absent. The condition is satisfied when both parts of the equality have identical dimensions, or expressed as an equality of some dimensionless variables. The relation between the two variables (z and l) of differing dimensions is only possible if a single dimensionless combination may be formed from them. Such a dimensionless combination may be formed if a fundamental physical constant of a transitional dimension is available. For example, length, l, and time, t, may be related via velocity, u, or acceleration g:

$$l = ut, \qquad l = gt^2. \tag{2.6.2}$$

A relation between velocity, length, and acceleration may be found from the above in the form of the Froude (Fr) number which does not include time:

$$\frac{u^2}{gl} \equiv Fr = 1 \qquad \text{or} \qquad u = \sqrt{g\,l}. \tag{2.6.3}$$

If a problem does not include such a physical constant of transitional dimension (scale-free allometric, self-similar or fractal and critical phenomena) such dimensionless combinations may be found exclusively from the ratio of the rate of change of variable dz (or dl) to that variable itself z (or l). In that case the relation between the changes of variables of differing dimensions dz and dl (which remain minor as compared to the variables z and l), may only have the following form (see Brody, 1945; Gell-Mann and Low, 1954; Hemmingsen, 1960; Kleiber, 1961; Stahl, 1963; Wilson and Kogut, 1974; Mandelbrot, 1982; Gorshkov, 1984c; Smirnov, 1986; Peng et al., 1992):

$$\frac{dz}{z} = \beta\,\frac{dl}{l}, \qquad d\beta = \psi(\beta)\,\frac{dl}{l}, \tag{2.6.4}$$

where β is a dimensionless coefficient of proportionality. The increment of a dimensionless value $d\beta$ may vary in proportion to the increment of the value dl/l (or dz/z), its proportionality coefficient being equal to an arbitrary function of a unique finite dimensionless value β, as shown by the second equation.

Any change in the variables may only be detected at the finite experimental accuracy available (the measurement error), which depends on the sensitivity of instruments attainable (Pipkin and Ritter, 1983). The relation between the minor relative increments (2.6.4) may also be tested empirically, provided the value of the relative increment exceeds that experimental accuracy. It follows from the above that a "nonlinear" relation between the two relative increments of the two variables is impossible: it would mean a lack of correlation. For example, forming dz/z and $(dl/l)^2$ one always may select the values dz and dl so as to keep dz/z within the measurement error, and the value $(dl/l)^2$ far below that limit. It is known that $dx/x = d\ln(x/x_e)$, where x_e is arbitrary. Therefore, $\ln(x/x_e)$ is a unique selected function, which has a dimensionless differential.

The general solution of (2.6.4) has the form:

$$\ln \frac{z}{z_e} = \phi \left(\ln \frac{l}{l_e} \right), \tag{2.6.5}$$

where the function $\phi(x)$ is uniquely expressed via the function $\psi(\beta)$:

$$\ln \frac{l}{l_e} = \int_{\beta_e}^{\beta} \frac{d\beta'}{\psi(\beta')} = f^{-1}(\beta), \qquad \beta = f\left(\ln \frac{l}{l_e} \right), \qquad \beta_e = f(0)$$

$$\phi(x) = \int_0^x f(x')\,dx'. \tag{2.6.6}$$

The symbol f^{-1} here denotes an inverse function, l_e is an arbitrary integration constant, and z_e and β_e are expressed via relations (2.6.5) and (2.6.6) at fixed

z and l. Such a relation is sometimes called a renormalization group. In the approximation of constant β, the solution of these two equations acquires a simple form:

$$y = \beta x, \qquad y \equiv \ln\left(\frac{z}{z_e}\right), \qquad x \equiv \ln\left(\frac{l}{l_e}\right). \tag{2.6.7}$$

Relations like (2.6.7) are called allometric in biology (Pardé, 1980; Peters, 1983). In what follows, the correlation of the form (2.6.7) at length l will be found for many variables z, so it appears convenient to express the slope, β, of the line, relating $\ln z$ to $\ln l$ ($y = \beta x$) by the symbol: z'

$$\beta = z' \equiv \frac{d \ln(z/z_e)}{d \ln(l/l_e)}. \tag{2.6.8}$$

The value l_e is an arbitrary dimensional constant. It is determined by the choice of the measurement unit (see index "e"). The value z_e is defined via the chosen value l_e and the measured values of z and l. The functional dependence (2.6.7) does not change when l_e changes (the so-called scale invariance).

Relations (2.6.7) can be rewritten in the form:

$$\frac{z}{z_e} = \left(\frac{l}{l_e}\right)^\beta \quad \text{or}$$

$$z = a l^\beta, \qquad a \equiv z_e l_e^{-\beta}. \tag{2.6.9}$$

Here the coefficient a (so-called "Hausdorf measure") has a complex fractal dimension if β is an arbitrary irrational number. Equation (2.6.9) is frequently used in the special biological literature (Peters, 1983).

We also show here the form of the functional dependence (2.6.5) for the case when $\psi(\beta_0) = 0$, and the function $\psi(\beta)$ may be expanded into the Taylor series over powers of $\alpha \equiv (\beta - \beta_0)$. We retain only the first non-vanishing term in that expression:

$$\psi(\beta) = \gamma_1 \alpha; \qquad \phi(x) = \beta_0 x + b_1(e^{c_1 x} - 1),$$

$$c_1 \equiv \gamma_1, \qquad b_1 \equiv \alpha/\gamma_1, \qquad x \equiv \ln\frac{l}{l_e}; \tag{2.6.10}$$

$$\psi(\beta) = \gamma_2 \alpha^2, \qquad \phi(x) = \beta_0 x + b_2 \ln(1 + c_2 x),$$

$$b_2 \equiv -\frac{1}{\gamma_2}, \qquad c_2 \equiv -\gamma_2 \alpha.$$

The terms of the function $\phi(x)$ retained in (2.6.10) may be considered corrections to the allometric formula (2.6.7) where b_1, c_1 and b_2, c_2 may be selected empirically, as may β_0. The constant β_0 may be either close to or equal to zero. In that case the correction terms acquire the leading role.

The relation of two variables via a single fundamental physical constant may also be presented in the form of (2.6.7) and (2.6.9). In that case, due to the linearity of the laws of dynamics, the slopes of the logarithmical direct lines for z' in (2.6.7) are expressed as simple rational numbers. For example, the dependence of the form $u = \sqrt{gl}$, relating the distance of the vertical jump l to take off velocity u may be written in the form of (2.6.7) at $u' = 1/2$, $u_e = \sqrt{gl_e}$ or in the form (2.6.9) at $a = u_e/\sqrt{l_e} = \sqrt{g}$.

Measurement units are prescribed by experimentalists from considerations of convenience. These units might never coincide for any two experimentalists, so they would never know that these two units were of one and the same dimension. What are the indications that meters and yards, years and hours coincide in dimension while, e.g., meters and years are of differing ones? We shall demonstrate that this question may only be answered experimentally.

Consider measuring length, which is the simplest case imaginable. We find that different quantitative estimates of that characteristic may be obtained, depending on the units used, e.g. yards vs meters. It is not known a priori whether both numbers describe one and the same characteristic of the object, measured in different units. That is only to be found empirically. One further finds that, to within experimental accuracy, the ratio of the number of yards to meters remains unchanged, independent of the actual length measured. Hence one may state that two such measurements do indeed describe one and the same characteristic of an object. It may be formally expressed in the form:

$$\frac{l_1}{1\,\text{m}} = c\,\frac{l_2}{1\,\text{yard}}, \qquad c = 0.914399, \tag{2.6.11}$$

where l_1 and l_2 always present one and the same characteristic of a measured object, that is its length l. We may formally reduce both parts of our empirically found equality (2.6.11) by $l \equiv l_1 = l_2$, finding the relation between yards and meters:

$$1\,\text{yard} \approx 0.91\,\text{m}, \qquad 0.91\,\text{m/yard} \approx 1.$$

Assuming the transitional constant to be identically equal to unity, we may completely exclude the yard from further consideration, proceeding to measure length in meters only.

Heat (Q) and work (W) were considered different characteristics of a system for a long time. Heat was measured in calories, and work in Joules. The discovery of the law of energy conservation demonstrated that work could transform into equivalent amounts of heat, i.e.

$$\frac{W}{1\,\text{J}} = c\,\frac{Q}{1\,\text{cal}}, \qquad c = 4.1855. \tag{2.6.12}$$

Equation (2.6.12) describes a law of nature, which always holds to within the achieved experimental accuracy. Thus, similar to the above, one may assume heat and work to be similar energy characteristics of the system, having identical dimensions. Treating both heat and work as energy, one may set: $Q = W$, eliminating the unit for measuring heat (calories), completely transferring to the use of Joules:

$$4.2\,\text{J} \approx 1\,\text{cal} \quad \text{or} \quad 4.2\,\text{J/cal} \approx 1.$$

One should not, however, forget that another characteristic is changed while work is transformed into heat. That is entropy (or information), a measurable, non-conserved characteristic; see Sect. 2.8.

Prior to discovery of Newton's second law, force (f), mass (m), and acceleration (a) were assumed to be unrelated. Force was measured in kilogram-force (kgF), mass in kilograms, and acceleration in m/s^2. Newton's law stated that when force f was applied to body of mass, m, acceleration, a, was generated, which was related to the force and body mass by:

$$\frac{m}{1\,\text{kg}}\,\frac{a}{1\,\text{m/s}^2} = c\,\frac{f}{1\,\text{kgF}}; \qquad c = 9.81. \tag{2.6.13}$$

(That is why if $a = g = 9.81\,\text{m/s}^2$, body weight (force) measured in kilograms-force numerically coincides with its mass, measured in kilograms, so that the relation is a consequence of Newton's law.) Because of the universal character of relation (2.6.13) which is always satisfied at velocities negligibly small in comparison with the speed of light, Newton's second law may be written in the form:

$$f = ma,$$

so that the force and the product of mass and acceleration are variables of one and the same dimension, and we may eliminate the unit for measuring force, the kilogram-force, from our expressions:

$$1\,\text{kgF} = 9.81\,\text{Newton (N)}, \quad 1\,\text{N} \equiv 1\,\text{kg\,m/s}^2, \quad \text{or} \quad 9.81\,\text{N/kgF} = 1.$$

The relation of energy, E, to body momentum, p, for bodies moving at velocities close to the speed of light, c, is also well known: $E^2 = m^2c^4 + p^2c^2$. At zero momentum the mass of a body is proportional to its energy. That mass characterizes the internal potential energy of the body at rest. When we move from one inertial reference system to another, both its energy and momentum change. They are transformed as constant vectors in the spatial-temporal continuum. Mass remains without change in all the reference systems. It is an invariant, a scalar. The total energy and momentum are conserved during body-to-body interaction. The mass is not conserved. E.g., the atom absorbing a photon of zero mass enters an excited state of higher potential energy and higher mass. Conservation of mass and of matter follows from the law of energy conservation only in the approximation of velocities low with respect to the speed of light. Since green plants use the energy of light for their life processes, lack of mass in light results in important ecological consequences (Sect. 5.5).

The body mass m is sometimes called its rest mass. The term mass in motion, M, is given to the variable related to energy via the relation $E = Mc^2$. In contrast to rest mass, m, the mass in motion, M, like the energy, E, is conserved within one and the same system of reference, but changes in a transition from one such system to another. However, introduction of an additional variable always related to body energy via a constant factor is physically irrelevant. Thus no mass in motion exists physically. Any body is only characterized by its mass m and the definition "rest" should be omitted (Okun, 1988).

The law of universal gravity in its nonrelativistic approximation of small velocities of two masses m_1 and m_2 at distance r from each other defines the force of their interaction:

$$f = G \frac{m_1 m_2}{r^2}, \qquad G = 6.670 \times 10^{-11} \frac{m^3}{kg \cdot s^2}. \qquad (2.6.14)$$

Since that law is universal and always holds, one can discard the dimension of mass altogether, assuming $G \equiv 1$. However, gravitational forces acting between two masses are negligibly small compared to electrodynamic forces, which control all the biochemical reactions and interactions between bodies studied by biology. The relative magnitude of gravitational forces may be defined by comparing the force of electrodynamic and gravitational interaction between two electrons. The Coulomb interaction between them is given by the well-known force of the form (2.6.14) in which m_1 and m_2 are substituted by the two electron charges, and the constant G is assumed equal to unity. (The dimension of the charges themselves is found from the Coulomb law.) The dimensionless ratio of gravitational, f_G, and electrodynamic, f_e, interactions is equal to (see, for instance, Allen (1955)):

$$f_G / f_e = \frac{G m_e^2}{e^2} = 2.3 \times 10^{-43}, \qquad (2.6.15)$$

where m_e and e are the electron mass and charge, respectively.

Thus gravitational interaction between the bodies around us which are of size comparable to the size of biological objects (individuals) is essentially switched off, as compared to electrodynamic forces. Only the interaction of all such bodies with the mass of the Earth remains noticeable, as expressed by the acceleration of free fall g, both on land and in the air. In the ocean gravitation is compensated for by the Archimedes force and is not manifested. If life failed to proliferate from ocean to land and air, or originated on minor planets of sizes comparable to those of artificial satellites, the existence of universal gravitational interaction would be unlikely to be discovered, and the motion of the planets would seem to follow its own exclusive laws, while all of life would run its course in the state of free fall, without any change in the nature of its biological and biochemical reactions.

In that sense, gravitational interaction is effectively not universal. The mass of 1 kg, a value typical in biology, has no relation whatsoever to the mass unit of $1 \, m^3/s^2 = 1.5 \times 10^{10}$ kg, which would have to be assumed were we to set $G \equiv 1$.

Thus only the empirically found universal relations between variables of differing dimensions make it possible to reduce the number of different units needed to describe measurable variables (Sedov, 1959, 1977). However, further reducing the number of different units does not depend on our wishes, but is controlled by the laws of nature, which are universal correlations. So why do the dimensions of mass, length, and time remain independent? That is because no universal correlations are found between these characteristics. Moreover, the very fact of processes occurring in the world around us demonstrates that no such universal relations exist.

Thus the choice of measurement units for mass, length, and time remains arbitrary in all the branches of science having to do with actual life and environment.

They may be fixed in some system of units, such as the International System of Units (SI). Fundamental constants appear to be more convenient for use in certain specialized studies (Okun, 1988). (E.g., the principal measurement units within the scope of the physics of high energies are usually the Planck constant, $\hbar$, the speed of light, c, and the mass of either the electron, m_e, or the proton, m_p.)

One may estimate the feasibility of introducing new terms and notions by the same reasoning. New terms should only be introduced when they include various non-correlated characteristics of an object. For example, the term "biota" describes living beings only, while "biosphere" embraces all the nutrients used by these beings as well. It also helps to make a distinction between such notions as theory and mathematical model. These are strict in the exact natural sciences (such as astronomy, physics, chemistry), but are not as accurately used in biology and ecology.

Theory is an empirically founded unique system of a limited number of correlations, describing a large spectrum of phenomena to an accuracy known from experimental practice. That accuracy is not necessarily too high, e.g. some theories are only capable of correctly predicting the order of magnitude of the value measured. Theory might well predict what is impossible. For example, everything which violates (2.6.11–14) is impossible within the estimated experimental accuracy. Anything at all may happen within the margin of these relations. The small dimensionless parameters (such as relative deviations from the equilibrium points $\Delta z/z_0$, see (2.7.9), or combinations including fundamental physical constants like the Froude number (2.6.3), fine structure constant $\alpha \equiv e^2/(\hbar c) = 1/137$ and others) are present in many theories. The Taylor expansion over powers of such small parameters (the so-called perturbation theory) permits step by step increases in accuracy of the result predicted by the theories. The nonperturbative approach should be used if the theory contains singularities near the zeros of small parameters.

No calculations within a given theory should be carried out to accuracies exceeding the empirically found margin of uncertainty of that theory's predictions. Calculations driven to higher accuracy are nothing but a gross blunder, which is called "exceeding the accuracy limit". For example, one should not sum inputs from various sources when estimating the global stores of fresh water or of biomass if such sources have different orders of magnitude, or cite a result which includes more decimal positions than the experimental error of the largest input.

In contrast to that approach, a mathematical model tries to reach some insight into the course of the process being considered. A model is constructed when no general theory is available. It merges together the known theories of separate elements of the overall phenomenon. Missing correlations, which are necessary for either deterministic or stochastic predictions, are either retrieved from the yet poorly tested empirical data or postulated. The accuracy of such postulated correlations remains unknown. When the accuracies of correlations included in the model are available, the mean square (MS) uncertainty of any prediction by such a model is proportional to the sum of such MS uncertainties of all the individual relations. Diverse models and various scenarios in every model, all of them describing one and the same phenomenon, are possible. They differ in the form of correlations used, their accuracies overlapping. Becoming gradually more and more complex as the number of correlations introduced into it grows, the model becomes capable of producing more and more predictions. However, the uncertainty of each such prediction also broadens with the growing number of these correlations. In this case the number of available mathematical models approaches infinity and the information obtained with the help of the models tends to zero. Testing enormous numbers of such scenarios with modern high speed computers does not in any way substitute for experimental testing of the accuracy of correlations introduced into such models.

2.7 Thermal Stability of Climate

The flux of short-wave solar energy absorbed by the Earth, I_e, heats the surface of the planet, resulting in terrestrial thermal radiation which is emitted back into space. As a result the budget of energy fluxes at the Earth's surface may be expressed in the form:

$$I_e = q_e + c \frac{\partial T}{\partial t}, \tag{2.7.1}$$

where I_e is the solar radiation absorbed by the Earth; it depends on the solar constant I_S, and the planetary albedo, A; q_e is the flux of effective thermal radiation emitted by the planet into outer space; c is the heat capacity of the planet; T is the absolute surface temperature. The last term in (2.7.1) describes the temporal change in the thermal energy of the Earth, Q. It is assumed that Q depends exclusively on the absolute temperature T. The planetary heat capacity $c = \partial Q / \partial T$ depends mainly on the heat capacity of the oceans (Mitchell, 1989).

We have in a stationary state: $T = T_0$, so that one may find for the surface of the planet:

$$q_{e0} = I_{e0} = I (1 - A_0). \tag{2.7.2}$$

The values of q_{e0} and A_0 depend on temperature T_0. Equation (2.7.1) is an implicit function of temperature T_0 and of the solar constant I_S ($I = I_S/4$, see (2.2.1)). Before studying the temperature dependence (2.7.2), we are going to clarify the principal form of the dependence of q_e on T_0.

The value of q_e may, to a good approximation, be described as blackbody radiation. That assumption determines the effective temperature T_e of the Earth's radiation escaping to space, which does not coincide with T_0. According to the Stefan-Boltzmann law we have:

$$q_e = \sigma T_e^4, \qquad \sigma = 5.67 \times 10^{-8} \, \frac{W}{m^2 K^4}. \tag{2.7.3}$$

The flux q_e is directly measured in outer space from on board artificial Earth satellites (Raval and Ramanathan, 1989). Thus the temperature T_e is well known. Using the value of I_e (see (2.2.2)) we find $T_e = 255\,K$ (or $-18\,°C$), see Table

Table 2.2. Planetary energy and temperature characteristics

Planet	Solar const. I_S $\frac{W}{m^2}$	Orbital parameters $(A = \alpha = 0)$		Thermal emission to space $(A > 0,\ \alpha = 0)$			Average values at planetary surface $(A > 0,\ \alpha > 0)$		
		q_R $\frac{W}{m^2}$	t_R, °C (T_R, K)	A	q_e $\frac{W}{m^2}$	t_e°, C (T_e, K)	α	q_0 $\frac{W}{m^2}$	t_0, °C (T_0, K)
Mars	589	147	−48 (225)	0.15	125	−56 (217)	0.07	134	−53 (220)
Earth	1367	342	+5 (278)	0.30	239	−18 (255)	0.40	390	+15 (288)
Venus	2613	653	+58 (331)	0.75	163	−41 (232)	0.99	16 000	+460 (730)

– A is the planetary albedo
– α is the planetary normalized greenhouse effect
– $q_R = I_S/4$ is the orbital planetary thermal emission at $A = 0$, $\alpha = 0$
– q_e is the observed planetary thermal emission into space
– q_0 is the observed average planetary surface thermal emission
– t_i, T_i are the respective surface temperatures

(Mitchell, 1989; Raval and Ramanathan, 1989)

2.2. The surface temperature, T, exceeds the temperature of escaping radiation, measured at the top of the atmosphere, T_e. Therefore the radiation of the Earth's surface q exceeds the escaping radiation q_e. That effect results from the greenhouse gases in the atmosphere, which trap a significant part of surface radiation and re-emit it downward. As a result, radiation of the Earth's surface, q, may be found from the equation:

$$q = I_e + \alpha q \quad \text{or} \quad q = \frac{I_e}{1 - \alpha}. \tag{2.7.4}$$

The reflection coefficient α describes the fraction of thermal radiation from the Earth's surface that is trapped by the atmosphere and "reflected" back to the surface. It is again absorbed there, additionally heating the surface then being emitted into the atmosphere, cf. Fig. 2.1. Emission from the Earth's surface may be described by the Stefan-Boltzmann law, which deals with temperature measured at the surface:

$$q = \sigma T^4. \tag{2.7.5}$$

Thus we have for a stationary state:

$$q_{e0} = q_0(1 - \alpha_0) \tag{2.7.6}$$

$$I(1 - A_0) = q_0(1 - \alpha_0), \qquad q_0 = \sigma T_0^4. \tag{2.7.7}$$

The reflection coefficient $\alpha = (q_0 - q_{e0})/q_0$ is often called the "normalized greenhouse effect". It may also be directly measured from on board artificial Earth satellites (Raval and Ramanathan, 1989). Having the surface temperature of the

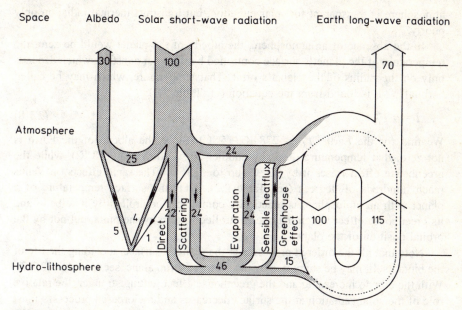

Fig. 2.1. The distribution of solar radiation. Shaded areas show the fluxes of free energy and of the ordered terrestrial processes. Blank areas show the long-wave thermal radiation of Earth. Numbers give the percentage of the incident solar radiation (Mitchell, 1989; Schneider, 1989a).

Earth, $T_0 = 288\,\mathrm{K}$ (15 °C) one may determine $q_0 = 390\,\mathrm{W/m^2}$ and find $\alpha_0 = 0.40$, cf. Table 2.2. The absolute value of the greenhouse effect is $\alpha_0 q_0 \approx 160\,\mathrm{W/m^2}$. Of that value approximately $100\,\mathrm{W/m^2}$ results from the activity of water vapor molecules in the air, which amounts to about 0.3% by volume of the Earth's atmosphere, and about $50\,\mathrm{W/m^2}$ from the atmospheric CO_2, its content being approximately 0.03%. The rest of the greenhouse effect results from such gases as CH_4, N_2O and O_3, their cumulative content in the atmosphere not exceeding 3×10^{-4}% (Mitchell, 1989).

The atmosphere producing the greenhouse effect is a multilayered stratified formation, similar to a fur coat. The flux of outgoing heat $q(z)$ at every layer at height z is proportional to the rate of change of temperature ∇T. With the external heat flux q_e and external temperature T_e given, the internal temperature, T_0, grows in proportion to that coat thickness; $T_0 = T_e + L_a \nabla T$. That "coat" turns part of the heat emitted by the body backwards. The Earth's surface temperature is determined by the temperature gradient actually observed in the atmosphere ($\nabla T = 5.5$ °C/km) and by the effective atmospheric thickness (atmospheric scale height $L_a = 6\,\mathrm{km}$). Up to $L \sim L_a$ the value of ∇T remains practically constant (Mitchell, 1989; Raval and Ramanathan, 1989). In contrast to a normal fur coat, the source of heat generating the greenhouse effect appears to be external: the atmosphere is transparent for solar radiation, but transmits thermal radiation only poorly.

In the absence of an atmosphere, the albedo of the planet would be zero, the temperature of the planet's surface controlled by the solar constant, which depends only on the radius of the planet's orbit. That temperature, which may be called "orbital", T_R is found from the equation (cf. Table 2.1):

$$I = \sigma T_R^4. \tag{2.7.8}$$

We find for the Earth: $T_R = 278$ K ($+5\,°C$). Since the albedo of the Earth is not zero, that temperature drops by another $23\,°C$ (down to $-18\,°C$), while the greenhouse effect raises it by $33\,°C$ (up to $+15\,°C$). The same effects on Venus reach hundreds of degrees (see Table 2.2). Thus the surface temperature of a planet with an atmosphere is practically completely controlled by its albedo and its greenhouse effect which may be controlled in turn by the biota, but not by the orbital position of the planet.

Note that all the ordered processes at the planet's surface, including the life of the biota itself, may be supported by the solar radiation alone, see term I in (2.7.7). With the albedo increasing and the greenhouse effect getting stronger, the relative role of the solar radiation at the surface decreases and the ordered processes must be extinguished. Thus planets removed far from the Sun might be warm, but life would still be impossible on them.

The flux of energy additional to solar radiation, which is produced by the combustion of fossil fuel, has reached 10^{13} W, or $0.02\,\text{W/m}^2$, see Table 2.1. At the same time the anthropogenic increase of the greenhouse gases, including CO_2, CH_4, O_3, N_2O, CFC − 11, CFC − 12 results in the greenhouse effect increasing by factor of 100, so that the additional thermal radiation of the Earth's surface now reaches $2\,\text{W/m}^2$ (Dickinson and Cicerone, 1986), corresponding to an additional global power of 10^{15} W. However the thermal power may only result in increasing the Earth's temperature, without changing the scale of the ordered processes on its surface, which are supported by the solar radiation and the additional power of combustion of fossil fuel.

To analyze the thermal stability of the $T = T_0$ state, we expand all the terms of (2.7.1) within the margin of the minor relative deviation from the equilibrium point:

$$\frac{T - T_0}{T_0} \equiv z.$$

Then, using the conditions in (2.7.7) at that equilibrium point $z = 0$ and accounting for the minor terms over z, we obtain:

$$\dot{z} + k_0 z = 0; \qquad k_0 \equiv \frac{\lambda_0}{c_0} \tag{2.7.9}$$

and

$$\lambda_0 \equiv \frac{q_{e0}}{T_0} \left(4 + \frac{A_0' T_0}{1 - A_0} - \frac{\alpha_0' T_0}{1 - \alpha_0} \right) \tag{2.7.10}$$

the notation introduced here being as following:

$$\dot{z} \equiv \frac{\partial z}{\partial t}, \qquad X_0' \equiv \frac{\partial X(T_0)}{\partial T_0}, \qquad X_0 = X_0(T_0); \qquad X = A; \alpha; q; c.$$

The sensitivity of climate λ_0 is a function of T_0. The stationary value of T_0 is a function of I, its implicit form defined in Eq. (2.7.7). Differentiating both parts of (2.7.7) over I we have (see North et al., 1981):

$$k_0 = \frac{1 - A_0}{c_0} \left(\frac{dT_0}{dI} \right)^{-1}. \tag{2.7.11}$$

The solution of (2.7.9) has the form:

$$z = z_0 \, e^{-k_0 t}. \tag{2.7.12}$$

It follows from (2.7.12) that at $k_0 > 0$ any deviations from the equilibrium point fade exponentially with a relaxation time k_0^{-1} so that the state $T = T_0$ is stable. Negative feedbacks prevail in such a system, suppressing minor perturbations in it. On the other hand, at $k_0 < 0$ any deviation from the point $T = T_0$ grows exponentially, and that state is unstable. Positive feedbacks prevail in such a system, strengthening any perturbations that arise.

Equation (2.7.1) may formally be rewritten in the form of (2.7.9) without expansion over z; one merely substitutes k_0 by the function $k(z)$, which is found from (2.7.1) if one knows the dependencies of all the terms in (2.7.1) on T (or on z). In that case $k_0 = k(0)$. If, unexpectedly, $k(0) = k_0 = 0$, higher order terms should taken account of in the expansion of $k(z)$ over z. If $k(z) \sim z^n$, we find $z(t) \sim t^{-1/n}$, i.e. tends to zero, but extremely slowly, with t growing, so that essentially there is no stationary solution of the problem. Besides, the form of the function $k(z)$ depends on numerous characteristics of the environment. With perturbations of these characteristics growing, the value k which characterizes the stability of the environment may also change. Therefore, we will call the value $k_0 = 0$ the "point of stability loss" in what follows.

Equation (2.7.1) and its form (2.7.9), in which the variable is substituted by $k(z)$, are often rewritten via the potential function (the Lyapunov function), which is given by the relation $k(z) = -\partial U(z)/\partial z$ at any z (North et al., 1981; Rapoport, 1986). The extremum of that function is at $z = z_0$ where $\partial U(z)/\partial z = 0$ characterizes the stationary point, while the second derivative $\partial^2 U(z)/\partial z^2$ characterizes the solution's stability. We have $U(z) = -(1/2)k_0 z^2$ at $z_0 = 0$, i.e. $-\partial U(z)/\partial z = kz$ and $k_0 = -\partial^2 U/\partial z^2$. In other words, $U(z)$ describes a stability trough at $k_0 > 0$, and an unstable peak at $k_0 < 0$. However, in actual problems of describing the state of the environment the behavior of all the terms of that equation (which describe conservation laws of the type (2.7.1)) far from the existing stationary state, remains unknown. Thus it is only of academic interest to consider the potential function. Our analysis of the environmental stability is limited to finding the stationary point (in our case the point $T = T_0$) as well as the rate of relaxation k_0 (which is the inverse time), and the perturbation threshold of the measurable environmental characteristics at which the system loses its stability, i.e. k_0 becomes zero.

In both physics and chemistry thermodynamic equilibrium is characterized by stability in any independent variable (such as pressure, volume, temperature, concentrations of the chemical elements in various physical states, etc.). Perturbation of any of these variables results in generation of the compensating processes, which return the system to its initial state. The property of equilibrium is well-known under the name of the Le Chatelier principle (see, e.g., Lotka, 1925). However, following strong perturbations, such as adding new substances, changing the volume of the system or its internal energy, the system finds a new stable stationary state at a new equilibrium point, different from the stable stationary state prior to that perturbation. In exactly the same way the stable states of dynamic equilibrium ("dissipative structures") may be described, within the external flux of energy (Nicolis and Prigogine, 1977). Physical and chemical states of lifeless planets in the solar system are particular cases of such dynamic equilibrium (Lovelock, 1982; Holland, 1984).

The very fact that a state of the environment fit for life has been sustained for billions of years, despite the constant forcing by strong geophysical and cosmic perturbations, testifies unequivocally to the stability of that state. That stability is characterized by temperatures (above the freezing and below the boiling points of water), pressures, and relative concentrations of chemical substances in their various physical states, which remained within the margin for life for geological time periods of hundreds of thousands or millions of years, despite the alternating glacial, interglacial, and ice-free periods (Broecker et al., 1985a; Broecker and Denton, 1990). The stability of the environment over periods of several thousand years or less is characterized by a strict constancy of practically every characteristic of the environment (Oeschger and Stauffer, 1986; Chappellaz et al., 1990; Barnola et al., 1991), so that no directional shifts of the environment take place. The question naturally arises whether such a stability is physical in nature (Holland, 1984; Holland et al., 1986), or results from the existence of life and of life processes (Gorshkov, 1985b; Lovelock, 1989).

First, if stability of the environment were to be exclusively explained by physical reasons, the equilibrium point would continuously drift, affected, as it were, by directed perturbations, external with respect to the terrestrial environment. Such a drift should have inevitably resulted in the system going outside the margin for life. For example, if organic carbon had not been deposited in sedimentary rocks, the content of inorganic carbon in the environment (in the form of CO_2 mainly) would have increased by four orders of magnitude, as compared to its present-day level, during the last 6×10^8 years (Ronov, 1976; Budyko et al., 1987). That would have resulted in a catastrophic runaway greenhouse effect, and an increase of the surface temperature past the boiling point of water. During the time life has existed on Earth (3.5×10^9 years) the solar radiation has increased by about 30% (Newkirk, 1980), which should have also resulted in an increase of the surface temperature above the upper limit fit for life (Lovelock, 1989). The atmospheric oxygen should have been spent on oxidizing volcanic products in about 10^8 years

(Budyko et al., 1987), and the atmospheric nitrogen should have been transformed into its bound soluble forms (Lovelock, 1988).

Second, the stationariness of the contemporary climate is evidently not stable, to within the error limit of the available measurements. To clarify that problem consider (2.7.10) and (2.7.11). Since the conditions

$$A_0 \leq 1, \qquad c_0 \geq 0$$

are satisfied for the albedo and the planet heat capacity, we find $k_0 > 0$ on condition that $dT_0/dI > 0$ (North et al., 1981), i.e. temperature should grow with I growing, and vice versa. However, since the dependence of $T_0(I)$ is unknown, and, by all indications, will never be measured directly, the last inequality may not be directly employed. Nevertheless, obvious conclusions may be drawn from (2.7.11), stating that the stability (the value of k_0) decreases 1) with $A_0 \to 1$, which happens if the whole planet is covered with ice; 2) when $c_0 \to \infty$, i.e. when water is evaporated in a runaway manner, so that temperature does not change. Further analysis of the stability of k_0 may be conducted by studying the feedbacks A_0' and α_0' in (2.7.10).

When $A_0' = \alpha_0' = 0$ climate stability is controlled by the first term +4 in round brackets of (2.7.10), which results from the negative feedback characterizing the Stefan-Boltzmann law (2.7.7). With temperature increasing, the escaping thermal flux grows, so that with the greenhouse effect and albedo remaining unchanged ($\alpha_0' = 0$, $A_0' = 0$) the Earth's surface cools. In that case the value of k_0 may be estimated, so that the relaxation time k_0^{-1} may be found. It follows from (2.7.10) that at $A_0' = \alpha_0' = 0$; $\lambda_0 = 3.3 \, \mathrm{Wm^{-2}K^{-1}}$. The average value of c_0 per unit surface area may be estimated by assuming that the principal input to c_0 is produced by the upper oceanic layer of depth H_s: $c_0 = (\rho C)_{H_2O} \, S_s H_s / S_E$, $(\rho C)_{H_2O} = 4.2 \, \mathrm{MJm^{-3}K^{-1}}$, where $S_s/S_E = 0.70$ is the ratio of the oceanic surface to the total Earth's surface area, $H_s \approx 300 \, \mathrm{m}$. To find both upper and lower limit of H_s we recall that H_s is larger than the depth of the mixed layer ($\sim 100 \, \mathrm{m}$) and is less than the depth of the principal thermocline ($\sim 1000 \, \mathrm{m}$): $100 \, \mathrm{m} < H_s < 1000 \, \mathrm{m}$. We find that $c_0 \sim 10^9 \, \mathrm{Jm^{-2}K^{-1}}$ ($3 \times 10^9 \, \mathrm{Jm^{-2}K^{-1}} > c_0 > 3 \times 10^8 \, \mathrm{Jm^{-2}K^{-1}}$). Recalling that $1 \, \mathrm{W} = 3 \times 10^7 \, \mathrm{J/yr}$, we find:

$$k_0 \approx 10^{-1} \, \mathrm{yr^{-1}}, \qquad k_0^{-1} \approx 10 \, \mathrm{yr} \, (A_0' = \alpha_0' = 0). \qquad (2.7.13)$$

Thus, when there is no greenhouse effect and the albedo is equal to zero, the surface temperature should relax back to its natural value in about ten years, provided the forcing perturbation ceases.

Actually both terms A_0' and α_0' in (2.7.10) present a thermodynamically positive feedback ($\alpha_0' > 0$, $A_0' < 0$): With temperatures growing the normalized greenhouse effect strengthens and the albedo decreases because both the snow and ice cover recedes (Mitchell, 1989). The last two terms in round brackets in (2.7.10) are negative, so they decrease the overall stability. The value α_0' is directly measured from on board the satellites by comparing the values of α_0 which correspond to different local surface temperatures (Raval and Ramanathan, 1989). According to these measurements $\alpha_0' T_0 \approx 1.0$, for cloud free skies. Taking account of cloud cover adds a term of the value of 0.6 to $\alpha_0' T_0$ (Mitchell, 1989). As a result we have $-\alpha_0' T_0/(1-\alpha_0) \approx -2.7$. The albedo reaction is calculated in various models of global circulation. According to them the value $A_0' T_0/(1-A_0) \approx -0.4$, which brings the negative sum of the last two terms in (2.7.10) to -3.1. Radiative properties of cloud cover are still obscure. If one assumes that the sign of the cloud cover feedback is also indefinite (Mitchell, 1989), the value of λ_0 remains indistinguishable from zero to within the measurement error, and may well be negative.

However, only physical and chemical feedbacks may be accounted for in all the measurements and calculations (the latter being neither too numerous, nor too important) (Holland et al., 1986; Kump, 1989). It has been definitely demonstrated by Raval and Ramanathan (1989) that the observed increase in the greenhouse effect is produced by the rising of water vapor concentration in the atmosphere at higher temperatures. Despite the enormous variability of water vapor content in the atmosphere, the relative humidity (i.e. the ratio of water vapor concentration to its saturating concentration) varies much less, and may, to a first approximation, be assumed constant (Mitchell, 1989). The dependence of the atmospheric water vapor concentration on temperature will then coincide with the behavior of saturating concentration. Such behavior is controlled by the Boltzmann exponent in (2.3.1), with the latent heat of evaporation L_W substituted instead of energy E in it ($L_W = 40.5\,\text{kJ/mole}\,H_2O$). That is the "activation energy" for evaporation in the Clausius-Clapeyron exponent. Using the numerical value of L_W we find that the concentration of water vapor approximately doubles ($Q_{10}^{H_2O} \approx 2$, see Sect. 5.1 below) if the temperature increases by $10\,°C$. That is the development resulting in a stronger greenhouse effect.

However the Clausius-Clapeyron exponent determines only the thermodynamic equilibrium water vapor content in the atmosphere. The evaporation temperature for water vapor $T_W = L_W/R = 4900\,K$ (here R is the gas constant, see (2.3.1)) is close to temperature of the Sun's surface, and is much larger than the Earth's surface temperature T_0. That is why the water cycle, including the evaporation driven by the radiation, the ensuing precipitation and run-off is an ordered process, which remains far from the equilibrium. Similar to other ordered processes at the Earth's surface driven by solar radiation, the water cycle would not speed up at higher temperatures, accompanying the stronger greenhouse effect. The only ensuing effect may consist in redistribution of evaporation and precipitation over the Earth's surface, their global average values, however, remaining unchanged. Speeding up of the water cycle may only result from a higher fraction of the solar energy being spent on evaporation, as compared to its present-day fraction, cf. Fig. 2.1. Consequently that would result in a change in surface temperature. Such an effect might only take place on land, precipitated by the land biota as it were (Shukla and Mintz, 1982, see Sects. 4.13 and 5.4).

As seen from Fig. 2.1 about one-half of the solar radiation is spent evaporating moisture. If a greater fraction of the solar radiation reaching the Earth's surface were spent on evaporation, that would result in a significant decrease in the Earth's temperature. Temperature does not rise in the course of evaporation. Water vapor is raised to higher altitudes in the atmosphere where it condenses, releasing the energy absorbed during evaporation. That energy escapes to outer space in the form of thermal radiation, and only an insignificant part returns to the surface, penetrating the reflecting screen of water vapor in the atmosphere, thus increasing the surface temperature. Clouds may simultaneously increase the reflectivity for both solar and thermal radiation, the latter coming from the surface, thus raising both the albedo and the greenhouse effect. The total effect of all those processes remains obscure as yet, because we still lack a satisfactory theory to describe processes which are far from thermodynamic equilibrium (Nicolis and Prigogine, 1977). That is essentially the problem of ambiguity of the radiative properties of clouds (Mitchell, 1989).

Other greenhouse gases (CO_2, NH_4, O_3, N_2O) are relatively homogeneously distributed in the atmosphere and to find the feedbacks between their concentrations and the Earth's surface temperature one has to address past epochs. More complete information on such feedbacks may be retrieved from analyzing the composition of ice cores of known age (Lorius et al., 1990), and from various mathematical models of global circulation (Cess et al., 1989; Mitchell, 1989). However, pursuing such studies, one may again only retrieve the physico-chemical feedbacks, as when studying the local differences in climate reactions. Possible control of the environment by the biota is still completely missing from such a treatment. Moreover, it is clearly impossible to identify all the degrees of freedom of the environment controlled by the biota, because the information power of the biota exceeds that reachable by civilization by 15 orders of magnitude (Gorshkov, 1991a, see the next section).

Thus stable states of complete ice cover (as on Mars) or of complete evaporation of liquid phases (as on Venus) are evidently not separated from the existing stationary state by any physical barriers, so that the matter of a sustained existing state of the environment remains unexplained (if we neglect the control by biota).

In contrast to physical stability, controlled, as it were, by the physical Le Chatelier principle, biological control of the environment does not result in any shift of the stable state, when affected by external forcings. Such a biological stability could be called the biological Le Chatelier limit, or threshold. However, throughout this book we are interested in biological stability only, and when speaking about the Le Chatelier principle we imply the biological negative feedbacks, which compensate completely for all the external perturbations, which then do not result in any shift of the position of the point of equilibrium.

2.8 Correlation Distances and Information

The ordered state of matter in an external flux of energy is characterized by the presence of correlated structures, featuring either unlimited or finite correlation distances. Both the atmospheric circulation and oceanic currents are structures correlated on a global scale by the rotation of the Earth and by the temperature drop from the equator to the poles. An unlimited correlation distance is typical for a river, to give another example: a dam set across its bed shows an effect practically up and down the whole stream. An unlimited correlation length is also typical for solid bodies. However many correlated structures only display strictly limited correlation lengths (such as in molecules composed of separate atoms); or these structures may be characterized by a certain distribution of the originating structures over the finite correlation lengths (such as the sizes of vortices in a turbulent flow). The volume in which such a state of matter exists, with correlated structures of finite correlation lengths, cannot be separated or divided into arbitrary macroscopic parts without losing the characteristics of that state. The vortex of a tornado or of a cyclone, as any other vortex in a turbulent flow, cannot be divided into its "parts". The same conclusion is valid for the Bénard cells, or for spatial domains, in which the states of periodic chemical reactions alternate. As to be demonstrated in the Section to follow, all forms of biological correlation can only display strictly limited finite correlation distances.

The degree of correlation and of order among the various entities may be quantitatively characterized by a distribution of correlation lengths, and by their entropy and information content. The correlation lengths may be described using various correlation functions and coefficients of the type of the second term from the expression (2.3.3). Entropy is a strictly defined function of state, valid for equilibrium thermodynamic states and for minor deviations from these states (Nicolis and Prigogine, 1977). Attempts to describe a system in dynamic equilibrium by employing a field of local microscopic values of entropy, which are defined for every point of space occupied by the system, meet with certain difficulties, because the characteristic of order should also include information on the spatial correlation of the system, which is of macroscopic size, so that a nonlocal description is needed (Prigogine, 1980).

To compute the degree of order in various correlated systems one may employ the definition of entropy and of information via the logarithm of probability for the given forms of correlation to start with (Brillouin, 1956). However, for such super-correlated entities such as living individuals and their environment, one fails to define all the complexity of their correlated parts in a concise manner. One then needs to compute the information content for some part of that entity, and ascribe some validity to that information, which may be defined as the ratio of the known amount of information to the total information describing the whole correlated entity.

Nevertheless the quantitative estimate of information may be used to compare the fluxes of information processed by the natural Earth biota with those information fluxes which are realistically attainable by all the computer power mankind possesses. Information may be characterized by the number of memory cells N. If each cell includes two equally probable values of some variable, the number of possible combinations of various values in all the cells will be 2^N. The logarithm to base 2 of that number is equal to N, that is to the number of cells. The number N presents the maximum possible amount of information (in bits, that is the memory volume) which such a system of cells may contain. If the state of N_1 cells in that system remains unknown, the amount of information is reduced to $N - N_1$. Finally, if the state of each cell remains undefined, the information becomes zero.

When the initial state of every cell is known, and certain erasure of memory takes place with time so that the state of all the cells become indefinite again, the loss of information is again defined by the number of cells, N. Increasing the number of the various states which each memory cell may occupy does not significantly change the maximum available amount of information: when that number is raised from 2 to n, the number of various possible combinations becomes equal to $n^N = 2^{N \log_2 n}$, and the amount of information increases to $N \log_2 n$. In other words, the amount of information linearly depends on N, and only logarithmically on n.

Elementary memory cells of the environment are the states of atoms and molecules: the ground states of atoms and molecules do not suffer decay. Photons may only interact with matter (photon to photon light scattering is negligibly small). Therefore, the decay of the short-wave solar photons into long-wave terrestrial thermal photons may only take place via excitation and decay of a cascade of molecular processes in the Earth's atmosphere and at the surface. The number of molecules with which the solar photons interact (the capacity of molecular memory of the planet Earth) coincides with the number of long-wave photons emitted into outer space. Since the average energy of a thermal terrestrial photon is of the order of $k_B T_e$, the flux N_e of long-wave photons per unit surface area of the Earth is

$$N_e = \frac{c_e q_e}{k_B T_e}, \tag{2.8.1}$$

where q_e is the effective flux of terrestrial thermal photons escaping to space, Eq. (2.7.3), see Table 2.2, and the dimensionless coefficient c_e is of the order of unity.

The terrestrial thermal radiation is close to the characteristic radiation of a blackbody at a similar temperature. Thus the number N_e in (2.8.1), characterizes the loss of information due to complete decay of the ordered molecular states, excited by solar radiation, and the disordered states, which had received no additional information in the process of their interaction with the solar radiation. If all the solar photons were completely ordered, as is the case with laser emission (or with the flow of molecules of a waterfall), all the terrestrial molecular memory cells would be excited in an orderly fashion, so that a total decay of their states into characteristic thermal radiation would take a certain time. In that case the flux of information coming from the Sun to the Earth would coincide with the number of excited memory cells, and would thus be given by the value from (2.8.1).

In reality solar photons are generated from characteristic black radiation at the surface of the Sun. The initial loss of information from the flux of the solar energy is characterized by the number of solar photons absorbed by the Earth. In a stationary state when the flux of solar energy, I_e, absorbed by the Earth coincides with the thermal radiation emitted by the Earth, q_e, the number, N_S, of such solar photons is equal to:

$$N_S = \frac{c_e q_e}{k_B T_S}. \tag{2.8.2}$$

Since both (2.8.1) and (2.8.2) characterize universal blackbody radiation, the proportionality coefficients in them (c_e) coincide with each other.

Each solar photon incident upon the Earth enters into interaction with terrestrial molecules. These terrestrial molecules are in chaotic thermal motion at an average energy $k_B T_e$. The chaos of thermal motion corresponds to continuous transfer of the molecule from one state to another (at the same energy) without of any selected position in the molecular memory cell, equivalent to information being erased. Having significantly higher energy, the solar photon is absorbed by the molecule, which proceeds to a state of high excitation. The molecular memory cell thus acquires certain information. The molecule, still remaining in that excited state and losing no information, may transmit part of that energy to other molecules, bringing them to a certain excited state, so that some information is present.The number of molecules acquiring information in that way will grow until the amount of energy transferred equals the initial thermal energy of terrestrial molecules, $k_B T_e$. Then the molecule which transmits energy suffers a backshock, so that the resulting state of the molecule is indefinite, and the information is lost. A cascade of such processes transforms the energy of solar photons into that of thermal terrestrial photons.

The process described may be envisaged as a cascade, in which the solar photon successively loses its energy to molecules acquiring information. To acquire additional information each molecule has to receive a portion of energy somewhat larger than the thermal energy $k_B T_e$. Apparently that transformation of energy will go on until the energy of the solar photon equals that of the terrestrial thermal photon. When that state is reached, the backshocks equal those the molecule delivers itself, and the molecule acquires no new information during collision. Each molecule carrying new information may then emit a photon of energy just exceeding the energy of the thermal photon, and returns to the disordered state of lost information. The number of molecules thus receiving information from the solar photon will equal the number of thermal photons, into which a single solar photon may decay, minus one, since the last downstep in that cascade is not accompanied by any transfer of information. If the process of discharge of molecular energy may be assumed slow enough, no loss of information (no decay) takes place along the whole of that cascade, so that such cascading is reversible. In other words the information, N, coming to Earth with all the solar photons it absorbs, is equal to the difference between the two numbers: N_e and N_S.

$$N = N_e - N_S = c_e \frac{q_e}{k_B T_e} \eta_e \tag{2.8.3}$$

$$\eta_e \equiv \frac{N}{N_e} = 1 - n_e^{-1}, \qquad n_e \equiv \frac{N_e}{N_S} = \frac{T_S}{T_e} \approx 23, \tag{2.8.4}$$

where n_e is the number of photons of terrestrial radiation into which a single solar photon decays, on average; η_e is the efficiency coefficient for the solar energy. The value of η_e gives the relative number of cells of molecular medium containing information, and $1 - \eta_e = n_e^{-1}$ is the relative number of molecular memory cells from which such information was initially erased. Since the value of n_e is quite large, $\eta_e = 0.96$, i.e. is close to unity, and the estimate of information coming to Earth practically coincides then with (2.8.1). However, at $T_S \to T_e$, $n_e \to 1$, $\eta_e \to 0$, and the information (2.8.3) turns to zero; as already stated above, the Sun having the temperature of Earth would send the same amount of energy to the planet, but would produce no ordered processes at the Earth's surface that way.

The total flux of the solar radiation is equal to $4\pi r_S^2 \sigma T_S^4$, where r_S and T_S are the Sun's radius and Sun's surface temperature. The Earth's solar constant is $I = 4\pi r_S^2 \sigma T_S^4 / 4\pi R^2$, where R is the Earth's orbital radius. Taking into account (2.7.2) and (2.7.3) we have $T_S^2 / T_R^2 = R/r_S$ provided the total flux of the solar radiation is assumed constant. Here T_R is the Earth's orbital surface temperature (at zero albedo and zero greenhouse effect). The angular size of the Sun in the Earth's sky increasing, the Sun's surface temperature T_S decreases. Were $T_S \to T_R$ ($r_S \to R$) the entire Earth's sky would be "filled up" by the Sun.

The Sun supporting ordered processes in the environment and in the biota is the physical basis of life existing on Earth. Therefore we consider (2.8.3) and (2.8.4) from different points of view: the solar photons are capable of generating ordered processes at the Earth's surface, transmitting all their energy down to that in equilibrium with the outgoing long-wave radiation, which escapes from the planet. Since the decay of a single photon into several long-wave ones during its interaction with molecules corresponds to an irreversible transformation of energy, the transformation of solar radiation not accompanied by any dissipation should leave the number of photons reaching thermal equilibrium with the thermal radiation of Earth, equal to the number of solar photons reaching the surface of the planet. These photons have the initial level of disorder implicit in solar energy, and they do not originate from decay in the course of the ordered terrestrial processes. If one assumes that all the ordered processes excited by solar energy decay into thermal photons as well, the Earth's temperature would be given by the expression $q_e = \sigma T_e^4$, Eq. (2.7.3). The number of solar photons is given by (2.8.2). The minimal flux of energy q_{min} of the long-wave terrestrial photons not related to generation of the ordered processes, i.e. to the effective work, satisfies the well-known Carnot condition:

$$N_S = \frac{q_e}{k_B T_S} = \frac{q_{min}}{k_B T_e}, \quad \text{or} \quad \frac{q_{min}}{q_e} = \frac{T_e}{T_S} = n_e^{-1}. \tag{2.8.5}$$

The efficiency of that work (the Carnot efficiency) is equal to $(q_e - q_{min})/q_e$ and coincides with (2.8.4).

The distribution of the solar energy into various ordered processes depends on the structure of the medium absorbing that solar radiation. It is apparent that the form of these ordered processes is different depending whether the biota is present or absent. The ordered processes are excited at an efficiency given by (2.8.4). However, the majority of these processes are not explained or described by equilibrium thermodynamics in which the efficiency (2.8.4) yields the maximum value, actually unattainable. Such a value may only be reached if no dissipation whatsoever takes place over long time periods such that thermodynamic equilibrium has enough time to set in. Actually the ordered processes have various dissipation times. Thus even processes with the longest dissipation times are generated at efficiencies below that given by (2.8.4). After such long dissipation times run out, the solar radiation completely decays into thermal photons. As a result the incident and the emitted (lost to space) radiation coincide with each other.

One may envisage a situation where the solar energy is mainly spent to generate ordered processes with practically unlimited dissipation times. For example, solar energy could be stored as potential energy·of synthesized organic matter or in the form of latent heat during continuous evaporation of oceans, etc. Such an absorbed energy would not transform itself into thermal radiation and would not bring about any heating of the surface of the planet. Then the thermal radiation of the Earth would be determined by that part of the solar energy q_{min}, Eq. (2.8.5), which would not be transformed into the energy of ordered processes. In this case the number of long-wave terrestrial photons would be equal to the minimal admissible value – the number of incident short-wave solar photons. Recalling that, with account of the Stefan-Boltzmann law $q_{min} = \sigma T_{min}^4$, and $q_e = \sigma T_e^4$ (cf. (2.7.3)), we find from (2.8.5) the value of T_{min}: $T_{min} = T_e(T_e/T_S)^{1/4} = 117\,\text{K}$ ($-156\,^\circ\text{C}$). The flux q_{min} per unit surface area of the planet would then amount to $11\,\text{W/m}^2$. In other words, such a hypothetical Earth would be totally covered with ice, devoid of life, and all the ordered processes at its surface would be completely different from those actually observed.

The surface temperature could then be raised via a stronger greenhouse effect. The additional chaotic thermal radiation accompanying the greenhouse effect is not associated with any decay of the ordered states of energy, and thus does not increase the flux of information. Moreover, the increase of surface temperature T_0 above the effective temperature of planetary radiation T_e decreases the efficiency of transformation of the solar radiation at the Earth's surface, which is given by (2.8.4), in which T_e is substituted by T_0. Thus the ordered processes generated by the solar radiation are transferred from the Earth's surface to the upper atmospheric layers. The ordered processes at the Earth's surface would completely stop at $T_0 \to T_S$. Such a tendency is found on Venus, see Table 2.2. To increase the flux of thermal photons from q_{min} to the observed value q_0, Eq. (2.7.7), one needs a level of the normalized greenhouse effect $\alpha = 0.97$, which is close to the value found for Venus. Hence, a complete overhaul of the present-day atmosphere would be needed for such a change, and life would then clearly be impossible. Therefore, to sustain the existing level of the ordered processes (including life) all such processes should necessarily decay, and their energy be dissipated within short enough times. That means that any organization may only be "mortal", and the produced "masterpieces" of order be continuously destroyed, so that they might be reproduced anew.

Finally the ratio of heat produced to the absolute temperature q/T of the system is equal to the entropy produced (Nicolis and Prigogine, 1977). Since the degree of order of processes at the Earth's surface is supported at a certain stationary level, the production of entropy due to decay of these processes is compensated by the influx of "negentropy" from the Sun, which, hence, is equal to the production of entropy, but with the opposite sign (Schrödinger, 1945; Brillouin, 1956). Due to the large temperature difference between the Sun and the Earth, the amount of entropy brought with the solar radiation is low as compared to its production on Earth, and hence to its retroflux from the Earth to outer space. As a result that net flux of entropy to the Earth is negative, and this is the origin of the term "negentropy". Thus, to the accuracy of a certain coefficient the flux of "negentropy" is given by the value q_e/T_e which coincides with the estimated amount of information, Eqs. (2.8.1) and (2.7.3), in the system of units where $k_B \equiv 1$. (Note, that the proportionality coefficients are well-known for blackbody radiation: at $k_B \equiv 1$ the entropy is $S = (4/3)(Q/T) = 3.7\,N$, where $Q = (\sigma/c)T^4$ is the thermal energy of radiation ($\delta Q = T\delta S$) and N is the average number of photons of thermal radiation (Landau and Lifshitz, 1964).)

If every molecular memory cell contains certain information, one may assume that one bit is proportional to one molecule. The condition $k_B \equiv 1$, Eq. (2.3.1), then corresponds to the relation 1 J/K $\approx 10^{23}$ bit. However, if only a fraction of molecules equal to η (see (2.8.3)) contains meaningful information, the condition $k_B \equiv 1$ corresponds to the relation:

$$1 \text{ J/K} \approx 10^{23} \text{ molecules} \approx \eta\, 10^{23} \text{ bit}. \tag{2.8.6}$$

This estimate is justified whenever the memory cells are objects of molecular size. All the absorbers of the solar energy in both the environmental media and the biota have such structures. As for the thermal energy associated with molecules in the thermal equilibrium state, in particular for all the thermal energy controlled by the greenhouse effect, the efficiency η, and, hence, the information contained in that energy, are equal to zero with very high accuracy of the order of 10^{-23}. However, practically all the forms of energy used by man and biota, including both the renewable and nonrenewable energy (such as solar energy, organic and fossil fuel, energy of wind and hydraulic energy) may be transformed into useful work at an efficiency, η, close to unity. Therefore one may use (2.8.6) to estimate the amount of information at $\eta \sim 1$.

Note that, in the case considered above when all the useful work is stored in the form of either potential or kinetic energy, and dissipation is absent, no production of entropy takes place: the flux of entropy from the Sun coincides with the backflux of entropy to space due to thermal radiation escaping from the Earth (i.e. the number of short-wave solar photons is equal to the number of long-wave terrestrial photons). Thus the flux of negentropy and information may in that case be estimated as the maximum of molecular and photon memory cells which may be excited in the course of decay of the accumulated potential energy, i.e. by the above expression (2.8.3).

Thus the total flux of information at the Earth surface in the course of ordered processes generated by solar radiation (2.8.3), may be estimated by the value of 10^{23} bit s^{-1} m^{-2}, or 10^{38} bit/s for the whole of the Earth's surface area (Thribus and McIrvine, 1971; Nicolis, 1986). The biota utilizes about 5% of the solar energy absorbed by the Earth, the principal part of that energy being spent on plant transpiration on land, and about 0.1% on photosynthesis (see Table 2.1). The fluxes of information used by the natural biota "computers" for transpiration and photosynthesis amount to 10^{36} bit/s and about 10^{35} bit/s, respectively. That information flux is directed to sustaining environmental stability by means of maintaining the life in natural biota.

The natural biota is capable of maintaining the stability of the environment up to certain thresholds of both environment and the natural biota, above which the stability of both is broken. The value of perturbation corresponding to such a threshold is of the order of 1% of the energy and information fluxes consumed by the biota (Chaps. 4 and 5), i.e. about 10^{33} bit/s. Mankind spends ten times more, about 10^{34} bit/s, for his energy consumption, see Table 2.1. That information flux supports civilization via destruction of the environment and the biota.

Note that molecular memory cells change their states with a definite probability in any operation (reading and duplicating the information etc.). As a result the information is erased and vanishes. In order to prevent the loss of genetic information programmed in DNA, life uses the catalytic system of DNA reparation and stabilizing selection based on competitive interactions of individuals in the population (Sects. 3.1 and 3.4). Apparently the information memory accumulated in the animal brain during its lifespan is also localized in the molecular memory cells. This information is expected to last during the finite time period of animal life (Chap. 5) and is much less stable compared to the genetic type. The collective interactions of molecules in the condensed matter of macroscopic memory cells conserve the information in modern computers for a long time. But that is why the memory capacity and the information fluxes in modern computers are rigidly restricted compared to the molecular memory cells used by the biota. The problem of suppressing spontaneous mistakes ("deleterious mutations") arises after the transition from macroscopic to molecular memory cells. The solution of that problem by future computers should be done by creating a catalytic repair system and other information-conserving mechanisms used by life (see Sect. 3.4).

Since memory cells in modern computers are objects of macroscopic size, the relation (2.8.6) is not applicable to them. The most advanced and powerful computers of the next generation will be able to process under 10^{12} bit/s of information (Foley, 1987; Weiser, 1991). Even if one assumes that all the people on Earth will have special personal computers of that capacity and power, mankind will not be able to process more than 10^{21} bit/s of information. To raise that information flux by another 15 orders of magnitude, up to the information flux flowing through the global biota, memory cells would need to be reduced to molecular size, and all the Earth covered with a continuous network of such computers, i.e. they should substitute the natural "computers" that have been in existence for billions of years.

Thus no mathematical models capable of describing the whole information fluxes in natural biota could ever be constructed.

The hereditary information of living individuals is contained in the polymer molecule DNA (Lewin, 1983), which includes about 10^9 monomer units (nucleotide pairs, i.e. memory cells), its information content reaching about 10^9 bit. The overall number of species in the biosphere is about 10^7 (Thomas, 1990). The hereditary information contained in all the species of the biosphere, with which each separate individual may interact, will thus include about 10^{16} memory cells. (Each nucleotide pair contains about a hundred atoms and is synthesized by the biota from inorganic molecules of the environment. Thus the number of molecular memory cells in the DNA molecule is a hundred times larger than the number of nucleotide pairs. Hence, the information content of a single mammal species may be given by the number of 10^{11} bit. However, most species in the biosphere are insects, and their DNA is a hundred times smaller, than that of the mammals. Thus the estimate of the total genetic information contained in the whole of the biosphere coincides with the value cited above.) The number of molecules (that is the number of memory cells in the environment) is about 10^{30} per cubic meter of that environment, so that the whole biosphere contains about 10^{48} such cells. It may be seen from these estimates that the environmental information with which the individual has to be correlated, exceeds its own hereditary information by many orders of magnitude.

Storage and processing of information should be related to its material carriers. Information contained in solar energy is processed by all of the biosphere, and is associated with spending all of the solar energy available. Information is processed and stored in either the animal or human brain tissue elements of molecular size which imitate the actual processes taking place in the environment. During such imitation the natural processes appear to be separated from their actual material carriers . Information in computers is also processed and stored in separate elements, which may be reduced to molecular size. That information may be transformed at an efficiency close to unity, practically without any energy expenditure (Robinson, 1984). Using adequate mathematical models one may attempt to imitate those processes which take place in the biosphere and the biota with such computers.

However biota already operates such "natural computers" built around the minimum possible molecular information carriers. The biota has already reached the highest possible efficiency of processing information. An embryo develops in an egg (within a natural "microprocessor") without absorbing any external energy (only the optimal temperature of such a development differs from species to species). In the course of development of either a fry or a chicken its egg may lose up to 20 % of its initial mass. The efficiency of information processing in such an egg thus exceeds 80 % (Kendeigh, 1974). In other words, all the energy absorbed by the biota is employed at a maximum possible efficiency level. In that case the actual processes taking place in the biota coincide with their best possible imitation models, that is such computers are merged with elements actually affecting the environment.

Hence, to approach the "technology" employed by the natural biota one would need some technical executing devices, driven by the solar energy and merged with computers running them, both simultaneously reduced to bacterial size, their computation programs made equivalent to genomes of several millions of the natural species in their information content. Thus one would need to completely reproduce the natural biota on a global scale, and consequently, the system already existing, that is the biota itself, is the only possible system capable of stabilizing the environment.

3. Stability of Life Organization

3.1 Biological Stability

All living beings exist by consuming part of the flux of external energy, i.e., by feeding. Similar to physical systems of the dynamic equilibrium type, consumed nutrients feed the reactions of directional biochemical decay of energy within the living body. The ordered character of such reactions of decay is induced by catalysts synthesized by the body itself. A catalyst is a chemical substance capable of speeding up certain chemical reactions without being spent in the course of the reaction itself. Reaction rate is proportional to the relative number of molecules having energy E above the potential barrier $A : E > A$, Eq. (2.3.1). A catalyst lowers that potential barrier A by a factor of several units, so that the reaction rate is increased by $\exp(A/RT)$. For most reactions their effective "barrier" temperature $T_A \equiv A/R$ exceeds the solar temperature: $T_A > T_S$ (see Eq. (5.1.1)). Thus we have $T_A/T > 20$ (see Eq. (2.8.4)), and

$$\exp\left(\frac{A}{RT}\right) \sim 10^8 - 10^{10}.$$

Hence, without a catalyst, the rates of respective biochemical reactions would have been many orders of magnitude lower, and spontaneous noncatalytic reactions would have been practically impossible. Thus, by synthesizing the necessary catalysts, the body controls all the biochemical reactions occurring within it, and strictly routes all the decay energy into prescribed channels. No quick spontaneous noncatalytic chemical reactions zeroing to thermodynamic equilibrium can be used by life.

After the physical death of the body when catalysts cease to be synthesized these controlled chemical reactions stop and a slow chaotic spontaneous decay of all the accumulated chemical energy proceeds via all possible channels. Decay of dead bodies is speeded up by the activity of bacteria and other organisms which use the available organic matter to sustain catalytic biochemical reactions within their own living cells. The synthesis of catalyzing molecules, specific for a given individual under constant conditions, as well as changes in the rate of that synthesis in response to change in the external conditions, are all written into its hereditary program as different parts – genes, of the polymer macromolecules of DNA (Lewin, 1983). The structure of the DNA molecules of the cell determines the genotype of the individual.

The rate of synthesis of various catalysts may also be influenced by an individual's experience (provided that individual possesses a nervous system). That experience is stored as various forms of extragenetic memory (the phenotype) during the lifespan of that particular individual. The information stored in all these other types of memory is not coded into the genotype and is not hereditarily transmitted. However, the very character of individual experience is prescribed by the genotype of the individual.

Each living individual functions in accordance with the laws of physics and chemistry. Every principle of physical self-organization, known today (Nicolis and Prigogine, 1977; Anderson, 1983; Schuster, 1984) and all the attractors, which may arise (Nicolis, 1986; Kaiser, 1990; Kauffman, 1991) may be used in various structures of the living individual. However, in accordance with rare physical fluctuations of high order, each individual decays in the course of time, losing its initial level of order. That decay of the individual takes place due to both aging and traumas of the individual, which take place during its lifespan (that is the decay of the phenotype), and because of the random decay changes (deleterious mutations) in the hereditary program of the individual (that is the decay of the genotype), the latter bringing about the decay of all the ensuing offspring of that individual.

As any other physical system subject to decay, the life of the individual is characterized by a certain time for decay (or the lifetime). The average time for decay of the individual phenotype is an easily measurable value. The average time for decay of the individual genotype may be obtained by measuring the time of appearance of deleterious mutations in the individual's offspring through several generations.

Within much shorter times than the time for their decay the living systems may, quite similar to rare physical fluctuations, be treated as stable systems of dynamic equilibrium. The stability of the internally correlated living systems means that the state of that system returns to its initial level after some external perturbation. Physiological reactions of the individual then arise to compensate for that perturbation, such as regeneration of damaged organs, etc. The destroyed parts of the DNA are repaired (Radman and Wagner, 1988).

All these reactions are programmed into the individual genotype and characterize physical stability of the individual. However, according to available observations, all these features of the individual are also subject to decay, and may be described by some finite measurable lifetime. Hence the life of a separate individual is a process of decay under complex control, which cannot be supported for an unlimited length of time, irrespective of the flux of external energy available.

Stability of physical systems over long observation times is equivalent to the existence of a deep potential well in some measurable variables of adequate choice (Sect. 2.7). No such well exists for decay systems. All the isolated live individuals and their genotypes are unstable in time, provided that time is of the order of or longer than their characteristic time for decay. In that sense the living organisms reside on top of a peak rather than in a well, and they constantly roll down that peak and perish. (Those peaks are qualitatively described in measurable variables below, see Sects. 3.5–9 and elsewhere.) The stability of life as a whole (instead of a separate individual) is based on a completely new principle, which places biology outside the scope of problems usually considered in physics and chemistry.

Life exists in the form of separate internally correlated individuals, (either as separate organisms or as correlated sets of such individuals, that is as social structures and communities), which have limited spatial dimensions – correlation lengths or distances (these are perceived as body size in case of separate individuals). The observed finite distance to which every type of correlation extends in every life form is, together with super-high organization, the most important difference between living individuals and the highly ordered physical fluctuations. As noted in Sect. 2.8, the latter may have arbitrary or unlimited correlation radii (such as cyclones, for example), and may also be globally correlated (such as the general atmospheric circulation or oceanic currents).

Internal correlation of individuals means that the numerous processes, such as biochemical reactions, taking place in different parts of the individual, are related to each other. A change in one process entails a certain, non-random change in the other. An increase in the level of order of an individual is related to increase in the number of such processes related to each other and of the number of types of correlations. The level of order of life processes is immeasurably higher than both the average level of order of the observed physical processes and of any complex spontaneous rare physical fluctuation, whatever its level of complexity.

The first observable feature of life is that life processes are never spontaneously generated, whatever the type and level of the flux of available energy. That is an empirical fact known from the times of Pasteur. Thus any living individual may be regarded as a superorganized physical fluctuation, the probability of it spontaneously arising in any flux of external energy (that is its physical self-organization) being equal to zero.

The second observable specific property of life is that, in contrast to rare highly ordered physical fluctuations, living creatures are never found in single numbers. They always exist in the form of a set (a population) of homogeneous individuals interacting with each other, each of them being of limited dimensions (body sizes). That property is retained independently of the mode of their breeding (either sexual or asexual). Individuals comprising the population are not correlated with each other: any one of them vanishing from that set in no way changes the state of the others. Hence, individuals in such a set interact competitively, instead of correlating with each other.

These observable properties of individuals unequivocally indicate that stabilization of the observed super-organization of live individuals is realized with respect to the set of non-correlated individuals, instead of any separate individual, and that is based on the stabilizing biological selection. As a result of such competitive interaction all the individuals are compared against each other. The individual already subject to decay is eliminated from the set, despite its life capacity still being retained. (Such individuals are called "decay individuals" below.)

That phenomenon expresses the essence of stabilizing biological selection. The remaining highly organized individuals (called "normal" below) fill the vacancy appearing in the set by breeding (replication-generation of their own copies), so that the stability of the set is sustained.

Competitive interaction should be continuous, independent of either presence or absence of limiting resources: the time interval between two successive acts of competitive interaction should always remain less than the time of spontaneous decay of the individual. The necessary condition for selection to take place is the absence of correlation between the individuals in the set (population). That means, in particular, that the spatial size of the individuals must necessarily be limited and that the population as a whole should have no overall government (control).

The term "population" is often used to denote the set of identical, weakly correlated components in one and the same individual, be it an organism or a social structure. We therefore speak about the population of blood erythrocytes or leukocytes, about the population of worker ants in an anthill or of bees in a beehive, about a population of animals in a herd or of leaves on a tree. Elements of competitive interaction may be encountered between such components of an individual, but nevertheless there is some level of partial correlation. Blood cells circulate in one and the same blood system. Worker ants belong to one and the same social structure and contain genetically pre-programmed information to that effect. There is no competitive interaction between various blood cells in an individual circulation system or between the worker ants in a single anthill. All the animals in a herd are correlated via the hierarchical structure of the herd, which, in contrast to those former structures, provides for a most efficient competitive interaction between these animals (Sect. 6.2). All the leaves of a tree grow from twigs connected to one and the same trunk. Leaves and twigs of the same tree compete for light among themselves.

Weak correlation between these components within an individual serves to lower the level of random fluctuations via the operation of the law of large numbers (Sect. 2.3). If a large number of weakly correlated erythrocytes are available, fluctuations in the influx of both oxygen and nutrients to organs and separate cells of a body remain low, which makes it possible for the whole body to function without a hitch. Similarly, fluctuations in the provision of food and of other substances necessary to anthills are kept low because of the large number of worker ants involved. An almost total lack of correlation in the functioning of separate leaves on a tree keeps fluctuations in the synthesis of organic materials by the tree itself low. Using the term "population" in these different meanings is sometimes quite confusing. Thus the term is used throughout the present book exclusively to indicate sets of competitively interacting completely non-correlated individuals of an arbitrary level of complexity.

The above definition of population completely covers the traditional definitions (Raven and Johnson, 1988). The expansion of the notion of population means that it now also comes to embrace the cases of asexual breeding, and social groups and communities.

Separate organisms (individuals) of either the same species, or of different species, may combine to form internally correlated social groups and communities in just the same way that cells and organs combine into a structure of a multicellular body. Such groups and communities may be envisaged as further extending the notion of an individual (called "hyperindividuals" below). The stable internal correlation within the social groups and communities may be supported via the stabilizing biological selection from among the set of competitively interacting social groups and communities (Wilson, 1975; Wrangham, 1977; Wilson, 1980; Wynne-Edwards, 1986). Such a set is called a "hyperpopulation" below. Communities are dealt with at more length in Chap. 4.

One should note that all types of internal correlation characterize an individual and not the population as a whole. No new types of correlation, absent in the individual, appear when one proceeds to population level. For example, it is the separate internally correlated community that the highly closed cycles describe at the highest accuracy, instead of arising as a new property of the large set of hyperpopulation of homogeneous communities or of the biosphere as a whole. Similarly the capacity to fly characterizes a separate bird or insect, instead of arising only as a property of a population of either birds or insects. The capacity to organize into an animal herd with a hierarchical structure may be supported via competitive interaction between different herds, which combine into a hyperpopulation of herds. A separate herd is then a generalized individual and does not represent a population of animals.

Individuals in a population may not in principle be correlated to each other. Competitive interaction and the stabilizing biological selection provide for a stable state of the population despite the continuous decay of these individuals in the course of their lives. The stability of a population is a new phenomenon which has no analogies in either physical or chemical systems. Thus this type of stability will be called biological stability in what is to follow. Note that biological stability characterizes a population and not a separate individual. The separate internally correlated individuals, be they organisms, social structures, or communities, do not feature such stability and decay with time. By definition, only individuals and not populations in general, are subject to stabilizing biological selection. Strictly speaking, genes responsible for controlling the life of an individual are subject to inclusive (resulting) selection (Hamilton, 1964; Dawkins, 1976). The functional meaning of the information written into genes is manifested in the course of an individual's life.

3.2 Differences Between Biological and Physical Stability

In this section we look into the principal differences between the notions of physical and biological stability, competition, and selection. Physical stability of the dynamic equilibrium of a system is controlled by the external flux of energy fed to that system, the decay of the level of order of that system being compensated by its regeneration. In other words, the ratio of the number of decays of the internally ordered correlated structures forming the system to the number of new generations of such systems is equal to unity. The number of such structures is of no importance. The physical state may be formed by a single structure, its correlation radius covering the whole state. When the external flux changes, physical stability is violated and the system enters a new state of dynamic equilibrium. One may only speak about competition between stable and unstable structures and about selection of one of these structures when the flux of external energy varies (Schuster, 1984). If the flux of external energy remains unchanged, the dynamic state of the system remains stable, and neither competition nor selection among the structures combining to form the system take place (Lima-de-Faria, 1988).

Selection of a more highly ordered physical state (physical self-organization) of the system only takes place when the organization of external flux of energy increases (Sect. 2.8). When the organization of that flux is diminished, a physical state of lower level of organization is selected. All the stable physical states of dynamic equilibrium are strictly determined by the level and character of their external fluxes of energy. If external conditions repeat themselves, precisely the same stable physically self-organized states of dynamic equilibrium originate. They naturally cannot compete among themselves nor with the average state of dynamic equilibrium. Decay of rare fluctuations is an act of physical selection taking place under conditions of constant flux of external energy.

In contrast to this situation, the set of living individuals supports the stability of its population in a constant flux of external energy only via continuous competitive interaction between a large number of mutually independent individuals and via the stabilizing biological selection. Living individuals are equivalent to superorganized physical fluctuations and decay irreversibly outside the population, independent of their breeding capacity, provided their offspring are also isolated and do not form a population. As will be demonstrated in sections to follow, the ratio between the number of decays of any type of biological correlation and the number of spontaneous generations of such types of correlation exceeds unity by many orders of magnitude, approaching the value of 10^{25}, and does not in practice depend on the level of the external flux of energy (Sect. 3.15). For the physical states of dynamic equilibrium that same ratio is unity.

The internal order in an individual is not limited to adaptation to existence in some prescribed environmental conditions. A most important characteristic in describing an environment is the flux of external energy. From that point of view the term adaptation could well be applied to physical states of dynamic equilibrium, which arise in the given flux of external energy, and which retain their stability within certain limits when that flux fluctuates (the so-called "physical tolerance", Kauffman, 1991). Beside adapting to their environment living individuals should be capable of stabilizing the conditions of that environment, and that necessity results in an incomparably more complex organization of these individuals, exceeding by far that of the physically self-organized systems. Stabilization of the conditions of the environment may take place via certain orientation (functioning) of the individual within its natural community. Both adaptation to the environment and work on stabilization of these environmental conditions are controlled by the respective informational genetic programs written into the individual. These programs will be called the adaptation program and the stabilization program below.

The only factors preventing decay of biological correlation are competitive interaction within the population and biological selection, but not the external flux of energy (as is the case with the physical systems). That decay consists of disintegration of the genetic programs of adaptation and stabilization. Thus a quantitative abyss, 25 orders of magnitude deep, exists between the states of common dynamic equilibrium and life, that abyss determining the principal qualitative difference between the two. One should stress once again that it is not the self-reproducing individual, but the population, which is a stable biological state of dynamic equilibrium with an unlimited life expectancy.

Completely different biological states of dynamic equilibrium may exist in the external flux of energy of a given level – various biological species featuring totally different level of organization are possible. This statement follows from the enormous diversity of the existent species, starting from the "poorly" organized single cell species to "highly" organized multicellular individuals and social structures. Indeed, the interaction between such contrasting species has resulted in differences between the fluxes consumed by each of them. However, the introduction of new species to new habitats and the observed process of forcing of the aboriginal species out of that habitat by the newly introduced ones proves that various species with varying competitive capabilities may well exist using the same fluxes of external energy. Paleontological data provide independent proof that species of various levels of organization had apparently existed within the same fluxes of energy during various historical periods (Raven and Johnson, 1988).

Thus the level of organization of living beings is not related to the level and character of the flux of energy they consume. Biological stability serves to maintain any existing superorganization of living organisms and contains the possibility of its evolution towards higher organization at the constant flux of energy feeding these organisms. In contrast, the physically stable organized state of dynamical equilibrium is completely determined by the character of the flux of external energy introduced to the system. The evolution of such a physical (or chemical) system towards higher organization is impossible at constant flux of external energy because the state of higher organization that may arise in the physical system will inevitably disintegrate.

Below we also focus on the notions of natural and group-stabilizing selection. The widely used term "natural selection" combines two essentially different phenomena: 1) biological selection (sometimes called "soft selection", Maynard Smith, 1978), which is based on competitive interaction between the individuals of one species and is switched off when the individuals are isolated from their natural population; and 2) physical selection (sometimes called "hard selection"), during which all the individuals devoid of life capacity are eliminated, independent of their competitive capacity, and that selection identically affects both the individuals within the population and those isolated from that population, provided all the other environmental conditions remain unchanged. The first type of selection operates independently of variations in the environment. The second is totally controlled by the actual environmental conditions.

The staggering diversity of internal organizations of individuals from different species works to correlate these species within the natural communities. Interspecies competition disrupts such a correlation, similar to competition between normal and cancer cells, which disrupts internal correlation in a multicellular body. Decay communities with their internal correlation between the disrupted species are eliminated from the hyperpopulation. When a new normal community is formed in their place, the species composition of that community is successively altered (the process of succession takes place; Horn, 1975; Finegan, 1984; Shugart, 1984; see Sect. 5.14). Interspecies competition is possible in a decay community, as well as during natural extinction (dying out) of the community, when foreign species are introduced into it, or when the external environment is perturbed. The interspecies competition presents a process of physical selection ending in elimination of one of the competing species (the exclusion principle of Gauze (Begon et al., 1986)).

By virtue of the definition of "population" there may be no competitive interaction between the two populations of the same species. If interaction between the two populations actually takes place, it means that individuals from both populations competitively interact, that is, both populations are merged into one. Competitive interaction between the internally correlated groups of species from either one or different species has a completely different meaning: such is the interaction between breeding couples of both sexes, between the nests of social insects, between the animal herds, or between the ecological communities of individuals (Wilson, 1980). Such an interaction strengthens internal correlation of those groups and may take place within the hyperpopulation of respective groups. The form of correlation in the enumerated groups of individuals does not differ, in principle, from correlation between the nuclear and cytoplasmic genes and organelles within the cell, or from correlation between the cells and organs in a multicellular body. As for the often used notion of group selection (see, e.g., Wilson, 1975; Wynne-Edwards, 1986; Maynard Smith, 1978), with respect to all those types of internal correlation it is identical to stabilizing biological selection among the hyperindividuals in a hyperpopulation. Note that in accordance with the above, the often used combination "group selection of populations and species" is a complete nonsense.

We now finally formulate the most important and unique principle of biology, which differentiates it from other sciences, and which will be subject to critical analysis throughout the rest of the book. All the types of biological correlations without any exception, are of decay-type in nature, and cannot be supported in arbitrary external fluxes of energy fed to the correlated entity for an unlimited time. The stability of any type of biological correlation is supported by the existence of a population – a set of the respective internally correlated objects, the individuals.

No new types of correlation appear when we proceed from individuals (assumed to lack such correlations) to populations of such individuals. All the individuals in a population are completely free of mutual correlation and live in a state of permanent competitive interaction, independent of the presence or absence of any limiting resources. Each individual is characterized by a certain probability of decay and of loss of the type of internal correlation typical of it. Decay individuals lose their competitive capacity and are forced out from the population by other individuals. Stability of population numbers is supported by copying (breeding) of individuals retaining their competitive capacity at a maximum level. In the absence of population and of competitive interaction between the individuals any type of internal correlation observed in isolated individuals is subject to inevitable decay and may never originate spontaneously again. All the aforesaid refers equally to every type of biological correlation, from the molecular level up to the level of communities in ecological systems.

3.3 The Quantum Nature of Life

A necessary condition for the stability of population is copying (breeding) of individuals. Being a superorganized decay state, life has already been existing for billions of years. It seems puzzling, at first glance, how copying of superorganized individuals may help to support the stability of the level of organization already achieved. Indeed, were we to try to reproduce technical achievements by copying mechanisms already in operation, such copies, produced following arbitrarily short lags after the actual start of operation, would inevitably include elements of wear and tear due to continuous aging and wear of the initial mechanism, so that such copies would necessarily feature a degree of order lower than the original (the initial mechanism) had had at the start. The same holds for any multicellular body. Objects changing noticeably over time periods considerably shorter than their possible copying times, may traditionally be called classical.

The unlimited conservation and growth of the level of organization of life resulting from Darwinian selection is well known to be possible only due to the quantum nature of molecular processes within the cell. Spontaneous and induced decay of molecules occurs by quantum jumps. The probability of the decay of a molecule per unit time is a physical constant, independent of either time or prehistory of the molecule. The permanency of the decay constant is a thoroughly substantiated empirical fact. That constant is proportional to the halflife period of these molecules, that is to the time needed for half the initially existing molecules to decay. The ground state of a molecule not yet decayed neither ages nor wears away. The copy of such a molecule, formed at an arbitrary instant of that molecule's life, is identical to the mother molecule taken at the initial moment of its history. In that sense the non-decayed molecule does not have any age. That non-trivial empirical fact serves as the basis of the quantum-mechanical theory (Schrödinger, 1945).

Identity is an experimentally tested characteristic, which refers to the fact that no increase in experimental accuracy may reveal any differences between two identical objects. If atoms and molecules were not identical to each other, chemical elements and substances would be incapable of conserving their properties. For example, gold would not be the same as it had been several hundred or thousand years ago. Two molecules not identical to each other may be experimentally resolved. For example, the two molecules of hydrogen, one of them containing two identical protons and another a proton and a deuteron (a nucleus consisting of a proton and a neutron) differ in their electronic energy levels and hence in their radiation spectra.

Functioning of single-cell individuals is controlled by the information-bearing molecules of DNA, their activity being regulated by trigger molecules of catalysts. The synthesis of the latter is also coded in the DNA. In the course of their life activities the molecules of DNA may suffer certain quantifiable decay changes. The residence time of most catalysts in living cell is very short and their structure completely determined by the existing DNA. Single-cell individuals are not immortal, they suffer decay as any other living organisms. Besides DNA and catalysts, the cell contains membranes, ribosomes and other cytoplasmic organelles that are a result of gene expression. Such macroscopic structures decay and age faster than DNA. After cell division about half of such structures should be newly synthesized in accordance with the information of the normal DNA in the daughter cells conserving the normal parent DNA. As a result the daughter cells contain a lower proportion of decay structures than the parent cell. Thus accumulation of decay structures in the parent cell can be compensated by creation of new elements in the daughter cells and a steady state in the succession of generations can arise. Therefore, over arbitrarily long time periods, one may always find a certain number of individuals not yet aged and worn, provided the set of the single-cell individuals is large enough, neither the DNA molecules nor catalyst molecules and cell organelles corresponding to them having had enough time to decay in these individuals. Replication of such individuals produces a certain number of copies identical in their level of organization to normal individuals at the initial moment thus restoring the initial number of normal individuals in the population. All the individuals with either their DNA or their triggering catalysts and excessive number of organelles already decayed are eliminated from the set via selection.

Clearly, only DNA molecules whose decay times exceed the time between two successive acts of DNA copying are fit for life, all the catalytic systems of reparation of that molecule naturally being taken into account (Ayala and Kiger, 1984). Such molecules may be called quantum. Were the DNA macromolecules to remain classical and decay faster than they were formed, the ordered nature of life could not be supported by biological selection (Eigen, 1971; Orgel, 1992).

Age changes are inevitable in any multicellular individual, and cells are present in it with their biomolecules already decayed. The support of level of organization of multicellular species is only possible by way of replication of one of the cells free of decay (that is of an unaged one), which such a multicellular individual might contain. These are germ cells in sexual breeding. Successive divisions of such a cell results in the formation of a new multicellular individual. It appears fundamentally impossible to build life on the basis of purely classical continuously aging multicellular individuals, without recourse to the quantum nature of a single cell, hence without passing through the periods of infancy, of development, and of ensuing death of each separate multicellular individual.

Bodies of multicellular plants and individuals of certain species (some invertebrates, and certain ectothermic vertebrates) grow throughout their entire lifespan. Cells of all of their organs divide continuously. Macroscopic structures containing normal DNA in their cells may be maintained in a steady state similar to that of the cells of unicellular individuals. However no selection of cells in a multicellular body is possible. Thus the DNA of its cells inevitably accumulates decay changes (deleterious substitutions). The gene expression and all the processes in cells are destroyed. As a result the individuals age and die.

The body growth of multicellular individuals of other species (insects, some ectothermic vertebrates and all endothermic vertebrates (birds and mammals)) stops by a certain age. Cell division is strongly suppressed in most organs of such adult individuals. Therefore their cells accumulate the macroscopic decay structures much faster than the decay DNA. As a result these types of individuals age rapidly and have a much shorter lifespan than species of the same average body size and metabolic rate which keep growing throughout their lives (Sect. 5.1).

3.4 The Nature of Genome Decay

The molecule of DNA is a double helix, an information-bearing polymer molecule consisting of the two mutually complementary spirals (they contain the genetic text of the properties of an individual). The monomers composing them are the four nucleotides (the letters of the four-letter alphabet of genetics). DNAs of higher order individuals are extremely large and consist of separate chromosomes (separate books, to continue the analogy). The complete text of all the properties of the individual is called its genome. Replication of DNA is performed by unwinding the double helix and building a complementary daughter strand of nucleotide pairs at each of the single parent strands, so that two identical copies of the parent DNA appear. However, errors are possible in the course of such copying (called mutations). Such errors include random change, insertion, or transposition of the nucleotide pairs or whole fragments of DNA (separate phrases, pages or whole volumes). Errors in nucleotide pairs (letters) are called point mutations. Errors in whole fragments (phrases) are called the chromosome mutations or macromutations (Ayala and Kiger, 1984; Lewin, 1983).

The probability of random mutation depends on the quantum characteristics of the polymer molecule, which are not correlated to the information written into that molecule. That probability is reduced by approximately a millionfold by a DNA-synthesis catalytic system such as proofreading and mismatch repair (Loeb and Kunkel, 1982; Radman and Wagner, 1986; Modrich, 1987), which is coded into certain parts of the DNA macromolecule. The proofreading and other repairing catalysts (enzymes) operate in the same way upon any section of the DNA molecule, independent of the information it contains. Thus the probability of random mutation, v, should remain identical for every section of the genome. In other words one may assume that the probability of random mutation, v, per single nucleotide site is a universal value typical for the whole genome.

The probability of random mutation in certain parts of the genome may increase in cases where special "mutator" genes are present, that is, coding enzymes which identify these particular parts of the genome and increase the probability of mutations in them, for example blocking the system of proof-reading (Drake, 1969, 1974; Drake et al., 1969; Ayala and Kiger, 1984). Hence, zones of higher mutability are also written into the general information in the genome. Decay of mutator genes results in the failure of synthesis of the respective enzymes and in the evening out of the rate of mutations in the genome as a whole. When affected by radioactive and/or chemical agents, the probability of induced mutations may increase evenly for every part of the genome, independently of information written into it. Higher mutability in certain parts of the genome in response to chemical forcing may also be programmed into some parts of the genome, their decay leading to elimination of the respective property. In what is to follow we envisage environmental conditions which are close to natural, and understand random mutations as spontaneous.

When synthesizing protein enzymes the information is first transcribed from the DNA to single-chain polymer molecules of the RNA, and is then translated to proteins, which are polymer molecules built of 20 amino acids (protein letters). These proteins play the role of catalysts of biological reactions. Autocatalysts of certain reactions in RNA are the RNA molecules themselves (Lewin, 1983). Genomes of certain viruses are built of RNA molecules directly. RNA molecules do not include any proofreading and mismatch repair systems. Thus the probability of random mutations in RNA viruses is a million times higher than that in individuals having their genetic information written into the DNA molecules (Holland et al., 1982; Gojobori and Yokuyama, 1987; Gojobori et al., 1990). The probability of random mutation in the RNA genome does not depend on the character of information written into it, and should be universal for all the RNA viruses, because of the universal structure of the RNA molecule. If we assume that the system of catalytic repair is also universal for any DNA genome, that is does not depend on either the size of the genome or the information written into it (Radman and Wagner, 1988), one may expect that the probability of random mutation, v, per nucleotide site is also a universal value for all the individuals containing such genomes. Such an assumption agrees satisfactorily with the experimental data available (Drake, 1969, 1974; Radman and Wagner, 1988), according to which such a probability, v, of random point mutation per nucleotide site per division is of the order of

$$v \approx 10^{-10} (\text{bp})^{-1} \, \text{d}^{-1}, \tag{3.4.1}$$

where the dimensions are denoted as follows: bp $\equiv$ base pairs; d $\equiv$ division. Deviations from (3.4.1) in either direction, observed in various species, do not usually exceed an order of magnitude (Drake, 1974).

Probabilities of mutual substitutions between the four nucleotide pairs differ slightly from pair to pair (Kimura, 1983; Jukes, 1987). Beside point mutations at a given nucleotide site, various macromutations are possible (these include transpositions, deletions, and insertions of certain sequences of nucleotide pairs from other parts of the genome). The cumulative probability of such events per nucleotide site does not exceed the average probability of point mutation (3.4.1) by more than a factor of five (Ayala and Kiger, 1984). Thus, recalling that the value of (3.4.1) is found to an accuracy of an order of magnitude only, we may further use that value as a representative estimate of the probability of a single random mutation (point plus macro).

A most important characteristic of genome stability is the average number of mutations per birth of a single individual, or per whole genome (which is actually the same) in a single generation. That characteristic is called the genome decay rate, μ, below. Let the size of the genome (that is the total number of nucleotide pairs in the genome) be M. The number of divisions of the embryo cell (of the parent zygote), that is the number of divisions per germ line, is denoted k_g. Then the dimensionless value of the genome decay rate is:

$$\mu = M \, v \, k_g. \tag{3.4.2}$$

We have for a bacteria: $M \approx 5 \times 10^6$ bp, $k_g = 1$ d, $\mu \approx 10^{-3}$. We further have for mammals: $M \approx 3 \times 10^9$ bp, $k_g \approx (20\text{--}40)$ d (the latter value is calculated by the number of doublings of the zygote needed to obtain from $10^6 \approx 2^{20}$ to $10^{12} \approx 2^{40}$ germ cells (Raven and Johnson, 1988; Vogel and Rathenberg, 1975; Vogel and Motulsky, 1979, 1982, 1986)), and $\mu \approx 10$ (Lewin, 1983).

The number of germ cells produced in women and men by the time of puberty (13 years of age) is equal, respectively, to $n_w = 7 \times 10^6$ and $n_m = 6 \times 10^8$ (Vogel and Rathenberg, 1975; Roosen-Runge, 1962, 1977). Accounting for ripening, their generation demands $k_{wg} = 23$ and $k_{mg} = 29$ dichotomous divisions. The daily sperm output is $u_s = 1.5 \times 10^8$ spermatozoa/day (Vogel and Rathenberg, 1975). In 50 years the number of ejaculations remains within $n_e \approx 1.8 \times 10^4$. So the total sperm output per male lifespan is about 10^{12} spermatozoa. Such an extremely high number is not needed for fertilization and is not usual for most species. It may be function similar to hormone-like injection to the female body in humans. There are two ways in which the daily sperm output may be achieved in the human male.

1) The number of stem germ cells does not change with age. Each stem (Ad) cell doubles. One of them remains in the unchanging store of stem cells. The second is transformed into 16 spermatozoa via four dichotomous divisions. Therefore the daily Ad output is $u_m = u_s/16 \approx 10^7$ Ad/day. To cover the annual sperm output $n_m/(u_m \cdot 365$ days/year$) = 23$ divisions/year of each Ad cells take place yearly (Vogel and Rathenberg, 1975). The value of k_{mg} grows linearly with a

male's age and reaches $k_{mg} = 1180$ by the age of 63. The ratio $\mu_m/\mu_w = k_{mg}/k_{wg}$ is equal to 51.

2) As in women, the number of Ad cells in men decreases with age. The number of stem cells used for the daily sperm output is $u_m = n_m/n_e = 3 \times 10^4$, each of them producing 4×10^3 spermatozoa by way of 12 dichotomous divisions. The value of $k_{mg} = 29 + 12 = 41$ does not depend on the male's age. The ratio $k_{mg}/k_{wg} = 1.8$ (instead of 51!). The number of Ad cells diminishes linearly with age at the rate of 1.1×10^4 cell/year. One may only distinguish between these two possibilities by measuring the actual rate of depletion of stem Ad cells with age, independent of natural degradation. Empirical data demonstrate that hereditary distortions in offspring increase approximately equally with the age of either parent. That fact testifies in favor of the second possibility, that is the level of decay is approximately equal in both males and females.

If $\mu > 1$, one should account for the probability of the appearance of several mutations. If multiple mutations remain completely uncorrelated, the probability of the appearance of n mutations is known to be described by the Poisson distribution (Arley and Buch, 1950; Sachs, 1972; Prigogine, 1978):

$$\left(\frac{\mu^n}{n!}\right) e^{-\mu}. \tag{3.4.3}$$

The Poisson distribution characterizes a multiplicity of mutually independent events. We have for average multiplicity $\bar{n}$, for variance (dispersion) $(n - \bar{n})^2$, and for standard (the root mean square) deviation $\sqrt{(n - \bar{n})^2}$, from (3.4.3):

$$\bar{n} = \overline{(n - \bar{n})^2} = \mu, \qquad \frac{\sqrt{(n - \bar{n})^2}}{\bar{n}} = \frac{1}{\sqrt{\bar{n}}}. \tag{3.4.4}$$

The second relation in (3.4.4) follows from the first one, and corresponds to the law of large numbers (2.3.4). Therefore, relations (3.4.4), may serve as criteria showing that we stay within the Poisson distribution (3.4.3). If several individuals are born, the average number of decay mutations is the same for each of them, the difference lying in the localization of those mutations in the genome. Therefore, when calculating the number of decay mutations one has to sum mutations in every individual, and consider μ to be the average number of mutations per single individual (instead of per generation), see Sect. 3.15 below.

Essentially, decay mutations are irreversible, as is every decay process in general. That irretrievably means that decay mutations result in an increase in the overall number of states of the genome. Probabilities of the direct and reverse mutations in any fixed nucleotide position (site) do not differ by more than an order of magnitude. However, these probabilities are lower than the cumulative probability of a decay mutation at arbitrary position in the genome per number of nucleotide sites in the genome. If the size of the genome is $M \sim 10^{10}$ bp, and $\mu \sim 1$, a decay mutation appears in some part of the genome in any individual born. Meanwhile a given reverse mutation appears only in one individual in every 10^{10} individuals, that is the probability of reverse mutation is ten orders of magnitude lower than that of the direct one. Conversely, the probability of reverse mutation in any two given nucleotide sites is twenty orders of magnitude less than that of the direct one, etc. Thus one may always neglect reverse mutations as compared to direct ones.

If direct and reverse mutations have probabilities coinciding in their order of magnitude, that means that such mutations are neither random nor do they decay, but are prescribed by a program written into the genome (Drake et al., 1969; Ayala and Kiger, 1984). Mutations featuring an anomalously high probability of appearance in a given local section of the genome (Ptashne, 1986, 1987) or those happening in a correlated fashion in certain differing parts of the genome (as mutations producing site-specific transposition of mobile gene elements, mutations producing a switch in mode from asexual to sexual reproduction in yeast (Hesin, 1984), and other such switches from one functionally sensible mode of cell operation to another) are also included in the program of the normal genome. These will occur until the part of the genome carrying that program decays. Meanwhile the decay of the program is a random process and follows the Poisson distribution too.

Generally speaking, neutral mutations (those not altering the phenotype and consequently the competitive capacity of an individual) and progressive ones (those increasing that capacity) are also possible. The latter quickly spread among all the individuals and are fixed in the population. They lower the level of inhomogeneity (or disorganization) in the genome, and hence are not decay in nature. The relative number of progressive mutations is much less than the total number of decay mutations (Sects. 3.8 and 3.15). Thus the value of μ (the decay rate) specifically controls decay of the genome. It is equal to the ratio between the number of offspring carrying hereditary mistakes to the number of offspring free of such mistakes in the genome, as compared to the parent genome.

3.5 Population: a Stationary State

Consider a population which initially consists of genetically identical individuals (clones). The clone genome may be considered a reference of genetic information, so that we calculate all the mutations taking place in that population with respect to that reference. For clarity, we also assume that such a reference genome is a normal one, containing all the information necessary for individual survival and for stabilization of the environment within the community to which that species belongs. The notion of the normal genome calls for a constructive definition, which would make it possible to differentiate, using some empirical procedure, the normal genome from the decay ones. That definition as well as the problem of degeneration of the normal genome (of the set of normal genotypes) is discussed in Sect. 3.6 below. To simplify our treatment, we consider the normal genome to be a unique one here, and all the deviations from it to be of a decay (deleterious) nature. Due to spontaneous separate decay mutations, new decay individuals featuring deviations from the normal genome will appear in the population during each successive generation of clone individuals. We denote the number of separate decay mutations existing in the genome as n. The number of individuals in the population having such a genome is N_n. Then, assuming that all the mutations are random and follow the Poisson distribution Eq. (3.4.3), we obtain the following equation to describe the change of the number N_n with time:

$$\dot{N}_0 = (B_0 - d_0)\,N_0,$$
$$\dot{N}_1 = (B_1 - d_1)\,N_1 + \mu B_0 N_0,$$
$$\vdots$$
$$\dot{N}_n = (B_n - d_n)\,N_n + \mu B_{n-1} N_{n-1} + \cdots + \frac{\mu^n}{n!} B_0 N_0,$$
$$\dot{N}_n \equiv \frac{dN_n}{dt}, \quad B_n \equiv b_n e^{-\mu}, \tag{3.5.1}$$

where N_0 is the number of normal individuals, b_n and d_n are the average birth rate (fertility) and death rate. We have $d_n = \tau_n^{-1}$ for the coefficient d_n, where τ_n is the average lifespan of an individual with n decay changes in its genome, the latter figure coinciding with the lifetime of a single generation in a stationary population. The coefficient b_n (fertility) is equal to the average number of offspring, generated by a single individual during the unit of time; B_n is the share of these offspring containing no changes in their genome, as compared to the parent genome. Accumulation of the deleterious decay substitutions in the genome results in a gradual erasing of information from the normal genome. We may thus assume that accumulation of deleterious substitutions goes as far as the lethal threshold $n_L : n < n_L$. At $n > n_L$ the number of lethal cases starts to increase quickly, and such individuals are eliminated from the population by physical selection.

A certain part of the genome of any organism, from 0.01 % to 1 % of the total size of the genome remains conservative and does not change from generation to generation, whatever the external conditions (Lewin, 1983). That means that any changes in that part of the genome, including any arbitrary point mutation, bring about a lethal outcome, that is, such individuals are immediately selected out physically. The rest of the genome is capable of accumulating decay substitutions up to the lethal threshold: $n \leq n_L$. Such accumulated decay mutations may be distributed randomly along arbitrary sections of the genome. Thus the limitation $n \leq n_L$ means limiting the average density of the number of decay substitutions per unit length of the genome: $r_L \equiv n_L/M$ or the value inverse to r_L, which is the average minimal length of the succession of nucleotide pairs, containing no deleterious decay substitutions: $l_L = r_L^{-1}$. Deviations from that average are described by the value of the Poisson variance (3.4.4). This aspect is discussed in Sect. 3.10 at greater length.

Lacking competitive interaction in the population (when it grows exponentially or exists under artificial laboratory conditions), both the birth and death rates of all the individuals may be assumed equal to each other ($B_0 = d_0 = B_n = d_n \equiv B$) when $n < n_L$. We have for arbitrary fluctuations of B_n and d_n

$$\overline{B_n - d_n} = 0, \qquad \sqrt{\overline{(B_n - d_n)^2}} \sim \frac{B_n}{\sqrt{N_n}}.$$

Thus the first term in (3.5.1) may be neglected at $\mu\sqrt{N_n} \gg 1$, which is always satisfied for all the species in the biosphere. The solution of (3.5.1) at $Bt \gg 1$ then has the form (Gorshkov 1989, 1990):

$$N_n(t) = N_0(\mu Bt)^n/n! \quad \text{at} \ N_n(0) = 0, \qquad N_0(0) = N_0. \tag{3.5.2}$$

Hence, if the number of individuals with the normal genome N_0 is constant, the total population number N grows exponentially due to an increase in the share of decay individuals:

$$N = \sum_{n=0}^{L} N_n \approx \exp(\mu Bt) \quad \text{at} \ N_n(0) = 0, \ N_0(0) = N_0. \tag{3.5.3}$$

If the population number remains constant, the number of normal individuals falls off exponentially. At $Bt \gg 1$ and $\mu Bt \ll n_L$ the frequency of occurrence $p_n \equiv N_n/N$ has the form of a Poisson distribution, its multiplicity $\bar{n} = \mu Bt$ growing linearly with time:

$$p_n \equiv \frac{N_n}{N} \approx \frac{(\mu Bt)^n}{n!} e^{-\mu Bt}, \qquad \bar{n} = \mu Bt \ll n_L. \tag{3.5.4}$$

As demonstrated below, the value n_L remains within $10^4 > n_L > 10^3$. Thus the latter condition (3.5.4) is satisfied for all the species over many generations. Therefore (3.5.1) does not have a stationary solution in the absence of competitive interaction, with $\mu Bt < n_L$.

When $\mu Bt \gg n_L$ one has to account for the finite number of terms in (3.5.3). In that case the frequencies of occurrence N_n/N are close to the lethal threshold and obtain the form of δ_{nn_L} functions (with the Kronecker symbol):

$$\frac{N_n}{N} \approx \left(\frac{\mu Bt}{n}\right)^n \left(\frac{n_L}{\mu Bt}\right)^{n_L} \approx \delta_{nn_L}, \text{ where } \delta_{n,m} = \left\{ \begin{array}{ll} 1 & n = m \\ 0 & n \neq m \end{array} \right., \tag{3.5.5}$$

so that the complete population consists of decay individuals, $N = N_{n_L}$ and the number of decay substitutions is $n = n_L$. Every following generation will shift population to the right beyond the lethal threshold, to the average of its decay rate μ. The number of individuals retaining life capacity after each generation is $N_{n_L} e^{-\mu}$. Hence, the stationary state may be supported when every individual produces e^μ offspring. However, any fluctuation of external conditions resulting in a lowering of the lethal threshold n_L may push the complete population beyond the limit for life. Thus the existence of the population in a state bordering on the very lethal threshold (3.5.5) is unstable and should result in the extinction of that species. Besides, for individuals with a large genome and low fertility, b_0, the condition $\mu Bt > n_L$ is reached in times, t, exceeding the average lifespan of the species $T_s \sim 10^6$ years (Simpson, 1944; Van Valen, 1973; MacFadden and Hubbert, 1988), that is $\mu BT_s \leq n_L$. The genome of such species should decay during the whole lifespan of the species according to (3.5.4).

Hence definite mechanisms must be acting in populations to stop the decay of the genome a long time before it reaches the lethal threshold n_L. The stabilizing program in the genome, necessary for correct functioning of the individual in its natural community, is erased much earlier than the lethal threshold is reached. This fact is testified to by the very possibility of selecting domesticated animal and plant species from the respective natural species via artificial selection and genetic engineering techniques. Domestic individuals are not capable of existing in natural communities and are completely devoid of the genetic information necessary to stabilize the environment. The most efficient functioning of a population within the community takes place on condition that the normal individuals in it comprise the overwhelming majority. The number N_n of individuals in a population may only be stationary while the number of normal individuals is at maximum, if either the birth rate is decreased, or the death rate is increased for the decay individuals, that effect being reached via interaction with normal individuals.

For purposes of convenience we introduce the relative birth and death rates for decay individuals:

$$\beta_n \equiv \frac{B_n}{B_0} = \frac{b_n}{b_0}, \qquad \delta_n \equiv \frac{d_n}{d_0}. \tag{3.5.6}$$

The stationary numbers of the normal individuals, $\dot{N}_0 = 0$, $N_0 = \text{const}$, is defined from (3.5.1) via the condition:

$$B_0 = d_0, \qquad b_0 = d_0 e^{\mu}. \tag{3.5.7}$$

To obtain a stationary state for the number of decay individuals $\dot{N}_n = 0$, $N_n = \text{const}$, all the terms $B_n - d_n$ in (3.5.1) should be negative, so that the appearance of decay offspring from parents of a lower level of decay be compensated. Hence, the death rate, δ_n, should always remain higher than the birth rate β_n. One may assume, without losing generality, that

$$\delta_n - \beta_n \gg \beta_n \geq 0, \qquad \left(\frac{\delta_n}{\beta_n} - 1\right)^{-1} \ll 1, \quad n > 0, \tag{3.5.8}$$

$$\beta_0 = \delta_0 = 1, \qquad \delta_0 - \beta_0 = 0.$$

Under condition (3.5.8) the stationary state has the form (Gorshkov, 1989a):

$$N_n = N_0 \left(\frac{\mu^n}{n!}\right) (\delta_n - \beta_n)^{-1}, \qquad N_0 = \text{const}. \tag{3.5.9}$$

It may be seen from (3.5.9) that the condition $N_n \ll N_0$ is satisfied at small levels of decay $\mu \ll 1$ if $\delta_n = 1$ and $\delta_n - \beta_n \sim 1$ (regulation of the relative birth rate of decay individuals), or if $\delta_n \gg 1$, $\beta_n \sim 1$ (regulation of the death rate of decay individuals). At $\mu \geq 1$ the condition $N_n \ll N_0$ is satisfied only for $\delta_n \gg 1$, $\beta_n \leq 1$ (that is the regulation of the relative death rate).

When a single normal genotype is in the population the relative birth rate regulation at $\mu > 1$ inevitably brings about an inverse condition $N_n \gg N_0$, that is the share of decay individuals in a population increases and its stability decreases. Then the total number of individuals in a stationary population is $N \approx N_0 e^{\mu}$ and hence the share of the normal breeding individuals in the population is $N_0/N \approx e^{-\mu}$. The number of breeding individuals in the population is called the effective size of the population, N_e, (Kimura and Crow, 1963). Hence, the decay rate μ being high, we have for birth rate regulation for decay individuals: $N_e = N_0 \approx e^{-\mu}N$. Each normal individual produces e^μ offspring in accordance with (3.5.7). All the offspring born are given identical expected lifespan, but breeding by all the decay individuals is prohibited. These conclusions are modified if the several normal genotypes are in the population, see Sect. 3.11.

For a species to function properly within its natural community the overwhelming part of the population should be constituted by normal individuals. Thus at low decay rate $\mu < 1$, regulation of both the death rate and birth rate are possible, that is the juvenile death rate may be relatively low. But at large decay rate $\mu \gg 1$ the number of decay individuals in the population may be held relatively low only if the death rate of decay individuals is regulated, that is if the juvenile death rate in the population is high.

The difference $\beta_n - \delta_n$ in (3.5.8) may be called relative competitiveness; it is at maximum in a stationary state, is equal to zero for normal individuals, and is negative for decay ones. It seems more natural to consider a value of the opposite sign:

$$\gamma_n \equiv \delta_n - \beta_n \equiv \text{noncompetitiveness}, \qquad (3.5.10)$$

which should then be called noncompetitiveness. The noncompetitiveness of decay individuals for both types of regulation of their numbers in a population remains $\delta_n - \beta_n \geq 1$. Hence, when we proceed from normal to decay individuals, their noncompetitiveness suffers a jump from zero ($\delta_0 - \beta_0 = 0$) to a value exceeding unity ($\delta_n - \beta_n \geq 1$). The noncompetitiveness of decay individuals cannot be much lower than unity; this corresponds to (3.5.9) remaining far from the pole appearing at $\delta_n - \beta_n = 0$.

The traditional variables of fitness and coefficient of selection differ from that of noncompetitiveness, γ. The absolute fitness, W, is defined as $W \equiv b - d$. Note that $W_0 = W_{\max} > 0$, as follows from the definition of the normal genome. Further, $W_{\max} = (dN_{0\to}/dt)N_0^{-1}$, where $N_{0\to}$ is the total number of offspring, including both the normal and decay ones, produced by normal parents, the share of the normal ones among the former being $e^{-\mu}$ and that of the decay $1 - e^{-\mu}$. The last value presents the mutation load (Kimura and Maruyama, 1966). The relative fitness is $w = W/W_{\max}$ (or $W/\bar{W}$), $w_{\max} = 1$, $1 \geq w \geq 0$. The coefficient of selection is $s = w_{\max} - w = 1 - w$. We have $1 \geq s \geq 0$ for stabilizing selection. It is assumed that the value of s may be small, e.g. $s = 0.01$ (Fisher, 1930; Haldane, 1954, 1957; Crow, 1958, 1970; Ohta, 1987).

The coefficient of selection, s_n, and the relative fitness, w_n, are related to relative birth rate and to noncompetitiveness, γ_n, by the relation:

$$s_n \equiv 1 - w_n = 1 - \beta_n + \frac{\gamma_n}{e^\mu - 1}. \qquad (3.5.11)$$

When only the death rate is regulated (i.e. $\beta_n = 1$) the values s_n and γ_n differ from each other by the factor $(e^\mu - 1)^{-1}$.

The use of the notion of relative competitiveness $\beta_n - \delta_n = (b_n - d_n)/B_0$ is stimulated by the fact that the maximum stationary value is $B_0 - d_0 = 0$, while

$B_n - d_n < 0$ for $n > 1$, that is the relative competitiveness $\beta_n - \delta_n \leq 0$. When the generation of offspring by all the decay individuals is zero ($b_n = 0$, $n > 0$) their numbers may remain stationary, because the rate at which decay individuals die is compensated by the rate at which they are born of normal parents. The latter produce decay individuals via decay mutations following the Poisson distribution. Then fitness of the decay individuals is $W_n \equiv b_n - d_n = -d_n < 0$, which is not accounted for by the traditional definition of fitness. For example, even if people with obvious genetic defects are prohibited from reproducing, such genetic deviations will still be present in the society because these will be produced by normal parents.

To regulate both the birth and death rates of decay individuals the possibility should be provided of identifying such decay individuals and of distinguishing them from the normal ones. That task is solved by combining all the individuals into a population and switching on competitive interaction between them. The difference between the normal and the decay individuals is only controlled by their competitiveness. Under natural conditions the number of decay individuals in a population is suppressed via their competitive interaction with the normal ones.

Superimposing conditions of stationarity, (3.5.8), which provide for the maximum competitiveness of the normal and for the noncompetitiveness of decay individuals, corresponds to the introduction of complex nonlinear relations between the normal and the decay individuals into (3.5.1). These relations may be prescribed in the form of the complex functional dependences $B_n(N_0, N_k)$ and $d_n(N_0, N_k)$, which describe the differences between normal and decay individuals and which are equivalent to introducing competitive interaction between them. However, such nonlinearities may be substituted by an analogue of the boundary conditions, (3.5.8).

Information on the necessity for individuals to join into a population, to switch on competitive interaction, and to reach the maximum possible competitiveness of the normal individuals must be written into the genomes of these normal individuals. That basic program of supporting the species stability should be safely insured against decay mutations (e.g., by multiple back-up); it should also decay itself if the number of decay substitutions becomes large and approaches the lethal threshold. As a result all the individuals, independent of their decay rate, still enjoy the capacity to join into a population and to interact competitively. These behavioral trends are prescribed by the internal program in the genome. Competitive interaction between the individuals in a population always occurs at a maximum intensity under the natural conditions of the specific ecological niche of a species, and does not depend on the "limiting resources" (Sect. 4.7).

When breeding is sexual the genetic material in the offspring presents a random mix of parental genetic material. Decay substitutions in the genomes of the offspring individual are then Poisson distributed (Maynard Smith, 1978; Kondrashov, 1982, 1988). Since decay of the genome results in a Poisson distribution anyway, the distribution (3.5.4) does not change when sexual breeding is switched on. (Sexual breeding broadens narrow peaks with low dispersion to that of the Poisson peak with a large dispersion (Kondrashov, 1988); it only shows in the states bordering on the very lethal threshold, Eq. (3.5.5), as discussed in Sect. 3.8.) The stationary state (3.5.8) and all the conclusions related to it also hold when sexual breeding is switched on. Besides, (3.5.1) and (3.5.8) may be envisaged as equations written not for individuals bearing decay genomes, but for inclusive numbers of genes with prescribed number of decay substitutions for the whole population, independent of separate individuals which bear those genes (Hamilton, 1964; Dawkins, 1976). Apparently the advent of sexual breeding changes nothing in either results or conclusions for the latter case.

3.6 Normal Genotypes and the Normal Genome

Determining competitiveness during the process of competitive interaction between the individuals in a population is actually a process of measurement. As any such process is characterized by some limited resolution, it is impossible to separate a normal individual from a decay one in the process of competitive interaction, if the genome of the latter contains n decay substitutions only, that number being less than the sensitivity threshold of competitive interaction $n_c : n < n_c$. The inverse value of that threshold, n_c^{-1}, may be called the resolution of competitive interaction. Thus competitive interaction is effectively switched on and active within the margin $n_c < n < n_L$. Here n_L is lethal number of decay substitutions. Similar to n_L the number n_c of the decay substitutions should be evenly distributed along the genome. The sensitivity threshold of competitive interaction is determined by the average density of decay substitutions per unit length of the genome, $r_c \equiv n_c/M$ or by the average length of the genome free of any decay substitutions $l_c = r_c^{-1}$. Deviation from the average density $(r - r_c)^2$ at certain sections of the genome of a given length is described by the Poisson variance (3.4.4). It may also be expected that r_c and l_c both appear to be universal characteristics of sensitivity of competitive interaction, which do not depend on the size of the genome within the large taxa. Estimates of the values of l_c and r_c for both haploid and diploid genomes are obtained in Sect. 3.11 from the analysis of empirical data.

All the genomes containing decay mutations in numbers $n < n_c$ possess the program of adaptation and stabilization necessary for individuals to function normally in the community, so that such genomes are genetically equivalent to each other. Various genomes found in the range $n < n_c$ will be called normal genotypes below. All the individuals possessing normal genotypes have equal competitiveness, which is at a maximum under the normal conditions (that is in a natural community, in natural environment, i.e. in a natural ecological niche). Indeed, $\gamma_n = 0$ in (3.5.10) for $n < n_c$, and that competitiveness exceeds that of any decay individual found in the range $n > n_c$ ($\gamma_n \geq 1$ in (3.5.10) when $n > n_c$). All the individuals with their genotypes remaining within the range $n < n_c$ are called normal below, and those with $n > n_c$ are decay.

The competitiveness has no absolute value and may only be described by some relative one. When comparing the competitiveness of any two individuals one faces only two possibilities. First, these competitivenesses may remain unresolved to within the resolution of competitive interaction. Neither individual is then capable of forcing the other from the population. Second, the competitiveness of one may exceed that of the other. The genotype of the first individual will then inevitably force that of the second one from the population, independent of the actual difference between the competitivenesses of the two. Thus the relative competitiveness appears to have a stepped nature. This nature is most vividly displayed during sexual selection. The female or the male may either accept or reject the mating partner. It is impossible to partly select mating partners, for instance with the selection coefficient $s \approx 0.01$, see Sect. 3.11 for details. That feature comprises the main difference between the notions of competitiveness and of fitness.

If the differences in competitiveness of two genotypes exceed the resolution of competitive interaction, one may assume, to a good approximation, that the genotype of higher competitiveness has a relative fitness of unity, so that it produces the most numerous offspring in the population

$$w_{n<n_c} = 1, \quad s_{n<n_c} = 0, \quad \beta_{n<n_c} = 1, \quad \gamma_{n<n_c} = 0,$$

while the genotype of lower competitiveness has a relative fitness close to zero, that is does not produce any offspring

$$w_{n>n_c} = 0, \quad s_{n>n_c} = 1, \quad \beta_{n>n_c} = 0, \quad \gamma_{n>n_c} \geq 1.$$

Thus noncompetitiveness $\gamma \cdot (e^\mu - 1)^{-1}$ coincides with the coefficient of stabilizing selection, s, and the value of $1 - \gamma(e^\mu - 1)^{-1}$ coincides with fitness in the case of truncating selection, see (3.5.11).

Assume that we managed to form a clone population of the normal genome with $n = 0$ at zero time $t = 0$. In accordance with (3.5.1) that clone will keep on decaying and accumulating decay substitutions up to $n = n_c$, since when $B_0 = d_0$ all the differences $B_n - d_n$ coincide with each other if $n < n_c$ and are also equal to zero. Similar to the considered case of decay down to the very lethal threshold n_L (when competitive interaction is totally absent) the population appears to be pushed to a value inverse to resolution n_c, and that happens in time $\mu B_0 t \gg n_c : \, N_n = 0, \, n < n_c, \, N_{n_c} = N$, see (3.5.5). Further increase of the number of decay substitutions is then stopped by competitive interaction, that is one may assume that $N_n \approx 0$ for $n > n_c$. The shape of the stationary distribution depends on the character of competitive interaction and may differ from a narrow peak at $N_{n_c} = N$. In particular, competitive interaction may stop the growth of the Poisson multiplicity (3.5.4) with time. In that case the stationary distribution will have the shape of a Poisson distribution with $\bar{n} = n_c$. Such a distribution always arises in the case of sexual breeding, Sect. 3.10.

Decay results in the formation of genetic diversity in a population. The genetic polymorphism – that is the number of different genotypes corresponding to n decay mutations of the initial clone – is equal to

$$4^n\, C_M^n \approx \left(4\,\frac{M}{n}\right)^n,$$

where M is the number of nucleotide pairs in the genome, C_M^n is the number of combinations from M by n, 4 is the number of different nucleotides (of genetic letters). Even with $n = 2$ the number of various genotypes reaches 10^{20} which by far exceeds the number of individuals in any multicellular species over the whole lifespan of that species. Thus no pair of individuals may randomly happen to be genetically identical to each other.

For small populations, a random drift of genes in which decay mutations have occurred takes place. A stable final state of that process is either loss or fixation of a given decay substitution in all the individuals of the population (Wright, 1932, 1988; Kimura, 1964, 1983; Ayala and Kiger, 1984; Altukhov, 1991). New substitutions appear in place of the lost decay ones, so that the total number of decay substitutions remains equal to n_c. Genetic drift results in a reduction of genetic polymorphism due to fixation of a certain part of decay substitutions with $n < n_c$ in certain sites of the genome in all the individuals in the population.

Localization of the deleterious decay substitutions in various populations originating from one and the same clone of normal individuals should be different due to the random nature of the process of decay and of the following genetic drift. When the value of n_c is high, genetic differences may also lead to the observed phenotypical (morphological, behavioral, etc.) differences between the populations, which are traced through many generations. Depending on the scope of these differences they may be perceived as either racial, national, or subspecies. However the races and nationalities thus originating remain genetically equivalent: various genotypes of individuals from all the races are normal, that is contain $n \leq n_c$ decay mutations, and still have the complete adaptive and stabilizing program of the species. Normal individuals from different races have equal competitiveness, which is higher than the competitiveness of all the decay individuals, the latter featuring different decay genotypes of $n > n_c$.

The phenomenon of splitting a population, initially formed from the clone of a normal genome, into different races and nationalities is similar to spontaneous breaking of symmetry of physical states, which, for example, takes place when a vertical beam is bent in a random direction, and is subject to a pressure exceeding its critical limit, or when ferromagnetic material is randomly magnetized (Haken, 1982, 1984; Nicolis, 1986; Goldanskii and Kuz'min, 1989).

Among the substitutions appearing during the decay of a clone of a normal genome both deleterious and neutral decay substitutions may occur (Kimura, 1989). These substitutions may be experimentally differentiated from each other in the following way. A given deleterious substitution in a given site of the genome can change the phenotype but does not change the individual's competitiveness in the range $n < n_c$, but the same substitution lowers that individual's competitiveness if it happens in a normal individual with $n = n_c$ or in a decay one with $n > n_c$. Neutral substitution never changes the phenotype and the competitiveness of an individual. There is no threshold for accumulation of neutral substitutions in a genome. Those sites of the genome in which such neutral substitutions may take place (if they exist at all) do not bear any information. Thus the sequence of nucleotide pairs in a normal genome may only be defined to the accuracy of such neutral sites.

The total number of neutral sites devoid of information content is apparently much lower than the overall number of information-bearing sites of the genome in which deleterious substitutions at $n > n_c$ are identifiable through the process of competitive interaction. Arguments in favor of such a statement are given below in Sects. 3.7 and 3.11.

The average number of differences between the nucleotide sites of the genomes of two individuals from different non-interacting natural populations may be taken as the sensitivity threshold of competitive interaction, n_c. The respective number of differences between the genomes of the two individuals from one and the same population should remain lower than n_c, since a certain portion of deleterious decay substitutions may be randomly fixed in the population if $n \leq n_c$. However, random fixation of one and the same decay substitution in different non-interacting populations is quite an improbable event. Therefore, if coinciding sequences are found in different populations, one may safely assume that these are fragments of the normal genome.

Hence, if several non-interacting natural populations of the same species are present, an experimental procedure may be capable of yielding, at least in principle, the sequence of genes in the normal genome to an accuracy exceeding the sensitivity of competitive interaction. To realize this, sections of the genome should be identified in individuals in each population which feature the lowest polymorphism, that is such sections of the genome in which the genotypes of all the individuals in the population feature the smallest mutual differences. In order to exclude the possibility of fixing deleterious decay mutations in the population one should further define the coinciding sections of the genome with the lowest polymorphism in a pair of non-interacting or weakly interacting populations. Such sections may be considered to be fragments of the normal genome of the species. If the overall number of non-interacting populations is large enough, that procedure might practically identify the whole sequence of genes in the normal genome. Thus the normal genome is characteristic of species. The normal genotypes are the characteristics of individuals.

The normal genome remains unique for each species. The information programmed in the non-transcribed nucleotide sequences of a normal genome should be correlated at large distances (Peng et al., 1992). The existing long-range correlation in nucleotide sequences of a normal genotype should be partly broken due to the presence of the permitted number, $n < n_c$, of decay (deleterious and neutral) substitutions, which are distributed with differing density per unit genome length in different parts of the genome.

Indefinite character (degeneration) of the genome is exclusively related to the number of neutral sites containing no information. The position of such neutral sites may be identified by comparing homological sequences in various individuals both within a single population and from population to population. Any pair of individuals with their normal genotypes residing within the $n < n_c$ range always has a large number of non-neutral sites with differing positions of nucleotide pairs, one of them being normal and the other decay. If different nucleotide pairs are found in the homologous sites of the genomes of three different individuals, these sites are neutral to a high probability. The probability of random coincidence may in that case be reduced by comparing the genomes of many individuals. Random fixation of a certain nucleotide pair or of a fragment of the genome in the neutral site of different individuals of the population may be detected by comparing homologous sites of the genome in individuals from several non-interacting populations. If fixed nucleotide substitutions in a homologous site are different in any two arbitrary populations, that site is neutral with high accuracy (Sect. 3.7).

3.7 Neutral Mutations

Let us consider truly neutral sites in the genome in greater detail. Assume that initially the frequency of occurrence of all the four nucleotide pairs in each neutral site is the same in all the individuals of the population (that is the state of thermodynamic equilibrium or of total degeneration). The genotypes with different neutral substitutions must correspond to identical phenotypes. So far we have neglected the mutation process. A random drift of nucleotide substitutions in neutral sites will then take place in small populations with sexual breeding, due to mixing of genetic material and to random dying out of individuals (Wright, 1931, 1988; Kimura, 1964). That process is described by the Fokker-Planck equation, which is a generalization of the common equation of diffusion. The final stable state of that random drift is fixation, of a certain substitution in the neutral site in all the individuals of the population (Kimura, 1964, 1983). Due to neutrality of states, and to the random character of the process of fixation the number of generations needed to fix a certain state is proportional to population number, N, (Kimura, 1983). In other words, fixation occurs in a time of the order of $N\tau$, where τ is the time between two successive generations, $\tau = \tau_g k_g$, where τ_g and k_g are the average times between two successive cell divisions, and the number of cell divisions to form gametes during the individual lifespan, respectively, see (3.4.2).

The probability of finding each nucleotide pair in a neutral site is identical, equal to 1/4. Assuming that the number of neutral sites in the genome is equal to n_0, we find that the total number of different sequences of nucleotide pairs in these sites is equal to 4^{n_0}. When the population number is $N \ll 4^{n_0}$, one may assume that these sequences are initially different in all the individuals of the population. The probability of finding one such sequences of nucleotide pairs in the neutral sites of individual genomes within the population is $1/N$ (Kimura, 1968, 1983, 1987). (If $N \gg 4^{n_0}$, the probability of fixing one of the sequences is 4^{-n_0}.)

The process of fixing one of the alleles, initially having one and the same frequency of occurrence, may be traced experimentally in vitro, when competitive interaction is effectively switched off (Ayala and Kiger 1984; Altukhov, 1991).

Now we account for the process of mutation. A neutral mutation is a particular case of a common decay mutation taking place with a probability v in a neutral (devoid of information) site of the genome, Eq. (3.4.1). The probability of occurrence of a new point mutation in a given site of the genome in a single generation is $vk_gN = N/N_u$, where $N_u = (vk_g)^{-1}$ is the number of members of such a population in which a neutral mutation occurs at a probability of unity in each single generation. The number of generations in which one mutation occurs in a population of N individuals is N_u/N. Correspondingly, the time interval during which such a mutation occurs is $\tau N_u/N$. The probability of fixing a specific neutral mutation in a whole population is proportional to $1/N$. Thus the probability of neutral substitution in a normal genome of the population per single generation is vk_g (Kimura, 1987). Hence, the resulting rate at which the mutation is fixed in the normal genome of all the individuals in the population does not depend on N and is equal to vk_g/τ.

The process of random fixation will only take place when the time of fixation τN is much shorter than the time of appearance of a new mutation $\tau N_u/N$, that is on condition that $N^2vk_g \ll 1$. That condition is satisfied for small populations of eukaryotes only, in which $N \ll 10^5$ individuals. The inverse condition $N^2vk_g \gg 1$ holds for practically all the single cell species, both prokaryotes and eukaryotes, as well as for many insect species. In that case no neutral mutation may become fixed. To a large extent the nucleotide sequences in neutral sites will not coincide for any two individuals arbitrarily chosen from the population.

Even when the initial thermodynamic equilibrium is absent, it should settle in the neutral sites as time goes on. For reasons of simplicity consider a single neutral site with two possible values of nucleotide pairs 1 and 2. The population numbers N_1 and N_2, valued at 1 and 2 in these sites satisfy the equations:

$$\dot{N}_1 = W_1N_1 + \nu_{12}b_2N_2 - \nu_{21}b_1N_1,$$
$$\dot{N}_2 = W_2N_2 + \nu_{21}b_1N_1 - \nu_{12}b_2N_2, \qquad (3.7.1)$$

where ν_{12} and ν_{21} are the probabilities of transition from state 1 to state 2 and back: $\nu_{12} \sim \nu_{21} \sim \nu \approx vk_g \sim 10^{-10}$ for bacteria and $\nu \sim 10^{-4}$ for RNA viruses (Holland et al., 1982); $W_i = b_i - d_i$ is the difference between the birth and the death rates (fitness), $i = 1, 2$. We have for neutral sites $\bar{b}_1 = \bar{b}_2$; $\bar{d}_1 = \bar{d}_2$. The stationarity of the total the population number $\dot{N}^+ = \dot{N}_1 + \dot{N}_2 = 0$ means that $\overline{W}_1 = \overline{W}_2 = \overline{W} = 0$, $\sqrt{\overline{W^2}} = b/\sqrt{N}$. When $\nu\sqrt{N} \gg 1$, that is when $N \gg 10^{20}$ (which is the case for practically every bacteria species, see Sect. 5.6), the first, diffusional term in (3.7.1) may be neglected. As a result, assuming, for simplicity reasons, that $\nu_{12} - \nu_{21} = 0$, we find:

$$\dot{N}^+ = 0, \quad \dot{N}^- = -(\nu_{12}+\nu_{21})bN^-, \quad N^- = N_0^- e^{-(\nu_{12}+\nu_{21})bt}, \qquad (3.7.2)$$

where $N^+ \equiv N_1 + N_2$, $N^- \equiv N_1 - N_2$.

When $\nu_{12} - \nu_{21} \neq 0$, the difference N^- tends to a finite limit, which is proportional to the difference $\nu_{12} - \nu_{21}$ (Jukes, 1987; Sueoka, 1988), its exponential relaxation rate being the same as in (3.7.2).

Thus the time period for settling thermodynamic equilibrium in that site is equal to $[(\nu_{12} + \nu_{21})b]^{-1} = \tau/(\nu_{12} + \nu_{21}) \sim 5 \times 10^6$ years, for $\tau \sim 10^{-3}$ years, and about 5 years for RNA viruses. Hence, equilibrium should settle in within the lifespan of a separate bacterial species, while for the RNA viruses all the neutral sites should always remain in the state of thermodynamic equilibrium. When the number of neutral sites in a bacterial genome would be 50 (which is one 10^{-5} part of the whole genome), the number of neutrally equivalent genomes (those having equal frequencies of occurrence) would reach $4^{50} = 2^{100} = 10^{30}$, that is, would be larger than the total number of individual bacteria in all the populations together, see Sect. 5.6. Nucleotide sequences in those sites would not have been species specific then, which is not actually observed (Lewin, 1983; Hesin, 1984). Hence, neutral sites in the genome are either negligible in number or remain totally absent from it. Section 3.13 presents independent arguments in favor of the assumption that neutral sites are as scanty in the eukaryote genomes.

Neutral sites are usually related to the observed level of degeneration of the genetic code (when several triplet-codons of nucleotide pairs correspond to one and the same amino acid in the protein), to the presence of non-transcribed sequences in the genome (those not coding the proteins, such as introns within the genes, spacers between them, repetitions of short sequences, etc.) (Ayala and Kiger, 1984; Lewin, 1983), to the presence of functionally inactive parts in the proteins. Degeneration of the genetic code may be neutralized by gene overlap (when different reading frames are used), and by the coding of synthesis of different molecules (such as tRNA) in other parts of the genome, each of these relating the amino acid to one of the possible degenerated anticodons (Grosjean et al., 1982; Kimura, 1983; Buckingham and Grosjean, 1986). The number of neutral sites is by far lower than the number of noncoding sequences in the genome. For example, the telomeres, the end sequences of chromosomes in the higher species, provide for the stability of chromosomes during their division, and do not change from generation to generation (Moses and Chua, 1991). The differences in physical and chemical properties of degenerated tRNA and of the proteins, differing in their functionally inactive parts, may be detected within the resolution of competitive interaction while remaining undetectable during laboratory experiments. Non-transcribed sequences probably play an important role in the process of development of a multicellular individual from an embryo.

Thus observation in vitro of neutral mutations does not necessarily mean that these correspond to identical phenotypes in natural populations. There is no absolute degeneration of genome in nature. The resolution of competitive interaction may be several orders of magnitude higher than that achieved in the laboratory. The problem of the existence of genome degeneration is actually the problem of threshold sensitivity of competitive interaction. Neutral substitutions can remain inseparable from deleterious substitutions within the range of $n \leq n_c$ in a single population (Kimura, 1983), see Sect. 3.6.

3.8 Normal, Decay, and Adaptive Polymorphism in a Population

The existence of finite threshold sensitivity of competitive interaction results in a genetic diversity of individuals which have the same or different phenotypes but feature equal competitiveness under the conditions natural for the given species. Such a polymorphism may be called normal, despite the fact that it is determined by deleterious decay substitutions, provided the number of those substitutions n satisfies $n \leq n_c$. As demonstrated above, the level of normal polymorphism in most species is extremely large, so that individuals with identical genotypes cannot be randomly found in practically any populations (Paune and Westneat, 1988). Even when neutral substitutions are totally absent, random drift of genes should take place in a population within the range where the deleterious character of mutations is not manifested. In small populations such a drift results in random fixation of a limited number of deleterious decay substitutions.

The sensitivity threshold of competitive interaction may differ from species to species. It is natural to expect that demands on the genetic program of all the individuals in a species should be the strictest in those species which exist under extreme environmental conditions. The sensitivity threshold of competitive interaction, n_c, in such species may be decreased to its minimal level. One can expect the lowest normal polymorphism in populations of those species. That is indeed the case for the polar bear – the largest carnivore living under the extreme conditions of the far North, and for the cheetah – the carnivore demonstrating the highest sprinting speed among all the land animals (Cohn, 1986; see also Sects. 3.11 and 3.14).

Neutral polymorphism not related to mutations may also be found. A typical example of such polymorphism is the right-to-left asymmetry in the bodies of individuals. For example, the river flatfish (*Pleuronectes flesus*) is found in two forms: one with both of its eyes on the right side of its body and the other a leftsided one (Andrijanov, 1954). Of the 215 individuals of the *P.f. bogdanovi* river flatfish subspecies caught by the present author in the Onega Bay of the White Sea, 21% were leftsided. The asymmetric shape of that fish is an adaptation to sea- and riverbed life. It is reached by a correlated change in the position of many of its organs. In a real environment the right form cannot have any noticeable advantage, since there is no right-to-left asymmetry there. The molecular stereoisomers in the cell are known to have identical symmetry in all the living beings and are the same for the right and the left forms. Thus both the formation and frequency of occurrence of the right and the left forms cannot be prescribed by the two different normal genomes, independently formed in the course of evolution, and should be programmed in one and the same normal genome. The actual configuration (the right and the left form) cannot be hereditary. The only hereditary characteristic programmed is the frequency of occurrence of the left form with respect to the right one. Frequency of occurrence is a neutral genetic characteristic which is randomly fixed in a certain position. That neutral characteristic should be subjected to random genetic drift with subsequent fixation in its alternative position. Due to random genetic drift in two non-interacting populations of one and the same species that frequency of occurrence may have different values (Andrijanov, 1954). In many species of the flatfish family such a drift has resulted in random fixation of either the right (*Hippoglossus vulgaris*) or the left (*Rhombus maximus*) form. When the body is formed along the somatic line or during vegetative budding a certain configuration should be preserved. Otherwise the correlation between the positions of separate organs would be broken, and the asymmetry of the body would be absent. At equal frequencies of occurrence of the right and left forms asymmetry might occur due to spontaneous breaking of symmetry (Nicolis, 1986). In that case the frequency of occurrence is not related to any program in the genome and should not suffer any genetic drift. Such a situation is found for duckweed (*Lemna minor* and *L.gibba*, Kasinov, 1968).

Due to the continuous process of decay of the normal genotypes a certain number of decay individuals with lowered competitiveness is always present in the population, their genotypes having $n > n_c$. Genetic diversity of the decay individuals results in the appearance of decay polymorphism in the population. In conditions of a natural ecological niche the number of such decay individuals may be kept at a level much lower than that of normal individuals. Thus the decay polymorphism is much lower than the normal one in those conditions and it may be safely neglected as compared to the latter.

However, adaptive genetic polymorphism is also present in any population. Non-decay "switching" mutations may take place in the normal genome. The changes of the genetic program which occur during such mutations may spread and get fixed within each population if it enters some new conditions different to the initial ones. Switching mutations does not contribute to higher levels of chaos or to erasing information of the normal genome. It is similar to switching to different TV programs and fine tuning of the image in each program. When a TV set ages and fails at random, no new possibilities for finer tuning or switching to new channels not envisaged in the design appear. The information on the types and number of possible switches, on the frequency of such switching mutations, and on all the functionally sensible modes of life of an individual are coded in one and the same normal genome. When the programs controlling such switching mutations in the normal genome disintegrate, the very possibility of such switching may vanish, and with it the functionally sensible mode of life of the individual corresponding to that switching.

Switching mutations may take place via site-specific transpositions of specific macrofragments of the genome, which are accompanied by either activation or inactivation of certain fragments of the genome. These include "latent genes": phenotypically dormant DNA sequences that are usually not expressed during the life cycle of an individual, but can be selected for, and have the capacity to be activated by, some genetic event such as mutation, recombination or insertion of a transportable element. Latent genes are distinguished from other pseudogenes by this potential for expression; in fact, these genes were first detected by the altered phenotypes resulting from reactivation of the latent sequences (Moody and Baston, 1990).

In contrast to decay mutations all these processes should be of catalytic nature, that is be performed by enzymes coded by separate parts of the genome. Individuals with their program switched acquire the highest competitiveness in the population and start to dominate it when environmental conditions correspond to that program. Stabilizing selection then proceeds to act as intensely as before, so that decay substitutions are not accumulated. Then switching mutations become reversible, that is a switch-back to the initial program occurs when the environment returns to its initial state, and individuals possessing such a program become dominant in the population once again. The whole set of external conditions, with respect to which their corresponding switching mutations are programmed in the genome, should be regarded as natural for the existence of the particular species. Both the adaptive and stabilizing programs of that species are retained under any of those conditions, these programs working to keep both the community and its environment stable. The process of adaptation via individual switching mutations to various programs of the normal genome will be called "programmed local adaptation" in what is to follow.

Switching mutations are similar to switching of genes in the course of an individual's life (Ptashne, 1986, 1987). However, in contrast to the latter, switching mutations are transferred to offspring and act throughout the whole of the population instead of in a separate individual only. Certain protein-induced multi-drug resistances in bacteria (Newbold, 1990), as well as transposition switching of sex in yeast (Hesin, 1984), changes of body and organ size in depending on habitation temperature (Bergman and Allen rules), changes in fat layer, in wing span, in clutch-size and in migration programs in the migrating bird species depending on their actual habitation area (Green et al., 1989; Greenwood, 1990; Yoshimura and Clark, 1991) may all serve as examples of such switching.

The whole possible set of species genome programs and the mechanisms used for switching from one such program to another, as well as any other genetic information, must inevitably decay when no stabilizing selection takes place. Thus all the possible genome programs are only saved when each of these programs is used by some population of species, the competitive interaction of individuals in it withholding the respective program from decay. Besides, to prevent the decay of these mechanisms, which switch from one sensible program in the genome to another, populations should continually exchange individuals, these following different programs from the normal genome of the species.

Due to the extreme complexity of all genetic programs, random local adaptation to changes in external conditions is improbable, be it a spontaneous appearance of a new functionally sensible regime via some single random decay point mutation or some macromutation, the information on that regime being initially absent from and not programmed into the normal genome. (Such a situation is quite similar to that when some classic masterpiece by a genius of composition or of performance is written onto a magnetic tape. One cannot really expect then that random erasure or wear and tear of tape would result in the appearance of a new masterpiece by another genius on that tape.)

It is particularly the absence of random local adaptation, which is confirmed by the observed stability and the discrete nature of all the biological species, that provides for the possibility of biological regulation and sustenance of environmental stability (see Chap. 4). The absence of such local random adaptation does not contradict the observed fact of species evolution, as discussed in detail in Sects. 3.15 and 3.16.

The frequency of switching mutations may be programmably changed depending on environmental conditions (Stahl, 1990). However, that frequency is different from zero in most cases. Thus, if the respective populations are large enough, few individuals may be present in them in which such switching mutations have indeed taken place, corresponding to some alternative functional mode. When conditions arise corresponding to that mode, individuals with their programs already switched enjoy a certain competitive edge over the rest of the population (provided no other switching mutations occur), so that the number of those individuals becomes the largest in the population (Rossi and Menozzi, 1990). Thus adaptive polymorphism exists in the population, programmed into its normal genome, in addition to the normal and decay polymorphism. Such adaptive polymorphism is incomparably narrower than either normal or decay polymorphism.

Broadening of such adaptive polymorphism increases the stability of the species (Fisher, 1930, 1958; Dobzhansky, 1951; Wright, 1988), as well as the number of communities in which the individuals from such species retain their stabilizing program necessary to support stability of that community and of its environment. Increase in decay polymorphism always results in shrinking the species habitation area and in lowering that species' stability. There are no natural variations of the external conditions at which decay mutations might result in increase of the number of decay mutants with a definite decay genotype. The notion of the normal genome retains its meaning if we include switching mutations. The normal genome, which includes all the possible functional modes for the individual pre-programmed into it, may be called "the inclusive normal genome". It is defined to the accuracy of neutral mutations and remains unique for all populations of the biological species.

Thus all the observed adaptive polymorphism may be attributed to one and the same normal genome of the population. Individuals with several different normal genomes may be present in the population only when they are correlated with each other, cannot exist without each other for long periods of time, and none of them can be forced out from the population due to competitive interaction between them. Several normal genomes, replicating independently of each other, are present in the nucleus-containing eukaryotic cells of higher organisms: one in the form of a set of nuclear chromosomes, and another as chromosomes of mitochondria and chloroplasts (in plants), which are found in the cytoplasm (Sager, 1972; Ayala and Kiger, 1984). Nuclear and cytoplasmatic genes cannot function independently of each other. Prokaryotic bacterial cells devoid of nuclei contain, beside their principal chromosome, autonomous cyclic genomes in the form of plasmids, which replicate independently (Ayala and Kiger, 1984). Plasmids can transmit from one bacterial cell to another. Some plasmids determine resistance to antimicrobial drag and toxic metal ions in bacteria (Foster, 1983; Newbold, 1990). The so-called coevolution in bacterial-plasmid population (Modi and Adams, 1991) may apparently be considered both as the transition between the different admissible states in the adaptive polymorphism and the increase of decay polymorphism in the perturbed natural conditions. Bisexual species have two normal genomes in their populations – the male and the female ones. Two different normal genomes may be present in individuals which are in a symbiotic relation to each other, as in case of the algae and the fungus in a population of lichen (Margulis, 1971). Finally the numerous normal genomes are mutually correlated in the community of different biological species, providing for biological regulation of the environment.

One may speak about the combined normal genome of all the individual species correlated in the community in exactly the same way as one speaks about the genome consisting of several non-homological chromosomes in the cell, or about the combined genome consisting of a nuclear and a mitochondrial DNA. The combined normal genome of a population of identical communities (similar to a community of lichen of a single species) remains unique for the given type of community. Rigid correlation between species in the community is often inadequately called adaptation. (Following such reasoning one should speak about mutual adaptation of different nuclear chromosomes.) Only rigidly correlated species in the community may feature the necessary wide range of reactions to changes in their environment. Such a community is characterized by a single combined normal genome with its minimal normal polymorphism, that is by the one corresponding to the largest genetic information of the community. It is as unthinkable to compose an artificial community of arbitrarily picked species as to compose a cell genome of arbitrarily chosen genes and chromosomes picked from the individuals of different species. All the deviations from the normal composition of species and from the normal population numbers of each given species in a given community are decay phenomena, which are eliminated in the process of competitive interaction and selection of homological communities in hyperpopulations (Gorshkov, 1985a, 1986a). Relative frequency of occurrence of such decay communities is controlled by the resolution of competitive interaction between various communities; it may be described by equations of the types (3.5.1) and (3.5.9).

3.9 Stability of the Biological Species

The resolution of competitive interaction reaches its maximum under natural conditions, and its threshold sensitivity drops to its respective minimum, which is much lower than the lethal threshold, $n_c \ll n_L$. The condition that competitiveness of the normal genotypes featuring the non-perturbed stabilization program (Sect. 3.2) is at its maximum under the natural conditions of that species, ecological niche is an independent one, providing for stability of the species, the community, and

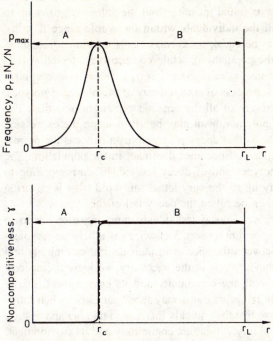

Fig. 3.1. Normal polymorphism and non-competitiveness in the natural environment. $r \equiv n/M$ is the density of decay substitutions, n, per unit genome length, M; P_r is frequency of occurrence of individuals with density r decay substitutions in the population; γ is non-competitiveness, see (3.5.9) and (3.5.10). The traditional variables of relative fitness, w, and of coefficient of selection, s, are related to non-competitiveness, γ, by a simple relation $\gamma = s = 1 - w$ provided the genome decay rate is $\mu = \ln 2 = 0.69$; $r_c \equiv n_c/M$ is threshold density defining sensitivity, n_c; $r_L = n_L/M$ is the lethal density, n_L is the lethal threshold of the number of deleterious decay substitutions. A is the range of normal polymorphism (the normal genotypes), and B is the range of decay polymorphism (decay genotypes).

the environment. As noted in Sect. 3.5 above, competitiveness, Eq. (3.5.8), measured for individuals within communities, does not coincide with fitness, which is measured for individuals isolated from the population, that is removed from the process of competitive interaction. Competitiveness should drop sharply under natural conditions, while non-competitiveness γ_n, Eq. (3.5.10), should simultaneously grow quickly from 0 to 1 with the number of decay mutations in the genome, n, entering the range $n > n_c$. Meanwhile fitness may remain practically unchanged in the range $n > n_c$ up to $n \approx n_L$, see Fig. 3.1.

When conditions deviate from the natural, the resolution of competitive interaction n_c^{-1} (that is the average length of the genome fragment containing no decay substitutions l_c) decreases, and the value of n_c (i.e. $r_c = l_c^{-1}$) increases, so that competitiveness of the normal and the decay individuals even out.

When conditions deviate strongly from the normal ones, the genetic information of normal genotypes loses its initial meaning, and the value n_c grows up to the lethal threshold n_L. For all the individuals within the whole range $n < n_L$ their competitiveness appears to be equal, on average (as is the fitness measured for individuals isolated from the population), while competitive interaction fails to perform its stabilizing functions ($\gamma_n \approx 0$ up to $n \sim n_L$). Decay polymorphism snowballs catastrophically in the process of such a decay of the normal genotypes, corresponding, as it were, to erasure of all the sensible genetic information. The quantitative measure of decay polymorphism may be given using the expression $(4M/n)^n$ (Sect. 3.7). When $n > n_c$ that decay polymorphism exceeds the normal one by many orders of magnitude and becomes dominant in the population. The rest of the possible decay genotypes and of decay individuals corresponding to them and retaining life capacity up to the very lethal threshold (that is covering the range $n_c > n \geq n_L$) may then be called the decay tail of the species.

Build-up of the relative number of decay individuals in a population results in erasure of the genetic stabilizing program (Sect. 3.2), which is otherwise responsible for correlated interaction between the species in their natural community and controls the mode of their behavior, that is the necessary work by the species contributing to the stability of both the community and its environment. Decay individuals devoid of their stabilizing programs may turn "gangster" when introduced into another community, so that they quickly increase in number and destroy the correlated interaction and stability within that community and its environment. Some well-known examples of such developments are given in Sect. 4.5. Formally such a situation corresponds to an increase in fitness but it cannot be considered a random local adaptation to altered conditions of the environment. After the community is destroyed and decays and the environmental conditions deteriorate, such "gangster" species are also eliminated. Such a situation cannot arise under the natural conditions of the natural community in its ecological niche, in which the natural genome and the normal genotypes of the species have originally formed.

Beside switching mutations programmed into the genome (Sect. 3.8) insensitivity to newly appearing diseases, poisons and other unnatural conditions may also appear due to decay of those parts of the genome which code fragments playing an important part in an individual's life under natural conditions, but also randomly encode susceptibility to various harmful substances and organisms not encountered in natural environments. Destruction of these parts of the genome, which may be inflicted in many different ways, as any other decay, randomly results in higher survival of such decay individuals under such unnatural conditions, as opposed to natural. Genetic information is only lost then, and no new genetic information is synthesized. (Similarly, a car with one of its tires burst regains some of its stability if another one is punctured – it "adapts".) It is apparent that in the overwhelming majority of cases there are no genomes and genotypes in the decay tail belonging to individuals with such random adaptation to prescribed change in the external conditions. It is known, for example, that artificial selection in any trait always reaches saturation (Mettler and Gregg, 1969; Raven and Johnson, 1988).

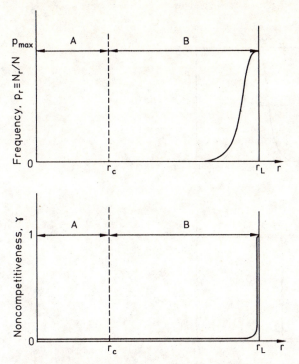

Fig. 3.2. Decay polymorphism and non-competitiveness in perturbed environment. For notation see legend to Fig. 3.1.

After returning to natural conditions the maximum competitiveness of the normal genotypes is restored, so that normal individuals force all the decay individuals from the population at an exponential rate. The rate of such exponential forcing out is defined by the maximum difference actually attainable $B_0 - d_0$ (which is the biotic potential of the normal individuals). When external conditions are perturbed for a sufficiently long time, the processes of decay embrace all the individuals in the population, so that no individual with its normal genome is left in it. The maximum frequency of occurrence for decay genotypes with n deleterious decay substitutions becomes $n \gg n_c$ and approaches the lethal threshold, see Fig. 3.2. In that extreme case the population may return to its initial state after the perturbation ceases and the conditions return to natural, provided competitiveness of decay individuals under the natural conditions monotonically increases with the number of deleterious decay substitutions decreasing in the range down to $n_c = n$. Then the maximum competitiveness goes to individuals surviving in the population with the number of such substitutions minimal: $n_{\min} > n_c$. They force all the decay individuals with $n > n_{\min}$ from the population at an exponential rate. In that case we have for noncompetitiveness, Eq. (3.5.10):

$$\gamma_{n_{\min}} = 0, \qquad \gamma_{n > n_{\min}} \geq 1.$$

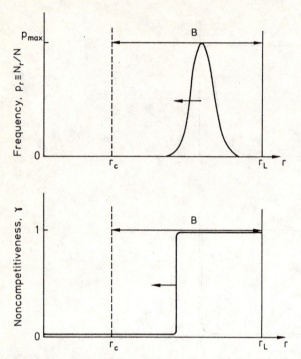

Fig. 3.3. Relaxation to normal genotypes after cease of perturbation in the natural environment. For notation see legend to Fig. 3.1.

Further progress back to the normal state of the population occurs via reverse mutations and genetic recombinations during sexual breeding, which decrease the number of deleterious decay substitutions in the genotype. Individuals thus appearing and having $n_{min} - 1$ deleterious decay substitutions in their genotype, acquire the highest competitiveness in the population and force individuals with n_{min} deleterious decay mutations out of the population. We then have

$$\gamma_{n_{min}-1} = 0; \qquad \gamma_{n>(n_{min}-1)} \geq 1$$

and so on, until the number of deleterious decay substitutions reaches the threshold n_c of sensitivity of competitive interaction (see Fig. 3.3). When all the fragments of the normal genome are retained in the population, spread, as it were, among the different decay individuals, genetic recombinations, considered in more detail in the next section, make it possible to reduce the number of decay substitutions by several units in each successive generation. Thus with genetic recombination operating it may be that there is no monotonic increase in competitiveness following a reduced number of deleterious decay substitutions.

All processes combine to produce genetic relaxation instead of genetic drift. The drift within the range of normal polymorphism does not disrupt either the stabilizing or the adaptive program of the species under natural conditions. Random drift within the range of decay polymorphism, taking place under unnatural conditions, cannot bring one back to the normal genome. Then such a drift is but a manifestation of further decay processes and should eventually lead beyond the lethal threshold, ruining the population.

Genetic drive, on the other hand, is related to random transpositions of macroscopic fragments of the genome (Dover, 1987). All the above statements on the drift of separate nucleotide pairs also refer to the random drive of the genome macrofragments.

After all the normal genotypes in the population are lost, genetic relaxation to the normal genotype may follow in different ways, related to various successions of reverse mutations and reparative recombinations. Thus the process of relaxation should depend on the pathway via which natural conditions of habitation are restored for the given species. When comparing decay populations at various stages of their relaxation it may appear that each population is best fitted to those perturbed conditions under which it exists. When transferring the decay population into different perturbed conditions it may happen to be less fitted to them than the aboriginal decay population. That phenomenon is observed in most domesticated animal and plant species which differ strongly from their natural predecessors (Begon et al., 1986). Such a phenomenon should not occur with species existing in their natural ecological niches, or during the process of decay of (instead of relaxation to) the normal genotypes of the population in cases of deviation from natural conditions.

Environmental conditions of the natural ecological niche fix the maximum competitiveness of the normal genome. The relative number of decay individuals is defined by the intensity of their competitive interaction with normal individuals instead of the limited resources of the ecological niche. Population density of normal individuals is prescribed by the information contained in the normal genome and may be held at a level much lower than that permitted by the available resources of the ecological niche. Such a situation exists particularly for most large animals (see Chaps. 4–6). That makes it possible to keep not only the species but its environment stable as well, including all the other species in the ecological community.

Within the picture described, the biological species is strictly determined within its ecological niche by the set position of the normal genome. When external conditions fluctuate, random oscillations take place around that normal genome without any shift in its position. The biological species cannot continually crawl away from that position adapting to changing environmental conditions. Only such genetically stable species and their communities are capable of satisfying the Le Chatelier principle in the biosphere and controlling the state of the environment.

Accumulation of decay individuals in any population accompanying deviation of environmental conditions from the normal should not disrupt the stabilizing program of the whole community. Even when a certain species in the community loses such a stabilizing program due to loss of the normal genotypes and to accumulation of an excessive number of decay individuals, such a decay species produces some additional perturbation with respect to other species in the community. The latter should retain their stabilizing program as well as the capacity to compensate environmental perturbations within some short time period, including the perturbation produced by the decay species. In that case such a decay species also returns to its normal state after the natural conditions are restored due to the compensating reaction of the community as a whole. If the situation is the opposite, the environment may go outside the scope of control, so that the whole community will be doomed. Thus excessive perturbation by the decay species is much more dangerous than complete extinction of any species entering the community from it.

Thus normal genotypes should be preserved in the populations of species consuming the principal part of energy fluxes in the community (Chap. 5), irrespective of the actual perturbation of the environment, so that after these natural environmental conditions are regained they capture the whole population at an exponential rate. Hence, prolonged deviations from the conditions of their natural ecological niches are prohibitive for small populations. Such populations may only exist under very stable weakly fluctuating external conditions. When the biomass of the whole community is fixed, an increase in the species diversity of the community results in a reduction of separate population numbers. Thus communities of high species diversity may only exist under quite stable external conditions. When these conditions are sharply perturbed, such communities must lose their stability together with the species forming them and disintegrate.

The highest species diversity is found in tropical forests on land and in the coral reefs at sea. Such communities and the species forming them may only exist under extremely stable environmental conditions, in the absence of any sharp perturbations. Stability of the environmental conditions is then supported by the communities themselves which quickly compensate all the fluctuations in the environment in agreement with the Le Chatelier principle (see Chap. 4). These communities feature the highest productivity and greatly provide for stabilization of the environment for the whole of the biosphere on the global scale. At the same time sharp anthropogenic perturbations of such communities result in their quick destruction, which destabilizes the environment for the whole biosphere.

Communities of the moderate and polar areas exist under strongly fluctuating environmental conditions. Contemporary terrestrial biota is apparently incapable of suppressing these fluctuations, stabilizing the environmental conditions in these zones to such an extent that communities with high species diversity, low numbers and low stability of each separate population would become possible. Communities in those zones feature low species diversity, high population numbers, and high stability of the genomes of all the species. These communities suffer strong perturbations, anthropogenic included, without losing their stability. However, their role in stabilizing the overall environment for the biosphere is significantly smaller than that of the tropical and subtropical communities, since their production contributes less to the overall production of the biosphere (Whittaker and Likens, 1975; see also Chap. 5).

We now demonstrate that all the known features of the genome structure, the characteristics of life cycle, the morphology and behavioral traits of individuals work to increase the genetic stability of the species and to increase the rate of relaxation back to normal genotypes and to the normal genome after external perturbation of the conditions of the natural ecological niche, so that competitiveness and stability of the community and of the environment both increase as a result.

3.10 Genetic Recombinations

Relaxation via reverse mutations occurs because lowering the number of decay substitutions by one results in a stepwise growth in competitiveness and in an exponentially quick capture of the whole population by the individuals with lowest decay level. For a reverse mutation to occur in a given site $(vk)^{-1} \sim 10^{10}$ individuals should be accumulated (under the condition of the subsequent accumulation of deleterious decay, mutation is stopped), i.e. 10^4 generations should pass in a population of 10^6 individuals. There are numerous programs in the genome which code enzymes speeding up the relaxation to the normal state of the genome. Among there are such features as "hot points" of higher mutability in vital parts of the genome, as well as multiple back-ups of the genome fragments with the ensuing random distribution of those fragments across different parts of the genome as mobile genetic elements (Ayala and Kiger, 1984). These programs increase the rate of relaxation due to reverse mutations to three orders of magnitude.

However, the relaxation rate is most accelerated by genetic recombination. Essentially recombination is as follows. Assume that there are two genomes containing one deleterious decay substitution in each of them. The probability that the locations of those decay substitutions coincide is negligibly small. Let us cut both genomes at some arbitrary but identical point and connect the righthand part of one to the lefthand of another and vice versa, see Fig. 3.4. As a result we obtain two new genomes. If then the cut (the chiasma) passes between the decay substitutions, one of the new genomes will contain no decay substitutions, that is it will be normal, while the second one will contain two decay substitutions. If both decay substitutions lie to the same side of the chiasma, recombination changes nothing, see Fig. 3.4. Several scores of such chiasmata occur in the process of each act of recombination in the process of specific cell divisions (meiosis) (Cano and Santos, 1990; Burt et al., 1991). Contact (syngamy) of two different genomes is always needed for genetic recombination to occur. That goal is attained via sexual breeding.

Note that in the course of the individual's life cycle there should be a period of diploid phase in which the haploid genomes (or haploid parts of the genomes as is the case with bacteria) of two different individuals combine into one. The principal period of existence during which the individual affects its environment the most may fall in either the haploid or the diploid phase (see Sect. 3.12, Maynard Smith, 1978; Bell, 1982; Kondrashov, 1988; Michod and Lewin, 1988; Dunbrack, 1989; Hedfick and Whittam, 1989; Kirkpatrick and Jenkins, 1989).

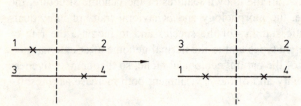

Fig. 3.4. Genetic recombination. Crosses indicate deleterious decay substitutions in the genome. When two genomes, each containing one deleterious decay substitution in its specific position (or containing different unspoiled fragments of the normal genome, which is essentially the same) merge, a single new genome may form containing neither deleterious decay substitution, as well as another genome containing both. That happens when the initial genomes are cut between the two substitutions, and the first half of the first is joined to the second half of the other one, and vice versa. If the cut happens to one side of both deleterious decay substitutions, recombination does not result in any changes. The probability of recovering the unspoiled genome is decreased with the distance between the two deleterious decay substitutions narrowing, and that effect serves as the basis for genetic mapping.

When the initial number of decay substitutions in both genomes is high, such recombination always results in the appearance of genomes with both higher and lower numbers of such decay substitutions. Recombination is a random process which should bring about a Poisson distribution of the number of decay substitutions in the offspring genomes forming after recombinations (Maynard Smith, 1978). The Poisson multiplicity, (3.4.4) and (3.5.4), should clearly coincide with the average number of decay substitutions in the genomes of the parent population. (If these decay substitutions already followed a Poisson distribution in the parent population, recombination would not change anything without reverse mutations.) If the parent population is characterized by a narrow peak in the $n > n_c$ range, recombination results in the appearance of normal individuals as early as the first generation of the offspring, having $n < n_c$. In other words recombination accelerates the process of genome relaxation by ten orders of magnitude, as compared to reverse mutations without any recombinations!

Sexual breeding and genetic recombination may result in a recovery of the normal individuals lost in the parent population, as early as the first generation of offspring only if all the fragments of the normal genome are present in their distributed form in the genome of the parent population. Recombination makes it possible to bring together all the fragments of the normal genome into a single genome of an individual in the offspring. If some fragment of the normal genome is lost from all the individuals in the population, return to the normal state of that fragment may only occur via reverse mutation. A gene consists, on average, of 10^3 nucleotide pairs. In accordance with (3.4.2) the decay rate of a single gene has an order of $\mu_{gen} \sim 10^{-7}$. The probability that some mutation takes place in a given gene in one single individual is $1 - e^{-\mu_{gen}}$. The probability for a mutation to occur in all the individuals of the population is equal to product of such probabilities for every individual, i.e. $(1 - e^{-\mu_{\text{gen}}})^N \approx \mu_{\text{gen}}^N$. That probability will be negligibly small for $N \geq 2$ so that no gene can be lost from the population within the species lifespan. Sexual breeding thus safely guards the population from the decay of its genome.

When breeding is asexual (parthenogenesis or budding) some decay of the genome takes place if a decay substitution occurs in some part of the genome in each normal individual of the population ($n = n_c$), that is if normal individuals vanish from that population altogether. The probability of such an event is $(1 - e^{-\mu})^N$, where μ is the decay rate of the whole genome, Eq. (3.4.2). At $\mu < 1$ that probability is of the order of μ^N. For example, if $\mu = 0.9$ and $N = 150$ we have $\mu^N = 1.4 \times 10^{-7}$, that is no normal gene will be lost from the population in $\mu^{-N} = 7 \times 10^6$ generations. (Separate individuals losing their normal genome are immediately forced out from the population under natural conditions.) Thus an asexual population of practically any population number keeps its stability under natural conditions within an almost unlimited time span, provided $\mu \leq 1$. However, no asexual population may enter a perturbed external environment for any sizeable time period, because competitiveness of the normal and decay individuals even out then and the normal individuals can be forced from the population. If conditions fluctuate to any noticeable extent, sexual breeding has to be switched on now and again in addition. Such a life cycle is typical for many insects (Williams, 1975; Raven and Johnson, 1988).

The probability $(1 - e^{-\mu})^N$ approaches unity for any N if $\mu \geq 10$, and several normal genes are lost in every generation from all the individuals of an asexual population, that is both normal genotypes and normal individuals vanish from the population. Since sexual breeding is absent (there is no recombination of genomes of different individuals), such genes cannot be recovered (10^{10} generations are needed to recover them via reverse mutations). Thus at $\mu \geq 10$ inevitable disintegration of an asexual population takes place. In other words, a stable state of a population with $\mu \geq 10$ is only possible in the case of sexual breeding (Muller, 1964). Sexual dimorphism, that is splitting of the population into males and females is not mandatory anyhow.

To support a stationary state of a permanently decaying genome condition Eq. (3.5.7) has to be satisfied. At low decay rate $\mu \ll 1$ that condition corresponds to each normal individual producing one normal offspring during its life span. In that case the population numbers will remain unchanged. However, to have at least one normal individual among the offspring of the normal parent at high decay rate ($\mu \geq 10$), the number of offspring should exceed $e^\mu \geq 2 \times 10^4$, see Fig. 3.5a. Such is indeed the number of offspring produced by many species. The number of seeds in many plants with high decay rate satisfies that condition (Wilson, 1975). The number of eggs spawned by a single fish during its lifespan (fecundity = average fertility $\times$ lifetime) often exceeds 10^6 (Wilson, 1975). (However, high fecundity is not necessarily related to high decay rate of the genome ($\mu \gg 1$). It may result from purely ecological factors, when the main work specific to the given species is carried out by the numerous juvenile individuals, while the few adult ones are

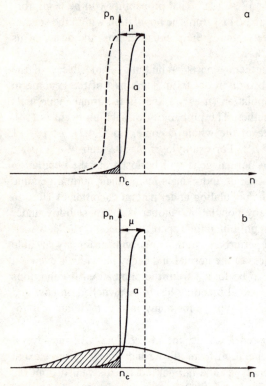

Fig. 3.5a,b. The Kondrashov effect: (**a**) Asexual breeding. n is the number of deleterious decay substitutions (contamination of the genome). p_n is the respective frequency of genotypes, n_c is the sensitivity threshold for competitive interaction (individuals are of equal competitiveness if $n < n_c$, while at $n > n_c$ their competitiveness is zero). The initial distribution of the parent population is shaded. Each parent produces e^μ offspring (see right dashed line). Due to accumulation of deleterious decay substitutions the distribution for offspring (the left dashed line) is shifted by the value of decay rate μ, Eq. (3.4.2) (the solid line). The offspring with $n > n_c$ are selected out. As a result the distributions for the surviving breeding offspring coincide with the parent one; (**b**) Switching on of genetic recombination. The distribution for offspring prior to selection (the solid line "a", see Fig. 3.5a) is broadened to the Poisson distribution (solid line "b"). The average values and areas enveloped by distributions "a" and "b" coincide with each other. After that the offspring with $n > n_c$ are selected out. As a result the number of offspring with $n < n_c$ (hatched area) appears to be much larger than the one for asexual breeding (the shaded area). When the Poisson width $\sqrt{n_c} \gg \mu$, one half of the offspring has the normal genotypes and the other half has the decay genotypes which are selected out.

only responsible for reproduction of those juveniles.) However, in both mammals and birds their progenies cannot be numerous because of their endothermic nature (see Sects. 5.2 and 6.2). For example, a woman cannot give birth to more than 20 children during her lifespan.

With of high genome decay rate, $\mu \geq 10$, and a low number of offspring are produced by the individual during its lifespan, $b_0/d_0 \ll e^\mu$, the stationary state may also be supported if sexual breeding takes place (Kondrashov, 1982, 1988). Assume that the distribution $N_n = N_{n_c}$ in parent genomes is characterized by an average number of decay substitutions $\bar{n} = n_c$ and a very low variance $\overline{(n - n_c)^2} \ll n_c$. The average number of decay substitutions in the genomes of the offspring shifts by $\mu \ll n_c$ to the direction of larger n, as compared to parent genomes. Let us assume that after a long period of asexual breeding the sexual process is switched on. Due to the random character of the process of genetic recombination, decay substitutions in the offspring genomes appear to be distributed according to Poisson, with approximately the same average $\bar{n} = n_c + \mu \approx n_c$ as the parents had, but a higher variance $(n - \bar{n})^2 = n_c + \mu \approx n_c$, as prescribed by (3.4.4) (Maynard Smith, 1978; Kondrashov, 1982, 1988). If $n_c \gg \mu$, approximately half the offspring appear to be normal and to have genomes with the number of decay substitutions $n < n_c$, so that they survive and breed, Fig. 3.5b. After that the distribution acquires the shape of a Poisson profile around its maximum, truncated on the right, and having a standard deviation of $\sqrt{n_c}/2$. If μ and n_c are related via $\mu \sim \sqrt{n_c}$, each subsequent generation shifts the truncated Poisson distribution beyond the threshold $n > n_c$ by a value of the order of distribution width $\sqrt{n_c}$. Up to that threshold, $n < n_c$ the distribution remains narrowed, with its variance $(n - \bar{n})^2 \ll n_c$. Sexual breeding broadens that distribution to the Poisson one and so on.

When $\mu \ll \sqrt{n_c}$ immediately after switching on sexual breading, offspring of normal parents appear to be normal, so they survive and breed. Hence, to support a stable population at $\mu \ll \sqrt{n_c}$ each individual should produce two offspring only, instead of the e^μ offspring in an asexual population (Kondrashov, 1982, 1988), see Fig. 3.5b. If $\mu \gg \sqrt{n_c}$ the share of surviving offspring drops off sharply.

To summarize, with the genome decay rate μ being high, that is the genome itself being large and containing much information, Eq. (3.4.2), the stationary state of the population may be supported via sexual breeding on condition that

$$n_c \geq \mu^2, \tag{3.10.1}$$

if the respective sensitivity threshold n_c is chosen for competitive interaction. Assuming $\mu \sim 10$, we obtain the estimate of the n_c value: $n_c \geq 100$. The actual value of sensitivity threshold for competitive interaction apparently exceeds that estimate so that $n_c \gg \mu^2$ for all existing species (see Sects. 3.11 and 3.13).

Note also that when $n_c \sim \mu^2$ in accordance with (3.4.2) and (3.10.1) the density of the acceptable number of deleterious decay substitutions per unit genome length $r_c \equiv n_c/M$ should increase for larger genomes: $r_c \geq (vk)^2 M$. When $n_c \gg \mu^2$ the value n_c does not depend on μ and r_c does not increase proportionally the genome size M and may be a universal quantity for all species.

One might call the genetic breeding strategy based on keeping the sensitivity threshold for competitive interaction excessively high $n_c \geq \mu^2$ (the Kondrashov effect) the strategy of a species with "hidden genetic information". In that case both the population of individuals of that species and the community in which that species exists gain something from the genome of that species being so large and featuring a large store of information in the normal genome and its high decay rate μ. At the same time the top limit on n_c, Eq. (3.10.1), prevents there being sufficient numbers of individuals in the population with their genotypes close to the normal genome. These individuals only randomly and rarely appear in the population and are not identified in the process of competitive interaction. They do, however, have enough time to produce the necessary "work" in both the community and the population of their own species, gaining some advantages over communities and populations lacking such individuals.

3.11 Sexual Dimorphism and Regulation of Birth Rate of Decay Individuals

All the considered advantages of sexual breeding relate to both single sex (hermaphrodite) and bi-sexual (sexually dimorphic) species. Only part of the population (the females) is capable of actually producing the offspring in the bi-sexual species, while in the single sex species all the individuals of the population are capable of producing offspring (such are the hermaphrodite species: sexual breeding exists in them but sexual dimorphism is absent – all the individuals are the same and combine the functions of both the male and the female involve; the asexual species rely on breeding by budding or parthenogenesis, so that the whole population consists of females only).

An equal number of males and females in the population results in halving the biotic potential of the population (that is of the maximum possible value of fitness, $W_0 \equiv B_0 - d_0$, which defines the maximum possible rate of exponential growth of the population), and that is considered a significant drawback of the bi-sexual strategy (Wilson 1975; Maynard Smith, 1978; Bell, 1982; Hamilton et al.,1990). Large non-productive losses of both pollen and sperm are considered another drawback of sexual breeding. However, no population ever increases its numbers at a rate close to the biotic potential under natural conditions. In some species of invertebrates the sex ratio of emerging adults can vary from nearly 100% males to nearly 100% females (Clutton-Brock, 1982). Therefore halving the biotic potential in a bisexual population with an equal number of males and females against that of a hermaphroditic monosexual or an asexual population can never manifest itself under the natural conditions. Energy losses associated with futile expenditure of either pollen or sperm are negligible in comparison with the natural variations of individual productivity. Besides, many bi-sexual individuals, such as ants, for example, are capable of using sperm at an efficiency close to 100%. Therefore, genetic recombination, based on monosexual (hermaphrodite) and bi-sexual (sexually dimorphic) modes of breeding are practically equivalent to each other in all the characteristics so far considered.

However, the bi-sexual strategy of genetic recombination is a much more complex system, which demands additional information to form two different types of individuals in the population – the male and the female (Partridge and

Harvey, 1986). As demonstrated in Sect. 3.5, preventing the genetic disintegration of the population and supporting it in a stationary state is only possible when the death rate of the decay individuals is forcefully increased or their birth rate is decreased.

Apparently, there is only one method for relative regulation of birth rate of decay individuals. That is polygamy based on sexual dimorphism, during which two normal genomes – of the male and the female – appear in the population. Sexual dimorphism is often understood as the apparent striking differences in body size and coloration, etc. between the male and the female. However, the main difference between them regarding sexual dimorphism is functional. The male is incapable of reproduction by himself. The female is only capable of reproduction after her contact with the male. In such a situation all the relations of competitive interaction and of stabilizing selection are transferred onto sexual relations, that is onto sexual selection. The male may prevent one female (a decay one) from breeding, while stimulating another (normal one) into it. The normal female may accept the normal male for mating and reject the decay male. Competitive interaction between the males is apparently aimed at winning the female, instead of environmental resources. In one way or another that interaction results in suppressing sexual activity of the decay males. As a result all the decay males and females are excluded from reproduction. Competitive interaction between the females appears to be either completely switched off or minimized (Partridge and Harvey, 1986). The expected lifespan of all the individuals (both normal and decay ones born of normal parents in the course of the inevitable processes of decay) is kept identical. In particular, a low juvenile death rate is sustained. The necessity vanishes for an energy consuming procedure of forced elimination of live decay individuals from the population (Gorshkov, 1989; Gorshkov and Sherman 1990, 1991). All these advantages have worked to make sexual dimorphism and sexual selection so widely spread throughout the animal world independent of species ecology (Emlen and Oring, 1977; Bradbury and Andersson, 1987).

Sexual dimorphism in plants (diclinous plants) also provides for regulation of birth rate of decay individuals: specific aerodynamic properties of pollen, specific structure of the female sexual organs to catch the normal pollen and other similar means are employed. However, that does not exclude competitive interaction between the individuals within the population of plants, so that the principal mechanism for genetic stabilization of the species in the plant world remains that of regulating the death rate of the decay individuals. Thus sexual dimorphism among plants is a feature much less developed than in the animal world. The relative number of diclinous plant species is equal to several per cent of the total number of plant species (Maynard Smith, 1978).

All the advantages of sexual dimorphism are only manifested in polygamy. They often reveal the difference between polygyny and polyandry within polygamy. However, as with monogamy, all the cases of polyandry should actually represent subvert polygamy: the decay males either totally or partially barred from sexual contact with the females are used to help the females to bring up the offspring

(Gorshkov, 1982a; Andelman, 1987), while the breeding females keep coupling with the normal males (that question is covered at more length in Chap. 6).

As indicated in Sect. 3.5 regulation of the birth rate and hence sexual dimorphism may only be completely effective at low decay rate, $\mu < 1$. The population will then always consist overwhelmingly of normal individuals, so that the presence of a small number of non-breeding decay offspring of normal parents does not perturb the normal genetic information of the population to any significant extent. In an opposite case, when $\mu \gg 1$, only regulating the death rate of the decay individuals may be effective. That is seemingly testified to by the data on most plants, for which the decay rate is $\mu \gg 1$ (Williams, 1975; Maynard Smith, 1978; Lewin, 1983). However regulation of the birth rate and, hence, sexual dimorphism become natural for the species with "hidden genetic information", based on the Kondrashov effect. The difference between regulating the death and the birth rates is then that, when regulating the death rate all the individuals belonging to the righthand part of the Poissonian peak, to $n > n_c$, Fig. 3.5, are extinguished during their youth and before puberty, whereas, when the birth rate is regulated, these decay individuals stay alive for a full lifetime, as the normal ones, but are excluded from breeding.

At large n_c the relative width of the Poisson peak is low, in compliance with the law of large numbers, Eq. (3.4.4), and the individuals with the smallest number of deleterious decay substitutions in their genomes ("hidden genetic information") are always a minority in the population in any breeding strategy. The genetic quality and competitive capacity of an individual in the population may be determined during its lifetime. The longer the life of the individual is extended, the better the quality of its genetic information may be defined. Therefore the strategy based on regulating the death rate via extinguishing juvenile decay individuals with their $n > n_c$, inevitably associated with energy, social, etc. losses, is less advantageous than the strategy of regulating the birth rate based, as it were, on sexual dimorphism, on preserving the lives of all the decay individuals, and on barring them from the process of breeding.

As it will be demonstrated in Sect. 3.13, the condition

$$n_c \gg \mu^2 \tag{3.11.1}$$

is met for most species. Such species are characterized by very high normal polymorphism, see Sect. 3.8. The condition (3.11.1) makes it possible to sustain the level of organization of individuals in the population of species with high decay rate $\mu \gg 1$ via bisexual breeding by means of suppressing the birth rate of decay individuals. With (3.11.1) the average steady state number of permissible decay substitutions in the Poisson distribution, $\bar{n}$, should be less than the sensitivity threshold, n_c, of competitive interaction: $\bar{n} \approx n_c(1 - 1/(2\sqrt{n_c}))$, see Fig. 3.6. The steady state share of decay individuals in the bisexual population is a small quantity of the order of $\mu/\sqrt{n_c} \ll 1$. Hence, no increase of the death rate of decay individuals is needed. Sexual dimorphism (that is separation of the population into males and females) makes it possible to remove decay individuals from

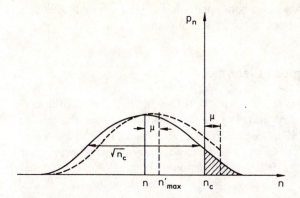

Fig. 3.6. The Kondrashov effect in sexual dimorphism. Solid line is the Poisson distribution of parent genotypes in the population. Individuals in the hatched area are excluded from breeding. The dashed line gives the distribution of the offspring genotypes when recombination is absent: the number of the offspring from parents with the normal genotype has increased, as compared to the parent population (see the solid line). It compensates for the non-breeding decay offspring in the hatched area, while the maximum distribution, n'_{max}, shifts to the right by the value of the decay rate μ. The average values of the decay substitutions, $\bar{n}$, and the areas under the envelope curves in both distributions coincide. Introducing recombination turns the dashed line into the Poisson solid line. See Fig. 3.5 for other notation.

further breeding through mating choices of normal individuals, i.e. of competitive interaction and sexual selection between all the individuals.

In contrast, when $n_c \sim \mu^2$, the share of decay individuals in a stationary bisexual population will be of the same order of magnitude as that of normal ones. Such a high load of decay individuals is apparently too large for an adequate functioning of the species within the community. To reduce the share of decay individuals in the population such species should turn to regulating the death rate, based on increasing the death rate of juvenile decay individuals. Consequently sexual dimorphism loses its advantages when $n_c \sim \mu^2$. That is why condition (3.11.1) is valid for the majority of bisexual species with high decay rate $\mu \gg 1$, the vertebrates in particular. No cases of hermaphroditism or parthenogenesis are found among birds and mammals. Parthenogenesis is only found in 25 vertebrate species (three fishes, two salamanders, and 20 lizards) (White, 1973).

In monogamous bi-sexual species, as well in hermaphrodite and parthenogenetic ones, only regulation of death rate is possible. Then the number of decay individuals in the population is reduced via more juvenile deaths. Monogamy loses all the advantages of sexual dimorphism. In its stabilization strategy for the species monogamy does not differ from hermaphroditism at all. Competitive interaction then goes on between the different monogamous couples (generalized individuals), similar to such interaction between regular hermaphrodite or parthenogenetic individuals. At low population densities hermaphroditism with its possibility of self-fertilization and parthenogenesis both appear to be more advantageous than monogamy, since there is no need to seek a sexual partner.

3.12 Diploid and Polyploid Genomes

Multicellular bodies contain up to $10^{15} \approx 2^{50}$ cells formed via divisions of the initial single embryonic cell (the zygote). The number of divisions along the somatic line k_s is, respectively $k_s \approx 50$ in case of dichotomic divisions (that is when each somatic cell then divides into two, etc.), and exceeds that number if we account for the fact that it is not all the cells which keep on dividing. However, one may assume for the majority of cases that $k_s \leq 2\,k_g$. That is why germ ($\mu = Mvk_g$) and somatic ($\mu_s = Mvk_s$) decay rates are of the same order of magnitude, so that we may henceforth neglect the differences between them.

All the cells of a multicellular body are correlated among themselves. There may be no strict selection of normal cells within the body. If the genome is large $M \sim 10^{10}$bp ($Mv \sim$ one division^{-1}) each division of the cell brings about some error (a somatic mutation). Each cell of the mature body thus contains in excess of 50 such errors. Thus, all the cells of such a mature body should contain about 10^{17} errors. That number is much larger than the size of the genome, so that any error, including those lethal for the body as a whole, should be found at least 10^7 times. Clearly, a body built that way cannot exist. The condition for building a body capable of life is the complete absence of somatic mutations in most of its cells.

Individuals whose genomes occur singly in each cell are called haploid (Ayala and Kiger, 1984). All the prokaryotes (bacteria and the blue-green algae) are haploid. Among the multicellular eukaryotes the haploid genome is typical for gametophytes, plants, which are always small in size (such are certain mosses and some algae) and some insects (such as the haploid drone among the bees) (Raven and Johnson, 1988). The largest haploid animals known (that is having strictly correlated bodies, insects mainly) have their genomes within $M < 5 \times 10^8$ bp (Lewin, 1983) and contain $10^{10} = 2^{30}$ cells, that is, their building takes $k_s = 30$ divisions. Hence, the condition

$$\mu_s \equiv Mvk_s \sim \mu \leq 1 \qquad (3.12.1)$$

is satisfied for haploid animals, and it may be considered the condition limiting the possibility of forming a haploid body (Gorshkov, 1989; 1990). The condition that more than 2/3 of body cells contain no somatic mutations has the form $e^{-\mu_s} > 0.67$, i.e. $\mu_s < 0.4$, which is principally the same as (3.12.1).

Large mammals contain up to $10^{15} = 2^{50}$ cells, which corresponds to $k_s = 50$ divisions, and have a genome of $M \approx 3 \times 10^9$ bp (Lewin, 1983). We have $\mu_s \equiv Mvk_s > 10$ for them, that is, mammals cannot be built on the basis of a haploid genome. The solution consists in a transition to diploidy, that is to duplicating of the genome. The idea that diploidy saves the process from somatic mutations is apparent and has been repeatedly expressed in many studies without any detailed discussion of that problem (Crow and Kimura, 1965; Gorshkov, 1990; Kondrashov and Crow, 1991).

The life cycle of all the diploid individuals implementing the sexual mode of breeding consists of two phases: the diploid and the haploid. In all the large plants and animals the life of their multicellular bodies takes place in the diploid phase while only their germ cells (the gametes) exist in the haploid phase. Merging together these cells form a zygote, which gives the start for the multicellular diploid body. Genetic recombination takes place between the two copies of the diploid set before the gametes are formed, during a special cycle of cell division, the meiosis. As indicated above, multicellular bodies may only exist in their haplophase in small plants and animals.

If the zygote contained no decay substitutions at all, the probability of co-incidence of the decay mutations in two homologic sites of the genome would constitute v^2, and the condition for building a multicellular body would have the form $Mv^2k_s \leq 1$, that is $k_s \leq 10^{10}$ divisions. (The dimension of an identical mutation in two homologic sites v^2 is bd^{-1} (b $\equiv$ base pair, d $\equiv$ division), respectively, so that the value Mv^2k_s is dimensionless.) In that case the number of cells that a multicellular body could contain would be

$$2^{10^{10}} \approx 10^{3 \times 10^9},$$

which would exceed by many orders of magnitude the size of the universe. However the limited sensitivity of competitive interaction results in a zygote necessarily containing several decay substitutions, the overwhelming majority contained in only one of the copies of the genome.

The catalysts (enzymes) of biochemical reactions are proteins. The structure of proteins is coded by parts of the genome, the genes (Watson et al., 1983). Beside the genes the genome contains large parts of DNA, whose functional meaning is still obscure (Lewin, 1983; Watson et al., 1983). The decay transformation of a gene together with the part of the genome correlated to it may bring about distortion of the biochemical reactions occurring in the body. As a rule, apparent decay features appear in the individual (either diploid or polyploid (Lewin, 1983)), if decay mutations affect the same gene in both (or every) copy of the genome.

Two differing nucleotide sequences in one and the same gene, which result in synthesizing two different sequences of amino acids in the protein coded by that gene are called the two alleles of the gene. Differences in the proteins are found by assessing the differences in their phenotypical features, in differences in their mobility during electrophoresis in gel, or via direct sequencing of the amino acid sequence in the protein. States with either coinciding or differing alleles of the genes situated in homologous sites (at the same locus) of the two copies of the chromosome are called homozygotic and heterozygotic, respectively. When studying a large number of genes positioned in paired chromosomes the majority are found in the homozygotic state, and a minority in the heterozygotic. The ratio of the share of heterozygotic genes to the total number of studied genes is called heterozygosity H (Ayala and Kiger, 1984). If one copy of the genome contains a normal (dominant) gene in a heterozygotic state, and the other a decay (recessive) gene, such a type of decay may not be manifested at all in the phenotype, or its manifestation may be significantly masked.

The dominancy of the normal gene is manifested in the enzymes it codes being dominant in controlling biochemical reactions, which are built into the correlated set of all the other normal biochemical reactions of the body. The recessive decay gene codes enzymes, which control biochemical reactions leading into a dead end, so that they do not fit into the general set of the normal biochemical reactions of the body. The decay may result from new decay mutations appearing in the heterozygotic part of the genome. In the case when the decay gene is dominant (e.g., when a chain of biochemical reactions controlled by the normal genome is blocked by a decay enzyme) the apparent decay is already manifested when only one copy of the genome decays, so that diploidy loses the above advantage. Thus such cases should only be encountered extremely rarely (Ayala and Kiger, 1984; Lewin, 1983).

To a first approximation the heterozygotic part of the genome of diploid bodies presents a set of normal genes in a single copy, and within that approximation it is an effective haploid part of the genome. Disintegration of the normal genome in its heterozygotic part cannot already be compensated by diploidy of the genome. Selection may only control preservation of the dominant gene. In the heterozygotic state recessive decay genes are not manifested in the phenotype. Further decay of recessive genes (even if one assumes that they had not been decay initially and had some functional meaning different from that of the dominant gene) cannot be prevented. Only blocking of such disintegration is possible for recessive genes when their homology with the dominant gene is strongly perturbed, far in excess of the threshold critical value. That happens due to a process of gene conversion during which homozygosis is restored along one of the two alleles of genes entering the heterozygotic state. However, both the normal and the decay gene may be found in the final homozygotic state with equal probability (Ayala and Kiger, 1984). Homozygotic decay states of $n > n_c$ are subject to selection.

Lack of any diploidy advantages associated with insurance against the deleterious decay mutations in the heterozygotic part of the genome results in possible occasional cooperative interaction between the two homologous genes, when the functions of one of them are complimented by those of the other (so-called interallelic complementation (Fincham, 1966)). That may, for example, lead to the appearance of a functionally sensible protein dimer coded by that cooperative pair of genes (Ayala and Kiger, 1984). In that case both cooperating genes are no longer decay, and the decay of each of them is selection controlled. Evacuation (or blocking, which somehow mutes the respective entity) of certain groups of genes or even whole chromosomes (such as, for example, sexual X,Y chromosomes) in one of the copies of the genome of diploid set, which might be lethal if simultaneously occurring in both copies, might also be considered a certain type of cooperation. Such cooperations are used to prescribe the sex of the individual and are apparently adaptive, unlike the decay changes in the genome. For example the male in most mammals contains the X,Y chromosomes, while the female has

X,X ones. In many invertebrates the male carries the (X,0) set with only one X chromosome (White, 1973; Hodgkin, 1990). By way of analogy with the common state the (X,X) state in the sexual chromosomes may be considered homozygotic, with the (X,Y) and (X,0) ones (the so-called hemizygotic state) as heterozygotic. These types of cooperation may be considered as particular cases of heterosis (Ayala and Kiger, 1984), i.e. the advantage of the heterozygotic state over both homozygotic ones (the individual containing no X chromosomes is not capable of life, that is the "homozygotic recessive" states (YY) or (00) are both lethal; an individual containing doubled X and Y chromosomes is abnormal).

When breeding is sexual and genetic recombination takes place too, the two copies of the diploid set of the offspring genome originate from the random combination of haploid gametes of the parents. Therefore the types of cooperation present in the parents may vanish in the offspring and be substituted by new ones. All these processes, including the above-mentioned chromosome prescription of the sex, may be envisaged as particular cases of switching, programmed into the genome, which increases the adaptive (functionally sensible) polymorphism of the population, as discussed in Sect. 3.7. All the types of the possible functionally sensible cooperations between the non-paired chromosomes and the non-paired fragments of the genome in both copies of the diploid set should be included into the common program of the normal genome. Random decay processes in the genome cannot result in a new functionally sensible cooperation, just as the male genome cannot originate from decay processes in the female genome and asexual species cannot originate from decay processes in the sexual ones and vice versa.

The random advantage of a heterozygotic condition as compared to both homozygotic ones in abnormal external conditions (to the exclusion of cases of cooperation), that is the random appearance of a "hybridizing force" usually results in destruction of the natural community of species and is therefore decay in nature. Typical examples of such developments are the hybrids appearing during artificial selection and the sickle cell anemia. In the latter case the point mutation, lethal in its homozygotic state, increases its frequency of occurrence in the heterozygotic state if the population enters a state of malaria infection (Ayala and Kiger, 1984; Vogel and Motulsky, 1979; 1982; 1986). These phenomena correspond to abnormal conditions, which are lethal (or unfavorable) for the normal genome but are randomly acceptable for some decay genomes of separate species. In the natural ecological niche in which the normal genome has formed, such conditions never appear. Any cooperation is principally impossible in the homozygotic part of the genome which insures it from decay changes. Homozygotic recessive states may be found in separate individuals. However, in a population with sexual breeding the decay recessive alleles in most individuals should be found in their heterozygotic state only.

3.13 Heterozygosity

A transition to diploidy decreases the effectively haploid part of the genome, vulnerable to decay mutations, to the value of $(M/2)H$, where $M/2$ is the haploid size of the genome (the average size of the genome in its haplophase, that is in the gamete), M is the total size of the genome in which the decay substitutions may accumulate, H is the heterozygosity, including the X and Y chromosomes, that is the ratio of the number of normal genes present in one of the chromosomes only to the total number of genes in both the paired and the non-paired chromosomes. The conditions for life capacity of the multicellular diploid individuals, similar to Eq. (3.12.1), then take the form:

$$\mu_{2s} \equiv \mu_s H \equiv M v k_s H \leq 1, \tag{3.13.1}$$

where the value of μ_{2s} may be called the diploid somatic decay rate, because it is particularly that value which controls the probability of phenotypically manifested mutations in the diploid genome. From these estimates we find that the heterozygosity of mammals (including the haploid sexual X and Y chromosomes in males) should not exceed 10–20%. Such an estimate of heterozygosity is given by the analysis of frequency of occurrence of the non-coinciding gene alleles in various locuses, which code different proteins and result in the observed phenotypical changes in individual features (Ayala and Kiger, 1984). The X chromosome in most mammals amounts to 5% of the haploid value of the genome $M/2$, while the heterozygosity of paired chromosomes is 4% (Ayala and Kiger, 1984). The Y chromosome is much smaller than the X. The length of the Y chromosome varies strongly among various populations and races of the same species. These variations are included in the normal polymorphism (Vollrath et al., 1992; Foote et al., 1992), see Sect. 3.8. As for the human species, the Y chromosome is longer in the Japanese, and shorter in Australian aborigines, than in Europeans (White, 1973).

Were the decay substitutions to have been distributed in a completely random manner through both copies of the genome, the relative number of the coincident (manifested) deleterious decay substitutions in both copies of the genome would be proportional to H^2. However manifested deleterious substitutions in the diploid individuals are subject to strict selection, so that their share is actually much smaller than H^2. In triploid bodies (those having three copies of the genome) selection only acts when the decay mutations simultaneously hit all three homologous fragments of the genome. The probability of the coincidence of such decay mutations in any taken pair of genomes is proportional to H^2. Thus the haploid part of the genome effectively vulnerable to decay mutations in triploid bodies is $(M/3)H^2$, and in the n-ploid ones its is $(M/n)H^{n-1}$, respectively, see Fig. 3.7, where M/n is the haploid part of the n-ploid genome.

The condition for forming a multicellular n-ploid body has the form:

$$\mu_{ns} = \frac{M}{n} v k_s H^{n-1} \leq 1. \tag{3.13.2}$$

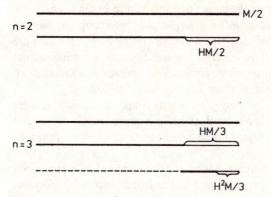

Fig. 3.7. Diploid and polyploid decay rates of the genome. The total length of all the chromosomes in the n-ploid genome is M. The haploid length of the genome (that is the length of the gametic genome) is M/n. Thick lines indicate the normal genomes. The diploid genome ($n = 2$) is formally indicated as the one in which all the deleterious decay substitutions are concentrated in only one (the lower) copy. Deleterious decay substitutions are however evenly distributed over both copies. It is apparent from such a presentation that the haploid part of the genome, unprotected from somatic mutations (the thin line) is equal to $HM/2$, and the non-paired X and Y chromosomes may also be included into it. As for the triploid genome ($n = 3$), the upper pair of chromosomes is presented the same way as is the diploid one. However, the section homologous to the thin line in the second copy contains only the share of decay chromosomes in the third copy. The rest of the genes of the lower chromosome (the thick part) are normal. As a result the part of the triploid genome, unprotected against somatic mutations is equal to $H^2M/3$. As for the n-ploid genome, that part is equal to $H^{n-1} M/n$, respectively.

The values of the decay rate μ_{ns} and the haploid genome M/n being the same, the heterozygosity in polyploid bodies may be much higher than in diploid ones, see (3.13.1). Denoting the total length of the n-ploid genome as M_n and its heterozygosity as H_n, we obtain that fulfilling conditions (3.13.1) and (3.13.2) at $M_n/n = M_2/2$ and $\mu_{ns} = \mu_{2s}$ corresponds to an equality:

$$H_n = H_2^{1/(n-1)}. \tag{3.13.3}$$

On the other hand, heterozygosities being equal to each other, the polyploid genome may be increased in length. We have at $\mu_{ns} = \mu_{2s}$ and $H_n = H_2 \equiv H$:

$$M_n = \frac{n}{2} M_2 H^{2-n}. \tag{3.13.4}$$

While the diploid heterozygosity is equal to $H_2 = 0.1$, the tetraploid one may reach $H_4 = 0.5$. In accordance with that, the number of deleterious decay substitutions increases sharply in the recessive genes of the heterozygotic part of the genome. We have $H_4 = H_2 = 0.1$ at equal heterozygosities. In this case the size of tetraploid genome may be increased to the ratio of $M_4/M_2 \sim 200$.

The value of heterozygosity in diploid and polyploid individuals is not an adaptive feature (except for the small number of cooperating genes), but characterizes the resolution (sensitivity) of competitive interaction instead. The latter fails to discern between the individual with a given level of heterozygosity and the supernormal one, in which both copies of the non-cooperating part of the genome are totally identical to the normal genome. If a population of such supernormal individuals is cloned at the initial moment, competitive interaction appears to be incapable of preventing the genome of those individuals from decay.

A "spontaneous breaking of symmetry" would then take place with respect to the normal genome, so that a given level of heterozygosity would set in and corresponding hidden deleterious substitutions would arise at arbitrary positions in the genome.

All the individuals with their heterozygosity H remaining below a prescribed threshold H_c have equal competitiveness and hence feature normal genotypes. Decay of the genome and increase of heterozygosity will apparently go on until H equals H_c. Further build-up in heterozygosity under natural conditions results in lowering of competitiveness and is cut off by stabilizing selection. Heterozygosity also includes part of the cooperating genes, which carry the functionally sensible information from the normal genome. That party of heterozygosity including the non-paired sexual X,Y chromosomes may be denoted by H_0. Then the observed heterozygosity in the natural population should vary within:

$$H_0 < H \le H_c. \tag{3.13.5}$$

The increase of heterozygosity above H_c results in a drop off of competitiveness of the individuals placed under the natural conditions of the ecological niche. Life capacity of the individuals is still sustained at up to the very lethal threshold $H = H_L > H_c$. That threshold is absent for species with small body size and small genome, that is $H_L = 1$, their multicellular individuals being capable of existing in the haploid phase, such as, e.g., insects and gametophytes (see Sect. 3.12). However, such a lethal threshold of heterozygosity is present in mammals with a large genome and large body size, which is much lower than unity: $H_L < 1$. Under natural conditions all the individuals with their heterozygosity staying within the limits

$$H_c < H < H_L \tag{3.13.6}$$

are decay and are eliminated from the population.

As demonstrated in Sect. 3.6, the sensitivity threshold of competitive interaction is characterized by the highest admissible density of the number of deleterious decay substitutions per unit length of the genome, $r_c = n_c/M$, or by a value inverse to it, $l_c = r_c^{-1}$, which is equal to the average length of fragment of the normal genome, free of deleterious decay substitutions. We assume that the values r_c and l_c are universal for all the fragments of the genome containing information, that is the competitiveness of all the individuals with $r \le r_c$ and $l \ge l_c$ is the same. Then the part of the diploid genome containing information, that is all the homozygotic states and the normal (or the cooperating) part of heterozygotic states should be characterized by the density r_c and the length l_c. Now the decay component of the heterozygotic state containing no information may have a density of deleterious decay substitutions much larger than r_c and, hence, the average length of its genome containing no such deleterious decay substitutions will be much shorter than l_c.

Hence, the average values of l_c for paired chromosomes (autosomes), in which originates the decay heterozygotic component free of information, should remain shorter that the respective value of the haploid (hemizygotic) part of the genome, that is of the non-paired X and Y chromosomes. That difference should quantitatively characterize the relative input of the truly neutral sites of the genome, free of information, into the total size of the genome. Were the neutral sites to constitute the dominant part of the genome, e.g., 90 %, the difference in l_c between the sexual chromosomes and autosomes would not exceed 10 %. If neutral sites were absent or constituted a minor part of the genome, the respective lengths would differ by a factor of several units and possibly by an order of magnitude.

The lengths of coinciding fragments of chromosomes may be determined either by directly sequencing homologic parts of chromosomes from different individuals of the population, or by using restrictase-enzymes which cut the DNA molecules in all the positions where the given sequences of four, six, or eight prescribed nucleotide pairs are found. The latter technique is widely used due to its simplicity and is called studies of the restriction fragment length polymorphism, RFLP (Ayala and Kiger, 1984; Hofker et al., 1986; Mandel et al., 1992).

Due to genetic recombination which mixes fragments of the genomes from different individuals in the population, the average lengths of the coinciding fragments in homological parts of the genome should be identical in autosome pairs in both a single and different individuals. The observed average lengths of coinciding fragments in a separate population may be somewhat longer than the lengths of the true fragments of the normal genome, devoid of decay substitutions only in the result of random fixation of a part of deleterious decay nucleotide substitutions. As indicated in Sect. 3.6, such fixed substitutions may be detected by comparing homological fragments of the genome in individuals of the different non-interacting populations, that is by determining the average length of coinciding fragments for different populations.

Studies of nucleotide sequences of the diploid chromosomes (autosomes) and of the haploid sexual X,Y chromosomes (in one of the sexes) demonstrated that the lengths of the coinciding nucleotide sequences of homological chromosomes, for the autosome (and the genome as a whole) both in a single individual and in different individuals, amount to several hundreds of (100–500) nucleotide pairs,

$$l_{1c} = n_{1c}^{-1} \approx (0.1 - 0.5)\,\text{kbp}, \tag{3.13.7}$$

while the lengths of coinciding fragments in X and Y chromosomes (in different individuals) amount to more than a thousand such pairs,

$$l_{2c} = n_{2c}^{-1} \approx (1 - 2)\,\text{kbp}, \tag{3.13.8}$$

i.e., are several times (and maybe an order of magnitude) larger (Sandberg, 1985; Hofker et al., 1986; Donnis-Keller et al., 1987, 1992; White and Lalouel, 1988).

The same should be true when comparing the lengths of coinciding DNA fragments of the related diploid and haploid species.

It means that the number of truly neutral mutations is far smaller than the number of deleterious decay mutations (assuming that the diploid and haploid chromosomes are equally important for the individual). It further means that the majority of deleterious decay mutations are concentrated particularly in the heterozygotic part of the genome. Finally, the value of the average length of coinciding fragments of the haploid part of the genome gives an estimate of the size of the decay tail of the haploid genome of the species, which is thus about 10^{-3} part of the haploid genome, that is the haploid genome of insects and the haploid part of the genome of mammals (the X,Y chromosomes) might suffer up to 10^5 point decay mutations without losing their life capacity. Most single mutations (about 80 %) occur due to transposition, deletion, or insertion of large fragments of the genome, which are several hundred times larger than the average size of a gene (10^3 bp) (Lewin, 1983; Ayala and Kiger, 1984; Finnegan, 1989). If one assumes that after averaging over all the point mutations and macromutations the average length of the fragment changing its position in the genome per single mutation is of the order of 10 kbp, then $n < n_{1c} \approx 10$. Such a number of single decay substitutions may occur in the haploid genome of insects or in the X,Y chromosomes of mammals, without any loss in competitiveness. Due to the presence of a heterozygotic part in the diploid genome of insects, that value may be almost an order of magnitude larger, that is $n < n_{2c} \leq 10^2$, see (3.13.7) and (3.13.8). As for the genome of mammals, which is an order of magnitude larger than that of insects, we obtain an estimate of $n_{2c} \leq 10^3$.

The data presented on the difference between the average lengths of restriction fragments are mostly available for the human genome. Man, however, has been far from his natural ecological niche for many thousands of years. The human species is the most polymorphic one within the biosphere. Normal competitive interaction between individuals in the human population is either weakened, or distorted, or completely switched off. Besides, for the last few hundred years the human population has been at a stage of exponential growth at a rate exceeding that of the accumulation of the decay substitutions μB in (3.5.3). Therefore the number of decay substitutions n, characterizing the genome of modern man, apparently lies within the decay tail, $n_c < n \ll n_L$, see Fig. 3.2, and the heterozygosity of man is $H > H_c$. The observed heterozygosity of the natural mammal species (excluding X,Y chromosomes) is $H \approx 4\%$. The respective observed heterozygosity of man is $H \approx 7\%$ (Ayala and Kiger, 1984). If we assume that $H = H_c$ for mammals, it may be concluded that $H_c < H < 2H_c$ for man. It follows that $H_L > 2H_c$. It is yet unknown how far it is from $2H_c$. However, these figures indicate that the obtained estimates for the X and Y chromosomes $n_{1c} \sim 10^2$ and for the whole genome $n_{2c} \sim 10^3$ give the upper limit, so that it may be expected that $n_{1c} < 10^2$ and $n_{2c} < 10^3$. The decay rate is $\mu \sim 10$ for mammals, see Sect. 3.4. Hence, the relation (3.11.1) is valid for mammals.

The total nucleotide heterozygosity is defined by the average length of co-inciding fragments in the diploid genome and has an order of 0.1–0.2 %. The gene coding the sequence of amino acids in the protein contains on average 10^3 nucleotide pairs (Lewin, 1983).

About one third of the nucleotide substitutions in a gene do not change any amino acid sequences in the protein due to degeneracy of the genetic code (synonymous substitution). Furthermore the catalytic properties of the protein are determined by the amino acid sequence of the active center, which comprises only a minor part of the protein polymer. Analyses of the nucleotide sequence of genes and non-transcribed parts of the genome adjacent to them indicate that most nucleotide differences in the chromosomes are accumulated particularly in those areas (Kimura and Ohta, 1974; Ayala and Kiger, 1984; Ohta, 1987).

Thus the average length of the effective sections (locuses) of the genome, their change in either of the two (diploid) copies of the genome of somatic cells perturbing the bodily functions, appears to be much less than the average length of the genome and is, by all appearances, within a hundred nucleotide pairs. The relative number of such non-coinciding effective sections in the two copies of the genome is what amounts to heterozygosity H, which should thus be of the order of 10–20 %, that is exceed by about two orders of magnitude the observed nucleotide heterozygosity. Simultaneous somatic mutations in the homologous functionally inactive parts of both copies of the genome appearing during the late stages of development of a multicellular body are not apparently manifested in its functions. However, those same mutations appearing in the initial germ cell (in either the gamete or the zygote) result in further perturbations of bodily functions, in its ensuing loss of competitiveness, so that it becomes subject to selection.

3.14 Stability of the Diploid Genome

As repeatedly stressed, all the observed functionally sensible morphological and behavioral differences between populations occupying different geographical regions lying in varying external environments should be programmed in the joint normal genome of the species. This contains the information on all the possible changes in the external environment which characterize the ecological niche of the species and all the necessary changes in both morphology and behavior correlated to them. The number of possible functional genetic differences between populations of the same species, related to switches from program to program, programmed into the normal genome, is much less than the randomly varying decay heterozygotic part of the genome.

The presence of high heterozygosity in the diploid species, in which most decay substitutions are concentrated, means that the diploid individuals may differ strongly from each other in the position of their heterozygotic part of the genome. The position of heterozygotic part of the genome may be kept at quite a conservative level in each population of the species inhabiting a certain territory (due to the slow nature of the process of change in heterozygosity) but differ strongly from that in another population. These differences may be perceived as subspecies (racial), so that they may be subjected to direct empirical testing. Another conclusion follows from that reasoning too, that the subspecies differences in the haploid species should be significantly less than in the diploid ones, and that statement might also be tested empirically.

If the subspecies differences are indeed mainly differences in the position of the heterozygotic part of the genome, while the value of heterozygosity is completely controlled by the need to build a multicellular body, that is remains one and the same in all populations, then it follows that all subspecies are genetically equivalent to each other. Indeed, all subspecies are positioned at an equal genetic distance from the normal genome (determined, as it were, by the constant value of heterozygosity), provided the number of individuals in the population is in excess of one thousand, that is fluctuations in deviations from the natural distribution, Fig. 3.1, remain within several per cent, as prescribed by the law of large numbers. The position of subspecies is defined by a spontaneous breaking of symmetry, related to the presence of heterozygosity. The increase in heterozygosity occurring during cross-breeding between the different subspecies, which brings it into the decay zone, Eq. (3.13.5), may hamper mixing of the sub-species even when their habitats overlap.

A typical example is given by the existence of the two European forms of seagull, *Larus argentatus*, and *Larus fuscus*. That species of seagull contains about ten subspecies, continuously transforming one into another as one proceeds along the Polar Circle from *L.argentatus* to *L.fuscus* (Green et al., 1989). All these subspecies feature normal genotypes with $n < n_c$. However the position of the admissible number of decay mutations, n_c, in the genome of the subspecies is constantly changing. When these subspecies are encountered in a European area of localization, the values of n_c for *L.argentatus* and for *L.fuscus* do not overlap. If individuals of both these subspecies breed, their offspring fall into the decay zone $n \sim 2n_c > n_c$ and cannot withstand competition with the normal individuals from either subspecies.

It is natural to determine the subspecies as different populations of the same species containing a small overlap of the normal polymorphism. Any subspecies may be converted from one to another by a succession of decay and reverse single mutations. The number of admissible deleterious substitutions, n_c, in the genome is universal for all the subspecies, and the total number of decay and reverse mutations should be equal to each other. On the contrary, however, the genome of one species cannot be transformed to that of another species in this manner, see Sect. 3.15. In that sense *L.argentatus* and *L.fuscus* should be considered as different subspecies but not as different species (Orr, 1991; Coyne, 1992; Kondrashov, 1992).

As described in Sect. 3.9, competitiveness of normal and decay individuals evens out under strongly perturbed external conditions, and an exponential increase of the relative number of decay individuals in the population starts then, see (3.5.4). The average heterozygosity of a population then increases up to the very lethal threshold H_L. The number of deleterious decay substitutions in the recessive genes of the heterozygotic part of the genome increases simultaneously, building up a genetic load of the population. Differences between the two gene alleles in one and the same locus of paired chromosomes is limited by the threshold at which gene conversion is switched on (enhanced) (Curtis and Bender, 1991). Return to the normal state of the population with $H \leq H_c$ is effected after conditions return to normal via higher competitiveness of normal individuals in the population.

If external conditions are perturbed for a long time so that all the normal individuals with their $H \leq H_c$ vanish from the population the highest competitiveness after the final return of those conditions to normal is assumed by individuals with the lowest heterozygosity in the range (3.13.6). Return to the normal state of the population with $H \leq H_c$ then proceeds via various mechanisms decreasing the heterozygosity. Among them are the processes of genetic conversion and inbreeding. Hermaphrodite self-fertilization and parthenogenesis, that is, asexual breeding, may be considered as such mechanisms if genetic recombination takes place between the two pairs of homologous chromosomes. Temporary switching to hermaphroditism and to parthenogenesis is observed in many invertebrates (White, 1973; Hodgkin, 1990). Inbreeding is apparently the principal mechanism reducing heterozygosity in mammals (more on this subject below).

With ploidy n increasing, the admissible level of heterozygosity increases under natural conditions, see (3.13.3), while the lethal threshold tends to unity: $H_L \to 1$. However, the return to normal heterozygosity H_c when external conditions are no longer perturbed is difficult for polyploid species typically characterized by long relaxation times and hence by lowered stability. Thus polyploidy should be found under constant external conditions.

All the above relates to the initial heterozygosity of a zygote, that is to heterozygosity in the germ line. Zygotes give rise to new individuals which are subject to stabilizing selection. However, selection does not function along the somatic line, so that deleterious decay substitutions are not eliminated. The processes of genetic conversion (of transition into the homozygotic state) keep on working, which results in the accumulation of homozygotic deleterious decay substitutions. That process may be one of the principal causes of individual aging (that idea was suggested to the author by M.V. Filatov). Heterozygosity of a multicellular body increases by a small value, about 1 %, during its lifespan (along the somatic line). (Assuming the total number of genes to be 10^4, heterozygosity H to be close to 10 %, the number of genes in the heterozygotic state to be 10^3, and the number of single mutations in the somatic line to be 10^2, we find $\Delta H/H \sim 1$ %.) Thus the increase in heterozygosity in the somatic line could hardly be responsible for individual aging.

Hermaphroditism with its capability for self-fertilization and parthenogenesis corresponds to monogamic inbreeding. Low heterozygosity is supported during hermaphrodite self-fertilization and parthenogenesis (White, 1973), so that the genome cannot be strongly contaminated with decay states (alleles) of genes, so characteristic for bi-sexual species and resulting in monogamic inbred depression.

Thus heterozygosity is almost always an admissible genetic load of decay genes, instead of the hidden treasury of possible adaptations to changes in the external conditions (Ayala and Kiger, 1984; Gorshkov, 1989). Transition to parthenogenesis with internal recombination of the genomes from a diploid set, and also to haplodiploid species (as in case of the haploid male and the diploid female; White, 1973; Trivers and Hare, 1976), and inbreeding in bi-sexual species diminishes heterozygosity and the genetic load of the population (instead of limiting the possibilities of adaptive reaction). Haploid genomes or haploid parts of diploid genomes (X,Y chromosomes and normal genes in heterozygotic states) must be contaminated by that load to a far lesser extent.

The presence of haploid non-paired chromosomes in the genomes of diploid species thus provides for a lower level of contamination of these chromosomes by decay deleterious substitutions than that of the diploid (paired) chromosomes. Mammalian males containing a single X chromosome clean that chromosome for the female lives, that female genome containing two X chromosomes. As a result the males have less mean lifespan than the females. Meanwhile the males of social insects (such as drones) of the honeybee feature a completely haploid genome. The death rate for drones is quite high so there must be many drones in the beehive, although only one of them is needed to fertilize the queen. The surviving drones feature the genome with the lowest number of decay deleterious substitutions. That genome is transferred to the diploid offspring consisting of working bees and the new queen, so that their genome is cleaned of decay deleterious substitutions.

The only way to clean the diploid parts of the genome from decay deleterious substitutions and to lower heterozygosity is inbreeding, which is invariably accompanied by frequent inbred depression. During inbreeding, deleterious decay substitutions in the heterozygotic state of parents may transfer to the homozygotic state of their offspring with high probability, which results in the offspring losing its competitiveness (inbred depression) so that they are eliminated from the population. However part of the offspring from inbreeding features a genome much cleaner of decay deleterious substitutions than that of the parents, due to genetic recombination taking place, Fig. 3.8. A population that does not inbreed cannot lower its heterozygosity and ease the load of deleterious decay substitutions.

Populations existing under extreme conditions may be subjected to even harsher selection. Sensitivity of competitive interaction in those species can be higher than the average value known for other species. Such species should have a lower frequency of decay individuals, lower heterozygosity, and hence, lower observed genetic diversity. As already noted above, such a shrinking in genetic diversity is indeed observed in such species as the polar bear (*Ursus maritimus*), musk-ox (*Ovibos moschatus*), Californian sea elephant (*Mirounga angustirostris*) and the cheetah (*Acinonix jubatis*) (Cohn, 1986; Yablokov, 1987).

Altruistic behavioral patterns and those which depend on the density of individuals in a population, including sexual breeding among others, are manifestations of correlations in the group of individuals. They may be supported via biological selection in a population of competitive groups of such individuals, which are

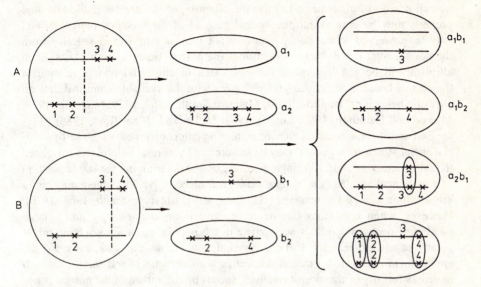

Fig. 3.8. The scheme of recombination during cross-breeding and self-fertilization. A and B are sexual diploid cells from which haploid gametes a and b form. Crosses indicate the positions of deleterious decay substitutions in the genome. It is assumed that parents have identical genotypes. Genome recombination in cells A and B take place at different positions (the vertical dashed lines), and ab are the diploid cells of the offspring which appear as a result of fusion of the gametes. a_1b_1 and a_1b_2 are cells with lower numbers of implicit deleterious decay substitutions in the genome (with lower heterozygosity) than that in the parent; a_2b_1 and a_2b_2 are cells with explicit (manifested) deleterious decay substitutions in both homologous parts of the genome (vertical ovals), absent in the parent (these are the cases of inbred depression or the recombination genetic load; Crow 1958, 1970).

essentially social individuals or hyperindividuals, see Sect. 3.2 (Wynne-Edwards, 1962, 1986). To give a few examples, an anthill, a beehive, or a herd of animals of definite species are internally correlated hyperindividuals and cannot be regarded as populations in exactly the same way as a multicellular body cannot simply be considered a colony of cells. Organization of anthills, beehives and herds is supported via competitive interaction between different anthills or different herds among themselves in a respective set (hyperpopulation) of such social structures (Wynne-Edwards, 1963).

Altruistic interrelations between relatives, either close or remote, within a single species, or between the individuals of different species (such as alarm calls among birds) are different types of correlation between the individuals in social groups of a single species or in communities of various species. Such types of correlation should be written into the normal genomes. Assume that two individuals – a normal and a decay one – have originated from individuals with a normal genome (it might be either the same original individual or different ones). If the decay individual is then prevented from further breeding under the drive of the normal one and further helps to raise the offspring of the normal individual, that property may be written into the normal genome of the breeding individual and may be preserved in the decay genomes not too far removed genetically from the normal one. It will be preserved until the normal genome itself exists. Such altruism will be equally typical for individuals in close and remote relation to the normal breeding individual, which agrees with the available empirical data on altruistic behavior (Hamilton, 1964; Maynard Smith, 1964, 1978; Manning, 1979; Michod and Hamilton, 1980; Lorenz, 1981; McFarland, 1985; Ross, 1986).

Self-sacrificial altruistic behavior increasing competitiveness of the self-sacrificial social structure in general may be manifested by normal individuals correlated to that structure as well. If a single normal genome determining the stable position of a biological species in its natural ecological niche is available, there may be no kin selection among the relatives (Hamilton, 1964; Maynard Smith, 1964, 1978). However, when conditions deviate from natural for long enough, and a large number of decay individuals accumulate in the population, a kin selection might greatly accelerate relaxation of the population to its normal state, provided the environment returns to normal. Kin selection with elements of self-sacrifice, which increases fertility of the closest relatives, speeds up the spread of the normal genes present in those relatives, throughout the population. The degree of relation in that case is proportional to the number of genes common to individuals embraced by that kin (Hamilton, 1964).

As already mentioned above, the queen in the honeybee species being diploid, haploidy of its drones provides for cleaning of their genome of decay genes, as in other haploid insects, and for decreased heterozygosity in the diploid worker bees. The latter contain all the genes of the drones and only half the genes of the queen. That result is achieved via increased death rate of the drones. The social behavior of honeybees is written into their normal genome, to which both the surviving haploid drones and hence the worker bees are closer than the diploid queen (Trivers and Hare, 1976; Brian, 1983). Similarly the male in mammals cleans the female's genome. Kin selection apparently has no relation to these processes of genome stabilization.[1]

All the existing correlations, both between normal individuals of the same species within the population, and between the normal individuals of different species within the community, may be considered altruistic: every individual restricts its reproductivity so as to maintain the normal reproductivity of it own and the other species, belonging to the community. Expulsion of the decay individuals (and of hyperindividuals, see Sect. 3.2) from the population (and hyperpopulation, see Sect. 3.2) by the normal ones in the course of competitive interaction is the general principle governing the existence of life. It may be considered egoistic behavior.

---

[1] I hope for the last statement will not be considered "the thirteenth misunderstanding of kin selection" (Dawkins, 1979; Maynard Smith, 1991).

The diploidy of the somatic cells in multicellular organisms and, similarly, the diploidy of the queen and workers in social insects prevent manifest deleterious substitutions from accumulation within the lifespan of such multicellular individuals and social structures, respectively. Recall that the major part of the haploid males are decay individuals. The relative number of normal haploid males is very small, see Sect. 3.12. On the other hand, the major part of the workers should be normal. Hence, workers have to be diploid individuals.

As for the genetically determined social structures, it is only the queen that can produce workers. The reason for that is very similar to the case of spermatogenesis, discussed in Sect. 3.4, and is as follows: The number of accumulated deleterious decay substitutions in the genome increases in proportion to the number of cell divisions, see Sect. 3.4. A queen in a social insect species produces about 10^9 eggs via 30 dichotomous divisions of the initial germ cell. Were workers capable of breeding, they would produce their progeny by means of several tens of additional divisions in each generation. The number of successive generations of workers over a single queen's lifespan would be much larger than one. Thus the number of deleterious decay substitutions in the progeny of workers would be much larger than in that of the queen. Therefore all the unusual traits of haplodiploid social insects (Trivers and Hare, 1976) can be explained without considering kin selection.

The presence of a large decay tail and the low relative number of truly neutral sites (that is of parts of the genome free of information) means that the normal genome features a large strength reserve. It is removed far from the border of life capacity (that is from the border of fitness of an isolated individual to environmental conditions) to a maximum possible distance. Except for a minor number of conservative (lethal) sites in the heterozygotic part of the genome, a series of decay mutations may occur in other parts of the genome without it losing its life capacity. The loss of competitiveness due to each such decay still permits a quick return back to the normal genome. The evolution of the genome, accompanied by growth in the individual's competitiveness, may, on average, remove the genome from the border of life capacity, without changing the isolated individual's fitness to the environment.

Artificial selection consists in the selection of such teratic states as are fit for efficient use by man (such as individuals with the anomalous production of meat, fat, milk, eggs, seed, flowers, etc.). Such special features are always accompanied by a loss of some other characteristics, which provide for the highest competitiveness of normal individuals. Without man's support all the domesticated breeds are immediately forced out from the natural community under natural conditions. Artificial selection in any trait always reaches saturation, which characterizes the limit in the decay tail (Calow, 1983; Raven and Johnson, 1988). Traits absent from the decay tail of populations of wild species (including their hybrids) cannot in any way be obtained via artificial selection (Raven and Johnson, 1988). Capabilities of gene engineering in constructing new artificial breeds are apparently even more limited due to the high probability of a lethal change outside the limits of the

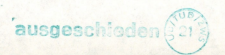

decay tail (Watson et al., 1983). Artificial selection is a change of environmental conditions which is lethal for normal genomes. Artificial support of certain decay genotypes, devoid of their stabilization program, turns the domesticated animal and plant breed into "gangster"-species, destroying the stability of the environment.

Conditions similar to artificial selection may exist under natural conditions too, when decay individuals randomly enter a state isolated from the normal ones (that means apparent decay substitutions of the same locuses in both copies of the genome and high heterozygosity). In that case the return to the normal genome in those species may only happen due to reverse mutations, so that it appears to be suppressed by ten orders of magnitude, as compared to normal relaxation back to the normal genome via recombinations. The diversity of such "decay" species is controlled by decay polymorphism (Sects. 3.8 and 3.9) and may be quite large (consider the number of genera of the fruit fly *Drosophila* in the Hawaii Islands and the number of Darwin's finches in the Galapagos Islands (Vitousek, 1988; Grant, 1991a,b) etc.). Such species might be devoid of their program of stabilization of the environment, so that they exert a perturbation load upon the functioning of the natural community. That effect should work to decrease the capacity of the community to compensate for external perturbations and also its competitiveness. Thus survival of species that have partially lost information from the genome of the normal species is only possible under narrower external conditions which do not vary as strongly (such as in the islands, lakes, or mountains). The natural habitat areas of all such species should always remain much smaller than the natural habitat areas of the normal species (Raven and Johnson, 1988; Grant, 1991a,b; Coyne, 1992; Kondrashov, 1992).

3.15 The Evolution of Species

All of the above refers to preserving the existing level of order in biological objects and to preventing their decay. Biological stability may work to sustain life at a prescribed maximum level of organization without any evolutionary changes. However, if that maximum level is either not reached or does not exist, the employed mode of stabilizing the level of organization of life based on Darwinian selection results in evolutionary changes in a certain direction. Random changes in genotypes, associated with loss of competitiveness, are eliminated. Provided they take place, random changes in genotypes associated with higher competitiveness are fixed and spread through the whole population.

As a rule, increase in competitiveness is associated with a higher degree of order in life processes. This factor controls spontaneous evolution of life towards its higher organization. The number of possible decay changes in genotypes resulting in the decrease of order in life processes is many orders of magnitude higher than the possible changes resulting in a higher degree of order. That is the very essence of the notion of order. It is why the rate at which life orderliness decays when competitive interaction and stabilizing selection are switched off should be many orders of magnitude higher than the rate of evolutionary changes. That difference may be found from the available empirical data.

The observed difference between the normal genomes of two related eukaryote species in the number of substitutions of nucleotide pairs is about 1 % of the size of the genome (Lewin, 1983; Ayala and Kiger, 1984). The difference between all the genotypes of the diploid individuals of one species due to normal polymorphism, over all their nucleotide pairs (see Sects. 3.8 and 3.13) is also of the order of 1 % of the genome size (Lewin, 1983; White and Lalouel, 1988). Hence, the observed difference between two species in the number of non-coinciding nucleotide pairs in their genomes does not characterize the genetic distance between those two species. Assuming that the genome of the two kin species contains 10^9 bp, we find that the difference in the number of nucleotide pairs between both the individuals from different species, and individuals within the same species amounts to $m = 10^7$ bp. The number of different genotypes, which may be built using that difference, is

$$4^m \approx 10^{6 \times 10^6}.$$

All those genotypes remain within the range of normal polymorphism, they are normal and correspond to individuals with full life capacity. Therefore, random coincidence between the genotypes of any two individuals (whether normal or decay), taken from the populations of the two kin species, is improbable. In other words, genotypes of the two species do not overlap each other, and therein lies the explanation of the observed discreteness of the species.

However evolution is an empirical fact, and transitions from the normal genome of an old species to that of new one still take place. If one assumes that the genome of the founder-individual is already at the border of the decay tail of the new species, then progressive transition to the normal genome of the new species takes place via single (point or macro) mutations. That process takes the same course as relaxation to normal genome described in Sect. 3.9, which goes via single reverse mutations after long-term perturbations of natural external conditions cease. In that case every single substitution driving the genome towards the normal one is associated with higher competitiveness, and it embraces the whole population exponentially in just a few generations (it is fixed). Such a process of approaching the new normal genome may be called microevolution.

The time t needed to fix that mutation is found from the equation $n_0^{t/\tau} = N$ or $t = \tau \ln N / \ln n_0$, where τ is the lifespan of a single generation, n_0 is the number of offspring produced by a single individual during its lifespan (fecundity), N is the number of individuals in a population. We have for a bacteria with $N \approx 10^{24}$, $\tau \sim 10^{-3}$ year, $n_0 = 2$: $t \sim 1$ month. As for mammals with their $N \sim 10^8$, $\tau \sim 1$ year, $n_0 \sim 100$, we find $t \sim 4$ years. For man the figures are $N \sim 10^9$, $\tau \sim 25$ years, $n_0 \sim 10$, and $t \sim 200$ years. In any case the time of fixation is negligible, compared with the time necessary to acquire a new functionally sensible substitution in any single individual from the population. Thus fixation will be considered instant in what is to follow. All the new progressive functionally sensible substitutions, leading to a formation of genes of the new normal genome, are initially absent from the population. Each new progressive substitution initially appears in just one individual in the population due to a single mutation (which is similar to reverse mutation in relaxation) and is instantly fixed in the population. Now, it is apparent that sexual breeding (that is the presence of genetic recombination) cannot speed up such microevolution as compared to the effect of asexual breeding. (Speeding up of evolution due to sexual breeding may only take place in extremely large populations, in which the time of appearance of a single progressive substitution (of reverse mutation) is of the same order of magnitude as the time of fixation of that progressive substitution. Hence, the appearance of two or more progressive substitutions is now probable (Crow and Kimura, 1965).)

Thus microevolution from the border of the decay tail of a new species to its normal genome (which is similar to relaxation to the normal genome in the old species) takes place due to single mutations during the relatively short time as compared to the species lifespan. The evolution from the border of the decay tail of one species into the decay tail of another one ("macroevolution") clearly cannot take place due to single mutations. If that were the case, individuals should be found driven by microevolution into either this or that species in quite a short time. That is not observed for the existing species: all the species retain their stability and discreteness. Thus there are no grounds to assume that transitions due to single mutations might be found even if we moved through time with the course of evolution.

Hence, all the observed microevolutionary changes among the presently existing species should be regarded as processes of relaxation to the normal genetic state of the population following the ceasing of external perturbations. These processes of relaxation, taking place due to altered frequencies of occurrence of the alleles for the genes to be found in the population, and due to single reverse mutations, are not related to evolutionary transitions from one species to another. To preserve the stability of a species the transition from one species to another should be prohibited to a high degree of certainty, as compared to permitted relaxation to the normal genome of the old species. In other words, there should exist a probabilistic barrier preventing the transition to a new species. That barrier is supported by the fact that the evolutionary transition goes via multiple mutations, their probability being proportional to the product of probabilities of the respective number of single mutations. It is particularly during such multiple mutations that the first new fundamental functionally sensible information may appear resulting in higher competitiveness of the individual, as compared to competitiveness of the normal genotypes of the former species. In other words the evolution is prohibited with high certainty. That is why the stabilization of the Earth's life and environment is possible. Let us look into that problem in more detail.

The new information distinguishing the genome of one species from that of another should be written as a certain sequence of nucleotide pairs, that is of "words" consisting of four different "letters". The total number of possible "words", which may be combined of n "letters", is 4^n. Since $4^5 = 2^{10} \approx 10^3$, we have $10^n = 4^{5n/3}$. Therefore, the genome containing 10^n "letters" may contain all the possible "words", each not longer than $5n/3$ "letters". The unique sequences in the genomes of most multicellular individuals (eukaryotes, their cells containing nuclei and of size about $50 \, \mu m$) contain no more than 10^7 bp, i.e. "letters". The rest of the genome is mere repetitions (Lewin, 1983). The genome of bacteria (that is of prokaryotes, their cells containing no nuclei and of size about $1 \, \mu m$) contain about 5×10^6 bp and practically consist of unique sequences only. Hence, "words" containing no more than ten "letters" may be present in the genome of any individual (for $n = 6$ we have $5 \cdot 6/3 = 10$). The genome of a virus contains about 10^5 bp. Therefore arbitrary combinations consisting of no more than 8 "letters" may be found in the virus genome. The number of fragments (primers or cohesive ends) actually existing in the genome among the arbitrarily chosen sequence of nucleotide pairs may be found empirically using the single primer polymerase chain reaction (Jones et al., 1990).

Since the probability of a random point mutation (that is, change of a single letter) in a given site of a cell genome is 10^{-10} per single division (and is about 10^{-4} per replication for RNA-viruses (Holland et al., 1982)), to obtain a definite change in a given site of the bacterial genome one has to accumulate 10^{10} individual cells (or 10^4 virus particles). The probability of two random errors is equal to the product of probabilities of the two separate errors. Accordingly, to change just two "letters" in two given sites one has to accumulate 10^{20} individuals, or 10^{30} if we are speaking about three sites (these figures for RNA-viruses are 10^8 and 10^{12} respectively). Elementary calculations show that the global population of a single bacterial species is about 10^{24} individuals (see Sect. 5.6). The time of reproduction for bacteria does not exceed a few hours, that it is of the order of 10^{-3} year. About 10^{27} individuals are generated annually in just a single bacterial species, that number growing to 10^{30} in about 1000 years. Hence, bacteria are capable of forming any three letter "words" (codons, Lewin, 1983) via single point substitutions. The number of viruses may be two orders of magnitude higher. Therefore, the RNA-virus genome is capable of simultaneously producing up to eight point nucletide substitutions.

The total number of individuals generated during the whole lifespan of any bacterial species or viruses is much less than 10^{40}. Therefore no specific word consisting of four letters or more in the bacterial genome and of nine letters or more in the RNA-viral genome may be formed that way. All the new functionally sensible fragments may only appear due to macromutations, that is random combinations of the already existent words and word combinations present in the genome (that process is called the molecular drive or DNA turnover, Dover, 1987). The probability of a random macromutation during which the fragment (word) already existing in the genome finds a new prescribed position does not exceed that of a given point mutation in its order of magnitude (Ayala and Kiger, 1984). Thus macromutation with given transpositions of no more than three fragments is possible for a bacterial genome (and one of no more than eight such transpositions in an RNA-virus genome). Since the maximum word length containing any combinations of letters is limited to ten letters (to eight letters in RNA viruses), a random formation of a new fragment is possible, composed of any combination of no more than 30 nucleotide pairs (of no more than 70 nucleotide pairs in the RNA-virus genome). Random macromutations accompanied by the formation of any given combination of 40 or more nucleotide pairs (that is of 80 or more such pairs in the RNA-virus genome) is already impossible. The very fact of evolution then means that the progressive properties of new fragments, formerly non-existent in the genome, which result in higher competitiveness, should originate at the level of arbitrary sequences containing up to 30 nucleotide pairs in the bacterial genome (or up to 70 such pairs in the virus genome). Naturally, the overwhelming majority of random macromutations are simply decay changes in the genome, or are within the decay tail (thus resulting in a loss of competitiveness), or drive the genome outside that tail (resulting in death).

The average lifespan of eukaryotes is about 10^6 years, according to paleo-data (Simpson, 1944; MacFadden and Hubbert, 1988). With the observed relative constancy of the number of species in the biosphere (Raup and Sepkoski, 1982; Wilson, 1989) extinction of every species should be compensated by the appearance of a new one, which, among the eukaryotes, would differ from the old one by a change of about 1 % of its genome. If the genome is 10^9 bp in size, that corresponds to a change of 10^7 bp. Estimating the number of individuals in a species as 10^9, and assuming the time of generation to be equal to one year, we find that there appears about 10^{15} individuals during that time. That is about 10^8 individuals fall for every positive (progressive) substitution. Following the analogy with decay rate the inverse value may be called generative rate (μ^+, its dimension being (+) substitutions/individual) of the genome. The value of genome decay rate μ, Eq. (3.5.1), that is the number of decay mutations per single individual (or per genome per generation, which is the same), denoted below as μ^- (its dimension being $(-)$ substitutions/individual) is of an order of unity for eukaryotes ($\mu^- \sim 1$ $(-)$ substitutions/individual). The single decay point and macro-mutations introduce inputs into genome decay rate, which are of equal orders of magnitude (Ayala and Kiger, 1984). The ratio of probabilities of the decay ($v^- = v$, see Eq. (3.4.1)) and positive (v^+) mutations per nucleotide site for the eukaryotes, κ_e, which is equal to the ratio μ^-/μ^+, is thus of the order of 10^8:

$$\kappa_e = \frac{\mu^-}{\mu^+} = \frac{v^-}{v^+} \sim 10^8. \tag{3.15.1}$$

That is, one positive mutation should appear every 10^8 decay mutations (if calculated per equal number of nucletide pairs affected by mutations).

Now we may estimate a similar value for prokaryotes, κ_p. The average lifespan of a prokaryote species is of the same order of magnitude as that for eukaryotes, that is $\sim 10^6$ years (Ochman and Wilson, 1987). The size of the bacterial genome is $\sim 10^6$ bp. Kin bacterial species differ by 10 % of nucleotide substitutions in their genome, that is $\sim 10^5$ bp, (Ochman and Wilson, 1987). The number of a single bacterial species is about 10^{24} individuals. The time of generation for bacteria is 10^{-3} year. During the lifespan of a single bacterial species about 10^{33} individual bacteria appear. Hence, there are about 10^{28} individuals per positive nucleotide substitution, that is the generative rate for bacteria is $\mu^+ \sim 10^{-28}(+)$ substitutions/individual.

The decay for bacteria is $\mu^- \sim 10^{-3}(-)$ substitutions/individuals, see Sect. 3.4. The ratio of probabilities of the decay to positive mutations for bacteria κ_p is of the order of

$$\kappa_p = \frac{\mu^-}{\mu^+} = \frac{v^-}{v^+} \sim 10^{25}, \qquad (3.15.2)$$

which is 17 orders of magnitude higher than the respective value for eukaryotes (3.15.1) (Gorshkov, 1987b, 1989, 1991e). Using the well-known value for probability of the decay mutation (3.4.1), we find from (3.15.2) the following estimate for probability of the positive nucleotide substitution, following from the observed rate of evolution for bacteria:

$$v^+ \approx 10^{-35} \ (+) \ \text{substitutions} \ (\text{bp})^{-1} \ \text{division}^{-1}. \qquad (3.15.3)$$

3.16 Evolution of Prokaryotes and Eukaryotes

Due to universal structure of the DNA molecule and of all the organization of life, it is natural to assume that the ratio of probabilities of decay and progressive mutations should also be of universal nature for the whole of life. In any case, these ratios cannot differ by those 17 orders of magnitude from eukaryotes to prokaryotes. Therefore we consider two possibilities: first that κ_e is universal, see (3.15.1), and, second, that κ_p is universal, see (3.15.2).

If we take the value of κ_e to be universal, we find for bacteria $(\mu^-)^{-1} \sim 10^3$ individuals/($-$)substitution, so that we find $(\mu^+)^{-1} \sim 10^{12}$ individuals/ (+)substitution. Recalling that any two bacterial species differ by the value of 10^5 (+)substitutions/species, we find that to transit to a new bacterial species 10^{17} individuals must be accumulated per single species. Hence a population consisting of 10^{24} individuals should actually include 10^7 various species, which exceeds the total number of species in the whole of the biosphere and which contradicts the observed discreteness of bacterial species.

Besides, positive point nucleotide substitutions would then take place for any species numbering more than 10^8 individuals, see (3.15.1). These would then occur due to any mutations at a probability of unity. The time for appearance of each subsequent mutation would then be controlled by the time of fixation of the preceding one. To within the approximation of instant fixation the rate of evolutionary changes would then tend to infinity. Such statements would hold for positive single macromutations as well. If one assumes that about 10^4 substitutions of nucleotide pairs take place for every single macromutation, the probability of such a macromutation would already reach unity for a population of 10^{12} individuals. Populations of that size are typical for many invertebrates. All such species would then be genetically unstable and would not be capable of preserving their discreteness for long enough periods of time, i.e. would not exist as biological species. Therefore such a possibility should be rejected. We are left with the second possibility.

The universal value may thus only be that of κ_p, Eq. (3.15.2). In that case, assuming that the evolution of eukaryotes occurs exclusively by the internal (endogenic) transformations of nucleotide pairs and of their macrofragments in the genome, we find that $(\mu^+)^{-1} \sim 10^{25}$ individuals/(+)substitution are needed if $(\mu^-)^{-1} \sim 1$ individual/(−)substitution. Such a number of individuals is not produced in any eukaryote species within the lifespan of that species.

Thus endogenic evolution of eukaryotes should be considered impossible. Evolution (and, apparently the origin of eukaryotes (Margulis, 1975)) may only be explained on the assumption of exogenic consumption of the functionally sensible "words" and "phrases" from the virus and bacterial genomes and from bacterial cellular structures by the eukaryote genomes and their cellular organelles (Margulis, 1975; Martin and Fridovich, 1981; Kordum, 1982; Hesin, 1984; Syvanen, 1984, 1987, 1989; Moses and Chua, 1988; Gorshkov, 1987b, 1989, 1991e; Amabile-Cuevas and Chicurel, 1992). There seems to be no possibility of explaining the observed evolution of eukaryotes without assuming such a genetic flow of information from viruses and prokaryotes. The long-range correlations in nucleotide sequences of the normal genome of the prokaryotes (Peng et al., 1992) should be conserved during transition of the genome's fragments from prokaryotes to eukaryotes.

Random genetic drift takes place in the range of normal polymorphism of any species $n \leq n_c$ (Sect. 3.8), which results in fixation of certain deleterious nucleotide substitutions within the small populations (Kimura, 1968, 1983, 1987; King and Jukes, 1969). Such substitutions cannot be identified in the process of competitive interaction, they do not decrease the competitiveness of individuals, and preserve that individual's genotype normal. Thus fixation of the deleterious decay substitutions in the range of normal polymorphism is not in any way different from fixation of the truly neutral substitutions, which characterize the degree of degeneracy of the genome (Kimura, 1968, 1983; Ohta, 1987). As demonstrated in Sect. 3.7 above the rate of generation of neutral substitutions in the normal genome of small populations does not depend on their population numbers and is of the order of $vk_g \sim 10^{-9}$ substitution (bp)$^{-1}$ generation^{-1} (Kimura, 1983). Assuming the time of generation for mammals $\tau \sim 1$ year, we find for the rate of substitutions $vk_g \sim 10^{-9}$ substitution (bp)$^{-1}$ year^{-1}. The time necessary for a substitution to arise is then equal to $\tau/vk_g \sim 10^9$ years. After a substitution is fixed, fixation of the next given substitution takes the same time. As a result, to fix $n \geq 2$ given substitutions needed to form a new progressive fragment of the genome, the time $n\tau/vk_g \geq 2 \times 10^9$ years is needed, which is several thousand times longer than the time of formation of any given species.

Nucleotide substitutions in mitochondrial DNA take place ten times as fast (De Salle et al., 1987; Cann et al., 1987), but it is still a process a hundred times slower than the rate of formation of species. As demonstrated in Sect. 3.7, random fixation of neutral substitution in a bacterial or viral genome is impossible due to large numbers of populations of bacteria and viruses. Therefore the observed rate of substitutions in RNA-viruses which is a million times as fast (Gojobori et al., 1990) may be explained by fixation of progressive (instead of neutral) substitutions, the latter occurring at the million times faster rate of v^+ in RNA-viruses, compared to (3.15.3). Hence, random fixation of substitutions in the range of normal polymorphism (Sect. 3.8) cannot explain the progressive evolution of a species.

However, the temporally uniform process of fixing random substitutions in the range of neutral polymorphism, which is independent of the numbers of populations, explains well enough the observed constancy of substitutions in the homologic genes of different eukaryotic species, i.e. the so-called "molecular clock" (Zuckerkandl and Pauling, 1965; Kimura, 1987; Ohta, 1987; Zuckerkandl, 1987). In many cases the time various contemporary species have taken to diverge from a common ancestor is known from paleodata. The observed differences in the nucleotide sequences of homologous sections of the genomes of two such species, divided by the time of their independent evolution, gives the doubled rate of molecular evolution of each species. Comparing several pairs of such species with differing times of divergence, one may find the average rate of molecular evolution during various time periods. These rates appear to be identical for every homologous section of the genome, and that effect is essentialy what the "molecular clock" is about.

The values v^+k and v^-k for bacteria present, respectively, the dimensionless probabilities of the positive and decay local mutations (including macromutations). Since $v^+k \sim (v^-k)^{3.6}$, the probability of a positive local mutation may treated as three to four given local decay mutations taking place simultaneously. As noted above, such mutations may lead to the generation of completely new sequences, formed of no more than 70 nucleotide pairs. Any macromutations are also possible with arbitrary transpositions of fragments of any length present in the genome. There is no mandatory duplication of the gene in which successive decay mutations take place; these are not manifested in the state of the individual due to the presence of the second copy of the normal (non-mutating) gene (Ohno, 1970). These three to four specific mutations in the genome increase the competitiveness of the individual, as compared to those having three to four arbitrary decay mutations in their genomes. The frequency of occurrence of individuals with such positive mutations increases against the background of the decay tail, see Fig. 3.1, and a secondary peak appears there.

The positive mutation does not, generally speaking, lead to a competitiveness higher than that of the normal genome (of the principal peak, see Fig. 3.1). Thus the secondary peak appears to be lower than the principal one of the species competitiveness. Step by step fixation of positive mutations in the secondary peak gradually shifts it outside the threshold of life capacity n_L, finally resulting in the formation of the normal genome of a new species. The old peak may meanwhile keep its initial position, if the new peak corresponds to the altered ecological niche. In that case sequential positive mutations only cover the part of the population occupying the secondary peak. That, however, does not change the estimates presented in (3.15.2) and (3.15.3), because they remain valid to the accuracy of two to three orders of magnitude, to which the number of individuals in a bacterial species N is known, as well as the lifespan for bacterial species.

The total number of bacterial species is of the order of 10^4 (Chislenko, 1981; Raven and Johnson, 1988). The bacterial genome consists of unique sequences and is about 10^6 bp in size. Genomes of the kin bacterial species differ by 10%, that is by 10^5 bp. The total number of unique sequences in all the bacteria in the biosphere is of the order of 10^{10} bp. The average lifespan of a bacterial species is 10^6 years. Hence we have for the rate of generation of progressive substitutions by bacteria $10^4(+)$ bp/year (that is one new species every ten years).

The total number of RNA viruses in the biosphere is of the order of 10^3 (Chislenko, 1981). The size of the viral genome is 10^5 bp (Lewin, 1983). Let us assume that the genomes of two virus species differ by 100%, that is by the same 10^5 bp. The total number of unique sequences in the genomes of all the RNA viruses in the biosphere is of the order of 10^8 bp. Assuming the lifespan of an RNA virus species to be 10^6 times less than that of a bacterial one (Holland et al., 1982; Gojobori et al., 1990) we find for the rate of generation of progressive substitutions by RNA viruses a value of $10^7(+)$ bp/year (a hundred species a year).

The number of eukaryotic species is of the order of 10^7, their overwhelming majority being insects (Raven and Johnson, 1988; Thomas, 1990). The average size of the eukaryotic genome is of the same order as the average insect genome, that is 10^8. Unique sequences comprise 1% of that total, that is amount to 10^6 bp (Lewin, 1983). Genomes of the two kin eukaryotic species differ by 1%, that is by 10^4 (by ten genes). The total size of the unique sequences in the genomes of all the eukaryotes in the biosphere is thus of the order of 10^{11} bp. The lifespan for eukaryotic species is 10^6 years. The rate at which the new progressive substitutions in eukaryotic genomes are acquired is, hence, of the order of 10^5 (+) bp/year (ten species a year), which is two orders of magnitude less than the rate of generation of progressive substitutions by the RNA viruses. And it is only 1% of these genes generated by viruses and bacteria which, upon entering the eukaryotic genomes via horizontal transfer, control their progressive evolution.

The evolution of each eukaryotic species within the 10^7 species existing in the biosphere is determined by one of the 10^9 genes generated by the RNA viruses and bacteria. It is assimilated by that species. Other genes either do not interact with individuals of that species, or effect some pathology, such as the AIDS virus, to give an example. On the average, each separate eukaryotic species assimilates one unique progressive sequence of about 10^3 bp long every 10–100 thousand years. The probability of simultaneous appearance of two progressive substitutions in a population of eukaryotes any population numbers is negligibly small. Therefore, sexual breeding is incapable of speeding up the evolution (Crow and Kimura, 1965).

The horizontal transfer of genes between different eukaryotic species is apparently not too large. Therefore the obtained estimate of the rate of evolution of eukaryotes based on the relative rate of evolution of the two kin species should be close to the absolute rate of evolution of each species. However, due to strong horizontal gene transfer between bacteria the given estimate of the rate of evolution of bacteria is undoubtedly underestimated. If the horizontal transfer of genes were extremely large, the relative rate of evolution of bacteria would tend to zero, despite the absolute rate for each separate species, which could then approach the rate of evolution of RNA viruses. Therefore the true absolute rate of evolution of bacteria is in between the observed relative rate of evolution of the two kin bacterial species and that of evolution of the RNA viruses, that is between $10^4(+)$ bp/year (that is one species in ten years) and $10^7(+)$ bp/year (that is 100 species a year).

The ratio of the residence time for viral (and retroviral) DNA in eukaryotic genomes to that in bacterial genomes should coincide with the inverse ratio of the absolute observed rates of evolution of eukaryotes to that of bacteria. On the other hand, that ratio should characterize the homology of genomes of contemporary eukaryotes and bacteria. The difference in the residence times for viral DNA in the genomes of eukaryotes and bacteria being large, that homology should be low. However, during exogenic, virus-controlled evolution, the younger eukaryotic species should feature higher homology with contemporary bacteria than the ancient species, "the live fossils". If the evolution were endogenic and independent for prokaryotes and eukaryotes, the homology of eukaryotes and bacteria should, inversely, increase for larger eukaryote ages.

As indicated above, the difference in the genomes of two kin multicellular species is of an order of 1 % (Raven and Johnson, 1988; Golenberg et al.,1990). Mostly that difference is related to normal polymorphism within each species (Sect. 3.8). The number of genes in the genome being of the order of 10^4 (Lewin, 1983) that means that less than 100 genes differ from each other in them. The lifespan of a species being of the order of 10^6, a new gene should appear in the genome within the time span in excess of 10 thousand years. Within the times of about several thousand years one may neglect the evolutionary processes. Within that approximation the normal genome may be regarded as a constant characteristic, and all the deviations from it as decay phenomena.

Note also that all the biological rules of an individual's structure and behavior are written into the normal genome. The necessarily present decay states in any population mean that, in contrast to physics, there are no rules without exclusions in biology (Dover, 1988).

3.17 The Rate of Evolution

New species originate in relatively small changes in the genome. That process (cladogenesis) is similar to that of formation of new branches in a tree or of new cells in a multicellular body. Assuming that each old species gives rise to two new ones, on average, and that the lifespan of each species is of the order of $T_s \sim 3 \times 10^6$ years (Simpson, 1944; Van Valen, 1973; MacFadden and Hubbert, 1988), we find that the time t needed to form all the presently existing species

$N \sim 10^7$ (Raven and Johnson, 1988; Thomas, 1990; May, 1990, 1992), is given by the equation

$$2^{t/T_s} = N \approx 10^7, \quad \text{that is} \quad t = T_s \frac{\ln N}{\ln^2} \approx 70 \times 10^6 \text{ years.}$$

Thus the whole complexity of species found today could have been formed within 70 million years, that is within a time of the order of a geological period. That is much shorter than the whole time of biological evolution ($T_e \sim 3 \times 10^9$ years) (Raven and Johnson, 1988). If the process of species formation were continuous during the whole of T_e, the number of species in the biosphere could have reached

$$2^{T_e/T_s} \approx 2^{1000} \approx 10^{300}.$$

It does not actually happen, however, since it is absolutely impossible to squeeze all those species into the Earth's biosphere.

Hence the existing number of species may be considered as the characteristic capacity of the biosphere, rather than the limit of the functionally sensible genetic variations. Therefore the presently observed number of species has apparently remained more or less constant over half a billion years (Grant, 1977; Raup and Sepkoski, 1982). According to paleodata the number of families in the biosphere has not changed by more than a factor of two (Raup and Sepkoski, 1982; Wilson, 1989). The change in the total number of species (which cannot be found from paleodata) has probably remained within a much smaller range. Now, the appearance of a new species is only possible when the old ones become extinct. Within the relatively constant environmental conditions supported by the biota there should be no spontaneous extinction of species. However, random generation of genes (such as in viruses, bacteria, etc.) should take place in the global biota, capable of destroying the normal (instead of only the decay) genome of certain species. The appearance of destroyer genes for certain normal genomes is equivalent to the transformation of an ecological niche into a condition unfit for the life of such species. The probability that the decay of a normal genome will compensate for the effect of destroyer genes is unimaginably small. Such a species should indeed become extinct. And only then can its place be occupied by the new species that has assimilated the progressive genes.

The rate of evolution should thus be controlled by the flow of destroyer genes. The observed constancy of the average lifespan for biospheric species, independent of their taxonomy and body size testifies to a universal character of that flow (Van Valen, 1973). The flow of progressive genes should be either larger or equal to the flow of destroyer genes. If it were smaller, all the species would alraedy have become extinct.

Along with exogenic destruction of the old normal genomes there may also be exogenic destruction of the old ecological niches. That should happen when new large taxa are formed (such as higher plants, insects, birds, mammals). In the course of these events certain species, having assimilated particular progressive gene fragments[2], acquire significant advantages in their competitive interaction with the old ones. Forcing out of large old taxa takes place, which is accompanied by massive extinction of the older species. Simultaneously the diversity of the new taxon increases (adaptive radiation takes place) (Raven and Johnson, 1988). The process of such radiation may occur due to assimilation of progressive genes, which do not significantly alter the structure of the species genome, while at the same time not weakening the advantages of the new taxon. If the formation of those new taxa results in significant changes in the structure of the communities, that is of species, through which the principal fluxes of matter and energy flow in the biosphere, such a restructuring of the biota may result in significant changes of the environment (see Sect. 5.6). The formation of new taxa and mass extinction of the old species has, on average taken place every 100 million years during the last half a billion years (Raup and Sepkoski, 1982; Raven and Johnson, 1988; Schneider, 1989b). In between those rare processes of the cardinal restructuring of the biota there apparently took place a smoother evolution, related to exogenic destruction of the genomes of older species.

The ordered state formed in either physics or chemistry may disintegrate into different channels. The probabilities of decay into each such channel are strictly determined by the ordered state itself. They may be measured for each such state and hence forecast in advance. Inversely, it is impossible to find from the decay state whether it stems from the disintegration of an ordered state (and what that state might have been) or remains within equilibrium interaction with other decay states.

The direction in which the level of order in living objects increases in the course of evolution could not have been programmed in the information contained in the preceding life forms of lower order, hence it is random and unpredictable (Erlich and Holm, 1963). If, on the other hand, decay of an already reached level of order takes place in the course of evolution (as is the case for parasites, for example), it occurs towards increasing the level of order in the community as a whole, and the course of that process is different from the one it had originally been formed by. The existing forms of life cannot intentionally and directionally select and support by selection properties that are not presently needed by individuals, but which might be of use in the future to some new species yet to evolve. Individuals cannot adjust to conditions yet non-existent, on which that individual has no information. In other words, biological selection cannot store bodily properties in advance, cannot choose the direction of selection, that is the present does not prescribe the future in biology.

All the features of life so far considered (such as sexual breeding, diploidy, etc.) could not have been designed to speed up the evolution or to choose its direction. On the contrary, all these features are aimed at increasing the rate of relaxation back to the normal state of the species, to block out the evolution,

---

[2] The treatment in this section does not depend on whether the destroyer or progressive gene fragments affecting the genome of the species are of exogenic or endogenic nature.

which makes possible disintegration of life, and to sustain the presently existing stationary state and environmental stability.

Biological selection provides for stabilization of the randomly achieved level of order and cannot affect the rate of evolution. That rate is determined by the characteristics of biological molecules, which do not in practice depend on the changes occurring in the environment. It may only vary randomly in a species with differing level of organization, and is inhibited in species of the "living fossils" type. Therefore, there is apparently no external moving force of evolution ("Red Queen Concept" (Van Valen, 1973, 1979; Hoffman, 1991)).

The ordered physical and chemical states occurring at a given flux of external energy cannot evolve towards higher organization when the flux and character of external energy does not change. Evolution towards higher organization of life is not related to the flux of energy that life uses, and in that sense it has nothing in common with physical self-organization, produced by the increased organization of external energy flux, the latter being the very external moving force for it (Anderson, 1983; Schuster, 1984; Kauffman, 1991). Random changes in fluxes of energy used by life do not alter the level of life organization on average. If certain species become extinct, they are never again resurrected, independent of possible changes in energy fluxes.

3.18 Is There Extraterrestrial Life in the Universe?

So far numerous attempts to find extraterrestrial life and intelligence have met with no success (Shklovsky, 1987; Kerr, 1992). The question arises, whether any proxy data might be available, based on the properties of life actually observed on Earth, which could testify either for or against the existence of extraterrestrial life. Among such properties of terrestrial life are the biological stability of populations of species and communities, discussed above, and the right-to-left asymmetry of macromolecules in the living cell (Gorshkov, 1982a).

The right-to-left asymmetry of the natural organic matter of biological origin, that is matter produced by living beings on Earth, is now disscussed.

Almost no complex multiatomic organic molecules possess a symmetry with respect to mirror reflection, so that after such an operation they cannot be returned into their initial state by any spatial rotations and transpositions of identical atomic nuclei. Thus a given molecule and the one produced by its mirror reflection differ from each other. They are called stereoisomers or enantiomers. A substance consisting of an unequal number of right- and left-hand molecules features some optical activity: it is capable of rotating the plane of polarization of light passing through it. (The mixture of stereoisomers containing an equal number of right- and left-hand molecules, called racemate, does not feature any optical activity). The biological enzymes which control the rate of every biochemical reaction (see Sect. 3.1) are also stereoisomers. Generally speaking, a left-hand enzyme may only affect the reaction between the organic molecules of a certain asymmetry sign, which may conditionally be called left-hand too. Now in case of a complete mirror reflection, that is of total substitution of all the left steroisomers participating in the reaction by their right-hand counterparts, the reaction will go on exactly as it did when only left-hand stereoisomers took part in it. That is the consequence of symmetry of the electromagnetic interactions with respect to mirror reflection.

It thus becomes clear that all the biological individuals and the organic substances serving as food to them, and hence the whole community as well, should be exclusively built of either left- or right-handed molecules: the presence of minor admixtures of the mirror-reflected molecules hampers biochemical reactions so that in the process of evolution these should have been selected out of the population via competitive interaction (Kisel, 1980, 1985; Gorshkov, 1982a). In the presence of excess oxygen, or during anaerobic breathing, the spatially superimposed right- and left-hand communities would have competitively interacted at the autotrophic level alone, competing for light and for the mirror symmetrical inorganic nutrient substances (CO_2, H_2O, NH_3, etc.) The right- and left-hand heterotrophs would occupy completely non-overlapping niches: the left-hand herbivores would not consume right-hand vegetation, and the left-hand carnivores would avoid right-hand prey. Since the formation areas for both the local community and the local ecosystem are comparatively small (Sects. 5.4 and 5.5), one could expect to find frequently alternating mutually mirror reflected communities.

Meanwhile the whole biosphere consists of left-hand organic stereoisomers (Lehninger, 1979). There are no indications of the existence of right-hand communities in the past, however far removed (Kisel, 1980, 1985). If life had initially developed with an equal number of the mutually mirror reflected communities, it becomes hardly likely that all the right-hand communities had been forced out of the whole of the biosphere by the left-hand ones. This becomes even less probable if life originated on the basis of its anaerobic feeding on organic matter of abiogenic nature. The organic molecules forming as a result of abiogenic photoreactions should have combined into a racemate. The spontaneously originating major statistical set of heterotrophs capable of replication should also have consisted of an equal number of the right- and left-hand individuals. Furthermore on the right- and left-hand communities should have developed completely independently of each other, without mutual competitive interaction for the food sources, incompatible, as it were, with each other. The random termination of all the right-hand local communities is as improbable as termination of life in general.

Life is based on the catalysis of biochemical reactions, on competitive interaction, and on stabilizing selection, which prevents disintegration of its organization. Thus there could have been no protoindividuals, their bodies built of an equal number of the left- and right- hand stereoisomers, and hence there could have been no spontaneous symmetry breaking (Nicolis, 1986) in such protoindividuals, leading to contemporary life forms. Quite the contrary, the body asymmetry in certain natural living beings, discussed in Sect. 3.8, may be treated as spontaneous symmetry breaking, originating in the process of evolution and adaptation to certain lifestyle. However, that body asymmetry appears without perturbation of the overall observed molecular asymmetry of life (Kasinov, 1968; Kisel, 1980, 1985), and does not have anything to do with the latter.

The differences between the properties of the left- and right-hand stereoisomers are only controlled by weak interactions, which produce infinitesimally small corrections (about 10^{-16}) to the respective electromagnetic values, thus resulting, for example, in the differences between the binding energies and the rates of chemical reactions for the respective molecules. Such differences lie far beyond the sensitivity of the biota and cannot be manifested within the ranges comparable to correlation radii of the natural local communities and to individual body sizes. For those weak interactions to result in vanishing of all the right-hand communities off the face of the Earth due to some random fluctuation, the correlation radii of such communities would have had to be enormous and comparable to sizes of the large ecosystems (that is to that of the whole hyperpopulation of the local communities) or to the size of the Earth itself. That contradicts the observed biological stability of life based on competitive interaction, see Sects. 3.1, 3.2, and 4.5. The left- and right-hand stereoisomers may function differently in the asymmetric abiotic environment. However, the observed relative degree of that asymmetry in the environment (such as, for example, the degree of circular polarization of solar radiation absorbed by plants) lies far beyond the sensitivity limit of competitive interaction of the biota, and cannot give any decisive advantage to either the right- or left-hand communities.

The biological stability described in Sects. 3.1 and 3.2 is an informational characteristic of life. It provides the conservation of any existing superorganization of life and contains the possibility of evolution towards higher organization. Biological stability is based on competitive interaction and is maintained by natural selection. Initially, however all the special features of biological stability of life should originate through random physical fluctuation in the prebiotic environment. Clearly, the non-informational chirally pure polymers capable of autocatalytic replication could be originated many times in the universe through a spontaneous breaking of mirror symmetry of the prebiotic environment (Morozov, 1978; Goldanskii and Kuz'min, 1989; Avetisov and Goldanskii, 1993). However, this physico-chemical ordered state is devoid of biological stability and cannot evolve towards higher organization, see Sects. 2.4, 2.5 and 3.2. The spontaneous breaking of mirror symmetry could originate and disintegrate randomly and independently in numerous local prebiotic environments due to fluctuation of the external flux of organized energy in the Earth and other part of the universe. The space and time averaged global prebiotic environment should be racemic, i.e. mirror symmetrical.

The absence of the right-hand community in the biosphere is evidence for the fact that the biologically stable informational content in chirally pure non-informational polymers could appear randomly only with extremely low probability (Eigen, 1971; Nicolis and Prigogine, 1977; Orgel, 1992).

To estimate the probability of the appearance of a similar system in the universe, certain assumptions on its molecular structure have to be made. It is natural to assume that the respective molecular structure could not be simpler than the proteins and genes already existing. To save oneself the trouble of accounting for the degree of degeneration of the genetic code, the estimate can be made for the simplest protein. The simplest proteins consist of a hundred amino acids (Ayala and Kiger, 1984). The number of possible combinations in a sequence of a hundred amino acids is $20^{100} = 10^{130}$: each of the twenty amino acids used by life may, with equal probability, occupy a position in each site of the protein chain (Eigen, 1971). The number thus obtained exceeds the overall number of possible interactions of all the atoms in the universe (about 10^{77} atoms) with an object of molecular size within the characteristic lifetime of atomic processes (about 10^{-17} s) during the whole lifespan of the Universe (about 10^{17} s), that number not exceeding 10^{110} (Allen, 1955). Thus spontaneous formation of an informational molecular structure capable of life could not have happened more than once in the whole universe. Moreover, if one imagines the process of multiple formation of universes similar to ours (with the same values of the basic physical constants, which make possible the formation of chemical elements, of stars, similar to our Sun, and of planets similar to Earth (Rosental, 1980; Shklowsky, 1987)), life could only have originated in very few such universes.

3.19 Biological Stability and Neo-Darwinism

The concept of biotic stability of the environment seems to contradict the principal biological paradigm, that has dominated science during the last hundred years, and which is now called neo-Darwinism (Dobzhansky, 1951; Mayr, 1963; Erlich and Raven, 1969; Stebbins, 1971, 1974). Following that paradigm, the biotic species are capable of adapting to practically any changes in the environment. Environmental changes due to abiotic factors also take place, but the rate of these changes is much less than the rate of biological adaptation. (Possibly, such a ratio has been violated during the industrial era for certain species.) Adaptation of the biota means that it is capable of changing under external environmental forcing. In its turn the biota alters the environment in the process of its functioning. However such a biotic effect upon the environment is random in nature and does not compensate for the abiotic changes.

Therefore, any environmental conditions are optimal for the biota adapted to them. There are no preferable optimal environmental conditions. The biotic regulation of such nonexistent preferable conditions is, naturally, impossible. A continuous adaptation of the living species to environmental conditions changing over the geological eras controls the observed evolution of the biota. The adaptation program for each species is optimized in the process of evolution. Adaptation and evolution are the two principal characteristics of life in general. In the process of evolution only the individuals more effectively adapted to environmental conditions survive and produce the more numerous progeny. All the useful hereditary information involves adapting to the existing environmental conditions.

The basis for the dominating paradigm is the observed genetic polymorphism, i.e., genetic nonidentity of the individuals in any given population, and the mutability, i.e., the appearance of new genetic options, not found in parental lines. It is assumed that parallel to detrimental mutations, which reduce the adaptive capacities of an individual, new useful mutations also occur, which increase the degree of their bearer's adaptation to practically any prescribed environment. The maximum adaptation is determined by the highest frequency of alleles (versions) found for each gene under various conditions. As a result most alleles feature some adaptive value in some environment. In other words, all the observed polymorphism is, basically, adaptive. The decay polymorphism is very small, particularly in perturbed environmental conditions.

In reality most decay traits (decay genotypes) are absent under normal conditions and consequently have a zero fitness. The new nonadaptive decay traits (new decay genotypes) inevitably arise in perturbed or highly variable conditions. Therefore these traits have, by definition, a finite nonvanishing fitness. Such events should traditionally (but erroneously) be considered as adaptations to perturbed conditions.

The total set of gene alleles composes the gene pool of the population. The genetically different individuals in the population carry unique adaptive capacities which may meet all the possible variations in the environment. The gene pool is continuously enriched by new alleles due to individual mutations. Mutations neutral under the presently existing conditions may appear useful under some new, formerly nonexistent conditions. The intraspecific mutational process (the sequence of single mutations) controls the evolution of separate species.

In such a traditional picture, the biological species cannot contain any information on sustaining the preferable optimal environmental conditions. The notion of a species is not genetically described or fixed. The genetic information contained in the population differs from environment to environment, i.e., the combination of occurrence frequencies for various genes changes. Following a change in the environment, such information would continuously shift from its initial level, according to the needed adaptation to new life conditions. Each individual is then adaptationally unique. Selection among the relatives displaying the elements of altruism with respect to their closest kin works to propagate their adaptive program. Because of the extremely high polymorphism, a return to the initial state of the genetic information in a population is improbable, even if the initial environmental conditions are repeated. This feature is indeed observed in the course of evolutional transfer from one species to another, close species (the Dollo principle of evolution irreversibility). However it contradicts the observed discreteness of contemporary species, the stability of morphological characteristics found in fossil species, and the lack of transitional fossil forms between these species.

The traditional concept is also in contradiction to the observed stability of the environment, which has remained fit for life during the last several billion years (see Sect. 2.7 and Chap. 4).

To accept the concept of biological stability, and of the environment optimal for life, it is necessary to reject the concept of random genetic local adaptation, which is the basis of neo-Darwinism, that is explain all the available empirical data which would make possible an unequivocal conclusion in favor of one of these two alternatives. Random local genetic adaptation should then be understood as the appearance of new functionally sensible adaptive changes in the genetic information in the population, not coded into the old genome, which appear when individuals enter new conditions. Such changes should appear due to the observed single (point and macro-) mutations and be manifested during time periods shorter than a thousand years, that is much less than the lifespan of a species according to paleodata, which is of the order of 3×10^6 years, see Sect. 3.17.

Following the analogy with the second law of thermodynamics a corresponding biological principle could be formulated stating that no new functionally and ecologically sensible genetic information can be created via sequential random decay single mutations in any existing species.

Neo-Darwinism has been repeatedly criticized from different sides (Ho and Saunders, 1984; Lima-de-Faria, 1988; Wesson, 1991), but also defended (Maynard Smith, 1991). It is demonstrated in the present chapter that all the available empirical data may be explained without introducing the concept of random local genetic adaptation. Moreover, all the contradictions related to use of that concept fall away. The necessity to involve the concept of Non-Darwinian evolution also becomes redundant (King and Jukes, 1969; Kauffman, 1991; Wesson, 1991). The theory of neutral mutations and of the molecular clock is saved (Kimura, 1983, 1987). However, the neutral theory appears to be irrelevant to the origin of species. The evolutionary theory of the origin of species on the basis of natural selection is preserved in practically the same form as had been suggested by Darwin. However, the priority of evolution is significantly decreased, as compared to priority of stabilization.

4. Stability of the Biosphere's Organization

4.1 Limitations to Expansion and Evolution of Species

As demonstrated in the preceding chapter, stable life is only possible when individuals compete with each other within the population. Formation of populations and competitive interaction between the individuals within them is a genetically fixed trait of all living beings. However, when external fluxes of energy and nutrients, fit for inclusion into the feeding cycle, are available and are not used by existing life, noncompetitive decay individuals, expelled from the population, may start using them, thus decreasing the average level of organization of life. To prevent such a development, competitive normal individuals should expand, that is claim all the external fluxes of energy and nutrients regenerating their own copies. Noncompetitive individuals are then expelled from the available niches (that refers to both the individuals of the given species and also other species which use the same fluxes of energy and nutrients, i.e. occupy the same ecological niches).

Expansion may occur both within the boundaries of a given territory, when the population density of a competitive species continuously builds up to reach its possible limit, and through expanding into the areas as yet unoccupied by that population. Evolutionary changes brought about by an increase in competitiveness also become fixed in the genotype in the course of expansion. During expansion the competitive interaction weakens, or even ceases. This implies that the competition capacity might remain unchanged only when expansion took significantly less time than such an acquired trait would take to deteriorate in the absence of competitive interaction. Expansion is a most general characteristic of life, observed in every species; it even covers such advanced forms of claiming new territories as space ventures by man.

Were the fluxes of free energy limitlessly available to life (i.e. in conditions of energy abundance), expansion would have been infinite; competitive interaction would then have been totally absent, so that stabilization and, consequently, life itself would have become impossible. Therefore, life may only exist on condition that fluxes of free energy are limited, i.e., there should exist some restriction of available energy (lack of energy abundance).

Separate biological species may exist stably outside their natural communities for lifespans of several thousand years, when the effect of evolutionary processes is not yet noticeable, provided the flux of external energy is limited. A population of a species with competitive interaction "on", may support stable numbers if the stationarity of a local environment is artificially supported, that is, if the necessary nutrients are introduced into that environment and the wastes are evacuated. Such is the existence of certain urbanized species (cockroaches, sparrows, rats, etc.) and of all domestic animals and plants.

However, separate biological species, isolated from their communities, appear to be unstable within lifespans of several millions years, when evolution takes its full force. Evolutionary processes may only work to increase the competitiveness of individuals. The increase in such competitiveness is not, generally speaking, associated with higher adaptation to the environment or with higher stability of the population.

For example, evolution in the direction of abnormally big antlers in certain extinct animals (McFarland, 1985), the appearance of exceptionally bright and excessive feathering in certain bird species (Zahavi, 1975; Manning, 1979; McFarland, 1985; Diamond, 1991), higher level of aggression, accompanied by lower vitality (Tinbergen, 1968; Lorenz, 1981) do not result in better adaptation to environment and may destroy the organization of life. The principal direction in which competitive capacities grow is dictated by larger correlation radii of individuals, that is by larger body size of individuals and by broader spatial sizes of various social structures. Evolution in that direction should have resulted in an unlimited growth of both the body size and dimensions of social structures, which would then expel all the other species from the environment.

Expansion of large individuals should have occurred both extensively, resulting in a general proliferation of large individuals, and intensively, resulting in a local expulsion of smaller size individuals from the environment, so that the larger size individuals would claim all the fluxes of nutrients available. Thus, finally, one or several groups of the most competitive species of the largest body size or social structures should have been singled out eventually resulting in a global correlation of the whole of biota (including both the flora and fauna), consequently stopping competitive interaction, selection, and life in general.

Tracing from paleontological data the evolutionary changes in certain animal species, we may satisfy ourselves that the evolution towards larger body sizes indeed takes place (Cope's rule (Stanley, 1973)). The same data show that expansion of large bodied individuals have indeed taken place, and large animals proliferated throughout the whole of the biosphere and could be encountered everywhere. However, paleodata fail to provide any conclusions on the population density of such large individuals, that is on the share of consumed nutrients per large individual. That conclusion may only be drawn by studying the presently existing biospheric communities. Such an analysis shows that no natural communities (that is communities not perturbed by anthropogenic impact) feature internal expansion of the larger individuals. Instead an opposite development is observed: with the body size of the species increasing the share of nutrients it consumes (the larger individuals consume in general) from the overall flux of nutrients decreases. The appearance of large animals in natural communities practically does not change the general structure of a community, which corresponds to fine tuning of that community's functioning.

On the one hand, proliferation of large individuals throughout all the communities of the biosphere means that communities including those individuals are more stable, hence more competitive, than communities devoid of large individuals. On the other hand, limitation of the number of such large individuals to a minimum in every observable community means that those communities in which the large individuals start to dominate in the share of their consumption of nutrients lose their stability and competitive capacities.

The only possible explanation for such a limitation of the role of large animals in the communities might be the necessity to close the cycle of matter, and support the stability of the environment, that is a close equality between the fluxes of organic synthesis and destruction under a compensating reaction of the biota to external perturbation. With the individual size (the correlation radius of individuals) growing, the number of noncorrelated functioning individuals falls off. Thus the law of large numbers is violated, Eq. (2.3.4), and large random fluctuations ensue in both synthesis and destruction, rendering impossible a close enough balance between the respective fluxes of matter. Under the conditions of limited availability of chemical components to living individuals (i.e., of nutrients), the communities disrupting the closed character of matter cycling adversely perturb the environment, which results in further perturbation of both the synthesis and destruction of the organic matter. As a result such communities lose their competitive capacity and are expelled by other communities which still keep the matter cycles closed, i.e., by such communities which predominantly consist of a large number of small individuals, among which the law of large numbers is still in force. That phenomenon is treated quantitatively in Sects. 5.5 and 5.6. It is particularly this force which prevents the evolution of the biosphere toward larger individual body sizes and social structures.

Were the fluxes of free energy or stores of nutrient unlimited, nothing would stop the evolution toward a global correlation ensuring quick decay of life in general. Thus stable life is only possible if, beside a limitation upon the flux of external energy (lack of energy abundance), the store of nutrients is limited as well, and there is no incessant flux of these nutrients from the outside, so that material resources remain short (lack of material abundance).

4.2 Closed Matter Cycles in the Biosphere

The following estimates demonstrate the necessarily closed character of matter cycles during both the biological synthesis and destruction of organic matter. The present day annual production of the whole biosphere in units of mass of organic carbon is estimated as 100 Gt C/year. Carbon amounts to only about one tenth of the overall live organic mass (Odum, 1983; Kendeigh, 1974). Thus the annual production of live organic matter may be estimated at 10^3 Gt/year. During the whole timespan of life on Earth, that is over 3×10^9 years that production should have reached 4×10^{12} Gt, that figure practically coinciding with the mass of the planet, equal to 6×10^{12} Gt (Allen, 1955). However the sphere available to life is only the biosphere, including the atmosphere, the ocean, and the thin soil layer on land, its overall mass being of the order of the total mass of oceanic water, which is 1.4×10^{9} Gt (Watts, 1982). The production of biota over its lifespan exceeds this latter mass by a factor of many thousands.

Hence, atoms of substance must have entered the synthesized organic matter many thousands of times, and for that process to be possible all the synthesized organic matter must have been decomposed into its inorganic components again and again. It also follows from that estimate that at least three decimal digits in the numerical expressions for the global fluxes of synthesis and destruction should coincide with each other. If only the orders of magnitude of these fluxes of synthesis and destruction were to coincide (as is the case in the contemporary land biota, perturbed by man), all the mass of the planet Earth would have quickly turned into pure organic matter if the synthesis were to dominate, and inversely, if destruction were to dominate, all the organic matter, and hence, all the biota would have ceased to exist long ago.

Since death is inevitable for every living individual, the organic matter contained in all the dead bodies should necessarily be destroyed by other living individuals. The competitive interaction between individuals results in developing specialization and in separating the individuals into various species following their different feeding habits. Some species synthesize organic matter, directly consuming the solar energy, others destroy that organic matter, using the energy contained in it. As a result correlated communities of different species must necessarily be organized to support life.

The closed character of the biochemical cycles of matter results in life being possible on the basis of organic substances, their energy available for use when these substances are destroyed. These limitations, following from the necessity to keep the cycles of matter closed, and imposed upon the Earth's biota, form the basis of ecology as a science. Meanwhile the observed distributions of living individuals and the abundance of species, which are sometimes considered to be the main study subject of ecology (Begon et al., 1986), only follow from such limitations. The principal task of ecology should thus be that of finding the causes of stable existence of life in the environment.

Lack of material abundance in the environment, as one of the necessary conditions of stable life, boils down to limitations imposed upon the external flux of nutrients entering the biosphere, and upon the stores of those nutrients within the biosphere.

The biological fluxes of either synthesis or destruction of organic matter should remain much larger than the external flux of nutrients entering the biosphere. For example, were that external flux to satisfy half the biological needs (provided a simultaneous evacuating flux of waste products were to exist so that the environment would remain stationary) no support of stable closed matter cycles would be possible. In that case half the biota would exist due to external fluxes, and the other half would strive to close the cycles of matter. Such a closure needs energy, and an active biota which would provide it. Thus the biota functioning through closing the cycle of matter would inevitably lose its competitive capacity, as compared to its other part, equal in size but functioning in the flux of external energy. That would result in the second part of the biota ceasing to function and to exist.

The remaining biota would reduce the biological fluxes of synthesis and destruction down to half their preceding levels, and would completely rely on the external fluxes of nutrients for feeding, without bothering to close the cycles of matter or to stabilize the environment. Such a biota could exist in the form of one or several species, not organizing into any ecological communities. Even with the external flux of nutrients remaining limited, that is with competitive interaction switched on (the latter preventing decay of populations) an evolutionary collapse to global correlation of the biota would inevitably take place in such a biota, within a time period of about one million years (that is the characteristic time of the formation of species), after which such a biota would cease to exist.

Besides, an environment not regulated by the biota would continuously change, deviating more and more from the state optimal for life. A random coincidence of the fluxes of nutrients and of evacuated wastes, which keeps the state of the environment stationary, cannot be stable. A random perturbation of such an equilibrium could bring about a destruction of the environment and extinction of the biota in significantly shorter time periods. Thus the biological flux of synthesis and destruction of the biota should exceed the external fluxes of synthesis and destruction to such an extent that the biota, functioning on the basis of communities and closed cycles of matter be, first, capable of compensating any significant fluctuations in the environment, and, second, appear much more competitive then the biota existing due to external fluxes of those nutrients. It is only in the latter case that such a biota may be expelled from the biosphere. It is particularly this situation that has so far been found in nature (see Fig. 1.3 and Sect. 1.7).

Now consider the problem of the amount of nutrients stored in the environment. The quantitative limitation on the amount of nutrients supporting the stable state of life is related to the rate of evolution and of progress. When absolutely no stores of nutrients are available outside the bodies of the living individuals, stable life, independent of the rate of evolution, is only possible if matter cycles are completely closed. Any community violating that closure of matter cycles would then immediately disintegrate and lose its competitive capacity.

Without external fluxes of nutrients, material abundance would correspond to such a situation, where the store of nutrients in the environment is much larger than their expenditure (or production) during the time of evolutionary change (or progress), or, in other words, when the time of evolution, T, is much less than the time of biological cycling of nutrients, τ. In a realistic situation, when the store of nutrients is limited as well as their fluxes through the environment, a stable life requires that the evolution be prohibited to a high degree, and the time T of evolutionary changes in the structure of communities remain much less than the time τ of any noticeable change of the store of nutrients in the environment: $T \gg \tau$, such that it would result in a loss of competitive capacity of the communities. The communities violating the closure of matter cycles would then be expelled from the population. In the opposite case, when $T \ll \tau$, such communities would spread throughout the whole population, expelling the communities which support the closure of matter cycle.

By definition, the environment includes stores of both organic and inorganic matter, which are involved in biochemical cycling. To maintain the fluxes of synthesis and destruction equal to each other in the biologically active chemical components (the nutrients), the stores of these components in both their organic and inorganic forms should not only be limited, but should also coincide in their order of magnitude. Otherwise either the synthesizing individuals (if inorganic matter is in excess) or the destroyers of the organic matter (when the organic matter is overabundant) would find themselves in conditions of relative material abundance, and the correlation between the synthesis and the destruction would inevitably be violated. As for the present-day environment (weakly perturbed by man) the stores of nutrients in their organic and inorganic forms are indeed of the same order of magnitude (Gorshkov, 1985a, 1986a; Gorshkov and Kondratiev, 1990). The time τ cannot exceed the time for biological cycling of nutrients stored in the environment, i.e., about 10 years (Gorshkov, 1987a). The time T is determined by the time of change of the community composition in species, which is of the order of 10^6 years (Simpson, 1944). Thus the condition $T \gg \tau$ is met in the non-perturbed natural biota by a factor of five to six orders of magnitude, and the appearance of communities destroying the closure of matter cycles is totally excluded.

Were the sedimented organic matter biologically active, the time for its biologic cycling would be four orders of magnitude longer than the time of cycling of environmental nutrients, i.e., would be of the order of 10^5 years. However, that time period would still be an order of magnitude shorter than the time of change of species, $T \sim 10^6$ years. Thus even if the sedimented buried organic matters were included into the biological cycle, conditions of abundance would not ensue over the time periods typical for the rate of biological evolution. Thus separate communities which violated the untouchable character of the buried organic matter and temporarily entered the realm of material abundance, thus destroying the environment, did not have time enough to propagate throughout the whole of the biosphere. They eventually lost their competitive capacity, and were ousted by communities sustaining the closed character of matter cycles.

The external flux of nutrients entering the biosphere is determined by the structure of the Earth's core and that of cosmic space. The Earth's biota is incapable of changing that flux. The necessary condition of life stabilization is achieved by the biota, which uses solar energy to develop powerful fluxes of synthesis and destruction of organic matter, these fluxes significantly exceeding the scale of external fluxes so that the necessary level of production is prescribed by the existing scale of external fluxes. The environmental stores of nutrients, entrained into biochemical cycles, should be sustained at a level significantly less than the biological production over the characteristic time of evolution. Despite the possibility of using various emzymatic means to increase the stability of the DNA molecule during information read-off from it and its replication, e.g. like proofreading and mismatch repair (see Sect. 3.4), evolution may only be prohibited to a certain limit, characterized by the observed time of evolution. That time is determined by the quantum characteristics of the molecules used in life processes, which cannot be changed by the biota either. Thus both the biotic production and the time evolution are determined by external conditions, which cannot be affected by the biota. Hence, only the stores of nutrients and their concentrations in the environment may be prescribed by Earth's biota and supported by it at a certain level. That is only possible if the Le Chatelier principle operates in the biota with respect to all the external perturbations (Sects. 1.4 and 2.6).

Thus no stable communities functioning in conditions of material abundance can exist in nature. However, locally, situations may quite often be encountered in nature, for example, immediately after some natural catastrophes, such as a volcanic eruption, glaciation, etc., where the biota has not yet had enough time to accumulate nutrients in the amount sufficient for building up the biomass of individuals capable of claiming all the available sources of energy. The communities of such a biota should be organized following the strictly closed cycles of the limiting nutrients, on the basis of strict correlation between the synthesizers and the destroyers of the organic matter. The cycling time, τ, of nutrients in such communities may be reduced to a few days (instead of the 10 years, typical for the biosphere as a whole). The drive for expansion in such a community should be about its typical spatial stratification. It should possibly stratify in a thin layer, providing for absorption of all the solar energy incident upon that community, and across a maximum possible surface, so that more such energy be intercepted. Such communities are indeed known: these are epilithic lichen, appearing at bare rock surface and organized as symbiotic individual algae and fungi (Farrar, 1976; see also Morneau and Payette, 1989; Gorshkov and Gorshkov, 1992), and Fig. 4.1.

To close this section, we consider a speculative way to stabilize complex systems of macroscopic processes without competitive interaction. That technique is based on centralized control, including a program of regeneration, that is of reproducing those parts of the system which have suffered decay. Destruction of the control organs themselves, which would render the whole system inoperative, may be practically completely excluded via multiple back-up of those organs. Such a totalitarian, unitary system would need no replication, would be free of the notion of competition, and would be capable of existing using even quite a small part of the available store of nutrients and external flux of energy. It would be capable of controlling its whole environment, compensating all the adverse perturbations and fluctuations via the Le Chatelier principle programmed into it, on condition that all the fluxes of information in that system reach some sufficiently high level. Such a system would lack the expansion drive. It could exist for an unlimited length of time in conditions of energy and material abundance outside any population as a single individual. ("The Black Cloud" by Fred Hoyle, and "The Ocean" in Stanislav Lem's "Solaris" are fictitious examples of such systems).

However, such a system would be foreign to progress, because, due to lack of competitive interaction, it would miss any preferable direction of change. Every possible change in the state of such a system would be equally probable. Since the number of decay states considerably exceeds the number of states corresponding to either an unchanged or increased degree of organization, change of that system would result in degradation, accompanied by loss of its ordered character. The stability of such a system may only be attained in its conservative state. Due to its high level of organization such a system could not have arisen spontaneously. It could only evolve via evolution based on competitive interaction.

All individuals include elements of regeneration. In the course of biological selection the stability of DNA molecules may be increased via the operating program of repair, that is restoration of the destroyed sections of the DNA molecule. Multiple back-up of the same genes via high polyploidization of the chromosomes and gene duplication within each chromosome makes it possible, in principle, to produce individuals with absolutely stable heredity, immune to decay. The program of regeneration of every biochemical perturbation arising in the course of life of an individual, together with genome polyploidization, makes it possible, in principle, to achieve an unlimited lifespan. However, either limitation or total liquidation of the decay DNA mutations also result in either decrease or complete stoppage of the progressive, non-decay mutations, because the ratio of the former to the latter, which is of the order of 10^{25}, as demonstrated in Sect. 3.15, may not depend on the stability with respect to decay mutations. Thus the transition to such a conditionally immortal, centrally controlled individual, existing outside any population, deprives such an individual of the possibility of further development, thus rendering it competitively inefficient, in contrast to the set of still evolving and competitively interacting, independent individuals.

As a result nature knows no immortal individuals, and no species exist in a state of correlated interaction among all the individuals of that species.

4.3 Biological Cycles

We now introduce quantitative characteristics of closed and non-closed matter cycles. The biologically active chemical elements are absorbed with certain ratios during the synthesis of organic matter. Thus knowing the masses and fluxes of certain nutrients other masses of nutrients may be retrieved from those ratios. In what is to follow we write all the quantitative ratios for carbon. We denote the respective masses of carbon stored per unit surface area in the biologically active reservoirs i ($i = a$ – atmosphere, $i = s$ – ocean, $i = l$ – land) in the organic and inorganic forms as M_i^+ and M_i^-; the fluxes of carbon during synthesis (production) and destruction of the organic matters in the ith reservoir will then be P_i^+ and P_i^-; net fluxes of the organic matter evacuated from the reservoir i as F_i^+, and that of inorganic matter imported into the reservoir i as F_i^-. Note that all the net fluxes

$F_i^{\pm}$ are equal to differences between the overall input $(F_{in}^{\pm})$ and output $(F_{out}^{\pm})$ fluxes. The law of matter conservation for any spatial domain is expressed by the equation:

$$\dot{M}^+ = P^+ - P^- - F^+; \qquad \dot{M}^- = P^- - P^+ + F^-, \tag{4.3.1}$$

where $\dot{M}^+$ and $\dot{M}^-$ denote the rates of change in the mass of organic and inorganic carbon, respectively, and the indices i are omitted from all the values entering that equation. The masses M^+ and M^- characterize the state of the environment. The equalities $\dot{M}^+ = \dot{M}^- = 0$ mean that the environment remains unchanged.

The degree of closure of the matter cycle is determined by the level to which the fluxes of synthesis P^+ and destruction P^- coincide with each other. The relative degree of closure of such cycles may be conveniently described quantitatively by their breach:

$$\kappa \equiv \frac{P^+ - P^-}{P^+}. \tag{4.3.2}$$

The relative fluxes F (or F_{in}) and P^+ describe how open the reservoir ν is with respect to external forcing. The ratios ν and ν_{in}:

$$\nu^{\pm} \equiv \frac{F^{\pm}}{P^+}; \qquad \nu_{in}^{\pm} \equiv \frac{F_{in}^{\pm}}{P^+} \tag{4.3.3}$$

may be called the net (ν) and the gross (ν_{in}) opennesses. When $\nu \ll 1$ and $\nu_{in} \gg 1$, external fluxes remain small with respect to synthesis P^+. The reservoir may be considered closed then and biological processes play a decisive role in it then. When $\nu \ll 1$ and $\nu_{in} > 1$, external fluxes are of the same order as, or are larger than, those of synthesis, but are carried through the reservoir without residing in it. The biological processes in a reservoir would still be decisive in such a reservoir. When $\nu \gg 1$ and $\nu_{in} \gg 1$, the reservoir is completely open, and the biological processes are insignificant in it. Since ν is small for the biosphere of the planet Earth as a whole, it presents a closed reservoir.

The times T^+ and T^-:

$$T^{\pm} = \frac{M^{\pm}}{|\dot{M}^{\pm}|} = \frac{\tau^{\pm}}{|\kappa - \nu^{\pm}|}, \qquad \tau^{\pm} \equiv \frac{M^{\pm}}{P^+} \tag{4.3.4}$$

are the times of complete extinction (if $\dot{M} < 0$) or of doubling (if $\dot{M} > 0$) of the stores of nutrients in a reservoir, i.e. of a complete restructuring of the environment, and $\tau^{\pm}$ are the times of biogenic cycling or residence times.

In a non-stationary case, when $|\kappa| \gg \nu$ we find from (4.3.1)–(4.3.4) that $T = \tau/|\kappa|$. In other words, if $|\kappa| \sim 1$, the reservoirs are destroyed in the time period of about τ years, and when $|\kappa| \sim 10^{-1}$, in about 10τ years, while $|\kappa| \sim 10^2$ yields the same time about 100τ years, etc. If the state is stationary $(\dot{M} = 0)$ we find from (4.3.1)–(4.3.4) that:

$$\kappa = \kappa_0 = \nu^- = \nu^+, \qquad (F^+ = F^-). \tag{4.3.5}$$

For the Earth as a planet, summing up over all the reservoirs the value of F^+ in (4.3.1) yields the organic carbon buried in sedimentary rocks, and F^- that of the difference between the emissions and sediments of inorganic carbon. According to paleodata, the observed ratios $F^{\pm}/P^{+}$ are close to 10^{-4}. The time of biogenic cycling $\tau^{\pm} = M^{\pm}/P^{+}$ is within 10–30 years (Gorshkov, 1987a). The time of geological cycling $M^{\pm}/F^{\pm}$ is about 10^{5} years (Budyko et al., 1987). The amount of organic carbon buried in sedimentary rocks is approximately four orders of magnitude larger that the amount of both the organic and inorganic carbon in the biologically active reservoirs. Thus, independent of the possible changes of both M^{+} and M^{-} by a factor of several units, one may state that the average fluxes F^{+} and F^{-} coincide with each other to the relative accuracy of about 10^{4} (see Eq. (4.3.5)).

Thus, for Earth as a whole, Eqs. (4.3.5) hold, and the value of stationary breach is positive, being of the order of 10^{-4}, supported by the biota at the relative accuracy of 10^{-4} too, see Fig. 1.1:

$$\nu^{+} = \nu^{-} = \kappa_0 \approx +2 \times 10^{-4}, \qquad \frac{|\nu^{+} - \nu^{-}|}{\nu^{+}} \sim 10^{-4}. \qquad (4.3.6)$$

The conditions in (4.3.6) mean that the biota is capable of supporting or holding the breach at a very low positive level, which provides for the burial of all the volcanic emissions in sediments, and for the strictly stationary concentrations of all the biologically active chemical substances in the environment.

The value of average perturbation of the environment F^{-} is defined by the structure of Earth's depths and cannot be regulated by the biota. The low value of $\nu^{-} = F^{-}/P^{+}$ is determined by the necessary value of P^{+} developed by the biota for the purpose of quick compensation of all the arising sharp fluctuations against the average perturbation of the environment. A breach of $\kappa_0 = \nu^{-}$, that is the equality of fluxes of synthesis and destruction to the accuracy of four decimal positions, is needed to keep the environment stationary in the absence of sharp fluctuations. Finally, the low relative difference between ν^{+} and ν^{-} points to a high level of average stationarity of the environment.

Thus, during long time periods of the order of several hundred million years the global biota has been, on average, controlling up to eight decimal positions in the values of production and destruction of organic matter. The coincidence of P^{+} and P^{-}, to the relative accuracy of the average breach, results from low random fluctuations of the values P^{+} and P^{-}. That result follows from a certain structure of communities, as discussed in Sects. 5.4–6. The value of breach may only be kept at the necessary level, Eq. (4.3.6), via the action of the Le Chatelier principle which is directed to compensate for any external perturbations of the environment. Thus the fact that fossil sources satisfy relations (4.3.6) (see Ronov, 1976; Budyko et al., 1987) serves as proof of the action of the Le Chatelier principle in the global biota throughout all of the Phanerozoi, because a random coincidence of ν^{+} and ν^{-} to the accuracy of the four digits is improbable.

When treating the land, l, and ocean, s, separately, one should account for the transport of organic carbon by the rivers. In a stationary state that process should work to increase the level of positive breach on land, κ_l, and should lead to negative breach κ_s in the ocean. Equations (4.3.5) and (4.3.6) may then be presented in the form:

$$\kappa_l \alpha_l + \kappa_s \alpha_s = \kappa_0 \ll \kappa_l \quad \text{or} \quad \kappa_l \alpha_l \approx -\kappa_s \alpha_s$$

$$\kappa_i \equiv \frac{P_i^+ - P_i^-}{P_i^+}, \qquad \alpha_i \equiv \frac{P_i^+}{P^+}, \qquad \alpha_s + \alpha_l = 1. \tag{4.3.7}$$

The difference $P_l^+ - P_l^- = F_{ls}^+$ which is equal to the run-off of organic carbon from the land, is compensated in the ocean $F_{ls}^+ = -(P_s^+ - P_s^-)$ so that as a result a stationary state of the environment is sustained in both reservoirs. According to modern estimates, the organic run-off is about 0.7% of the land production, $\nu_l = F_{ls}^+/P_l^+ \approx 0.007$ (Watts, 1982; Schlesinger, 1990), which is 30 times as high as the estimated global average breach, Eq. (4.3.6). That effect is largely a result of anthropogenic eutrophication of rivers, along which most of the global human population resides. Thus the given value is only the ceiling of the stationary breach of land. The lowest estimate of that value may be obtained from the annual rate of carbon storage in the soils of the formerly glaciated ecosystems. That value reaches 0.07% of land production (Schlesinger, 1990), thus approaching the estimated value of κ_0, Eq. (4.3.6). It may also be concluded from those data that the relative fluctuations of the annual average values of κ_0 do not exceed that of κ_0, Eq. (4.3.6).

4.4 The Le Chatelier Principle in Natural Biota

We shall traditionally call the chemical element X either organic or inorganic nutrient, according to whether it enters an organic or an inorganic substance (e.g., the organic carbon enters the organic molecules within a living cell). We denote the fluxes of synthesis (the net primary productivity) and of destructivity of the organic nutrient X as P_X^+ and P_X^-, respectively. The dimension of these values is kg X m^{-2} year^{-1}. We denote the environmental density of mass of organic and inorganic nutrient X per unit land surface as M_X^+ and M_X^-, respectively (their dimension is then kg X m^{-2}).

The Le Chatelier principle in natural biota, which keeps the environment in homeostasis, means that any change ΔM_X^- in the environment will be accompanied by the appearance of a breach in matter cycles, that is of the difference $(P_X^+ - P_X^-)$ directed to compensate for that change. The correlation between any two variables of differing dimensions may not be provided via any fundamental physical or chemical constant, a transitional dimensionality (see Sect. 2.6). Due to the extreme complexity of the interaction between the individuals in a natural community, the biota "forgets" the values of such constants. Thus the only possible correlation between those variables is a scale-invariant proportionality between the dimensionless ratios of the increments of these two variables to their initial values (see (2.6.4) and (2.6.7)):

$$\frac{P_X^+ - P_X^-}{P_{X0}^+} = \beta_X \frac{m_X^-}{M_{X0}^-}, \qquad m_X^- \equiv M_X^- - M_{X0}^-, \tag{4.4.1}$$

where M_X^-, M_{X0}^- and P_X^+, P_{X0}^+ are the perturbed and the nonperturbed values of the mass of nutrient X in the environment, and of the net primary production of the biota, respectively. Below the "X" indices are omitted in both formulae for simplicity's sake.

Due to the law of matter conservation (4.3.1), the natural physical fluxes $F^\pm$ in any reservoir remain, on average, much less than $P^\pm$, $\nu_i^\pm \ll 1$. Thus when considering significant fluctuations and external perturbations of the environment, these values may be neglected in (4.3.1). Then, taking into account that $\dot{M}^- = \dot{m}^-$ one may rewrite (4.4.1) and (4.3.1) in the form:

$$\dot{m}^- = -km^-, \quad m^+ + m^- = 0, \quad k \equiv \frac{\beta}{\tau}, \quad \tau \equiv \frac{M_0^-}{P_0^+}, \tag{4.4.2}$$

where τ is the time of biological cycling or residence time of inorganic nutrient in the environment.

The condition for operation of the Le Chatelier principle and for biological stability of the environment has the form (see Sect. 2.7):

$$\beta > 0, \qquad k > 0. \tag{4.4.3}$$

The construction of a mathematical model capable of describing the whole information fluxes in natural biota is impossible, see Sect. 2.8. But such a mathematical model is not needed if we apply the Le Chatelier principle. The particular validity of the Le Chatelier principle is that its quantitative presentation needs no intimate understanding of the structure of the system. Due to the extreme complexity of all the entangled interactions between the species in any community, the values β and k may only be obtained empirically. The values of k and β are, together with P_0^+, P_0^- and $M_0^\pm$, the principal characteristics of nonperturbed systems. They remain constant, and the relations (4.4.1) and (4.4.2) are linear at low perturbations, m^-, provided all the other characteristics of the biota and the environment remain weakly perturbed as well. The solution of (4.4.2) for constant k has the form:

$$m^- = m_0^- e^{-kt},$$

i.e. $k^{-1} \equiv \tau/\beta$ presents the characteristic time of system relaxation back to the normal state of the environment. Note that, after perturbation ceases, the environment returns to its former, that is initial (instead of a new) stable state. For example, after excessive CO_2 enters the atmosphere from external sources, the natural nonperturbed biota should transfer it into organic forms of low activity (such as soil humus, peat, and the dissolved organic matter in the ocean), thus retrieving the former concentration of CO_2, optimal for the biota in the atmosphere.

When the organic matter of living individuals is synthesized, certain ratios should be followed between the fluxes of production (and destruction) of the organic nutrients P_X^+, which correspond to the ratios between those same nutrients in living cells. For example, phytoplankton cells are synthesized and oxygen is

released by them in the ocean following the generalized Redfield molar ratio
(Redfield, 1958; Redfield et al., 1967; Broecker, 1982; Takahashi et al., 1985):

$$P_C^+ / P_N^+ / P_P^+ / - P_{O_2}^+ = 130/16/1/175, \tag{4.4.4}$$

where C denotes carbon, N denotes nitrogen, P denotes phosphorus, O_2 denotes
oxygen, and the productivities P_X^+ have the dimensions of $X\,m^{-2}\,year^{-1}$. A significant proportion of single-cell algae also have $CaCO_3$ shells, which increases the
share of carbon in (4.4.4) by approximately 20 % over the world ocean (Broecker,
1982; Neshyba, 1987). Random perturbations of the environment may occur independently in each nutrient. Thus for biological control of the environment the
natural biota (more precisely the repearing species, see Sect. 5.15) should be capable of producing the differences $P_X^+ - P_X^-$ in arbitrary ratios between the nutrients
(Peng et al., 1987). That effect is achieved via synthesis of extracellular excretions
of the organic matter (Khailov, 1971; Platt and Rao, 1975; Fogg, 1975; Gorshkov,
1982c) and of the metabolically inactive parts of plants (such as wood trunks or
shells of marine organisms), in which the ratios between the nutrients are different
from those in living cells, and also via selective destruction of the dead organic
matter.

Equations (4.4.2) with constant coefficients k and β are hold if a separate
component of the environment X is independently perturbed in each reservoir.
Formally, Eqs. (4.4.1) may be written for various mutually related reservoirs and
interrelated nutrients X_i. Then the values β_X and k_X in (4.4.1) and (4.4.2) may,
as a general case, be presented as complex functions of all the variables characterizing the concentrations of nutrients X_i in each reservoir. When each such
nutrient suffers a low perturbation, these functions may be expanded into a Taylor
series, from which we then exclude the nonlinear terms. As a result one arrives
at a system of linear equations, relating the temporal derivatives $\dot{m}_{Xi}$ and the increments m_{Xi} of nutrients X in reservoir i to increments m_{Yj} of nutrients Y in
reservoirs j. The matrix of the resulting system of equations may be diagonalized
via a linear transformation (a linear substitution of the variables), and then finding
the eigenvalues (Lotka, 1925) the system may then be presented in the form of
noncohesive set of equations of the type of (4.4.2). In that case all the statements
set forth above hold for each equation. Below, the relations between the reservoirs
is demonstrated for the example of the global cycle of carbon (see Sect. 4.12).

All the surrounding species in the community may be treated as components
of the environment for each given natural species of the biota. Perturbation of
the community structure may then be described by the same equations, (4.4.1)
and (4.4.2), treating the values m^- as the relative changes in the measurable
characteristics of the community. One may consider the number of individuals of a
separate species as such a variable, or the fluxes of matter and energy, consumed by
that species, which are uniquely related to the former. The synthesis and destruction
of organic matter, that is the consumption of energy and matter may be treated
as part of the useful work performed by the given species within the community,
which is aimed at stabilizing both the biota and the environment. A characteristic
universal for all natural communities is the distribution of the consumed fluxes

of matter and energy versus individual body sizes of the consumers, independent of their taxonomic properties, Fig. 1.3, which is often called the size spectrum (Sheldon et al., 1972). The deviations from that distribution within each interval of the histogram of Fig. 1.3 may be regarded as perturbation of the community and be described by (4.4.1) and (4.4.2).

It is apparent that compensation of both the biotic perturbations and perturbations in the environment may only be pursued up to a certain threshold level, that is the Le Chatelier principle may only be sustained that far. For example, after the natural biota is annihilated or is substituted by artificial communities, the biological regulation of the environment stops. The values of β should be at maximum for natural biota not yet perturbed. With that perturbation growing in magnitude, the value of β ceases to be constant, and starts to decrease, that is Eqs. (4.4.1) and (4.4.2) become nonlinear over the perturbation. The value of perturbation at which β becomes zero, may be considered the threshold beyond which the stability of the system of biota plus its environment is destroyed (Sect. 2.7).

The threshold values of the admissible perturbations are the most important characteristics of the natural biota together with the optimal concentrations of substances in the environment, M_0, the relaxation times, $k_0^{-1} \equiv \tau/\beta_0$, and the fluxes of production, P_0^+ and destruction, P_0^-. Finding those thresholds becomes especially important because of the growing anthropogenic forcing of the biota and its environment.

As follows from the distribution in Fig. 1.3, the principal work in stabilizing the environment is carried out by microscopic individuals in the community. After averaging over the periodic seasonal oscillations, that part of the distribution in all the communities apparently suffers only quite small fluctuations (Gorshkov, 1981; Kamenir and Khailov, 1987; Kamenir, 1991). No more than 1 % of the total flux of energy and matter in the community is due to consumption by the larger individuals of the community, the mammals, despite the fact that the biomass of the mammals may constitute a significant part of the total biomass of all the animals of the community. Hence, mammals under natural conditions only form the superfine structure of the community. Mammals, like dinosaurs in the past, have and had never been the lords of the biosphere, as they are sometimes considered (Alwarez and Asaro, 1990; Courtillot, 1990). Extinction of the dinosaurs at the C-T border 65 million years ago had not driven the biosphere outside its stability threshold, and had not practically affected its capability to compensate for adverse fluctuations of the environment (Raup and Sepkoski, 1982).

If a threshold of stability is exceeded locally, local perturbations of the biota ensue and pollutants begin to accumulate in the environment. Diffusion fluxes of these pollutants into the neighboring regions appear. The size of the perturbed area is defined by the active distance over which the concentrations of pollutants fall to the stability threshold of the nonperturbed biota. If the level of perturbation is fixed, a stationary state sets in with a maximum perturbation of the environment in the center of that local pollution. The concentration of the pollutants may be lowered in that local center either proceeding to a partially closed technological cycle (a local perturbation of the biota then remains present), or increasing the diffusion or evacuation of the perturbing substances outside the local area. The usually prescribed level of the maximum admissible concentration is determined as the threshold effect upon human health, which has nothing to do with the stability threshold of the biota. Within that area of perturbation the biota ceases to execute its stabilizing functions and may be substituted by any artificial communities or be totally annihilated.

With the perturbation strengthening the affected area expands. A stationary global state of the environment may only be sustained so far as the remaining nonperturbed part of the natural biota is still capable of compensating for all the anthropogenic perturbations, i.e., so long as the stability threshold is not exceeded globally. The past glaciations were not global catastrophic events. The ice cover area to total land area ratio was 20% in the last glacial period and is 13% now (Schlesinger, 1990). Thus only 7% of total land area was additionally covered by ice during the last glaciation. The fact that conditions fit for life were sustained during the periods of glaciation, triggered by astronomical factors alone, proves that such perturbations had not exceeded the global stability threshold. During each geological period the biota and the environment retained their stationary stable state over thousands of years (Oeschger and Stauffer, 1986; Hansen and Lacis, 1990; Lorius et al., 1990). The presently observed global perturbations of the environment (Hansen and Lacis, 1990; Lorius et al., 1990) occurring over the period of a few decades, unequivocally point to the natural biota on a global scale exceeding the stability threshold.

4.5 Biospheric Communities

High levels of closure of matter cycles and biological sustaining of the state of the environment optimal for life via controlling the level of breach, all result in the need for having spatially limited internally correlated communities of various species, capable of both synthesizing and destroying organic matter. Within the spatial domain of such a community the concentration of biologically accumulated substance differs from such concentrations outside that community. Thus together with the environmental domains that they change, the communities form local ecosystems of finite sizes.

The correlation among the individuals of the community is provided by the exchange of matter and energy fluxes, which fade at larger distances between those individuals. The highest degree of such correlation is possible for local ecosystems of minimal size. According to proxy estimates the size (that is the maximum radius of correlation) of the local ecosystems apparently varies from $100\,\mu$m to 10 m, not exceeding the overall size of higher plants (see Sects. 5.4–6). Another characteristic of the size of the community is also the distance at which the number of species consuming the principal part of the fluxes of energy in the community (Sect. 5.6) is saturated. One should stress that the usually employed saturation distance of the number of species, which is independent of the fraction of energy fluxes they consume (see, e.g., Giller, 1984) yields a highly overestimated radius for the community.

The community is an internally correlated system, much more complex than any individual from any species entering it. The structure of the community is determined by and combined from the gene pools of populations of a strictly prescribed combination of species entering that community. That structure cannot be changed, nor the principles along which the community functions, without a cardinal restructuring of all the genomes of all the species in it, and that may only happen in the course of long evolution.

The appearance of any additional form of correlation means a higher level of order. Random (fluctuational) rise in a physically stable correlation is less probable, the higher the level of order associated with it. As demonstrated in Sect. 3.1, the adaptation of the individual to its environment and a stable correlation within any individual of any species (i.e., the adaptation genetic program), may only result from biological selection within the population of individuals of the given species. Correlation of any level among the individuals may only result from and be supported by the biological selection within the population, that is selection among the competitively interacting hyperindividuals of the respective level (such as a set of social structures, or communities). Correlation among the local ecosystems, which supports a high degree of closure of matter cycles and regulates the level of breach, so as to compensate for external perturbations of the environment (that is how the Le Chatelier principle acts, i.e., the stabilization genetic program) may only be supported via competitive interaction between the communities populating the local ecosystems (these are the hyperindividuals), all taking place within a respective population of the local ecosystems (that is a hyperpopulation). Such a population of local ecosystems usually occupies a large area homogeneously vegetated, which is usually simply called an ecosystem (Whittaker, 1975; Odum, 1983).

The neighboring local ecosystems are not correlated to each other. Thus with the size of the local ecosystems diminishing, the spatial distribution of the biota becomes the more chaotic. That chaos is a typical observed trait of virgin nature.

The decay community may be expelled from the ecosystem, i.e., hyperpopulation of communities via excessive destruction, so that decay biota exceeds synthesis within the perturbed local ecosystem, and the erroneously functioning biota (both flora and fauna) are then destroyed. After that the normally functioning biota from the surrounding normal local ecosystems may enter the perturbed area, resurrecting the perturbed environmental zone, and combining into a new competitively capable community.

Thus only those species are retained in the community which have written in their genome, beside the program of adaptation to the environment (that environment includes all the other species in the community too), another program, which is actually much more important, and that is the program for stabilizing the environment at a state optimal for life, i.e., "the stabilization program", see Sect. 3.2. Both programs are written into the normal genomes of all the species of the community. The stabilization program includes information on feeding habits, on general behavior, the density of population of the species, etc., such that together they provide a most efficient and quick compensation for all the adverse external perturbations of the environment. The normal densities of population of the majority of species having such a stabilization program and functioning within the boundaries of a natural community, are not prescribed by the available limit of nutrients compatible with the given energetics of the individuals of such a species, but always remain far below those limits (cf. Chap. 5). Supporting the normal population number of a species is the responsibility of the genetic stabilization program, either carried by that species itself, or run by the other species, which control the population number of that first species within the community. The stabilization program is evidently much more complex than the adaptation program, and that is why the stabilization program is the one which suffers decay first.

The existence of such a stabilization program imposes certain limitations upon the adaptation program too. Thus species devoid of such a stabilization program (that is the situation occurring when foreign species are introduced into alien communities, or when that program somehow decays in native species), may happen to be better adapted to the local environment than the species containing such a program in their genomes. Then proliferation of such species takes place up to the very limit prescribed by the availability of nutrients (Parker and Maynard Smith, 1990), and then these species oust the native local ones and the community is destroyed. The environment deteriorates then, the whole community loses its competitiveness and is ousted, in its turn, by the normal communities in which all species feature stabilization programs. By way of example one may mention the phenomenon of algae cluttering the rivers of the Old Continent, when certain hybrid individuals of the New Continent algae are introduced into them (Barrett, 1989).

Numerous species that are quite well adapted to prescribed conditions of the environment may exist. However only those of them which carry stabilization programs may exist for long enough time periods. One may thus state that the sole meaning of life consists in producing the work necessary to stabilize the environment within the respective community. The normal community cannot include "gold-brick" species, which perform no such work; moreover gangster species, which interfere with the work of the others, and which break up the inner correlation within the community, are also impossible. Communities, randomly picking up such species, lose their competitive capacity and are ousted by normal communities.

Direct experimental proof of the existence of a hyperpopulation of communities would need laborious and costly measurements of the boundaries of local ecosystems, within which the matter cycles are closed at a minimal breach. That may be achieved by actually measuring the circulation of radioactive markers of non-volatile elements, introduced into a local ecosystem without perturbing its natural structure. However, the boundaries of such local ecosystems may be visually found in the simplest local ecosystems of epilithic lichen, see Fig. 4.1. They are found to remain identical in both Fig. 4.1a, where the lichen of a definite species does not merge into a continuous cover, so that the circulation of its nutrients takes place within each autonomous patch, and Fig. 4.1b, where those patches merge to produce a continuous cover, and the resulting picture reminds one of the political map with borders of the neighboring independent states shown. The borders may then be envisaged as the areas of competitive interaction between the adjacent local ecosystems. However, as long as we still lack tests of closed circulation of nutrients, which would be available using those radioactive markers, such an interpretation of Fig. 4.1a,b remains nothing but a plausible hypothesis.

Establishing and maintaining a correlation of a higher level is stimulated by the higher competitive capacity associated with such a correlation. Such correlations cannot spring up randomly, due, for example, to physical decay of the preceding life forms. Correlated systems of the type "Predator–Prey" or "Parasite–Host", as well as all the diverse forms of symbiosis between the various species, may only appear and be supported via generation of the internally correlated communities and their populations, which include such systems. There is no competitive interaction between either predator and its prey, or parasite and host, or any species entering a symbiosis arrangement, just as there is no such competition between the various organs in a single individual. Supporting the newly originated type of correlation may only be the task of competitive interaction between various non-correlated communities, including such correlated systems.

Any "selfish" (Dawkins, 1976, 1982; Cavalier-Smith, 1980; Doolittle and Sapienza, 1980; Orgel and Crick, 1980; Reid, 1980) or "neutral" (Kimura, 1983) individuals, not entering any type of correlation between other individuals as an intrinsic component (similar to organs in a separate body), which do not combine into a natural population and do not take part in competitive interaction among themselves, should quickly decay, and, thus, cannot exist under natural conditions. To clarify that point we consider certain examples at length.

Certain plasmids are present in the cells of some bacteria, which are ring-shaped extrachromosomal DNA molecules, capable of autonomous replication and of free transition from one cell to another (Lewin, 1983; Ayala and Kiger, 1984; Hesin, 1984; Modi and Adams, 1991). If we stick to the principle formulated above, the level of order in those plasmids may at first only be supported via competitive interaction between the cells containing them. Cells with decayed plasmids, that have lost certain characteristics of their functional activity should lose competitive capacity and be ousted by cells with normal plasmids. In that case the plasmid functioning is correlated to functioning of the cell as a whole. Such a correlation (a symbiosis) is no different from correlation between the body and one of its organs, in that its loss does not bring about immediate death of the individual. Second, plasmids may play a significant role in supporting some pan-cellular level of correlation of the type of the community of cells of various forms. Then the communities containing cells of that type with their plasmids decayed will lose their competitive capacity and be ousted by the communities containing cells with normal plasmids. Finally, the third possibility is that there exists a population

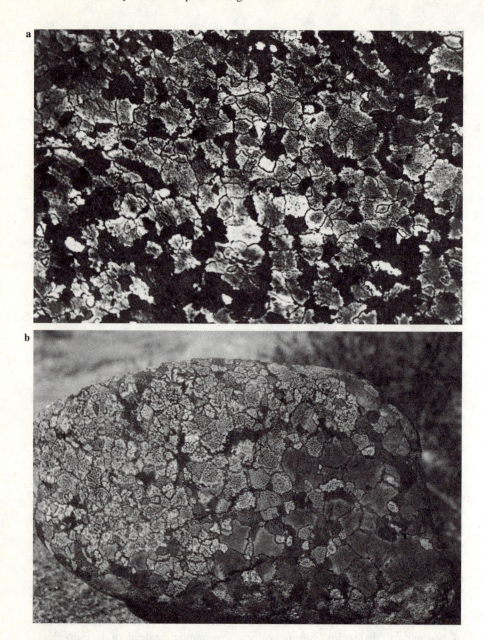

Fig. 4.1a,b. Spatial distribution of the epilithic lichens in White Sea islands: (**a**) local lichen communities (fungi + algae) of different species (*Lecidea spp.* and *Rhizocarpon spp.*) are divided by boundary lines; (**b**) different local lichen communities of the same species (*Lecidea spp.*) are divided by the same visible boundary lines.

of competitively interacting plasmids of the same cell. In that case the plasmids would use their cell as their environment, in which the existence of the population of plasmids is supported. The existence of separate selfish neutral plasmids, not correlated to either separate cells or their communities, and not organized into an internal community is impossible, since such plasmids should decay quickly and lose some vital trait, such as, for example their capacity for replication. The same conclusions are related to any DNA apparently selfish whose existence within the cell, its nucleus or cytoplasm may so far appear parasitic and functionally obscure. Experimental testing of every one of the above alternatives appears possible, and would also serve to test the basic biological principle (see Sect. 3.2).

One may similarly treat the presence of parasites in the bodies of higher organisms. Naturally, the malfunctioning individual containing parasites in its body features lower competitive capacity as compared to the healthy one. Thus decay of the organization in parasites, and decrease of their functional activity should have led to higher competitive capacity of their hosts and, hence, to their higher numbers. However, that is not actually the case, and no complete degradation and extinction of parasites is observed. Even when losing some of their inner organization, parasites only do so in the direction of increasing the efficiency of their functioning in the host body. The loss of their own respiration and distribution systems by some of the parasites which had formerly possessed these, only works to increase their competitive capacity within the host body, as compared to those species that have retained such morphological features. One may ask how is the most efficient organization supported, and how is the decay of organization prevented in parasites residing in their host's body?

If a whole population of competitively interacting parasites exists either within the host body or on its surface, their functional organization may be supported via biological selection among them, taking place within the limits of each separate host. However, the loss of competitive capacity of a host affected by parasites should result in decreasing the number of such deficient individuals and in their further exclusion from the population together with their parasites. In the opposite case, when the body of a single host is not large enough for a population of parasites to live in, the process of expulsion of the host affected by parasites from its own population might only be retarded via the decay of the organization of parasites, that is via the extinction of the phenomenon of parasitism itself. Thus in every conceivable case one appears unable to explain the stability of the phenomenon of parasitism by considering only the correlation between a separate host and its parasites.

The only possible way to explain the phenomenon of parasitism is by envisaging the community of the species, which includes the host species of the parasites. The complex nature of correlation between the species in the community results the community, in which a sufficient number of individuals from a given species contain such parasites, appearing to be more competitive than communities in which the individuals from the same species host no such parasites. Competitive interaction between communities in a population of communities results in selection and support of those communities which include parasites. The cause for higher competitive capacity of such communities may be related (Sects. 1.7, 5.5 and 5.6) to resulting limitations upon and control of the number of individuals of large body size in these communities. Otherwise the uncontrolled growth of that number could disrupt the closed matter cycles. Higher degree of correlation between the host and its parasites should also work to improve the competitive capacity of a community. That may be the reason for complex successive change of host during the life cycle of most parasites (Dogel, 1975; Raven and Johnson, 1988).

For our last example we shall consider the correlated interaction between the predator and its prey. That type of correlation has been repeatedly treated using various mathematical models (Lotka, 1925; Maynard Smith, 1974). If one considers the interaction between the predator and its prey alone, to the exclusion of all the other interactions, it appears extremely difficult to reach even a dynamic stability of the system, and remains impossible to explain the sustained genetic stability of correlation of such kind. Thus it may be assumed plausible that predators are supported, similar to parasites, via competitive interaction between the various communities. The presence of predators in a community increases the efficiency with which that community functions, as well as its competitive capacity, the overall task of the community remaining to keep the matter cycles closed. Periodic oscillations in the population numbers of predators and their prey should be controlled by the characteristic time for the community as a whole, instead of the times describing the physiology of both the predator and prey. That effect is indeed observed for interaction between the lynx and the hare (Keith, 1963) and between pests (insects) and plants (Kendeigh, 1974; Holing, 1978; Isaev et al., 1984). The oscillation periods appear to be of the same order of magnitude then, and they all differ quite strongly from the typical lifespans of either the lynx, the hare, or the insects, the latter differing by several orders of magnitude from each other. Apparently, the observed oscillation periods in predator activity are defined by the characteristic times describing the cycles of plant-edificators functioning and dominating in these communities (see also Sect. 4.10).

If decay individuals are accumulated in the population of prey, the correlated character of interaction between the prey and their parasites (predators) may be disrupted. That would, in its turn, lead to lower ratio of the number of parasites (predators) to that of prey. However, such a decay polymorphism, advantageous for prey, would result in perturbation of the program of community stabilization and to deterioration of the environment. Thus high polymorphism in the prey species, sustained via sexual breeding (the so-called "Red Queen Hypothesis", Rosenzweig, 1973; Williams, 1975; Maynard Smith, 1978; Bell, 1982; Lively et al., 1990; Hamilton et al., 1990; Moller, 1990; Hoffman, 1991) destroys the level of correlation in the community, and thus may not serve as the reason explaining the widespread sexual mode of breeding, see Sect. 3.11.

Selection among the communities, which stabilizes correlated interaction between the seemingly selfish DNA and the cell, between the parasites and their hosts, the predators and their prey, also works to drive the parallel evolution of such correlated components of the community. Random coincidence in evolution rates of these separate components, their correlation simultaneously sustained at every step, seems to be absolutely improbable.

Under the conditions of anthropogenic perturbation of the environment, when the closed character of matter cycles appears to be destroyed, such communities, working to close the cycles of matter, seem not to be necessary any more. The "predator-prey" system loses its stability. One may mention the populations of sparrows, urban blue rock pigeons, and anthropogenic mallard ducks, their stable existence not accompanied by any stable existence of predators, which would feed off them. There are practically no anthropogenic predators, except for cats and dogs, directly supported by man, which is a well-known empirical fact. (At the same time the uncontrolled activity of cats and dogs in urbanized areas may result in practically total extinction of their prey species.) In principle the anthropogenic species, not included in any natural communities, should evolve toward complete freedom from parasites. However, the time elapsed from the start of their isolation from the natural communities is still insufficient to experimentally observe such a tendency.

Artificial combination of several species originating from different communities would be devoid of any intrinsic coordinated program of stabilization, so that combination would fail to merge into a community capable of sustaining the environment in a state fit for life for long enough time periods. It would be quite similar to taking various organs from different species trying to combine them into a single individual capable of life. Moreover, such a program of stabilization should inevitably decay with time in any isolated local ecosystem, initially including all the necessary species from a natural community and a properly functioning stabilization program. Eventually gangster species would appear in such a system, so that the community would then decay, and both that community and its environment would be destroyed. It is only when surrounded by hyperpopulation of identical communities, that such a decay community might be ousted and substituted by the new community still retaining its stabilization program. Thus, first, no isolated local ecosystem, either natural, or artificially organized, may sustain closed matter cycles for any unlimited length of time; and, second, the artificially constructed sets of local ecosystems, arranged from the arbitrarily chosen species, cannot combine into self-sustained "populations" of competitively interacting local ecosystems, which would be capable of closing matter cycles over unlimited time periods.

It has become fashionable lately to construct artificial communities of plants and heterotrophic individuals, welded into glass balloons of several liters in volume. These communities have stores of nutrients sufficient to keep the plants functioning together with heterotrophs for several years, with the synthesis and destruction of the organic matter within such communities remaining completely uncorrelated. Random partial closure of matter cycles at the level of breach of 0.1 bring such communities into the range of several dozen years. However, the inevitable processes of aging and decay must eventually destroy that random closure of matter cycles within the community, terminating its existence.

It is of undoubted interest to stage an experiment similarly isolating a set (a population) of competitively interacting natural communities, such as, for example, lichens. The number of such correlated communities in such a population being sufficiently high, the lifespan of that population may appear to be practically unlimited, despite the limited lifespans of separate communities in it. Such an experiment would obviously produce certain information on the correlation radius (size) of separate communities.

Repeated attempts were also undertaken to construct a closed system including both higher plants and man (Lisovskii, 1979; Allen and Nelson, 1989). The concentration of oxygen in such systems was kept at a level acceptable for man and his need for water was also satisfied. These experiments failed in stabilizing the mass of organic matter. To keep the concentration of carbon dioxide constant, the cellulose stored before the start of the experiment had to be burned, and instead straw was accumulated from higher plants, etc. According to the estimates by the present author, who followed the published data on that experiment (Lisovskii, 1979) the breach of such a system was $\kappa \approx 0.5$, that was at a level not less than that of the modern agricultural systems.

Various sets of local ecosystems exist under various environmental conditions (such as shelf, pelagic waters, mountains and plateaux on land): forests, steppes, reefs, open ocean communities, which combine into the Earth's biosphere. Thus the biosphere is a major set of noncorrelated local ecosystems, not exceeding several tens of meters in size, devoid of any centralized control.

4.6 Biological Regulation of Matter Cycles

The notion of a local ecosystem implies that a difference exists between the concentration of nutrient X inside, $[X_{in}]$, and outside, $[X_{out}]$, the local ecosystem: $\Delta[X] = [X_{in}] - [X_{out}]$. That difference in concentrations should exceed the sensitivity threshold of the biota, $\Delta[X_{min}]$: the change of concentration remaining below $\Delta[X_{min}]$ does not alter the functional state of the biota. The value $\varepsilon_{min} \equiv \Delta[X_{min}]/[X]$ is to be called the resolution of the biota with respect to nutrient X: the biota may only react to the relative change in the concentration X such that $\varepsilon \equiv \Delta[X]/[X] > \varepsilon_{min}$. The value of ε_{min} should clearly be of the order of or less than the breach κ_0. The sensitivity limit of the biota is obviously higher than the natural fluctuations in the same nutrient:

$$\varepsilon_{min} < \left\{ \overline{([X] - \overline{[X]})^2} \right\}^{1/2}.$$

The existence of such a difference in concentrations results in the appearance of diffusion fluxes F, which tend to equalize the concentrations. Such a difference may only be supported if the diffusion fluxes are compensated by biological transport of nutrients (the fluxes of synthesis, P^+, and of the ensuring destruction, P^-, of the organic matter).

The borders of local ecosystems are prescribed by those surfaces at which both the gradients of concentration and the diffusion fluxes, averaged over fluctuations and over their diurnal and annual changes, go to zero to the accuracy of about $\varepsilon_{\min}$. The principal biochemical transport of nutrients in land biota is by higher plants. Thus the size of the local ecosystem should be of the order of the largest plants in the community (to be more exact, of the order of maximal distance between the correlated parts of such higher plants). Within the areas occupied by separate higher plants, autonomic local ecosystems of smaller size may be found (e.g., lichen).

The environment is described by the concentrations of nutrients within the local ecosystems, that is within the life domain. The external environment is characterized by concentrations of nutrients outside the local ecosystems.

Due to natural selection among local communities, the neighboring local ecosystems in uniform localities should feature identical characteristics (to within the sensitivity of the biota). Thus the differences in concentrations and the diffusion fluxes in the horizontal, y, directions should be much less than in the vertical, z, direction, as well as biochemical fluxes compensating them: $\Delta[X]_{\min} \leq \Delta_y[X] \ll \Delta_z[X]$. The diffusion fluxes in the vertical direction within the neighboring local ecosystems are equal to each other and are the same in the total ecosystem (i.e., in the hyperpopulation of the local ecosystems). They are proportional to the concentration gradient and are expressed as:

$$F = -D\left(\frac{d}{dz}\right)[X] \approx \frac{\Delta[X]}{R_e} = F_{\text{in}} - F_{\text{out}}$$

$$R_e \equiv \frac{H_e}{D}, \quad F_{\text{in}} = \frac{[X_{\text{in}}]}{R_e}, \quad F_{\text{out}} = \frac{[X_{\text{out}}]}{R_e}$$

$$\Delta[X] \equiv [X_{\text{in}}] - [X_{\text{out}}], \tag{4.6.1}$$

where H_e is the vertical size of the local ecosystem; D is the coefficient of either the molecular or the eddy diffusion of the nutrient; F_{in} and F_{out} are the nutrient fluxes of export outside and import into the local ecosystem; R_e is the external resistance of diffusion transport. Conductivities or exchange coefficients $k_e \equiv (H_e R_e)^{-1}$ may be used instead of the resistances R_e.

While the external environment remains intact, the concentrations of nutrients inside the local ecosystem do not change, and the net fluxes of nutrients into the system becomes zero. If these external conditions change, the concentrations of nutrients inside the local ecosystem may start to be directionally changed by the biota (the same is also true for the external environment), altering the fluxes of both the synthesis and destruction of the organic matter. Stationary average environmental conditions fit for life may only be supported on condition that the changes in processes taking place in the biota affected by external perturbations are directed to compensate such perturbations and to return the system to its unperturbed condition. Using the language of control, that would correspond to the presence of negative feedback in the biota. As already noted above, the processes that arise to compensate for external perturbations of a stable system is called the Le Chatelier principle (Lotka, 1925; Landau and Lifshitz, 1964).

Within the local ecosystem the concentrations of biologically active substances may be either supported by or changed by the biota on condition that the fluxes of synthesis and destruction of organic matter exceed the net fluxes of physical transport, that is when:

$$F \leq P^+ \quad \text{or} \quad \nu \equiv \frac{F}{P^+} \leq 1. \tag{4.6.2}$$

Introducing the internal resistance to synthesis

$$R_i \equiv \frac{[X]}{P^+} \tag{4.6.3}$$

on the grounds of convenience, we obtain the following relationship between the net and gross openness (see Eq. (4.3.3)):

$$\nu \equiv \nu_{in} \varepsilon, \quad \nu_{in} = \frac{R_i}{R_e}, \quad \varepsilon \equiv \frac{\Delta[X]}{[X]}. \tag{4.6.4}$$

The resistances R_i and R_e are defined by (4.6.1) and (4.6.3) and may be directly measured similar to ε, Eq. (4.6.4). Three distinctly different situations are possible:

1. The physical fluxes of export and import of nutrient out of and into the ecosystem are less than, or are of the order of, the biological fluxes of synthesis and destruction of the organic matter. In that case the difference between the concentrations inside and outside the local ecosystem may be of the order of the very concentration of the nutrient inside the ecosystem, that is enrichment is possible of the local ecosystem by that nutrient, its concentration in the external environment remaining arbitrary. Qualitatively such a situation is expressed by:

$$\nu \sim \nu_{in} \leq 1 \quad (\varepsilon \sim 1, \ \nu_{in} \varepsilon_{min} \ll 1). \tag{4.6.5}$$

Such nutrients may be called biologically locally accumulated. Practically all the biologically active substances in land soil enter that group (Gorshkov, 1986a). The ratio between the mass of such a nutrient in its organic form M_X^+, taken over all the local ecosystems, and that of its organic form M_X^- in the external environment may be then arbitrary: $M_X^+ \ll M_X^-$, $M_X^+ \sim M_X^-$, or $M_X^+ \gg M_X^-$. The biota is capable of regulating the concentrations of biologically locally accumulated nutrients in local ecosystems, i.e., in the environment of the biota, at arbitrary concentrations of those nutrients in the external environment.

Certain communities in the biosphere appear to be constantly and directionally (instead of fluctuationally) affected by the external flux of either organic or inorganic nutrients ($F_{in}^{\pm}$). Among such are the communities of many lakes with high import of nutrients by the rivers flowing into those lakes, or those of the marine estuaries, as well as certain seas of the world ocean. For example, such fluxes of nutrients and of heat enter the Barents Sea with the Gulf Stream. To keep the environmental conditions stationary there, such communities should compensate for these external forcings, and the way to do so is to function at a significant breach of their matter cycles. Perturbations that such communities may suffer are deviations of those directional fluxes from their average values. Environmental conditions in the local ecosystems of such communities may only be conserved if the conditions in (4.6.2) are met, that is when the production P^+ or destruction P^- exceeds the difference between the import and export of nutrients $F^\pm = F_{in}^\pm - F_{out}^+$ found in the environment external with respect to those communities.

2. Physical fluxes of import to and export from a local ecosystem are much larger than the biological fluxes of synthesis and destruction of organic matter. The difference between the concentrations of nutrient inside and outside the local ecosystem is then much less than its concentration inside the local ecosystem, the latter practically coinciding with its concentration in the external environment. However, the relative difference between the concentrations (ε) then exceeds the biological sensitivity threshold (ε_{min}). In such a case the biota is capable of changing concentrations of inorganic nutrient in local ecosystems and in the external environment by redistributing the stores of that nutrient in its states M_X^+ and M_X^-, provided the mass of the organic nutrient M_X^+ remains of the order of the mass of biologically active inorganic substances containing that nutrient in the external environment, M_X^-, having taken over all the local ecosystem of the biosphere: $M_X^+ \sim M_X^-$.

If the concentration of inorganic nutrient in the external environment decreases below the optimal level, i.e. the level providing the highest competitive capacity of that community within the local ecosystem, the biota speeds up destruction of organic matter, raising it above the level of synthesis, and increases the concentration of inorganic nutrient in the local ecosystems. The difference of concentrations is then produced in that nutrient between the immediate environment of the biota and the external environment, so that a diffusion flux of that nutrient into the external environment appears. That process must inevitably take place in all the natural (nonperturbed) local ecosystems of equal competitive capacity. Those local ecosystems which lack such a feature lose their competitive capacity and are ousted by the other local ecosystems. As a result the store of organic nutrient M_X^+ in local ecosystems is diminished, and the store of that nutrient in the external environment is increased. The process stops when the concentration of inorganic nutrient in the external environment reaches its optimal level. That optimal level is determined by the characteristics of the existing biota.

Inversely, when the concentration of the nutrient in the immediate environment of the biota is above the optimal level, the biota works to reduce that concentration as compared to that in the external environment, via higher synthesis, which then begins to dominate. We also see that the flux of nutrient then reverses and enters local ecosystems from the external environment, so that the mass M_X^- decreases, and the mass M_X^+ increases.

If the mass of nutrient in the external environment, M_X^-, significantly exceeds that in the ecosystems, $M_X^+ : M_X^- \gg M_X^+$, the biota seems to be incapable of changing the concentration of that nutrient in either environment or, respectively, its immediate environment. An inverse ratio: $M_X^- \ll M_X^+$ is impossible; the organic matter may only be accumulated via functioning of the biota itself, and that process stops when the optimal concentrations of both organic and inorganic nutrient are reached in the environment. The excess mass M_X^+, not needed for regulation of M_X^-, will be inevitably withdrawn from the biotic cycle via storage in the biotically inactive reservoirs, for example in sedimentary rocks.

Those nutrients that are biotically regulated in the external environment may be called biologically globally accumulated. They are quantitatively described by:

$$\varepsilon_{min}\nu_{in} \le 1, \quad M_X^+ \sim M_X^-, \quad (\nu_{in} \gg 1, \ \nu \le 1, \ \varepsilon_{min} < \varepsilon \ll 1). \quad (4.6.6)$$

Among such nutrients are the atmospheric carbon dioxide and the water-dissolved oxygen (Gorshkov, 1986a, 1987b), as well as fresh continental water (the notation $M_{H_2O}^+$ should then be understood as free water in the bodies of living beings, and in the soil, and $M_{H_2O}^-$ as atmospheric water). Biological regulation of CO_2 is observed in internal atmospheres of vegetation cover.

3. Finally, if the physical fluxes of nutrient are so large that the biota is incapable of producing any concentration differences in excess of its own sensitivity against the background, the concentrations of such nutrients clearly cannot be regulated by the biota. Such nutrients may be called biologically non-accumulated. They obey the equations:

$$\varepsilon_{min}\nu_{in} > 1 \ \text{or} \ M_X^- \gg M_X^+, \quad (\varepsilon < \varepsilon_{min} \ \text{at} \ \nu \le 1, \ \nu > 1 \ \text{at} \ \varepsilon = \varepsilon_{min}). \quad (4.6.7)$$

Among the biologically non-accumulated nutrients are free oxygen and free nitrogen in the atmosphere. The biota functioning in an air environment is evidently incapable of regulating the concentrations of O_2 and N_2 in the atmosphere. Among the non-accumulated nutrients are also the nutrients in flowing waters and in the upper oceanic layer, where eddy diffusion at average sea roughness is extremely high. Nutrients become biologically accumulated in these environments in local ecosystems only, these ecosystems formed of particles not exceeding $100\,\mu m$ in size (Sieburth and Davis, 1982), since eddy diffusion is substituted by molecular diffusion there. At the oceanic surface layer, the nutrients become biologically accumulated in the absence of currents and in still weather (Gorshkov, 1986a).

4.7 Biological Stability and Limiting Nutrients

The concentrations of biologically non-accumulated nutrients in the external environment do not coincide with those optimal for functioning of the biota. However, concentrations of biologically non-accumulated nutrients may be regulated by the biota when the reservoirs of these biologically non-accumulated nutrients are in either chemical or physical equilibrium with those of the biologically accumulated nutrients. Consider oxygen by way of an example.

The biologically non-accumulated concentration of oxygen in the atmosphere is in physical equilibrium with the oxygen dissolved in soil water and the ocean. The equilibrium concentration of water-dissolved oxygen is 40 times less than that in air. Furthermore, the coefficient of diffusion of that gas in water is four orders of magnitude less than in air. Thus physical fluxes of oxygen in water are six orders of magnitude less than the physical fluxes of O_2 in air. The dissolved oxygen appears to be locally biologically accumulated and its concentration is subject to regulation by the biota. Due to physical equilibrium between the concentrations of oxygen in the atmosphere and that dissolved in water, the former also appears to be subject to regulation by water biota although the resulting concentration of oxygen in the air may appear not to be optimal for land biota. Since the store of biologically active organic matter is three orders of magnitude lower than the store of O_2 in the atmosphere, the concentration of the latter cannot be biotically reduced by more than several hundredths of a per cent (Ryther, 1970). However, biota is capable of compensating the depletion of atmospheric oxygen (taking place via oxidation of products of volcanic eruptions) by synthesizing additional organic matter, which is accompanied by the emission of additional CO_2, and by subsequent deposition of organic carbon in sedimentary rocks.

The biological processes in natural communities may only be limited by the biologically non-accumulated nutrients. The concentrations of all the biologically accumulated nutrients must be supported at a level close to optimal by the aboriginal biota, so these cannot take part in limiting the functioning of the biota. In the absence of biologically non-accumulated nutrients, the biotic productivity may only be limited by the attainable rates of chemical reactions and by the solar radiant power. In natural communities the productivity of many plants actually reaches those limits. That is a testimony in favor of lack of limitations upon the biotic productivity from non-accumulated nutrients. Hence, if such non-accumulated nutrients exist, their concentrations should remain within those optimal limits, to which the biochemistry of contemporary biota is actually tuned.

It is, however, easy to see that the last statement is improbable. The concentrations of biologically non-accumulated nutrients are not regulated by the biota. Biochemical transformations of such non-accumulated nutrients cannot follow closed cycles, since the communities with closed cycles of non-accumulated nutrients are in no way advantaged, as compared to those with their cycles open. (The closed character of cycles of non-accumulated nutrients may be associated with the closed character of such in accumulated nutrients, if certain stoichiometric relations between the former and the latter hold. However such stoichiometric relations may change in the process of evolution.) As a result, the concentrations of non-accumulated nutrients appear to be unstable and cannot remain within the limits optimal for functioning of the biota. During long time intervals such concentrations should drift, finally getting outside the margin fit for life. Thus concentrations of all the chemical substances used in life cycles must clearly be subject to biotic regulation. The limiting nutrients (cf. the so-called Liebig principle, Lotka, 1925; Odum, 1983) may only be found in strongly perturbed or artificial communities.

The fluxes of nutrients accompanying the process of synthesis of organic matter should agree with the stoichiometric relations characterizing the relative content of those nutrients in organic matter and the amount of oxygen necessary to destroy the given amount of organic matter:

$$P_{X_1}^+ / P_{X_2}^+ / \ldots / P_{X_n}^+ = (X_1 / X_2 / \ldots / X_n)_{org}. \qquad (4.7.1)$$

The ratio of nutrient concentrations in the organic matter, $(X_i)_{org}$, to those in the environment, $[X_i]$, are related via internal resistance R_i, Eq. (4.6.3), to consumption of nutrients from the environment:

$$[X_1]/[X_2]\ldots = (R_{iX_1}/R_{iX_2}\ldots)(X_1/X_X\ldots)_{org}. \qquad (4.7.2)$$

The ratios of nutrient concentrations in the organic matter and in the environment may only coincide with each other when all the internal resistances are equal to each other: $R_{iX_k} = R_i$.

For compensation of all the external perturbations of the environment to be quickest, the productivity developed by the biota should be at its maximum (cf. Sect. 4.2). That would correspond to minimal internal resistance, depending exclusively on the internal structure of the living bodies. Hence, the ratios of concentrations of nutrients are prescribed by the righthand parts of (4.7.2) for the environment. Now, what is the controlling factor for the absolute values of nutrient concentrations in that environment? Apparently, there exist certain minimal concentrations $[X]_{min}$ for each nutrient X, below which life becomes impossible. The maximum concentration $[X]_{max}$ of that nutrient may be related to the maximum productivity of the biota at a prescribed incoming flux of external energy, which is the solar radiant energy: $[X]_{max} = R_{iX} P_{X\,max}^+$. The maximum concentrations of nutrients may not, however, necessarily correspond to the optimal values of other characteristics of the environment, such as its temperature, pressure, etc. The biotic regulation of the environment means that concentrations of all the nutrients accumulated in the environment are supported by the biota at levels intermediate between those maxima and minima. Thus, if one assumes the concept of biological regulation from the start, the notion of limiting nutrients becomes void for natural conditions. No environmental nutrient may be consumed by the biota at the level of saturation, when both the productivity and destructivity of the biota become independent of changes in concentrations of the consumed nutrient, while the resistance R_i changes in proportion to that concentration. It is only in this case that the natural biota appears capable of reacting to external perturbations of any nutrient in accordance with the Le Chatelier principle, compensating those perturbations. Its internal resistance R_i should then change non-linearly, following (4.4.1); see also (2.6.4), (2.6.7) and (4.12.4). In the particular case $\beta_X = 1$ (see (4.4.1)) these internal resistances should remain constant.

However, when any species is introduced into the unnatural environment the ratios (4.7.2) may noticeably deviate from the respective ratios typical for the natural conditions of existence of that species. In that case the nutrients with the lowest concentrations may appear to play the limiting role (the Liebig principle, Lotka, 1925; Odum, 1983). The concentration of limiting nutrient prescribes the productivity of the biota. Changes of other concentrations do not affect that productivity, and the respective internal resistances change in proportion to those concentrations. All the cultivated agricultural species exist in such conditions.

Thus the principal condition for biological regulation of the environment is the capability of the biota to react to external perturbations of the environment. That means that such perturbations should enter the sensitivity margin of the biota. In other words, the components of the environment subject to biotic regulation should be biologically accumulated. Concentrations of nutrients (that is of the components of the environment regulated by the biota) are kept at levels intermediate between the maximum and the minimum possible. The information on such intermediate concentrations, which are optimal for biota, is written into the normal genomes of all the species combining into natural communities. Such information (that is the stabilizing program) may suffer decay, similar to any other genetic program (such as the program of adaptation). This program of stabilization (and, hence, the program for keeping environmental conditions in a state fit for life) is supported by competitive interaction between the communities combining into the hyperpopulation (into the ecosystem). Communities with their decayed programs of stabilization (decay communities) work to deteriorate their enviromental conditions, lose their competitive capacity, and are ousted by the normal communities, which are capable of supporting, and do support, the locally optimal environmental conditions.

It is the existence of the hyperpopulation of competitively interacting internally correlated communities that is the basis for supporting life itself. Competitive interaction and natural selection among the internally correlated communities is similar to selection among any internally correlated living structures (single-cell, multicellular, etc.), and does not correspond to the repeatedly discussed group selection of populations and species (see Sect. 3.3). Competitive interaction among the separate communities does not go in the direction of the quickest assimilation of nutrients (resources from the environment) by the "normal" communities, thus depriving the less operative "decay" ones of their resources of existence. Such a strategy of competitive interaction would have led to quick degradation of the environment and to extinction of the whole hyperpopulation (i.e. the ecosystem). The normal communities are those which are capable of balanced consumption and use of environmental resources, so that the optimal life conditions are preserved. Conversely, communities capable of the maximally quick degradation of environmental resources are the decay ones, featuring lower competitiveness. The principles of extremes do not provide a true understanding of the way in which a natural community functions.

Preservation of the stabilization program for each species in the community only occurs due to internal competitive interaction within the species. To preserve that stabilization program within the species it is necessary that normal individuals featuring such a program have a maximum competitiveness. Only such species are capable of providing the highest competitiveness of the community in general. Thus, generally speaking, competition is not for the limiting nutrient, or for energy resources, or for the maximum population, but for keeping the relative number of normal individuals (those carrying in their genomes the program for sustaining an optimum population number density of the given species) at maximum.

Competition for the limiting nutrients and energy resources springs up among the individuals within species introduced into communities unnatural for those species. The stabilizing program in such species loses its meaning. Decay individuals, devoid of the stabilization program but capable of using the limiting environmental resources and at a high rate and of reaching the highest possible population density, happen to be the most competitive ones. Extremum principles may correctly describe the ecology of populations of such individuals extracted from their natural communities (Parker and Maynard Smith, 1990).

4.8 Productivity and Immigration in the Community

The principal condition for the existence of an internally correlated community of finite size is the relative constancy of the individual composition of those species which control the principal part of both energy and matter fluxes, that is of those species which account for the major part of the productivity P^+ and of the destructivity P^- in the community. The community may efficiently eliminate its decay individuals and reproduce its normal individuals only when both immigration and emigration of individuals of these main species in the community are small, as compared to reproduction within the community itself. For the community to function adequately, in agreement with its prescribed stabilizing and adaptive genetic programs of each of its species, the relative number of decay individuals with distorted programs should be low in all the species. To satisfy that condition the immigration of decay individuals into the community and emigration of the normal individuals from it should remain less than both their elimination and reproduction within the community itself. Since immigration may occur from the neighboring decay communities, which contain decay individuals in large numbers, the only way to support the level of organization of any species in the community via internal competitive interaction within the species, is to keep immigration small, as compared to reproduction of these individuals within the community itself.

The productivity (birth rate), P_α^+, and destructivity (death rate), P_α^-, the immigration, $F_{\alpha\,\text{in}}^+$, and emigration, $F_{\alpha\,\text{out}}^+$, of individuals of the species α are related to change of their total biomass via equations of the type (4.3.1):

$$\dot{M}_\alpha^+ = P_\alpha^+ - P_\alpha^- + F_{\alpha\,\text{in}}^+ - F_{\alpha\,\text{out}}^+. \tag{4.8.1}$$

The biomass, M^+, productivity, P^+ and destructivity, P^-, are equal to the population density number, birth rate and death rate, respectively, if the mean individual's body mass and surface area are equal to unity (see Sect. 2.6). The condition that immigration remains low as compared to reproduction (which is equivalent to the condition of "enhanced local accumulation", see (4.6.5), of normal individuals within the community), has the form (the stationary case $\dot{M}_\alpha^+ = 0$):

$$\nu_{\alpha\,\text{in}}^+ \equiv \frac{F_{\alpha\,\text{in}}^+}{P_\alpha^+} \ll 1. \tag{4.8.2}$$

We denote the volume number density of individuals of the species α as $[\alpha]$. Then the biomass (or the number of individuals, which is proportional to it) of the individuals of the species α in the community is $M_\alpha = [\alpha]H_\alpha$, where H_α is the vertical dimension occupied by the species α in the community. The productivity

P_α^+ is $P_\alpha^+ = [\alpha]H_\alpha/\tau_\alpha$, where τ_α is the characteristic reproduction period (that is the time lapse between the two generations in a stationary population). Immigration is characterized by a horizontal flux and may be defined via the horizontal diffusivity D_α in the form $F_{\alpha\,in}^+ = D_\alpha[\alpha]/L$, where L is the horizontal size of the community. Then (4.8.2) takes the form:

$$\nu_{\alpha\,in}^+ = \frac{D_\alpha \tau_\alpha}{L H_\alpha} \ll 1. \tag{4.8.3}$$

The diffusivity D_α may be determined by eddy diffusion for those planktonic, free-floating, both motile and immotile species which cannot keep pace with water movement, that diffusion being typical for the environment of the local ecosystem. As for the motile nektonic animals, their D_α is determined by their random wanderings. We have in the latter case $D_\alpha \sim u_\alpha L_\alpha$, where u_α is the speed of movement, and L_α is the linear size of the feeding ground (home range) of the motile animal (Gorshkov, 1982a, see Sect. 5.10).

The conditions in (4.8.2) and (4.8.3) should be met for the principal species in the community. These species (called "general edificators") are charged with elimination of the decay individuals from the community in both their own and some subordinate species. They perform that function via interspecies competitive interaction. The competitive interaction within subordinate species may be slackened or even completely switched off. In that case the principal species in the community conduct "artificial" selection among the subordinate species, leaving the normal individuals in them (that is individuals commanding the necessary adaptive and stabilizing programs) and eliminating the decay ones (those devoid of such programs). Such subordinate controlled species are clearly incapable of existing outside the given community. Their genetic program may be free of information on the necessity of competitive interaction, that is the individuals of those species may be incapable of discriminating between the normal and the decay individuals. The information on such differences may only be contained in the normal genomes of the dominating controlling species, which are charged with conducting such "artificial selection" among the subordinate controlled species. (Such interactions are similar to interaction between the nuclear and cytoplasma genomes in eukaryotic cells.)

Certain environmental conditions make the existence of subordinate controlled species inescapable. For example, photosynthesis is only possible in the upper euphotic oceanic layer, penetrated by the solar light. Even the most transparent oceanic waters completely absorb that light at depths in excess of 100 m, so that photosynthesis becomes impossible there. The most active photosynthesis is restricted to the first 25 m of oceanic depth, where up to 90 % of solar light is absorbed (Neshyba, 1987). Destruction of organic matter does not need the presence of solar light and may go on at arbitrary oceanic depths. The aerobic decomposition may only occur at those depths to which oxygen may penetrate. An anaerobic decomposition may occur independent of the availability of oxygen.

What could be the possible structure of the communities, closing the matter cycles and supporting conditions fit for life? Keeping their buoyancy positive, it is physically possible to hold all the living beings close enough to the oceanic surface. Multicellular algae contain special organs with air bubbles in them, which keep their buoyancy positive. One might imagine a community, consisting of individuals with positive buoyancy in all their excretions, even after their individuals' deaths. In that case all the decomposition of synthesized organic matter could also be concentrated within the euphotic layer, limiting sinking of the organic matters to a minimum of breach of matter cycles, given by the value κ_0, Eq. (4.3.6). Life would be absent below the euphotic layer in such a hypothetical ocean.

However, due to extremely strong wind mixing of the euphotic oceanic layer, all the components of the environment of the community appear to be biologically non-accumulated locally. The eddy diffusion coefficient in the surface layer approximately 100 m deep averages $D \sim 10^6 \, \text{m}^2/\text{year}$, reaching as high as $10^{11} \, \text{m}^2/\text{year}$ during storms (Ivanoff, 1972, 1975). The reproduction time constant for phytoplankton is $\tau_\alpha > 10^{-2}$ year (see Table 5.1). Assuming $L \sim H_\alpha < 100 \, \text{m}$ we find that $\nu^+_{\alpha \, \text{in}} > 1$. Hence, immigration of the individuals of phytoplankton algae exceeds their production in the surface layer, and no community can be formed there with a constant composition of its individuals.

This, however, becomes possible at depths below 100 m, where the eddy diffusion coefficient drops by three orders of magnitude to $10^3 \, \text{m}^2/\text{year}$ (Broecker et al., 1985b; Lewis et al., 1986). However photosynthesis is impossible at those depths and a only community of heterotrophs may be organized there (that is bacteria and animals feeding off the organic matter). Those heterotrophs should perform the function of the controlling species via the necessary "artificial selection" of algae, predominantly eating away the decay individuals among them. The heterotrophs should also be capable of eating out live decay algae, which is apparently realized via cyclic vertical displacement of the heterotrophs into the euphotic zone and back (Ehrhardt and Seguin, 1978). Hence, a considerable part of matter cycles must necessarily be closed within the euphotic layer, particularly via eating away of live, instead of dead individuals and their excretions. According to observational data, the share of primary production in the ocean actually consumed by the microconsumers (which eat live cells of phytoplankton) amounts to about 10 %, while that share does not exceed 1 % on land (Whittaker and Likens, 1975) (see Table 5.1). However, that does not violate the distribution (Fig. 1.3) in the ocean, since the major part of the oceanic heterotrophs is composed of the smallest invertebrate individuals (Neshyba, 1987; Kamenir, 1991).

The major part (about 90 %) of all the primary product of the ocean is absorbed however in the detritic channel as dead particles and dissolved organic matter (Khailov, 1971; Toggweiler, 1990). Hence, to support the existing hereditary organization (the genetic information) in the phytoplankton, the decay level of its genome (that is the relative number of individuals in the following generation containing new deleterious decay substitutions, absent in the preceding genera tion) should remain below 0.1 (that is with respect to the number of individuals in algae, eaten alive by heterotrophs). That situation is provided for via the small size of the algae genome, see Sect. 3.4. The single cell algae have a genome which is significantly smaller than that of the multicellular algae (Lewis et al., 1986). It follows then that oceanic phytoplankton should consist mainly of single cell algae, which agrees with observations. In those few areas of oceanic pelagial where the algae consist mainly of multicellular individuals (e.g., in the Sargasso Sea) and feature a larger genome and, hence, higher decay levels, the share of algae eaten alive by the small size heterotrophs should be significantly larger (see Fig. 1.3).

The condition in (4.8.3) is satisfied for heterotrophs by their vertical migrations, because their reproduction time is increased an order of magnitude, as compared to algae (Whittaker and Likens, 1975), because they spend little time at the surface, and also because they may rise to the surface in calm weather, when the surface eddy diffusivity decreases.

Advantages related to the predominant eating out of the decay individuals in algae may only be manifested when it results in an improvement of state of the environment (within the sensitivity, or resolution of the biota) in the range occupied by the given community. That improvement should refer to organic food of heterotrophs, to inorganic fodder of algae, to chemical composition of the environment, etc. Quite similar to the situation with both inorganic and organic nutrients, this requires the condition of global accumulation (4.6.6) to be satisfied. At large values of $\nu_{\alpha\,in}^+$ zooplankton cannot change the population number density of either decay or normal individuals of phytoplankton to such an extent that it would differ by a factor of several units within and outside the local ecosystem. However, if it is capable of lowering the density of the decay individuals, and, hence, to increase the density of the normal individuals by the relative value of $\varepsilon_\alpha \equiv \Delta[\alpha]/[\alpha]$, such that the environment is improved by a value exceeding the threshold sensitivity of the biota, $\varepsilon_{\alpha\,min}$, that would effect a net flux outside the local ecosystem consisting of normal individuals (that is the difference $F_{\alpha\,in}^+ - F_{\alpha\,out}^+$). That condition may be written, similar to (4.6.6):

$$\nu_{\alpha\,in}^+\varepsilon_{\alpha\,min} \leq 1, \quad \nu_{\alpha\,in}^+ \gg 1, \quad \varepsilon_{\alpha\,min} < \varepsilon_\alpha \equiv \frac{\Delta[\alpha]}{[\alpha]}. \tag{4.8.4}$$

To organize a community of a horizontal size $L \sim 10\,$m, a vertical size $H \sim 100\,$m, at a value of $\nu_{\alpha\,in}^+ \sim 10$ in the open ocean, it is enough to satisfy the condition $\varepsilon_{\alpha\,min} \leq 10^{-1}$. That means that a decrease in the number of decay individuals by 10% should bring about a noticeable improvement in the local environment. Actually the sensitivity of the biota is apparently much higher, and we have $\varepsilon_{\alpha\,min} \sim 10^{-4}$ (Sect. 4.6). Therefore a value $\nu_{\alpha\,min}^+ \leq 10^4$ is enough to satisfy the condition (4.8.4). Thus the condition of global accumulation of phytoplankton is satisfied in the ocean to a good safety margin (up to mean surface diffusivity $D \sim 10^9\,$m^2/year).

Thus the individuals of algae phytoplankton do not belong to any definite community and are not contained in any given domain occupied by any given local ecosystem during their lifespan by all appearances. Intraspecies' competitive interaction and stabilizing biological selection are completely switched off within each species of phytoplankton. Only rigid physical selection is left, accompanied by elimination of lethal mutations, incapable of supporting correlation relations with other species, that is of supporting both stabilization of the environment and of the community. Correlated interaction between the zooplankton belonging to a given local ecosystem and the phytoplankton results in purifying the physical flux of algae passing through the local ecosystem of the decay individuals. As a result each local ecosystem is a source of normal individuals of phytoplankton, which is the factor supporting the level of organization of the global population of algae in the ocean. The decay communities of zooplankton, incapable of eliminating the decay individuals from phytoplankton, locally perturb the environment, lose their competitive interaction and are ousted by the normal communities.

The mechanisms of stabilization of the organization of life, of the type of "artificial selection", are encountered during interactions of the "predator-prey" type, and the controlling species may then be both the predator and the prey (see Sect. 4.5). (The well known Lotka-Volterra model of self-regulation predator-prey population numbers (Lotka, 1925; Maynard Smith, 1974) do not contain the controlling species and apparently have no connection with the real natural community.) Besides, the support of the stabilization program, which is responsible for preservation of the environment, lies with the controlling species for all the major animals. These consume the major portion of energy and matter fluxes in the community. Among such controlling species are the edifier plants, bacteria, fungi, and minor invertebrates (cf. Sects. 5.5 and 5.6, and Fig. 5.3). Major animals have feeding grounds (home ranges) exceeding by far the size of local ecosystems. Thus a large animal cannot belong to any one single community. The organization of large animals (Chap. 5) is supported along the same principles which govern the concentration of the globally accumulated nutrients, and the organization of phytoplankton in the open ocean.

4.9 The Biological Pump of Atmospheric Carbon

As demonstrated in Sect. 4.8, the support of genetically stable life in the ocean is based on absorption by heterotrophs, i.e. by zooplankton and nekton (that is by locomotive individuals) inhabiting the oceanic depths, of a considerable portion of dead organic matter synthesized in the euphotic layer. As a result, the two domains – of synthesis of the organic matter, and of its destruction – are spatially separated in the vertical, which results in typical profiles of all the nutrients in the ocean. To keep the matter cycles closed and concentration profiles stable in both organic and inorganic matter, the flux of organic matter precipitating into oceanic depths should be compensated by a back flux of inorganic matter brought up into the euphotic zone. That is why that part of primary production, which originates from consumption of nutrients entering the euphotic zone from below, is called "new production" (Dugdale and Goering, 1967). The rate of total ("gross") photosynthesis, less phytoplankton respiration, is called the net production. The ratio of new production to total (gross) production is called the f-ratio. Recycled nitrogen in the euphotic layer exists as ammonia (NH_4^+), whereas the "new" nitrogen exists in the form of nitrate (NO_3^-), so the f-ratio is traditionally measured as the relative

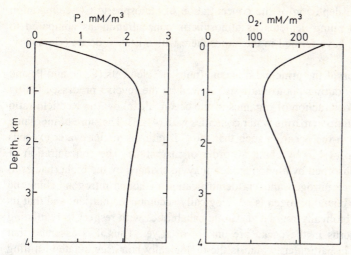

Fig. 4.2. The observed change in oceanic concentrations of dissolved inorganic phosphorus and oxygen with depth. Observational data averaged over the world ocean are given (Takahashi et al., 1981; Levitus, 1982; Bolin et al., 1982, 1983; Sarmiento et al., 1988).

phytoplankton uptake rates of the ^{15}N-labelled nitrate and ammonia (Dugdale and Goering, 1967). Prediction of the 'f-ratio following either first principles or empirical observations is still elusive (Eppley and Peterson, 1979; Platt et al., 1989; Sarmiento et al., 1989).

The upflux of inorganic nutrients into the euphotic zone is mainly supported via eddy diffusion, i.e., via the emergent gradients in concentrations of all the nutrients, see Fig. 4.2. The concentrations of the N and P nutrients upwelling into the euphotic zone from below increase downward. In contrast, the concentration of oxygen, penetrating the zone of oxidation from the above, drops off with depth, Fig. 4.2.

In the absence of life, the nutrients would have been evenly distributed within the whole oceanic depth, and their surface and deep concentrations would have eventually evened out. Hence life operates as a biological pump, which brings inorganic nutrients into the oceanic depths from the surface. The term "biological pump" is associated with the name of Roger Revelle (see, for example, McElroy, 1986). However, no specific reference is usually given. The action of that pump is related to "new" production. Were the whole community to stratify within the well mixed euphotic zone, the action of that biological pump would have stopped. As demonstrated below, the latter presumption is actually impossible, due to the inevitable decay of the community, of life, and of the environment as a whole.

Nonvolatile dissolved inorganic nutrients in the form of NO_3^- and PO_4^{3-} are redistributed by the biota within the ocean only. Meanwhile the inorganic carbon dissolved in the oceanic surface layer is at physico-chemical equilibrium with atmospheric CO_2. Following Henry's Law, the depletion of CO_2 dissolved in surface water results in a depletion of the concentration of atmospheric CO_2. Operation of the biological pump depletes its atmospheric concentration, as compared to that which would have formed in the atmosphere with a lifeless ocean (Gorshkov, 1979, 1983a).

The absorption of the principal biogenic (nutrient) elements (C, N, and P) and the release of O_2 during photosynthesis, as well as the reverse processes taking place during the destruction of organics in the ocean, all follow the Redfield ratio (4.4.3). The N/P ratio in marine water coincides with (4.4.3). The store of inorganic matter dissolved in the ocean is such that the C/P ratio in marine water exceeds the Redfield ratio (4.4.3) by about an order of magnitude. The concentration of bound nitrogen absorbed by phytoplankton may be changed by the biota (bacteria) via fixation of free nitrogen and via denitrification of bound nitrogen. Thus one may assume that bound nitrogen is a biologically accumulated nutrient and that its concentration is biotically regulated. Biotic capabilities with respect to regulating the total phosphorus in the ocean are unknown as yet. Thus it is assumed that it is phosphorus in particular, which is the biologically non-accumulated limiting factor. The total nitrogen in the ocean is accumulated by the biota following the Redfield ratio (4.4.3), while the total dissolved inorganic carbon is in excess and hence cannot be regulated by the biota either.

If this is the case, the net primary production should be proportional to the concentration of phosphorus in the euphotic layer. The principal step in concentration of phosphorus is observed at depths within 500 m (Neshyba, 1987). Thus uniform mixing of the ocean would not have resulted in any significant difference of concentration of phosphorus from its present concentration at depths. Were the new production absent ($f = 0$) and were all the nutrients there homogeneously mixed, the net primary production in the ocean would have settled at a level controlled by the concentration of phosphorus at depths, which is an order of magnitude higher than the observed surface one. The net oceanic production would then also become an order of magnitude higher than is observed, and would have reached the level compatible with the maximum observed photosynthesis efficiency (see Chap. 5). Hence, the store of phosphorus in the ocean is such that the limiting factor in the absence of new production is light instead of phosphorus. The very fact that there is just as much phosphorus as the biota needs, instead of an order of magnitude more or less, testifies that the store of phosphorus in the ocean has apparently been formed by the biota and is still controlled by it, although the exact mechanism of that control is not presently known. Thus there are no grounds for assuming that phosphorus is a limiting factor, or that the maximum production by the biota is limited by the store of phosphorus. On the contrary, it is natural to assume that, being limited by the availability of solar light alone, it settles at a level, optimal and different for each specific environment (such as land, the open ocean, the shelf, the zones of upwelling, etc.), which yields the most efficient biotic control of environmental conditions liable to such control at all. The concentrations of all the nutrients are biologically accumulated then and are kept at levels that the biota prescribes itself.

The new production and the biological pump are switched on by the biota owing to the need to support the biological stability of the genetic structure of communities of the open ocean, which control the state of the environment. Switching on the biological pump lowers the surface concentration of phosphorus and the net primary production. There is no ground for assuming that the level of that new production reaches its maximum everywhere, compatible to that minimal concentration of phosphorus in the euphotic layer, at which the oceanic biota is still capable of functioning. Most probably the relative value of new production (that is, the f-ratio) may be changed by the biota within rather a wide margin (Eppley and Peterson, 1979), within which an efficient stabilization is provided of both the genetic structure of the communities and of the optimal environmental conditions.

We are going to demonstrate, in what is to follow, that the store of dissolved inorganic carbon in the ocean is also not excessive for the existing biota, but is supported by it at a certain level, which apparently provides for an optimal functioning of the oceanic biota, including such parameters as the atmospheric concentration of CO_2, and, hence, the temperature of the surface euphotic layer.

The inorganic carbon dissolved in the ocean mainly enters it as bicarbonate (HCO_3^-) and carbonate (CO_3^{2-}) ions. The surface concentration of the dissolved carbon dioxide (or the partial pressure of CO_2 molecules, which is proportional to the former) reaches only half of one per cent of the total concentration of inorganic carbon, denoted as ΣCO_2 (Ivanoff, 1972, 1975; Keeling, 1973):

$$\underset{2.0}{\Sigma[CO_2]} = \underset{1.8}{[HCO_3^-]} + \underset{0.2}{[CO_3^{2-}]} + \underset{0.01}{[CO_2]} \quad \text{mol C/m}^3. \tag{4.9.1}$$

Typical values of the respective concentrations are shown here for the surface oceanic layer, see Fig. 4.3. All the compounds of the dissolved organic carbon are in a state of chemical equilibrium and suffer certain changes when the concentration $[CO_2]$ changes, the latter being in a steady state and in physical equilibrium with the atmospheric concentration of that gas, $[CO_2]_a$.

The relation between the relative changes of $[\Sigma CO_2]$ and $[CO_2]$ is of the scaling character (see (2.6.4) and (2.6.7)) in which the proportionality coefficient ζ is called the buffer factor (or the Revelle factor, see Keeling, 1973):

$$\frac{\Delta[CO_2]}{[CO_2]} = \zeta \frac{\Delta[\Sigma CO_2]}{[\Sigma CO_2]}. \tag{4.9.2}$$

The buffer factor ζ may be calculated from the conditions of chemical equilibrium and of electric neutrality of a macroscopic volume of sea water. It may also be measured directly. According to these measurements the buffer factor ζ varies from about 9 to 15 in various regions of the world ocean, dependent on water temperature, deviating by no more than 30 % from its average of $\zeta = 10$ (Broecker et al., 1979).

Thus, a 10 % change in $[CO_2]$ entails a 1 % change in $[\Sigma CO_2]$ only. Such an inertia of change in $[CO_2]$ is explained by the fact that electrical neutrality of sea water is supported by a certain concentration of positive ions A^+ (by alkalinity),

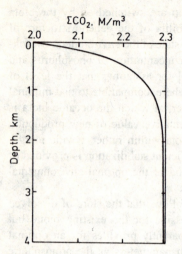

Fig. 4.3. The observed profile of the dissolved inorganic carbon $[\Sigma CO_2]$ in the world ocean. See legend to Fig. 4.2.

which does not change with changing CO_2 concentration in water. The carbonate alkalinity A_C^+:

$$A_C^+ = HCO_3^- + 2\,CO_3^{2-} \tag{4.9.3}$$

amounts to more than 70 % of the total (titrated) alkalinity A^+ in the ocean.

The concentration of hydrogen ions H^+ is five orders of magnitude lower than A^+ (Keeling, 1973). Thus the change in ΣCO_2 may principally occur due to redistribution of concentrations of HCO_3^- and CO_3^{2-}, with the total negative charge of molecules remaining intact. For example, following the addition of a given number of molecules of CO_2, an equal number of CO_3^{2-} ions may vanish, with a doubled number of HCO_3^- ions appearing in their place according to the reaction:

$$H_2O + CO_2 + CO_3^{2-} = 2\,HCO_3^-. \tag{4.9.4}$$

Due to the low value of the $[CO_3^{2-}]/[HCO_3^-]$ ratio the concentration of $[HCO_3^-]$ increases but only quite weakly, and that illustrates the fact that the buffer factor ζ is indeed quite large.

Redistribution of all the other ions (among which the borate present in sea water plays the most important role) does not contribute more than 20 % to all the measurable values (Maier-Reimer and Hasselmann, 1987). According to the Le Chatelier principle, extracting the ions of CO_3^{2-} from the surface water shifts the reaction to the left and the concentration of CO_2 in water increases. The ions of CO_3^{2-} vanish via formation of $CaCO_3$, which is used by the biota to form shells (Neshyba, 1987). That process results in lower alkalinity, A^+. (A significantly weaker change of alkalinity accompanies fixation of the NO_3^- and PO_4^{3-} ions by phytoplankton.) Inversely, at those large depths where the concentration of CO_2 builds up, individual shells consisting of $CaCO_3$ are dissolved, which shifts reaction (4.9.4) to the right, depleting the concentration of CO_2 and raising alkalinity A^+. That process describes the biological alkalinity pump. It works to decrease alkalinity at the surface and to increase it at depth. Simultaneously it operates against the biological pump of carbon: it decreases the concentration of CO_2 at depth and builds it up at the surface. However, its contribution to the total consumption of carbon remains below 20% of the total consumption of carbon during the synthesis of new production. Thus the relative change of alkalinity during biological reactions is approximately five times as low as the relative change of ΣCO_2 (see, for instance, Sarmiento et al., 1988).

The whole chemistry of carbon in the ocean is characterized by two independent variables, the total (titrated) alkalinity, A^+, and ΣCO_2 usually being selected. The concentration of CO_2 is thus a unique function of ΣCO_2 and A^+. If A^+ remains constant, ΣCO_2 appears to be a unique function of CO_2 only, and hence of atmospheric CO_2 (Degens et al., 1984).

The change in concentration of CO_2 may be calculated either from its known functional dependence on ΣCO_2 and A^+, or via the buffer factor (4.9.2). To the accuracy of terms of the order of 20%, the dependence of buffer factor ζ on ΣCO_2 and A^+ may be expressed via expansion into the inverse ratio $[HCO_3^-]/[CO_3^{2-}]$, see (4.9.1) (Gorshkov, 1979, 1986b):

$$\zeta = \frac{[HCO_3^-]}{[CO_3^{2-}]} + 5 + o\left(\frac{[CO_3^{2-}]}{[HCO_3^-]}\right). \tag{4.9.5}$$

The observed concentration of ΣCO_2 at large depth is 15% higher than in the surface oceanic layer. In the approximation of constant buffer factor ζ we have:

$$\frac{[CO_2]}{[CO_2]_0} = \left(\frac{[\Sigma CO_2]}{[\Sigma CO_2]_0}\right)^\zeta \approx 1 + \zeta \frac{\Delta[\Sigma CO_2]}{[\Sigma CO_2]_0}, \tag{4.9.6}$$

where $\Delta[\Sigma CO_2] = [\Sigma CO_2] - [\Sigma CO_2]_0$, and concentrations in the surface oceanic layer are indexed with "0". Hence, with the increase of $[\Sigma CO_2]$ by 15% the concentration of $[CO_2]$ increases by a factor of 2.5. The dependence of the buffer factor on CO_2 concentration somewhat increases the last figure. Thus the deep layer concentration of the dissolved carbon dioxide is several times higher than the surface one. At the same time the surface concentration of CO_2 is at equilibrium with the atmospheric value. If life in the ocean ceased, all the concentrations in both the surface and deep layers would even out. Then the concentration of CO_2 in both the surface oceanic layer and the atmosphere would increase severalfold! That could well bring about a catastrophic change in the level of greenhouse effect and in climate within the mixing time of that oceanic layer, in which such gradients of nutrients are observed, see Fig. 4.3. This mixing time is of the order of several hundreds of years (Degens et al., 1984). Hence, the oceanic biota keeps both the atmospheric concentration of CO_2 and the surface temperature at a level fit for life.

The store of inorganic carbon dissolved in the ocean in the form of bicarbonate and carbonate ions, residing at chemical equilibrium with the dissolved CO_2, is

60 times as large as its store in the preindustrial atmosphere, see (4.9.1). Thus terminating oceanic life, while at the same time keeping the total carbon in both the atmosphere and ocean intact, and tripling the atmospheric concentration of carbon would result in only a 3 % decrease in the average concentration of CO_2 in the ocean.

The store of dissolved organic carbon in the ocean coincides with the store of atmospheric carbon (Toggweiler, 1990, Sect. 4.11), and hence is 60 times lower than the store of ΣCO_2. At first glance that violates the condition in (4.6.6) for biologically regulated nutrients. However the considered chemistry of the ocean indicates that the store of inorganic carbon available for biotic use appears to be significantly less than the total store of ΣCO_2, and is of the same order of magnitude as the store of organic carbon, so that the relation in (4.6.6) still appears to be satisfied. If a given mass (m_s^+) of the dissolved organic carbon goes through decay, the emerging inorganic carbon is distributed between the atmosphere (m_a^-) and ocean (m_s^-).

The ratio of change in concentration of the atmospheric CO_2 to ΣCO_2 in the ocean is equal, in agreement with (4.9.2):

$$\frac{\Delta[CO_2]_a}{\Delta[\Sigma CO_2]} = \xi \zeta \approx \frac{1}{20}, \qquad \xi \equiv \frac{[CO_2]_{a0}}{[\Sigma CO_2]_0} \approx \frac{1}{200}, \tag{4.9.7}$$

which accounts for the fact that the average solubility (that is the ratio between the equilibrium CO_2 concentrations in air and water) $b \equiv [CO_2]/[CO_2]_a$ is close to unity (Broecker and Peng, 1974). The volume of atmosphere scaled to surface average air pressure ($V_a = 4.2 \times 10^{18} \, m^3$) is three times as large as that of the ocean ($V_s = 1.4 \times 10^{18} \, m^3$). Thus after an equilibrium settles between the ocean and the atmosphere, the distribution of either excess or deficit of carbon will hold at a ratio of 1/6 (Oeschger et al., 1975; Siegenthaler and Oeschger, 1978; Gorshkov, 1982c):

$$\frac{m_a^-}{m_s^-} \approx \frac{1}{6}, \quad m_a \equiv V_a \Delta[CO_2]_a, \quad m_s \equiv V_s \Delta[CO_2]_s. \tag{4.9.8}$$

The absorption of inorganic carbon from the atmosphere into the ocean follows the same ratio when the store of the dissolved organic carbon is built up via its excess biological production.

Thus the oceanic biota affects the atmospheric concentration of CO_2 in two different ways. The first is related to change in the intensity of the biological pump at a constant ratio between the masses of organic and inorganic carbon in the environment. The second is related to possibility of the partial transfer of organic carbon to inorganic and back. Both are apparently used by oceanic biota to support environmental conditions at a level optimal for life.

4.10 Atmospheric Concentration of CO_2 and New Production by the Ocean

Increase in atmospheric CO_2, entailed by the depletion of new production, may be quantitatively estimated from the data on the gradient of ΣCO_2 and from the value of the buffer factor, ζ. The possible depletion of atmospheric CO_2 accompanying increased new production is related to observed concentrations of phosphorus and nitrogen via the Redfield ratio (Gorshkov, 1982c, 1984a).

One may average the studied oceanic region over seasonal variations and over large enough area of water, such that the horizontal transport of nutrients becomes small compared to the total vertical transport. Then all the variables entering our relations will depend on depth Z alone. We denote net fluxes of both organic and inorganic nutrient X (either C, N, or P) through a unit horizontal plane at depth Z as $F_X^+(Z)$ and $F_X^-(Z)$, respectively. Depth Z increases from the surface down. The downward flux of organics goes along the positive Z coordinate, and the upward flux of inorganic matter goes against that coordinate. An equality should be satisfied for the case of constant annual average masses of organic and inorganic carbon within arbitrary oceanic volumes at every depth Z (cf. (4.3.1)):

$$F_X^+(Z) + F_X^-(Z) = 0. \tag{4.10.1}$$

The flux of inorganic nutrient is mainly of diffusive nature and is controlled by its concentration gradient:

$$F_X^-(Z) = -(D(Z))\frac{\partial}{\partial Z}[X(Z)], \tag{4.10.2}$$

where $D(Z)$ is eddy diffusivity, averaged over the surface and over seasonal oscillations; it may be assumed identical for every dissolved substance.

Assuming that all the synthesis of the organic matter is concentrated at the surface at $Z = L^+ = 0$ (note that the actual distribution of photosynthetic activity with depth is accounted for in studies by Gorshkov (1982c, 1984a) and Lewis et al.(1986), which does not affect the treatment to follow), we find that the change of $F^-(Z)$ following the passage through a layer of unit thickness is equal to the density of destruction of the organic matter in that layer $b(Z)$:

$$-\frac{\partial}{\partial Z}F^-(Z) = b(Z) = \frac{\partial}{\partial Z}F^+(Z). \tag{4.10.3}$$

The new production of the ocean per unit area of water, P_n^+, and the flux of the newly generated "new" inorganic carbon, P_n^-, equal to the former (see (4.11.5)), is described by:

$$P_n^- = P_n^+ = fP_g^+ = \int_0^H b(Z')dZ' = F^+(0), \tag{4.10.4}$$

where H is that depth at which these concentration gradients become zero, P_g^+ is the gross (total) primary production of the ocean. Measuring $b(Z)$ and $F^-(Z)$ at various depths, eddy diffusivity $D(Z)$ may be found (Oeschger et al., 1975), and the values of new production P_n^+ and of the f-ratio may be estimated.

The average depth at which new production is destroyed is given by:

$$L^- = \frac{1}{P_n^-} \int_0^H Z' b(Z') dZ'. \tag{4.10.5}$$

We assume that the destruction of new production is completely localized at depth L^-:

$$b(Z) = P_n^- \delta(Z - L^-), \qquad F^-(Z) = P_n^- \vartheta(L^- - Z), \tag{4.10.6}$$

where $\delta(Z) = \frac{\partial}{\partial Z} \vartheta(Z)$ is the Dirac delta-function, $\vartheta(Z)$ is the step function: $\vartheta(Z) = 1$ for $Z \geq 0$, and $\vartheta(Z) = 0$ for $Z < 0$.

That approximation corresponds to constant flux of inorganic nutrients in the ocean (that is a flux independent of Z), such that the observed change in the gradient of nutrient X is compensated by a respective change of eddy diffusivity:

$$F_X^-(Z) = -D(Z) \frac{\partial}{\partial Z} [X(Z)] = \begin{cases} P_n^+, & L^- > Z > 0 \\ 0, & Z < L^-. \end{cases} \tag{4.10.7}$$

Integrating (4.10.7) we find:

$$P_{nX}^+ = \frac{\Delta X}{R_e}, \quad \Delta[X] \equiv [X]_d - [X]_s; \; [X]_s \equiv [X(0)], \; [X]_d = [X(L_-)], \tag{4.10.8}$$

$$R_e = \int_0^{L^-} \frac{dZ}{D(Z)} \approx \frac{L^- - L_s}{D_e} + \frac{L_s - L^+}{D_s} \approx \frac{L_e}{D_e}, \tag{4.10.9}$$

$L_e = L^- - L_s \approx L^-$; $L^- \sim 200\text{--}500\,\text{m}$, $L_s \sim 75\,\text{m}$, $D_s \gg D_e$, $D_e \approx 6 \times 10^3\,\text{m}^2/\text{year}$, $R \sim 30\,\text{m/year}$, where L_s is the depth of the well mixed surface layer, D_e and D_s are eddy diffusivities in deep and surface layers, respectively (Ivanoff, 1972, 1975; Oeschger et al., 1975; Broecker et al., 1985b; Neshyba, 1987), [X] is the concentration of nutrient X at depths, L_e is the effective depth above which the gradient of nutrient concentration is observed (Neshyba, 1987).

The gross P_{gX}^+ and new P_{nX}^+ primary productions may, as a general case, be written as (cf. (4.6.3)):

$$P_{gX}^+ \equiv \frac{[X]_s}{R_{gX}} = f^{-1} P_{nX}^+, \quad P_{nX}^+ = \frac{[X]_s}{R_{nX}}, \quad R_{nX} \equiv \frac{R_{gX}}{f}, \tag{4.10.10}$$

where (4.10.10) is a definition of the internal resistances R_{gX}, and R_{nX} which may be a function of concentration $[X]_s$. When the concentration $[X]_s$ is far from saturation, the value of R_{gX} is constant. In saturation mode R_{gX} is proportional to concentration [X], so that production does not depend on concentration (Hochachka and Somero, 1973).

Equating P_{nX}^+ in (4.10.10) and (4.10.8) we have:

$$P_{nX}^+ = \frac{\cdot [X]_d}{R_e + R_{nX}}, \quad \left([X]_s = [X]_d \frac{R_{nX}}{R_e + R_{nX}}\right). \tag{4.10.11}$$

Concentrations of inorganic nutrients in oceanic depths, $[X]_d$, are defined by the total store of nitrogen and phosphorus at those depths. The biota is incapable of changing concentration $[X]_d$ via changing the intensity of the biological pump (working at constant mass of the dissolved organic matter). If one assumes a constant internal resistance R_{gX}, independent of surface concentration $[X]_s$ (Lewis et al., 1986), the biota appears to be capable of changing $[X]_s$ via changing the average depth at which the heterotrophs reside, L_e, hence changing external resistance R_e (see (4.10.11)). With L_e increasing at constant eddy diffusivity, the external resistance increases, and the diffusional flux of nutrients, the new production, and the intensity of the biological pump all decrease. The surface concentration falls too. The f-ratio being constant, the gross production is also bound to drop. The latter refers to phosphorus as well. If one assumes that new production of nitrogen is controlled by the absorption of NO_3^-, while the gross production is controlled by cumulative absorption of NH_4^+ and NO_3^- at different internal resistances $R_{gNH_4^+}$ and $R_{gNO_3^-}$, then, at lower surface concentration of NO_3^- and decreasing new production, the gross production may only insignificantly change at a constant concentration of NH_4^+. The f-ratio should then decrease in proportion to the concentration of NO_3^- (Lewis et al., 1986). The surface concentration of nutrient $[X]_s$, that is the level of water oligotrophicity is regulated by heterotrophs residing at depth. Hence, water oligotrophicity at constant deep water diffusivity is controlled by the biota, instead of abiotic conditions at the oceanic surface, such as temperature, solar radiation, etc.

Biotic regulation of surface concentration $[X]_s$ is also possible via transfer to a saturation regime, controlled by the phytoplankton, when resistance to nutrient consumption R_{gX} varies in proportion to its concentration. If $R_{gX} \ll R_e$ and f is constant, such a situation should result in both new and gross production by phytoplankton remaining constant. The depth at which heterotrophs reside, and the intensity of the biological pump, should then also remain without changes.

Thus in every case both the oligotrophicity of oceanic surface waters and the surface concentrations $[X]_s$ of nutrients are completely controlled by oceanic biota.

New production of nitrogen and phosphorus has the form (4.10.8), (4.10.10), or (4.10.11), since phytoplankton in the surface layer consumes the same compounds, which are transported within the oceanic depths by eddy diffusion. However, ΣCO_2 is also transported in the ocean by eddy diffusion but, similar to land biota, phytoplankton consumes molecules of CO_2 (Degens et al., 1968; Gorshkov, 1987a). That conclusion follows from the fact that atmospheric and oceanic dissolved CO_2 have identical $^{13}C/^{12}C$ ratios. In oceanic and land biota that ratio is 18% lower, and in ΣCO_2 it is 9% higher than in the atmosphere. Were the oceanic vegetation to use ΣCO_2 for photosynthesis, the $^{13}C/^{12}C$ ratio in it would have to be 9% higher than in land biota, which is not the case (Gorshkov, 1987a). Shells of marine animals (e.g., mollusk shells, lime coral skeletons, etc.) are built without the process of photosynthesis, directly from ΣCO_2, and thus their $^{13}C/^{12}C$ ratio is higher than in organic matter (Druffel and Benavides, 1986).

Thus one should set $X = CO_2$ in (4.10.10) and $X = CO_2$ in (4.10.8):

$$P_{Cn}^+ = \frac{[\Sigma CO_2]_0 - [\Sigma CO_2]_s}{R_e} = \frac{[CO_2]_d - [CO_2]_s}{\xi \zeta R_e}; \quad \xi \equiv \frac{[CO_2]_s}{[\Sigma CO_2]_s} \quad (4.10.8a)$$

$$P_{Cn}^{+} = \frac{[CO_2]_s}{R_{nC}}, \qquad R_{nC} = \frac{R_{gC}}{f}. \tag{4.10.10a}$$

Equating (4.10.8a) and (4.10.10a) we find:

$$P_{Cn}^{+} = \frac{[CO_2]_d}{(\xi\zeta R_e + R_{nC})}. \tag{4.10.11a}$$

For $X = N$ and $X = P$, the concentrations at depth are about ten times as high as at the surface. That means that the external resistance to diffusion R_e is about ten times as high as the internal one, R_{nX}. The coincidence of surface concentrations of N and P means that their internal resistances coincide with each other: $R_{nN} = R_{nP}$. The observed ratio C/N/P is 40/16/1. Hence, the concentration of CO_2 is approximately three times as low as that necessary to satisfy the Redfield ratio (4.4.4). That means, in turn, that the internal resistance to CO_2 consumption is the lowest, i.e. $R_{gC} \approx (1/3)(R_{gX})$, $(X = N, P)$, so that sensitivity of the biota to changes in CO_2 concentration is the highest. The effective external resistance to "penetration" of CO_2 is decreased by a factor of $\xi\zeta \approx 1/20$, as compared to external resistance to penetration of ΣCO_2, N, and P, and becomes of the same order of magnitude as internal resistance R_{nC} in (4.10.11a). Under natural conditions all the internal resistances R_{gX} should be close to constant, while the difference between productivities and destructivities should alter following the law given by (4.4.1), the dimensionless constants β_X being of the order of 1. At $\beta_X = 1$ resistances R_{gX} are strictly constant. Specific values of β_X depend on the biota and on particularities of the natural environment. No nutrient may be considered limiting in that case: concentrations of all the nutrients are then supported by the biota at a level optimal for its functioning. It is only under environmental conditions drastically differing from the natural ones that particular nutrients may become limiting.

Under natural conditions the surface, and hence the atmospheric, concentration of CO_2 is uniquely related to surface and deep concentrations of N and P because the Redfield ratio is satisfied. Using (4.10.10), (4.10.11), and (4.10.11a) we have (see Gorshkov, 1982c; Gorshkov and Kondratiev, 1990):

$$[CO_2]_a = \frac{1}{b}\left(\frac{C}{X}\right)\frac{[X]_d R_{nC}}{R_e + R_{nX}}, \quad [X]_s = \frac{[X]_d R_{nX}}{R_e + R_{nX}} \approx [X]_d \frac{R_{nX}}{R_e}$$

$$[CO_2]_a = \frac{1}{b}\left(\frac{C}{X}\right)\frac{[X]_s R_{gC}}{R_{gX}}, \quad X = N, P; \quad R_{nX} = \frac{R_{gX}}{f}, \tag{4.10.12}$$

where $b = [CO_2]_s/[CO_2]_a$ is the solubility of CO_2, and the ratio C/X corresponds to (4.4.4). With concentrations of both nitrogen and phosphorus at depth (they practically coincide with average concentrations of these elements in the ocean), and external resistance (which is controlled by eddy diffusivity) all remaining fixed, the concentration of atmospheric CO_2 is controlled by the f-ratio and by the internal resistance R_{gC} to absorption of CO_2. At $f \to 0$ we have $[CO_2]_a = [CO_2]_{max}$, while at $f \to 1$ we have $[CO_2]_a = [CO_2]_{min}$:

$$[CO_2]_{a\,max} = \frac{1}{b}\left(\frac{C}{X}\right)[X]_d\frac{R_{gC}}{R_{gX}},\tag{4.10.13}$$

$$[CO_2]_{a\,min} = \frac{1}{b}\left(\frac{C}{X}\right)[X]_d\frac{R_{gC}}{(R_e+R_{gX})} \approx \frac{1}{b}\left(\frac{C}{X}\right)[X]_a\frac{R_{gC}}{R_e},\tag{4.10.14}$$

The maximum scope of changes in $[CO_2]_a$ is:

$$\frac{[CO_2]_{a\,max}}{[CO_2]_{a\,min}} = \frac{R_e+R_{gX}}{R_{gX}} = \frac{R_e}{R_{gX}}+1 \approx \frac{R_e}{R_{gX}} \approx 10.\tag{4.10.15}$$

With eddy diffusion growing, R_e falls and $[CO_2]_a$ increases respectively. If both the f-ratio and R_e remain fixed the change in $[CO_2]_a$ may only take place due to the change in inner resistances. The decrease in R_{gX} entails lower surface concentrations $[X]_s$, $X = N, P$. However bringing those values down to zero can only lower $[CO_2]_a$ by 10% maximum, since the observed ratio is $[X]_s/[X]_d = R_{nX}/R_e \sim 0.1$.

If one assumes the surface concentration $[X]_s$ fixed, $[CO_2]_a$ appears independent of R_e and f:

$$[CO_2]_a = \frac{1}{b}\left(\frac{C}{X}\right)[X]_s\frac{R_{gC}}{R_{gX}} = \frac{1}{b}\left(\frac{C}{X}\right)R_{gC}P_{gX}^+.\tag{4.10.16}$$

Instead it is controlled exclusively by internal resistances, that is by gross primary production. In reality, surface concentrations do not vary at low latitudes, where most of the ocean surface is found. The concentration $[CO_2]_a$ at low latitudes may only be increased (via lowering of the f-ratio).

Thermohaline overturning results in submergence of large masses of cold water to depth in high latitudes of the Antarctic circumpolar ocean ($\sim 10^{15}$ m^3/year, which is about 30 Sverdrups, 1 Sverdrup = 10^6 m^3/s, Stuiver and Quay, 1983; Neshyba, 1987), these masses then being distributed and upwelled to the surface over the whole world ocean surface area. The average rate of such upwelling is of the order of 2 m/year over the whole world ocean surface area, which is much less than the inverse external resistance: $R_e^{-1} \sim 30$ m/year, see (4.10.9). Thus transport of nutrients due to water upwelling is low compared to diffusional transport and may be neglected in (4.10.2). Surface concentrations of N and P in cold waters are almost five times as high as those in warm waters. Quick submergence of cold surface waters results in higher f-ratio in these waters (Eppley and Peterson, 1979).

Assuming the relative surface of cold waters to be equal to 10% of the total surface of the world ocean we find that a fivefold lowering of the surface concentration of nutrients in cold waters would result in the average surface concentration of nutrients globally lowering by a factor of 1.5. That would result in a respective increase of oceanic gross production at fixed internal resistances, and, in accordance with (4.10.16), would bring about a lowering of $[CO_2]_a$. If one assumes the concentration of nutrients at depth to be constant, the surface concentrations of nutrients in warm and cold waters may only differ due to differences in internal resistances. In that case $[CO_2]_a$ may decrease due to lowering of internal resistances, R_{gX}, to increasing of f-ratio, and also to lowering of eddy diffusivity in cold waters, see (4.10.9) and (4.10.12).

Gorshkov (1979, 1982c) (see also Chen and Drake (1986)) commented on the possibility of stronger action of the biological pump for atmospheric CO_2, and hence of lowering of the concentration of atmospheric CO_2, due to decreases of the average surface concentrations of N and P in the ocean. The possible effect of higher oceanic productivity in subpolar ocean working to lower the concentration of atmospheric CO_2 was later noted by three separate study groups (Knox and McElroy, 1984; Sarmiento and Toggweiler, 1984; Siegenthaler and Wenk, 1984; see also McElroy, 1986; Sarmiento et al., 1988). They related the 30% decrease in atmospheric CO_2, as compared to its preindustrial level during the last ice age, to that particular process. Inversely, the drop in productivity of the polar ocean should have led to an increase in atmospheric CO_2 up to its observed preindustrial level. If one assumes that productivity increases with solar radiation, that would correspond to satisfying the Le Chatelier principle for oceanic biota: stronger solar radiation brings higher temperatures, and the increased production of the polar ocean lowers the concentration of atmospheric CO_2, so that temperature growth is compensated for.

4.11 Changing Production of Dissolved Organic Matter in the Ocean

The new production by oceanic biota keeps both the atmospheric and oceanic environment of living beings in a state which is strongly offset from its equilibrium, both physically and chemically. New production may vary, following the Le Chatelier principle, in response to variations in the solar activity (Berger, 1988). If matter cycles are closed, the balance between the synthesis and destruction of organic matter remains unchanged: change in new production is compensated by a respective change in its destruction, so that the mass of organic matter in the ocean remains unchanged. If one assumes that production in the ocean is limited by concentrations of nitrogen and phosphorus in the surface layer, and possibly by solar radiation in the subpolar oceanic surface area, while consumption of CO_2 occurs at saturation, then one concludes that oceanic biota is incapable of reacting to the observed increase of atmospheric CO_2. That popular opinion resulted in excluding oceanic biota from the possible candidates for the sink of atmospheric CO_2 (Degens et al., 1984; Prentice and Fung, 1990; Tans et al., 1990; Schlesinger, 1990; Falkowski and Wilson, 1992).

Discarding the concept of limiting nutrients and considering concentrations of all the nutrients as both formed and supported by the biota at levels optimal for it, call for a revision of that opinion. As demonstrated in the preceding section, the sensitivity of the biota to changes in concentration of CO_2 in the surface water is higher than its sensitivity to changes of concentrations of nitrogen and phosphorus, which are believed to be the limiting ones. It may thus be expected that the biota should react more efficiently to a relative perturbation of the atmospheric CO_2 at constant concentrations of nitrogen and phosphorus, than to equal relative perturbations of nitrogen and phosphorus at a constant concentration of CO_2. Here one should understand perturbation as external forcing, similar to anthropogenic distortion of the environment, instead of seasonal and geographic variations to which the natural biota should be adapted.

An enormous mass of dissolved organic carbon (DOC) is present in the ocean, which is one thousand times higher than the cumulative mass of all the living beings of the open ocean (Table 5.1) and which approximately (by order of magnitude) coincides with the mass of atmospheric carbon (Toggweiler, 1990; Druffel and Williams, 1990). While the state remains stationary, the dissolved organic carbon is very slowly destroyed to inorganic components and is as slowly produced. Its preindustrial production did not exceed 1 % of the net primary production of the ocean (Gorshkov, 1991b). So far the functional role of DOC in the ocean remains unclear. It is natural, however, to suggest that DOC is a reservoir controlled by oceanic biota, using which that biota is capable of sustaining optimal concentrations of inorganic nutrients in the environment.

The present-day mass of total oceanic DOC is about 2 Tt C, here the prefix tera $T \equiv 10^{12}$ (Sugimura and Suzuki, 1988; Druffel et al., 1989; Ogawa and Ogura, 1992; Martin and Fitzwater, 1992). The total DOC store ties up about 30 % of inorganic stores of phosphorus (~ 20 Gt P, see Fig. 4.2) and nitrogen (~ 700 Gt N, see (4.4.4)) in the world ocean and less than 5 % of the dissolved inorganic carbon (DIC or $\Sigma CO_2 \sim 40$ Tt C). It follows then that the biota of the ocean is capable, in principle, of increasing DOC by almost three times, at the same time keeping the ratios in (4.4.4) intact. The store of DIC should then decrease by about 20 %. In accordance with the buffer relation, (4.9.12), that would lead to a multiple decrease of atmospheric CO_2. Inversely, shrinking DOC the biota is capable of increasing the atmospheric concentration of CO_2 by more than 100 %.

All the gross primary production by phytoplankton may take part in changing production of DOC. Thus the reaction of oceanic biota to change in production of DOC appears to be amplified by the factor of f^{-1}, as compared to the reaction of the ocean to change of the new production described in the preceding section. It all gives one grounds for assuming that the change in both production and mass of the DOC gives the biota a chance to control the state of the environment most efficiently (Gorshkov, 1979, 1982c, 1984a).

The oceanic measurements (Williams and Druffel, 1987; Druffel et al., 1989; Druffel and Williams, 1990) have made available vertical profiles of changes in radiocarbon in dissolved organic (DOC) and inorganic (DIC) carbon, see Fig. 4.4. Such data offer the possibility of finding the ratio between the preindustrial and present-day production of DOC in the ocean.

During the preindustrial era (and into the industrial era up to the start of nuclear tests) radiocarbon in both the organic and inorganic molecules had remained in stationary equilibrium. Its decay in the ocean was compensated by its inflow from the atmosphere. Carbon enters the ocean with molecules of $^{14}CO_2$ and $^{12}CO_2$

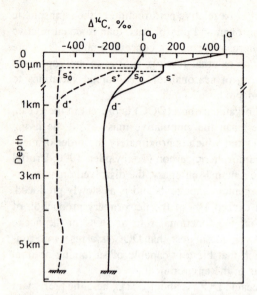

Fig. 4.4. The present-day and the preindustrial profiles of oceanic $\Delta^{14}C$. The solid line shows the dissolved inorganic carbon $(-)$, the dashed line dissolved organic carbon $(+)$. Symbol "s" indicates the present-day surface values, symbol "d" the values at depth. Symbol "a" stands for the atmospheric value, and "s_0" and "a_0" are the respective preindustrial values for carbon (Druffel and Williams, 1990; Gorshkov, 1991b, 1993a,b), see Appendix A.

across the air/sea interface about 50 μm thick by way of molecular diffusion (Degens et al., 1984). The CO_2 molecules flowing through the surface oceanic layer separate into two channels which are parallel to each other: in one the DIC is generated via various chemical transformations, while in the other DOC is biologically synthesized. The dissolved radiocarbon then penetrates into deep layers by eddy diffusion. The range of that diffusion is characterized by a certain gradient in radiocarbon. In deep waters radiocarbon is mixed at a rate quicker than that of its decay, and its concentration remains practically constant.

Note that DIC is in local chemical equilibrium with the dissolved CO_2 but DOC is not. This is the reason for the observed discontinuity of the $\Delta^{14}C$ profile for DOC.

The concentration of radiocarbon in the atmosphere doubled after nuclear tests began. The difference between the radiocarbon concentrations in the atmospheric and surface layer oceanic CO_2 had increased by almost an order of magnitude, as compared to the preindustrial era, bringing a respectively higher influx of radiocarbon into the ocean, see Fig. 4.4. However, concentration of the surface dissolved inorganic radiocarbon in the ocean increased by 13%, on average. Were the production of DOC to remain at its preindustrial level, the gradient of concentration of dissolved organic radiocarbon should have increased by some similar margin. Actually, though, the gradient of organic radiocarbon concentration, and hence its diffusional flux into the oceanic depths has increased by almost an order of magnitude, Fig. 4.4. The present day rate of accumulation of organic radiocarbon in the surface waters exceeds its diffusional flux into deep water. That is why the concentration gradient has been quickly increasing with time. It is thus apparent that the production of DOC must have increased by more than an order of magnitude compared to its preindustrial level.

Such an increase could only have resulted from the reaction of oceanic biota to the observed build up of atmospheric CO_2, which in itself resulted from deforestation and from combustion of fossil fuels. The net primary production by oceanic biota and the nutrient ratio (4.4.3) in all the synthesized organic matter apparently remain at their preindustrial levels. What has actually increased is the share of the produced "long-lived" dead organic matter, while the share of production and the biomass of the "short-lived" live cells decreased at every trophic level, including fish. That was equivalent to an effective decrease in the rate of decay of organic matter, which resulted in a growth of the mass of organic matter in the ocean, provided total primary production remained constant. As a result one observes biological pumping of the excess atmospheric CO_2 into refractory dead organic matter in the ocean.

Appendix A treats that phenomenon quantitatively, starting from data published by Druffel and Williams, (1990) (see Gorshkov, 1991b). The preindustrial production of DOC by the world ocean, P_0^{+DOC}, equal to destruction, P_0^{-DOC} was:

$$P_0^{+DOC} = P_0^{-DOC} = 0.24 \text{ Gt C/year.} \tag{4.11.1}$$

The present-day DOC production by the world ocean, averaged over the years 1955 to 1986 (elapsed since the beginning of nuclear tests and up to the start of measurements) increased by a factor of 20 and constituted, see Appendix A:

$$P^{+DOC} = 4.2 \text{ Gt C/year.} \tag{4.11.2}$$

The net primary production by the world ocean is estimated at the level of 42 Gt C/year (Fogg, 1975; Platt and Rao, 1975; Whittaker and Likens, 1975; De Voogs, 1979; Vinogradov and Shushkina, 1988; Platt et al., 1989, see Table 5.1). Hence, preindustrial production of DOC (4.11.1) was approximately 0.2 % of the net primary production, and its present value has increased to 8 % of that value. The change of concentration of atmospheric CO_2 during the industrial era only affected the state of the surface oceanic layer, in which photosynthesis of organic matter took place. The total store of DOC ($\sim$ 2000 Gt C, see Appendix A), was mainly concentrated in oceanic depths. During the last 200 years, the mass of DOC store should have increased by less than 20 %, see Appendix A. Besides, the rate of decay of DOC should be controlled mainly by the concentration of oxygen, and its distribution has not changed during the industrial era (Gorshkov, 1984a). Thus the present-day rate of decay of DOC should coincide with its preindustrial value. As a result we have for the rate of increase of DOC, $\dot{m}^{DOC}$, taking the average for 1955–1986, see Appendix A:

$$\dot{m}^{+DOC} = P^{+DOC} - P^{-DOC} = P^{+DOC} - P_0^{+DOC} \approx 4 \text{ Gt C/year.} \tag{4.11.3}$$

There are two ways for excess atmospheric CO_2 to be absorbed by oceanic biota at permanent concentrations of nitrogen and phosphorus. First, the gross oceanic primary production may increase via extracellular excretion of the hydro-carbon-type organic matter, containing no nitrogen and phosphorus (Khailov, 1971; Fogg, 1975; Platt and Rao, 1975). These are the particular substances produced as primary photosynthetic products. If nitrogen and phosphorus are lacking, no new cells may be built from that organic matter, so that such products must be excreted to the external environment from the cell, thus adding to the store of oceanic DOC (Gorshkov, 1982c, Chen and Drake, 1986). The store of DOC in the ocean during the industrial era should have been complemented by organic matter devoid of nitrogen and phosphorus, so that the C/P ratio in DOC should have increased by about 10%. In particular, that ratio in DOC should significantly differ between the new surface and the old deep waters, which is apparently not observed.

Second, the production by oceanic biota may be treated as a sum of cellular production and production of DOC. During the preindustrial era these two forms of production amounted to 99.4% and 0.6% of the total production, respectively, and were compensated by an equal rate of decay. With net primary production and the chlorophyll concentration remaining unchanged (Falkowski and Wilson, 1992) the biota may, in reaction to the increased atmospheric CO_2, increase the share of DOC produced, reducing, accordingly, the share of cellular production. Since the rate of destruction, which depends on concentrations of organic matter and of oxygen, remains practically the same for DOC, while decreasing in proportion to production by cells, such a possibility corresponds to an effective reduction of destruction. As a result the store of DOC in the ocean should start to increase. The C/P ratio in DOC may then remain unchanged. Apparently, it is this second possibility which is actually realized in nature: the biota increases the production of DOC in response to CO_2 build-up in the atmosphere, and, conversely, reduces such production when the atmospheric concentration of CO_2 drops. In the latter case the organic carbon is transformed into its inorganic atmospheric and oceanic forms (Gorshkov, 1991b), provided the rate of destruction of DOC remains the same.

Thus the dynamics of change in production and total store of DOC in the ocean during both the industrial era and the postglacial period agrees with the Le Chatelier principle, as applied to oceanic biota. It works to keep the concentration of CO_2 in the atmosphere constant by compensating (damping) adverse perturbations.

4.12 Changes in the Global Cycle of Carbon

According to measurements taken from 1958 onwards by many observatories both on land and at sea, see Fig. 1.2, the concentration of atmospheric CO_2 keeps growing. The analysis of gas composition of air bubbles from Antarctic ice cores (Friedli et al., 1986, Staffelbach et al., 1991; Leuenberger et al., 1992; Raynaud et al., 1993) yields information on the atmospheric concentration of CO_2 from the very start of perturbation at the end of the eighteenth century, see Fig. 1.2. It also follows from ice core data that, to within the error margin, the "preindustrial" concentration of atmospheric CO_2 had approximately been equal to 280 ppmv (Siegenthaler and Oeschger, 1987) and had remained constant for the last few thousand years (Oeschger and Stauffer, 1986). At the end of the last glaciation 15 000 years ago it had lowered to 180 ppmv (Barnola et al., 1991). Today the atmospheric concentration of CO_2 has reached 350 ppmv (Trivett, 1989; Starke, 1987, 1990), which is 25 % higher than the preindustrial level.

The observed global change of the carbon cycle is mainly due to anthropogenic perturbation of the natural land biota which exceeded its stability threshold by the middle of the eighteenth century. Perturbations of land biota are superimposed by direct anthropogenic perturbations of the environment, principally due to combustion of fossil fuel. The oceanic biota remains stable and keeps on compensating perturbations of the environment. However that oceanic biota already fails to cope with global anthropogenic perturbations, so that the end result is global change of the environment in both the atmosphere and the ocean.

As repeatedly noted elsewhere, it is the enormous power of the production and destruction of organic matter developed by the natural biota which is implicitly dangerous and may precipitate a quick disintegration of the environment, should the closed matter cycles be disrupted beyond the Le Chatelier principle (see Sect. 4.4). Present direct measurements of both biotic production and destruction are only conducted with large errors, which exceed several tens of a per cent. Thus, due to the extremely high level of natural closure of matter cycles it remains practically impossible to detect any breach of these cycles.

By analyzing the practices of land use one obtains data on the ecological state of the areas used: arable lands, pastures, intensely exploited forests, etc., on which one may find clear cut statistical data (Houghton et al., 1983, 1987; Houghton, 1989). However the ecological state of other areas cannot be estimated using that technique. The parts of those areas still totally outside man's activities (most of the open area of the world ocean and a small part of the remaining virginal land surface) should react to the global increase of CO_2 concentration in the atmosphere, absorbing, in accordance with the Le Chatelier principle, excessive CO_2 from the atmosphere. However, perturbed biota with its altered composition in species, covering areas not accounted for in land use analysis, may by itself violate the Le Chatelier principle and emit additional CO_2 into the atmosphere.

The principal change in CO_2 content occurs in four media only: the atmosphere, the fossil fuel, the ocean, and the land surface part of the biosphere. As noted above, the atmospheric concentration of carbon has been directly measured from 1958 on, and is also available from ice core data. Emissions from fossil fuel are well estimated from the very start of the industrial era. Now such emissions of carbon from fossil fuel occur at the rate of 5.8 Gt C/year (Watt, 1982; Marland et al., 1988; Starke, 1987, 1990). Of that amount 3.5 Gt C/year is accumulated in the atmosphere (Trivett, 1989). Land use results in additional emissions of up to 2.5 Gt C/year (Houghton, 1989). Thus the known sum of carbon emissions into the atmosphere from areas of active industrial activities is 8.3 Gt C/year. Of that amount 3.5 Gt C/year is accumulated in the atmosphere. The remaining 4.8 Gt C/year (Trivett, 1989) may be absorbed by either the ocean or that part of the land surface biota which remains outside the scope of industrial activity (Sundquist, 1993). If the ocean absorbs more than 5 Gt C/year, that means that the remaining land surface biota also emits CO_2 into the atmosphere, that is violates the Le Chatelier principle and is beyond the threshold of admissible perturbations. The carbon-storage potential of soils of strongly perturbed biota in perturbed environment is unknown. The analysis of the carbon-storage potential of natural soils in natural environment indicates that soils are incapable of accumulating carbon quickly, so that when such accumulation of carbon by land biota takes place, it may only result from changes in the distribution and in the biomass of terrestrial vegetation (Schlesinger, 1990). At the same time destruction of soil organic matter may occur at an arbitrary rate. Mean loss of soil carbon following agricultural conversion reaches about 30% in various ecosystems. In certain tropical forest areas that value may reach a maximum of 70% (Schlesinger, 1986; Bouwman, 1989).

To envisage the difficulties of detecting carbon emissions by land biota, one may compare the figures cited above with primary production by the biota (that is with the rate of synthesis of organic carbon). The net primary production on land is estimated at 60 Gt C/year (Ajtay et al., 1979), and that in the ocean at about 40 Gt C/year (Mopper and Degens, 1979; Platt et al., 1989; Falkowski and Wilson, 1992; Falkowski and Woodhead, 1992; Holligan and Boois, 1993). The error in both these estimates may well exceed 30% (Whittaker and Likens, 1975). An independent estimate of the rate of destruction of the organic matter is burdened with an even larger error (Gorshkov and Sherman, 1986). Meanwhile if the rate of destruction exceeds the rate of synthesis by only 10%, that means an annual reduction of biomass of the land surface biota of 6 Gt C/year. Carbon emissions due to soil use are directly estimated from the rate at which biomass is reduced in these areas, although lack of accurate data on production and destruction results in large errors of those estimates.

Carbon mainly penetrates into the ocean via diffusion through the air–sea interface. The net flux of carbon either into or out of the ocean is proportional to the difference between the atmospheric and oceanic partial pressures of carbon dioxide (pressure is taken in a limited air mass in equilibrium with the surface water layer, to be more exact). That difference between the two partial pressures varies strongly across the world ocean, even changing its sign in going from high to low latitudes, and displays absolute maxima which exceed the total increment of atmospheric CO_2 over the industrial era, see Fig. 4.5. Thus attempts to estimate the global net air-to-sea flux of carbon via averaging the local data (Broecker et al., 1986; Tans et al., 1990; Etcheto et al., 1991; Watson et al., 1991) are associated with large errors and cannot even claim a correct order of magnitude of that flux (Broecker et al., 1986; Gorshkov, 1986b, 1992a; Robertson and Watson, 1992; Gorshkov, 1993a,b). Studying penetration of carbon through that interface one

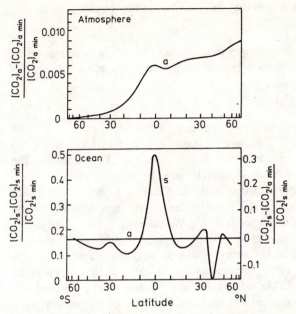

Fig. 4.5. The observed latitudinal variations of CO_2 concentration in the atmosphere and the ocean. "a" are changes in the atmosphere; "s" are changes in the ocean. Within the scale of changes in the ocean (the lower curve) the observed changes in the atmosphere (upper curve) degrade into a horizontal line (Broecker et al., 1979, 1985b).

may only estimate the top limit for the net flux of carbon into the ocean, assuming that the ocean is kept in its non-perturbed state by sea biota, and that the average annual increment of CO_2 concentration in the surface waters is equal to zero.

That maximum flux amounts to 20 Gt C/year, that is exceeds the rate of emission of fossil carbon by a factor of three (Gorshkov, 1986b, 1992a).

The only way to obtain the rate of absorption of carbon by the ocean at an acceptable accuracy is to use radiocarbon data on the distribution of ^{14}C in both the atmosphere and the ocean (including both the organic and the inorganic dissolved carbon) prior to and after atmospheric nuclear tests (see Sect. 4.11, Appendixes A and B). These data make it possible to estimate the temporal change of the rate of carbon emissions by land biota and to identify the moment when the Le Chatelier principle was violated in that part of the biota, thus estimating the threshold for such a perturbation.

Due to the law of matter conservation carbon may be distributed between the four above-mentioned active global reservoirs: the fossil fuel (f), the atmosphere (a), the biosphere (b), and the sea (s). Indeed, as already mentioned above, all the other existing reservoirs are either inactive, or feature a negligibly small capacity for storing carbon (Degens et al., 1984). Thus getting accurate enough data on the rate of change of at least one such reservoir, either the biosphere or the ocean, would be sufficient for describing the whole situation with the carbon cycle.

The law of matter conservation may be described in the following form:

$$\dot{m}_a + \dot{m}_s + \dot{m}_f + \dot{m}_b = 0, \tag{4.12.1}$$

where the m_i denote respective changes in the mass of carbon in these reservoirs, each being given by the difference between the present-day mass, M_i and its stationary (non-perturbed) value, M_{i0}:

$$m_i = M_i - M_{i0}.$$

As usual dots denote rates of change ($\dot{m} = dm/dt$, t is time).

Note again that the rates of change of mass of carbon in fossil fuel ($\dot{m}_f$) and in the atmosphere ($\dot{m}_a$) are known from the very start of perturbation. The ocean reacts to changes in the atmospheric CO_2 (in both its weakly perturbed biota and its physico-chemical state) according to the Le Chatelier principle. The rate of absorption of carbon by the sea ($\dot{m}_s$) depends on the relative increment of the mass of carbon in the atmosphere, that is on m_a/M_{a0}. We have $\dot{m}_s = 0$ in a steady state, when $m_a = 0$. While the relative deviation remains small $m_a/M_{a0} \ll 1$, one may expand the rate ($\dot{m}_s$) into a Taylor power series over m_a/M_{a0}, in which only its linear term is actually retained. The respective proportionality factor ((k_s)) is found in Appendix B from the available radiocarbon and ^{13}C data. That coefficient (the stability coefficient) is a fundamental characteristic of state of the non-perturbed ocean (referring both to its biota and to its physico-chemical state). It characterizes the rate of relaxation of the environment to its natural state (Sects. 2.7 and 4.4). That coefficient should remain constant over millennia and may only change during an evolutionary transition of the environment from one steady state to another (for example, when it transits from an ice age to an interglacial period and back). We then have (see Appendix B):

$$\dot{m}_s = k_s m_a, \qquad k_s = 0.054 \text{ year}^{-1}. \tag{4.12.2}$$

The rate of absorption of carbon by the ocean, ($\dot{m}_s$) is equal to the sum of rates of absorption of carbon in its organic ($\dot{m}+_s$) and inorganic ($\dot{m}-_s$) forms. We have, respectively, for the k_s factor (see Appendix B):

$$k_s = k_s^+ + k_s^-, \qquad \dot{m}_s^\pm = k_s^\pm m_a, \qquad k_s^+ = 0.038 \text{ year}^{-1}.$$

The rate of absorption of carbon in its organic form by oceanic biota, $\dot{m}_s^+$ may be presented in the form (4.4.1). The rate of change of the organic matter, $\dot{m}_s^+$ is equal to the difference between the change in its production P_s^+ and destruction, P_s^- (see (4.4.1) and (4.11.3)):

$$\dot{m}_s^+ = \Delta P_s^+ - \Delta P_s^-, \quad \Delta P_s^\pm \equiv P_s^\pm - P_{s0}^\pm, \quad P_{s0}^+ = P_{s0}^-, \tag{4.12.3}$$

where $P_{s0}^\pm$ are stationary non-perturbed values. Using (4.12.3) one may rewrite (4.12.2) for the organic carbon in the form of a scaling relation, (4.4.1):

$$\frac{\Delta P_s^+ - \Delta P_s^-}{P_{s0}^+} = \beta_s^+ \frac{\Delta[CO_2]_a}{[CO_2]_{a0}}, \tag{4.12.4}$$

$$\frac{\Delta[CO_2]_a}{[CO_2]_a} = \frac{m_a}{M_{a0}}, \quad \beta_s^+ = k_s^+ \tau_s^+, \quad \tau_s^+ = M_{a0}/P_{s0}^+,$$

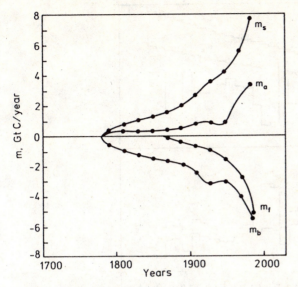

Fig. 4.6. Changes in the global carbon cycle. $\dot{m}_i$ are rates of change in the ith reservoir: $i = a$ for the atmosphere, $i = s$ for the ocean, $i = f$ for fossil fuel, $i = b$ for land biota. Points for the atmosphere ($\dot{m}_a$) and fossil fuels combustion ($\dot{m}_f$) are the observed two-decade averages: ice core atmospheric data before 1958 (Friedli et al., 1986; Staffelbach et al., 1991) and direct atmospheric measurements after 1958 (Watts, 1982; Gammon et al., 1986; Trivett, 1989; Starke, 1987, 1990; Reviere and Marton-Lefevre, 1992; Murata, 1993); fossil fuel combustion data after 1860 (Watts, 1982; Marland and Rotty, 1984; Starke, 1987, 1990). Points for ocean ($\dot{m}_s$) and land biota ($\dot{m}_b$) are calculated from (4.12.1) and (4.12.2), (Gorshkov, 1992b, 1993c).

where $\tau_s^+ = 14$ years is the time of atmospheric carbon turnover through oceanic biota, see Table 5.1. The expression (4.12.4) differs from the often used scaling relation, called "fertilization of biota by excessive CO_2" (see, for instance, Kohlmaier et al., 1987; Bazzaz and Fajer, 1992) in containing, in addition to change in production (ΔP_s^+), destruction (ΔP_s^-) as well. Both such possibilities were discussed in Sect. 4.11, where it was demonstrated that destruction seems to be weakened in the ocean ($P_s^- < 0$, $P_s^+ = 0$), instead of stronger fertilization ($\Delta P_s^- = 0$, $\Delta P_s^+ > 0$).

Thus the unknown rate of reduction of mass of carbon in land biota, $\dot{m}_b$ may be found from the equation of global budget of carbon (4.12.1), see Figs. 4.6–8. Numerically we have $\dot{m}_b + \dot{m}_s^+ \approx 0$, i.e. the total (land + ocean) organic carbon of the biota is not changed, see Appendix B.

The non-perturbed natural land biota should have reacted to the external perturbation of the environment in a manner similar to the non-perturbed ocean. Thus one may write:

$$\dot{m}_b = k_b m_a, \tag{4.12.5}$$

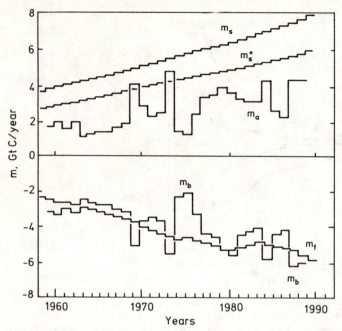

Fig. 4.7. The global rates of change in the carbon cycle over the period of systematic atmospheric observations. For notation see Fig. 4.6. $\dot{m}_f$ and $\dot{m}_a$ are the observed values (see Watts, 1982; Trivett, 1989; Starke, 1987, 1990). $\dot{m}_s$ and $\dot{m}_s^+$ are calculated from the observed values of m_a from the formulae: $\dot{m}_s = k_s m_a$, $\dot{m}_s^+ = k_s^+ m_a$, $k_s = 0.054$ year^{-1}, $k_s^+ = 0.038$ year^{-1}, see Appendix B; $(\dot{m}_b)$ are calculated from (4.12.1) (Gorshkov, 1992b, 1993c).

where the coefficient k_b for the non-perturbed biota is characterized by its non-perturbed constant positive value k_{b0}. It is natural to assume that due to the universality of the biochemical organization of life the dimensionless scaling coefficient β_s^+ in (4.12.4) is the same for land and sea biota. Taking into account that $k_s^{\pm}$ did not change appreciably during the industrial era, i.e. $k_s^{\pm} = k_{s0}^{\pm}$ and setting $\beta_s = \beta_b$ we have

$$k_{b0} = k_{b0}^+ = \frac{k_s^+ \tau_s^+}{\tau_b^+} \approx 0.055 \text{ year}^{-1}, \tag{4.12.6}$$

where $\tau_b^+ = M_{a0}/P_{b0}^+ = 9.8$ years is the atmospheric turnover time through the land biota (see Table 5.1). Note that the unperturbed relaxation coefficient k_{b0} in land biota coincides approximately with the total relaxation coefficient for the ocean: $k_s = k_s^+ + k_s^-$. This fact may be explained as follows. Land biota has larger productivity than sea biota (see Table 5.1). But only biota can react to the perturbation of environment on land. On the other hand the physico-chemical processes in the ocean also tend to equilibrium with the atmosphere.

The value k_b begins to drop off in the perturbed land biota and becomes zero when the biotic stability is broken (Sects. 2.7 and 4.4). To analyze changes of

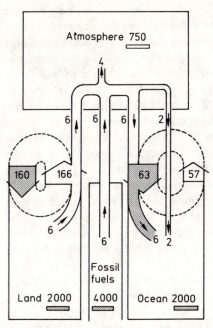

Fig. 4.8. Present-day state of the carbon cycle. Shaded arrows give the fluxes of synthesized organic carbon. Open arrows give the fluxes of destroyed organic and inorganic carbon. Numbers give the fluxes of carbon in Gt C/year. Net primary production (NPP) to gross primary production (GPP) ratio, NPP/GPP, are 0.37 for land biota and 0.67 for sea biota (Whittaker, 1975; Whittaker and Likens, 1975). Thus GPP is 160 Gt C/year for land and 63 Gt C/year for ocean, see the values of NPP in Table 5.1 below. The stores of carbon are underlined: thick shaded lines for organic carbon, thin blank lines for inorganic carbon, Gt C (Gorshkov, 1992b, 1993c).

state of the anthropogenically perturbed environment it is convenient to use the variables k_i in (4.12.1):

$$k_a + k_s + k_f + k_b = 0, \qquad k \equiv \dot{m}_i/m_a, \tag{4.12.7}$$

where k_i for fossil fuel ($i = f$) and the atmosphere ($i = a$) are formal values found from the empirical data on $\dot{m}_i$ and m_a, while the same value for the ocean ($i = s$) is the rate of relaxation of the non-perturbed system, independently found from the data of radiocarbon analysis. The behavior of k_b for land biota is found from (4.12.7), see Fig. 4.9. With the signs of k_i coefficients thus defined (see (4.12.7)) the atmospheric stability corresponds to $k_a < 0$, and the stability of the ocean and land biota is described by $k_s > 0$, $k_b > 0$. Therefore, the conditions for satisfying the Le Chatelier principle have the form:

$$k_a < 0, \quad k_s > 0, \quad k_b > 0. \tag{4.12.8}$$

It may be seen from Fig. 4.9 that the stability of land biota and of the atmosphere started to change from the middle of the seventeenth century ($k_b < k_{b0}$). By the middle of the eighteenth century the stability of land biota was completely violated ($k_b = 0$). Starting from that time and up to the beginning of the nineteenth century stability of the atmosphere was only supported by sea biota. The carbon exchange between the land biota and the ocean may take place only via the atmosphere. The observed absence of atmospheric perturbation means that the net carbon fluxes between the land biota and the ocean were equal to zero up to the beginning of the nineteenth century, see Figs. 4.6 and 4.9. From the beginning of the nineteenth century destruction of land biota exceeded the critical level of $k_a = 0$, after which biota of the ocean already failed to cope with stabilizing the atmosphere, and the process of global change of the environment had started ($k_a > 0$). As the natural land biota is destroyed, the relative rate of emission of carbon from it (k_b) gradually starts to drop off, although the absolute rate ($\dot{m}_b$) keeps on growing (Fig. 4.6). Apparently, with the total destruction of natural land biota and its substitution with domesticated complexes (man controlled agri-, silva-, and aquacultures), the stabilizing potential of land biota will become zero, and the rates k_b and ($\dot{m}_b$) will fluctuate randomly around their zero values. That tendency is observed in Figs. 4.9 and 4.10.

The start of the global change of composition of the atmosphere is estimated from the ice core data (Friedli et al., 1986; Siegenthaler and Oeschger, 1987). According to these, up to the middle of the present century the relative rate of growth of the atmospheric concentration of CO_2, $k_a \equiv \dot{m}_a/m_a$ (see Fig. 4.9) was approximately twice as low as it presently is. If one assumes that the value of k_a remained intact, and coincided with its present value for the whole period of global change and that the ice core data yield an overestimate of m_a up to the middle of the present century (Jaworowski et al., 1992), then the moment the global changes started (Fig. 4.6) and the values of thresholds in Fig. 4.9 all shift approximately one century to the right (Gorshkov et al., 1989).

The absolute rate of absorption of carbon by the ocean, $\dot{m}_s$, Eq. (4.12.2), grows linearly with m_a at constant k_s. Thus setting emissions of fossil carbon at a certain level $\dot{m}_f$ (after complete extinction of natural land biota) one could expect that concentration of atmospheric carbon would rise to a certain fixed level, at which the rate of absorption of carbon by the ocean, $\dot{m}_s$ would be equal to $\dot{m}_f$, ($\dot{m}_f = k_s m_a$), $\dot{m}_a = \dot{m}_b = 0$. However, if one assumes that absorption of carbon by the ocean occurs mainly by an order of magnitude increase in the production of the dissolved organic carbon and by a 10% decrease in the production of live cells (which is equivalent, at unchanging reproduction times, to a respective reduction of their biomass), further increase of oceanic absorptivity appears impossible at a constant k_s. The process of absorption is particularly controlled by live cells. That is why such a process may hardly be sustained if the live biomass of the ocean is reduced by more than 10%. Hence anthropogenic perturbation of the biosphere at its present level brings the natural land biota to complete disintegration, while the oceanic biota is close to its maximum compensating capabilities in coping with perturbations of the environment.

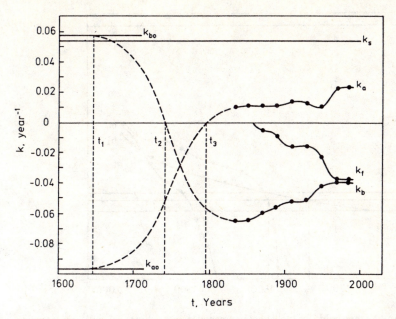

Fig. 4.9. Environmental stability (relaxation) coefficients. $k_i = \dot{m}_i/m_a$, see Fig. 4.6 for notation of $\dot{m}_i$, $m_a = M_a - M_{a0}$; M_a and M_{a0} are the varying (perturbed) and the stationary (non-perturbed) mass of atmospheric carbon; $k_{f0} = 0$, k_{b0} and k_{a0} are non-perturbed stability coefficients of fossil carbon, of land biota and atmosphere. Points show two-decade averages, plotted from ice core data up to 1958, and from atmospheric measurements after 1958. Dashed lines interpolate between the observed and the non-perturbed values. Vertical dotted lines denote: $t = t_1$ the margin of the highest stability of environment (the maximum non-perturbed relaxation rate), $k_b = k_{b0}$ at $t < t_1$; $t = t_2$ loss of stability by land biota, $k_b = 0$; $t = t_3$ loss of atmospheric stability, $k_a = 0$, and beginning of global changes in the atmosphere. In the region $t_1 < t < t_2$ stability of land biota decreased, and in the region $t_1 < t < t_3$ atmospheric stability decreased (Gorshkov, 1992b, 1993c).

Were we able to return land biota to its unperturbed state, it would absorb about $\dot{m}_{b0} = k_{b0}m_a \approx 9$ Gt C/year from the modern atmosphere. Here we use the present-day increment of atmospheric carbon mass, $m_a = 160$ GtC, see Fig. 1.2, and assume that non-perturbed land biota retains its non-perturbed relaxation coefficient, k_{b0}, Eq. (4.12.6), at such a value of m_a. Hence at the present-day level of fossil fuels combustion, $-\dot{m}_f = 6$ Gt C/year, the atmospheric CO_2 concentration would decrease at a rate $\dot{m}_a = 11$ Gt C/year and the preindustrial equilibrium state could be restored in several decades.

Anthropogenically perturbed land areas now amount to 61% of the total land surface area. The areas of wilderness constitute 39% of that area (World Resources, 1988; Turner et al., 1993). The biota of that wilderness might absorb $\dot{m}_{bw} = \dot{m}_{b0} \times 0.39 \approx 3$ Gt C/year if we assume its primary productivity to coincide with average land primary productivity. Overall, the land biota currently emits about $-\dot{m}_b = 6$ Gt C/year to the atmosphere, see Fig. 4.8. That means that the biota in

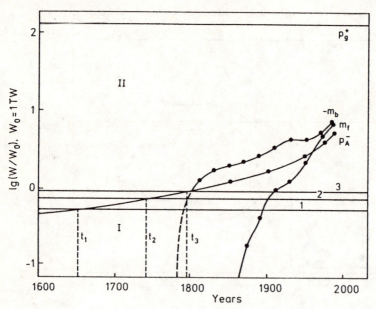

Fig. 4.10. Energy thresholds for global environmental stability. Lines $\dot{m}_f$ and $-\dot{m}_b$ coincide with those in Fig. 4.6 ($\dot{m}_b$ sign changed, logarithmic scale, power units); p_A^- is the fraction of net primary production in power units consumed by man (food (man plus livestock) and wood consumption is assumed to reach 1 kW/person). Values $\dot{m}_f$ and $-\dot{m}_b$ are assumed to be unique functions of p_A^-; vertical dashed lines t_1, t_2, t_3 coincide with those in Fig. 4.9. Horizontal lines are as follows: line 1 gives the maximum permissible value of p_A^- compatible with the maximum stability of the global environment; line 2: p_A^- threshold, marking global violations in stability of land biota; line 3: p_A^- threshold marking global violations of environmental stability (of the atmosphere). Range I is ecologically permissible (stable biota and environment); range II is ecologically prohibited (both biota and environment are destroyed). Horizontal line p_g^+ is the power of gross primary production in the total biosphere.

the perturbed land areas emits about $-\dot{m}_{bp} \approx 9$ Gt C/year. Were the land biota completely perturbed it would emit about $-\dot{m}_{bpt} = -\dot{m}_{bp}/0.61 \approx 15$ Gt C/year so that the atmospheric CO_2 concentration would increase at a catastrophic rate of $\dot{m}_a \approx 14$ Gt C/year. The complete abandonment of the combustion of fossil fuels would reduce the last number only to 8 Gt C/year. These estimations demonstrate the great importance of conservation and enlargement of the areas of wilderness.

4.13 The Water Cycle

Water is the principal body and metabolic component in all living beings. The whole of terrestrial life exists within a narrow temperature margin in which water is found in its liquid phase. Enormous stores of water in the biosphere distinguish

Earth from all the other planets of the terrestrial group in the solar system (Allen, 1955; Prinn, 1982). These stores are mainly concentrated in the world ocean, containing 1.4×10^9 Gt of H_2O. At their present rate the processes of water outflow into the hydrosphere from the Earth's depths may be responsible for the appearance of no more than one tenth of the contemporary hydrosphere. Sedimentary rocks are 2 km thick, on average (Allen, 1955). They are formed from matter fluxes rising from the Earth's depths. The relative water content in matter surfacing in rift zones and erupted by the volcanoes, which form the sedimented layer and the hydrosphere, does not exceed 10 % (Lvovitsh, 1974; Degens et al., 1984; Baumgartner and Reichel, 1975; Henderson-Sellers and Cogley, 1982; Shukla and Mintz, 1982). The share of water in the counterflow of matter into terrestrial depths must be at least as high. Hence, the average depth of the hydrosphere should not have exceeded 10 % of the average depth of the sedimentary layer, that is 200 m (instead of the actually observed 3 km (Allen, 1955; Watts, 1982)).

Many biochemical reactions are accompanied by the formation of free water. As follows from Table 5.1 below the production of the biosphere is about 200 Gt/year of dry organic matter, one tenth of that amount being organic carbon. It is natural to assume that productivity of the paleobiosphere had been of the same order of magnitude. Assume that only 1 % of paleobiological production had synthesized free water (e.g., from CH_4 and CO_2, which could have been present in the Earth's paleoatmosphere (Allen, 1955; Budyko et al., 1987)). Then the whole of the hydrosphere could have been formed by the living beings in less than 10^9 years, that is within about one quarter of the whole timespan of life on Earth. It means that, in accordance with geological data, the hydrosphere could have been formed about 3×10^9 years ago (Baumgartner and Reichel, 1975; Henderson-Sellers and Cogley, 1982). Biochemical reactions could have changed at some later stage to acquire their contemporary form. Thus the possibility may not be excluded that the Earth's hydrosphere is of biological origin.

The present-day store of oceanic water exceeds the store of organic matter in the whole of the biosphere by many orders of magnitude. In the sense defined above, water in the ocean is a biologically non-accumulated material over time periods less than 10^9 years. Water evaporation in the ocean cannot be biologically regulated. Atmospheric moisture above the ocean and its effect upon the magnitude of the greenhouse effect cannot depend on the functioning of oceanic biota.

The time of complete latitudinal mixing of the atmosphere is of the order of a few months (Palmen and Newton, 1969). The turnover time for atmospheric moisture (that is the ratio of the atmospheric store of moisture to rate of evaporation) is of the order of ten days (Brutsaert, 1982). That results in the observed inhomogeneity of the atmospheric distribution of moisture, so that the moisture regime (including the atmospheric store of moisture, precipitation, and evaporation) strongly differs from sea to land. Evaporation in the ocean exceeds precipitation (Lvovitsh, 1974; Baumgartner and Reichel, 1975). The difference between evaporated and precipitated moisture is transported to land, where that flux is precipitated and runs off to the ocean, in agreement with the law of matter conservation, as river

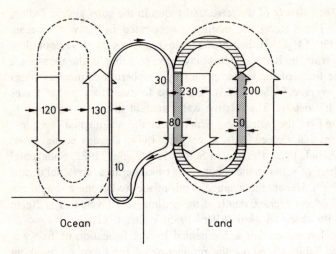

Fig. 4.11 The effect of biota on the water cycle. Figures indicate the rates of: evaporation (arrows up), precipitation (arrows down), and river runoff (horizontal arrows), cm/year (Lvovitsh, 1974; Baumgartner and Reichel, 1975; Chahine, 1992; Table 2.1). Evaporation and precipitation in the ocean, sea-to-land moisture transport, equal to the river runoff, cannot be regulated by the biota. (The ratio of the rate of river runoff (cm/year) to sea-to-land moisture transport (cm/year) is equal to the ratio of surface areas of sea and land.) In the absence of land biota precipitation would have transferred to underground waters, and evaporation would only take place from the surface of rivers and lakes (which constitute only 2% of the total land surface), that is precipitation at land would have been completely controlled by moisture transport from the ocean, and would have approximately coincided with the river runoff. Plant transpiration approximately triples the water cycle, as compared to lifeless land (small blank arrows). If all the solar energy incident upon the land was spent on plant transpiration, the water cycle could be potentially increased by a factor of nine (large blank arrows). A situation close to this extreme is found in tropical forests.

runoff (Lvovitsh, 1974). On average, that part of the moisture flux on land may not be biologically regulated.

However, in addition to that precipitation brought from the ocean, evaporation on land also takes place and precipitation follows in a land-closed cycle. In the absence of land biota that additional precipitation should have been much less than precipitation brought from the ocean. Precipitated moisture is quickly transferred to underground waters, which feed rivers and lakes, occupying about 2% of the land surface. Evaporation from the surface of rivers and lakes is negligibly small in comparison with precipitation brought in from the ocean. Fluctuations of oceanic precipitation would have triggered sharp changes in the river runoff.

It is only the formation of vegetation cover and soil which results in high levels of evaporation from the whole of the land and in smoothing out of the random oscillations of river runoff. After vegetation is formed, part of the river runoff is spent on storing moisture in soil, in green plants, and in the continental atmosphere. The increase of that mass steps up the land water cycle. Water on land is a biologically accumulated substance. According to available measurements, precipitation presently exceeds river runoff on land by about a factor of three (Lvovitsh, 1974; Shukla and Mintz, 1982; Chahine, 1992). Hence only one third of precipitation is brought from the ocean and more than two thirds come from the closed water cycle on land. That principal part of the land moisture regime is formed by its biota and is subject to biological regulation, Fig. 4.11.

It is routinely assumed that the moisture regime of the continents is completely controlled by the regular circulating air flows, which depend on the latitudinal and seasonal distribution of the solar radiation, on continental relief, and on the relative distribution of continents and oceans (Palmen and Newton, 1969). However the data on distribution of the solar energy (see Table 2.2) indicate that the power of evaporation by leafage, regulated by the biota, that is the transpiration power, exceeds the power of dissipation (and hence of generation) of wind energy over the whole of the Earth. Irregular atmospheric circulational fluxes, such as cyclones and tornadoes, are produced by latent heat of evaporation, released during condensation of atmospheric moisture. Thus, from the energy point of view, change in the regime of transpiration by land surface plants may completely change the regime of irregular circulational air flows in the atmosphere and the regime of precipitation on land related to it, that is the moisture regime of the continents.

Since cumulative leafage surface greatly exceeds that of bare soil (the ratio of those surfaces is called the leaf index, and is of the order of 10 in forests, while not exceeding 5 for land surface on average (Whittaker, 1975; Whittaker and Likens, 1975; Table 5.1), transpiration by vegetation may significantly exceed evaporation from the areas devoid of vegetation cover, and even from open water surface area. Apparently the level of transpiration is limited to a certain maximum, which corresponds to a situation when all the available solar energy is used exclusively for transpiration. According to available observations, up to 90% of the incident solar energy is intercepted by leafage and is spent on transpiration in virginal forests unperturbed by man (Duvigneaud, 1974; Odum, 1983), while the same figure does not exceed 40% in man-transformed cultivated lands (Duvigneaud, 1974). Thus man's forcing of the natural forest communities during the whole of history could more than halve the evaporating power of vegetation on a global scale.

Nowadays deserts occupy about 20% of the total continental surface (Whittaker, 1975; Whittaker and Likens, 1975). Desert flora and fauna testify by their very presence that the deserts had existed even before humanity originated (Kendeigh, 1974). However, areas occupied by deserts of natural origin could have been tens or even hundreds of times smaller than those they occupy today. Slow formation of deserts over periods of tens and hundreds of thousands of years took place with the Le Chatelier principle still acting: desert communities were only gradually spreading into areas formerly occupied by their predecessors. The drop off in productivity of desertified areas only slightly weakened the action of the Le Chatelier principle. In that sense modern attempts to use artificial irrigation to turn deserts into "blooming gardens" of cultivated species, devoid of stabilization programs (see Sect. 4.5), are much more dangerous, since these feature high productivity, run completely open matter cycles and totally disrupt the Le Chatelier principle.

After the 1960s many American ecologists tended gradually to think that fires, repeated every few decades, are a normal state of the natural ecosystems (Odum, 1983; Romme and Despein, 1989). Actually, however, it is practically impossible to identify the true cause of a fire, because the latter annihilates all traces of its origin, as a rule. Attributing many fires to lightning discharges remains unsubstantiated. By an overwhelming majority the fires are probably of anthropogenic origin. Natural fires do take place, of course, as triggered by volcanic eruptions, to give an example, and that could even have started the use of fire by man. However, recalling that the moisture regime of the land surface could have been regulated biotically, natural fires might have been an extremely rare event, repeated no more frequently than once every few hundred years or even millennia. In contrast to the present day desert fauna and flora, which are particularly adapted to such desert conditions, there are no organisms found with clearly manifested features of adaptation to high temperatures (the thick bark of some trees at trunk base or cone opening at high temperature in certain pine species may be explained by many other causes). It is particularly the extremely rare character of forest fires in the natural environment which can support durable climax communities, and that is a prerequisite necessary to explain the high degree of closure of matter cycles and the stability of the environment, as based on the Le Chatelier principle acting in the biota (Gorshkov and Gorshkov, 1992).

The biological destruction of organic matter in the natural communities is a very complex process. It cannot be achieved by a fire. Frequent fires in modern national parks (Romme and Despein, 1989) may be caused by the anthropogenic perturbation of the natural biota and of the moisture regime it regulates over extended areas, surrounding these parks.

4.14 Competitively Interacting Communities and the Gaia Hypothesis

The analysis of empirical data conducted in Chaps. 2–4 indicates that life is based on internally correlated local communities, capable of controlling their local environment. Similar to any other living individual these communities have finite size (the finite correlation radius), occupy limited spatial areas and may thus be envisaged as superindividuals. Mutual correlation of the gene pools of the various species combining into a community is similar to mutual correlation between the genetic information contained in the nuclear DNA and mitochondrial DNA, DNA of chloroplasts and other cytoplasmatic genes and organelles. Mutual correlation between the individuals of various species entering the community is similar to such correlation (to "altruistic interaction") between the organs in a living body. In that sense one may speak about the existence of physiology of a community (Margulis, 1971, 1975; Lovelock and Margulis, 1973; Lovelock, 1988).

However the normal community, that is sustaining of the stable superorganization of the local ecosystem occupied by the community (by all the individuals of all the species entering that community and acting in a correlated manner, together with their environment) can only be supported via competitive interaction between the noncorrelated homogeneous communities entering a respective hyperpopulation (the ecosystem). That ecosystem does not organize into a superindividual and has no physiology of its own. That is the main difference between the approach outlined in the present book and the Gaia hypothesis (Lovelock, 1982, 1989). Internal correlation between the individuals cannot embrace the whole of the biosphere. In the latter case competitive interaction needed to support such a global correlation would be absent. Hence the global correlation should have inevitably and quickly deteriorated (Sect. 4.2). Thus there can be no "physiology of the biosphere", as there can be no physiology of a population or of a species, so that the Gaia cannot be envisaged as a global superindividual (Lovelock, 1989).

A set of hyperpopulations of various communities combines into the global Earth biota. The set of ecosystems corresponding to them and the environment interacting with them combine into the biosphere. The global biota is nothing but a set of noncorrelated local communities. It is particularly due to competitive interaction between such communities which is possible because of their lack of correlation, that the biota is capable of controlling its environment on the global scale (Sects. 4.6 and 3.1). From that point of view the term Gaia introduced by Lovelock (1972) could be identified with the notion of the global biota or with that of the biosphere (Sect. 2.6). Envisaging Gaia as a globally correlated superindividual, in which no natural stabilizing selection is possible, precipitated most critical comments with respect to that concept (Doolittle, 1981; Dawkins, 1982; Kirchner, 1989; Barlocher, 1990; Barlow, 1991).

However, despite the fact that Gaia cannot be a superindividual, statements of the type "life has the capacity to regulate the temperature and the composition of the Earth's surface and keep it comfortable for living organisms" (Lovelock, 1988), and "biological processes homeostatically maintain on a planetary scale geochemical and climatic conditions favorable for life" (Kirchner, 1989), remain true within the concept presented herein (Sect. 4.6). The initial idea put forth by Hitchcock and Lovelock (1966) is that the observed deviation of the non-equilibrium state of terrestrial atmosphere from that of the atmospheres of lifeless planets (also driven out of physico-chemical equilibrium by solar radiation) points to the existence of life as a specific biological mechanism which controls the stability of the particular unstable state of the Earth's atmosphere. The present work attempts to clarify the main principles by which that mechanism functions.

The principal difference between the concept considered here and that of Gaia (which is equivalent to a globally correlated superindividual; Lovelock, 1989) is that biotic control of the environment is only possible when the biota affecting its environment, is capable of producing noticeable local advantages which increase the competitive capacity of the local internally correlated community. It is only in that case that decay communities, which "erroneously" affect the environment, may be forced out of the hyperpopulation. If no such advantages result from forcing certain components of the environment, these components cannot be controlled by the biota (Sects. 4.6 and 4.7).

It is apparent that the biota cannot control the value of the solar constant (Sect. 2.7), the geothermal power, the rate of continental drift, or the global transport of matter and heat precipitated by inhomogeneous heating of the Earth's surface and by the rotation of the Earth. Biota has to adapt to these cosmic and geophysical factors. However, changes in the course of these processes (which are in themselves always adverse to biota adapted to certain average conditions) may be compensated by that biota via affecting certain biologically controlled components of the environment. In particular, temperature changes due to cosmic and geophysical processes may be compensated by the biota via change of the concentration of the greenhouse gases and of the albedo of the Earth's surface (Sect. 2.7).

The surface temperature is regulated essentially via changes in evaporation, in concentrations of the atmospheric water vapor and of CO_2, and via the albedo. Land biota may change temperature within a local area occupied by a single community by altering transpiration (i.e., evaporation of water accumulated within the plant through its leaf surface), and by changing the albedo of leaf cover. The latter process has been considered in detail for the model community "Daisy World" (Lovelock, 1989). Changes in the regime of transpiration by land biota may change the budget of solar radiation on land by several ten per cent, alter the regime of atmospheric moisture and precipitate a change in surface temperature by several tens of degrees (Sects. 2.7 and 4.12). Therefore the complete restructuring of land biota due to modern practices of land use may affect the temperature regime on land an order of magnitude more than would be achieved by the doubling of CO_2 concentration in the atmosphere.

Biota is apparently capable of detecting local changes in temperature (the local greenhouse effect) related to local changes in the concentration of water vapor within the region of space occupied by a single community. That may only take place in land surface communities, since the oceanic biota is clearly incapable of regulating evaporation and concentration of water vapor in the atmospheric column. However, the local changes of concentration of CO_2 produced by a single community are only very weakly correlated with local changes of temperature, since temperature in general is controlled by the homogeneous concentration of CO_2 within the whole atmospheric column. If such a sensitivity lies outside the scope of the biotic sensitivity, biological regulation of temperature via altering the concentration of atmospheric CO_2 is impossible. In that case the atmospheric concentration of CO_2 sustained by the biota is not related to environmental temperature and is dictated by other needs of the biota. In other words, the biota consisting of a set of minor, mutually noncorrelated communities, "cannot be aware" that CO_2 is a greenhouse gas. The situation is similar with ozone (can the biota be aware of the ozone layer and its role as a screen against the UV radiation, protecting the whole of the land life?): the concentration of ozone near the Earth's surface which is strongly correlated with concentration of ozone in the higher atmospheric layers, may be held by the biota at a certain level for some other reasons, so that communities could be formed on land, including species sensitive to UV radiation.

The assumption that the oceanic biota is totally incapable of regulating the surface temperature contradicts the relative thermal stability of climate during the past epochs, as indicated by paleodata referring to periods when life was only found in the ocean (Lovelock, 1989). It follows then that oceanic biota should feature a sensitivity high enough to detect the correlation between local temperature changes and the local concentration of CO_2. The possible explanation for such higher sensitivity may lie with the observed accumulations of plankton which form patches up to 50 km in diameter (Cushing, 1975). Such patches naturally include many different communities of individuals and may be compared to animal herds consisting of numerous individuals. If one assumes that at least a temporal correlation is achieved within such patches between all the communities entering it, synchronous changes become possible in line with the chemical composition of the atmosphere, CO_2 in particular, at horizontal distances significantly exceeding the effective height of the atmospheric column. Then the diffusion flux of CO_2 in the atmosphere appears to be of the same order of magnitude as the production of carbon within the water surface area occupied by the patch of plankton, see (4.6.1), (4.6.2) and (4.8.3). Then the change in concentration of CO_2 within the whole atmospheric column, and hence the change of temperature correlated with it (that is the local greenhouse effect (Raval and Ramanathan, 1989)) appears to lie within the margin of the biotic sensitivity. The reaction of the biota in the "correct" direction should then be found in the process of competitive interaction between the various patches of plankton.

The impossibility of detecting the local correlation of the type "temperature–CO_2 concentration" within a single community might mean that for the last few hundred or thousand years the bulk CO_2 concentration in the atmosphere, sustained by the biota, has been controlled not by temperature, but by the necessity to keep biotic productivity at an optimal level. Such an assumption means that the present-day regulation of surface temperature is mainly conducted by the non-perturbed land biota via biological control of transpiration and of the albedo of vegetation cover. Extinction of natural land vegetation and its substitution by a set of cultivated species will then result in a loss of biological regulation of environmental temperature and in perturbation of the thermal stability of climate (Sect. 2.7).

The lack of a relationship between the surface temperature and the concentration of atmospheric CO_2 within the sensitivity margin of a separate community possibly explains the depletion of atmospheric CO_2 (regulated by the biota) that had, according to ice cores, taken place during the ice ages. Were the biota to regulate the atmospheric CO_2 only as greenhouse gas, one would expect an increase in CO_2 during those times, which would agree with the Le Châtelier principle and would let the biota damp the occurring temperature drop. One of the possible principal causes for such drops in temperature during the ice ages had been the change of oceanic equator-to-poles transport of hcat (the change in thermohaline overturning), produced by variations of the solar constant of cosmic origin, which had resulted in expansion of continental ice cover (Broecker et al., 1985a; Broecker and Denton, 1990; Lehman and Keigwin, 1992). Such transport of heat is a globally correlated process and cannot be regulated by the biota.

Were Gaia a single globally correlated superorganism, having its internal physiology, it could possess the information on all the global correlations and command a mechanism for compensation of any global perturbation. However, the existence of such a globally correlated Gaia contradicts the observed stability of natural communities (Sects. 3.2 and 4.5) and the observed evolutionary processes (Sect. 4.2).

Meanwhile, it is particularly due to that process of evolution that the notion of Gaia may be attributed a certain meaning. As noted above, the cosmic and geophysical conditions of the external and internal environment change in a direction unfavorable for the biota. The biota is capable of compensating such unfavorable changes by affecting the components of the environment within the scope of its control. However, as the changes in environmental conditions outside the scope of biological control proceed, the compensating action of the unchanging biota may gradually lose its efficiency. Evolution should lead to such a change of the biota that should provide the most physically efficient control of the environment possible during every geological period. The subsequent evolutionary change of the Earth's global biotas, sustaining environments optimal for life at all times, despite the progressive change of both the geophysical and cosmic conditions, could in that sense be called Gaia. Such a notion of Gaia would agree with the biota evolving as competitively interacting communities, which make possible the action of the stabilizing natural selection, being at the same time free from contradictions related to the global correlation of the biota.

Co-evolution of the global biota and the environment (in the form of Gaia) may be called sustainable development of the biosphere. That process only takes place during geological time periods, which are prescribed by the rates of progress of geophysical and cosmic abiotic processes. For the biotic compensation of life-unfavorable changes of the environment to remain efficient the rate of biological evolution (which is the principal characteristic of Gaia) should be at least as quick as abiotic processes. The observed fact that the environment has remained fit for life for 3.5×10^9 years indicates that such a condition is met. The maximum rate of evolution of the biota should be many orders of magnitude lower than the rate of genetic relaxation (Sects. 3.9–14), which defines the stability of the biota in the given environmental conditions at an arbitrary moment of geologic history (Sect. 3.9). The minimal rate of evolution is determined by the degree to which the evolutionary processes are prohibited with the available molecular structure of the information bearing molecules, provided the external conditions remain unchanged (Sects. 3.15–17). During quickly progressing abiotic changes of the environment the biota may apparently adapt its own evolution rate within the indicated margin. When the rates of abiotic processes go outside that margin, the biota cannot catch up with them, that is, the Le Chatelier principle weakens in its action. The very fact that the external conditions have never gone outside the margin fit for life (Sect. 2.7) means that such a weakening had never been too bad. Hence the Le Chatelier principle has never been violated in the biota throughout the whole of the history of life, and the environment has at all times retained its biological stability. In other words, abiotic processes catastrophic for the biota and its environment have never arisen in nature.

One should note that there can be no sustainable development of the biosphere, i.e., coevolution of the natural biota and the environment perturbed by man (Clark and Munn, 1986) over periods much shorter than the characteristic period of evolutionary change, which is of the order of 10^6 years, that is over tens, hundreds, or even thousands of years. During such short time periods (which characterize the duration of anthropogenic perturbations) either random fluctuational oscillations may take place around a single stable state of the biosphere (when both the biota and the environment it controls remain stable), or the biosphere, the environment, and life as a whole may completely disintegrate (if stability of the biota is violated).

5. The Energetics of Biota

5.1 Metabolic Power of the Individual

All the biochemical processes in the biosphere may be reduced to synthesis and destruction of organic matter. During synthesis of organic substances from inorganic ones energy is absorbed from the environment. Conversely, energy is released in the process of destruction of organic matter. The energy content of organic substances (calorific coefficient), including hydrocarbons, fats, and proteins naturally differs from substance to substance. However, on average, the energy content per unit mass of organic carbon is approximately constant for most individuals in the biosphere and constitutes (Odum, 1983):

$$K_C = 42 \text{ kJ/g C}. \tag{5.1.1}$$

The mass of living individuals exceeds, by a factor of ten, the mass of organic carbon in biota as a whole, if we account for free water. This relationship is used in all the computations below. Thus we may assume an energy content of a unit live mass $K = 4.2 \text{ kJ/g} \cong 1 \text{ kcal/g}$. Deviations from this average may, in the extreme, reach a factor of two (Whittaker, 1975; Winberg 1979; Odum 1983).

The energy content coefficient, K, for living individuals has a simple meaning. Its dimension kJ/g coincides with that of squared velocity. Therefore it is convenient to write:

$$K \equiv \frac{\omega^2}{2} \approx 4.2 \text{ kJ/g} = 4.2 \times 10^6 \text{ m}^2/\text{s}^2, \tag{5.1.2}$$

$$\omega = 3 \times 10^3 \text{ m/s}.$$

The velocity ω is a velocity of body movement such that its kinetic energy becomes equal to the energy content of all its bodily substances, or to the average velocity of all the body molecules reached during instant combustion of all its organic matter. Recalling that about 3/4 of living organisms' body mass is water, we may relate that velocity to temperature, following standard relationships from kinetic theory of gases (Levitz, 1962):

$$\frac{3}{2} RT = M \frac{\omega^2}{2}, \quad R = 8.3 \text{ J K}^{-1} \text{mol}^{-1}, \quad M = M_{H_2O} = 18 \text{ g/mol}$$

and obtain the maximum possible efficiency η, of energy expenditure for living individuals, as given by the Carnot cycle (see (2.8.4)):

$$\eta \approx \frac{T^+ - T_0}{T_0} \approx 0.95, \qquad\qquad\qquad\qquad (5.1.3)$$

$$T^+ = M \frac{\omega^2}{3R} \approx 6000\,\text{K}, \quad T_0 \approx 288\,\text{K} \approx 15\,°\text{C}.$$

Such a temperature coincides with that of the Sun's surface, and the maximum energy expenditure efficiency (5.1.3) with the maximum efficiency at which the solar energy may be used (Sect. 2.8).

To support biochemical reactions within the living body each individual uses the energy released during decomposition of organic matter. This leads to exchange of substances between the individual and its environment. The rate of food consumption by an individual, Q, kg/year, and the rate of consumption of organic carbon, Q_C, kg C/year, may be called metabolic rate (Brody, 1945; King, 1974). The rate of energy consumption by an individual (respiration) may be called metabolic power q. Variables q, Q, Q_C are interrelated via $q = QK = Q_C K_C$. Using the calorific coefficients K and K_C we find that the exchange rate of $1\,\text{kg C/year}$ or of about $10\,\text{kg}$ of food per year corresponds to a power of $1.3\,\text{W}$.

In agreement with the Arhennius-Boltzmann molecular energy vs temperature distribution (2.3.1), the metabolic rate grows exponentially with the known coefficient Q_{10}, which shows the degree of increase in metabolic power per $10\,°\text{C}$ of temperature increase. Assuming $T = T_0 + \Delta T$ we have:

$$q(T) = q(T_0) \exp(k \cdot \Delta T),$$

$$k \equiv \ln \frac{Q_{10}}{10\,°\text{C}}, \quad Q_{10} \equiv \frac{q(T_0 + 10\,°\text{C})}{q(T_0)}.$$

For most species the value of Q_{10} is close to three (Winberg, 1976).

The individual's metabolic rate may vary within quite wide margins. However, it cannot drop below a certain minimum value, found some time after food consumption, when the individual is at optimal temperature and relaxes in a state of complete rest. This is called the basal metabolic rate q_0 (Brody, 1945; Winberg, 1976; McNab, 1983). The maximum power produced by an individual per unit body mass is determined by the maximum rate of biochemical reactions in the living cell and should be universal for all kinds of living beings. Under natural environmental conditions the average daily power expenditure for almost every species reaches $(1.5–2.0)q_0$ (Calder, 1974; King, 1974; Winberg, 1976).

The potential daily energy expense or potential rate q_p in extreme environmental conditions is determined by the maximum possible rate of consumption of external food by the individual. The potential rate usually does not exceed four times the basal rate (Kendeigh et al., 1977).

For an average-sized man his basal metabolic rate is around $80\,\text{W}$ and the daily energy expenditure about $140\,\text{W}$, while a sprinting man may put out power in excess of $10\,\text{kW}$ (Brody, 1945). The metabolic power q produced by an animal is conveniently related to basal rate q_0 via a dimensionless total activity A:

$$q \equiv (A + 1) q_0. \tag{5.1.4}$$

If the existence rate is about $2q_0$, the mean total existence activity is $\bar{A} = 1$.

5.2 Body Size Limits

Metabolism must support biochemical reactions in all the living tissues of an individual. Of principal importance is the value of metabolic rate per unit mass or weight of an individual (the mass-specific rate) (Brain and McNab, 1980). Using weight (mg, where g is the free fall acceleration) instead of mass (m) is convenient because the metabolic power per unit weight (the weight-specific rate) has the dimension of velocity, and this power completely controls the possible movement rate of a land surface animal (Gorshkov, 1981, 1982b).

Since all the external energy enters the individual's body through its surface, it is also convenient to consider metabolism per unit area of the average living body projection upon the Earth's surface. We therefore introduce the "effective vertical size of an individual", l, and its "projection area at the Earth's surface", s:

$$l \equiv \frac{m}{\rho s}, \tag{5.2.1}$$

where m is the metabolically active mass of that individual, in which biochemical reactions occur (wood of tree trunks, in which biochemical reactions are practically absent, must not be included into the plant mass m); ρ is the density of living tissues, which we shall always consider equal to that of water, $\rho = 1\,\text{t/m}^3$. For the green plants and fungi their vertical (l) and horizontal ($\sqrt{s}$) sizes differ by an order of magnitude. Green plants are characterized by another dimension, their height H_0 which is usually of the order of $\sqrt{s}$, and also by the leaf index, d_0, which is equal to the ratio of cumulative leaf surface to plant projection area, s. For locomotive animals their projection area, averaged over the interval of movement, is $s \simeq l^2$.

Metabolic powers per unit projection area (j), weight (λ), and volume ($\hat{\lambda}$) of an individual are given by:

$$j \equiv \frac{q}{s},$$

$$\lambda \equiv \frac{q}{mg} \equiv \frac{j}{\rho g l}, \quad g = 9.8\,\text{m/s}^2,$$

$$\hat{\lambda} \equiv \frac{j}{l} \equiv \rho g \lambda. \tag{5.2.2}$$

All the relationships in this chapter would look much simpler in a system of units where $\rho = g = K = 1$, see Sect. 2.6. However, in such a system we have a distance unit $K/g = 430\,\text{km}$, a time unit $\sqrt{K}/g = 210\,\text{s}$, and a mass unit $\rho(K/g)^3 = 8 \times 10^{22}\,\text{g}$, which would be extremely inconvenient. In biology it is convenient to use the system of units where water density and free fall acceleration are equal to unity: $\rho = g = 1$. In such a system the dimensions of volume, mass and weight are identical and the specific rates per unit volume, mass and weight are equal to each other. But this system is incompatible with SI, unfortunately. Therefore we stick here to the SI system, in which these three constants have to enter all relationships. We have to differentiate between the values of λ and $\hat{\lambda}$, which have different dimensions but characterize one and the same variable. Lower case characters will also denote variables expressed in energy units, and capital ones, the same variables in mass units. They are all related to each other via

$$y = KY = K_C Y_C, \tag{5.2.3}$$

where y is a variable expressed in energy units, and Y or Y_C is the same variable in units of living mass or of organic carbon, respectively, see (5.1.1) and (5.1.2).

Were the densities of energy and matter fluxes, consumed by an individual, determined solely by environmental conditions, e.g. by physical diffusion, the value of j would be the same for individuals of any body size, and hence the metabolic power per unit volume $\hat{\lambda}$ or weight λ would decrease with growing body size l as $1/l$. Meanwhile it is natural to assume by virtue of the basic biochemical organization of life that it is the power of biochemical reactions in a unit volume of the living body, i.e. $\hat{\lambda}$, which is approximately constant for all the living beings. With environmental conditions dictating the value of j, and the value of $\hat{\lambda}$ remaining biochemically fixed and universal, we could then have organisms of only the strictly determined size $l = \hat{\lambda}/j$.

In fact, the metabolic power per unit body volume may vary within quite wide margins depending on the species. However by all appearances, these margins are universal for all the living world, since body size may only vary within strictly determined limits for a given j, see Fig. 5.1. Second, the majority of species that play an important role in the biosphere gravitate to an optimal value of λ, universal for life as a whole. Therefore, at fixed j one may speak about an optimal body size for living beings, see Fig. 5.1.

Heterotrophic individuals, which only consume organic matter synthesized by other individuals, may significantly change their j by radically altering the organization of their bodies: they may transit from consumption based on physical diffusion (as is the case for bacteria, fungi and plants) to active mechanical consumption of food, using digestive and distributing system of their bodies (as the locomotive animals do).

In the process of evolution several fundamental possibilities of increasing the value of j were discovered, and consequently the optimal body size increased. Animals which made that leap include non-vertebrates, ectothermic ("cold-blooded") vertebrates, endothermic ("warm-blooded") and passerine birds (*Aves passerines*), Fig. 5.1. Each of these groups is characterized by its own value of j, and by an optimal body size at fixed optimal value of λ_{opt}, Fig. 5.1. In each of these groups the body size may vary from λ_{min} to λ_{max}, see Fig. 5.1. Empirical data available for presently and previuosly existing animals of a given taxonomic group give grounds for stating that the values λ_{min} and λ_{max} are universal for life as a whole.

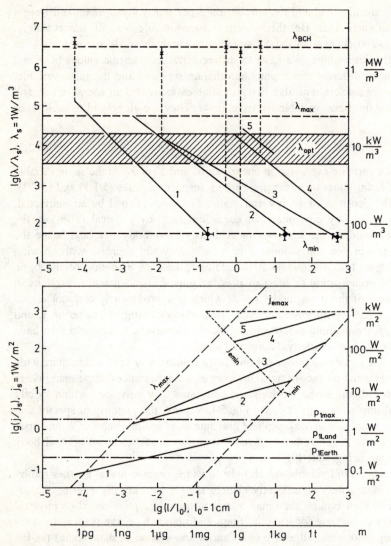

Fig. 5.1. The dependence of the basal metabolic power (the basal rate) on individual body size. Solid lines (Brody, 1945; Hemmingsen, 1960; Kleiber, 1961; Winberg, 1976; McNab, 1983; Gorshkov, 1981, 1982b, 1984c; Kanwisher and Ridgway, 1983): 1 – plants, bacteria, fungi, protozoa (without infusoria); 2 – infusoria and multicellular invertebrates; 3 – ectothermic vertebrates and cephalopodae; 4 – endothermic animals; 5 – passerine birds. Top: The mass-specific rates correspond to unit body volume.

$$\hat{\lambda}_0 \equiv q_0/l\,s.$$

q_0 - the basal rate of an individual (the dark respiration power for plants (Govindjee, 1982)); $l = m/(\rho s)$, (s – the individual projection area upon the Earth's surface, for animals $s = l^2$) m – individual body mass. The hatched band $\hat{\lambda}_{opt}$ includes more than 95 % of all the species in each taxonomic group (Chislenko, 1981). Separate points present the

If the metabolic rate per unit surface area of the body or per its projection upon the Earth's surface, j, were constant for each group, the metabolism of a unit volume would have decreased as $1/l$ with individual body size increasing, see (5.2.2). Actually, a slight growth of j is observed in each taxonomic group which, with individual body size increasing, slows the decrease of λ at larger l. That way individuals of larger body size may originate within each given taxonomic group (Fig. 5.1). It has been empirically found that all the dependencies of j (and, consequently, of λ) upon body size l are governed by allometric relationships (Sect. 2.6), and they may thus be presented as straight lines in bilogarithmic scales. The slopes of these lines depend on the morphological features of multicellular individuals in each given group (similar to critical indices and anomalous dimensions in physics (Haken, 1982; Schuster, 1984)).

The minimum values are obviously determined by the respective existence or basal metabolic rate. These values limit the maximum possible individual body size in each taxonomic group, Fig. 5.1. Extending the obtained basal metabolic rate lines at their known slopes to maximum known body size of both living and extinct individuals of a given taxonomic groups (the latter available from paleodata), we find that the values of λ_{min} for three such taxonomic group (see lines 1, 2, 3 in Fig. 5.1) coincide. This fact prompts one to assume that the value of λ_{min} found, is indeed the sought admissible universal limit of mass-specific metabolic rate (metabolic power per unit body weight).

In the course of their life animals sometimes have to use their maximum possible metabolic power. This power cannot exceed a certain biochemical limit (λ_{BCH}), which must, by all appearances, be universal for life in general. The maximum power outputs are produced by locomotive animals during their highest or longest jump and also by dividing bacteria, if the time lapse between the two successive divisions is minimum (amounting to about 15 min (Lewin, 1983)). (The time of dividing (doubling), τ, is approximately equal to the ratio of the individual body mass, m, to its metabolic rate measured in mass units, $Q \equiv q/K$, and may be

---

observed maximum body size both in the presently living and extinct individuals, sitting upon extrapolated lines for respective taxonomic groups (Gorshkov, 1981), which determine the minimal power $\hat{\lambda}_{min}$. (Compare with these data the "metabolism" of a unit volume of the Sun, which constitutes $0.27 \, W/m^3$, i.e. $0.05 \, \hat{\lambda}_{min}$ (Allen, 1955).) Crosses show the observed maximum metabolic power (bacteria division (Gorshkov, 1981), animal jump power per unit volume of the driving muscle (Gorshkov, 1982b), determining the biochemical limit $\hat{\lambda}_{BCH}$.

Bottom: – power per unit projection area, $j_0 = q_0/s$. Dashed lines: the minimal ($\hat{\lambda}_{min}$) and maximal ($\hat{\lambda}_{max}$) power per unit projection area for endothermic animals (Gorshkov, 1982a; McNab, 1983) Dash-dotted lines show the power of the net primary productivity:
$p_{1 \, max}$ – maximum (Ivanoff, 1972, 1975; Whittaker and Likens, 1975)
$p_{1 \, Land}$ – the average continental (Whittaker and Likens, 1975)
$p_{1 \, Earth}$ – the Earth as a whole (Whittaker and Likens, 1975).

expressed via $\lambda \equiv q/mg$, the constant K, Eq. (5.1.2), and $g : \tau \approx K(g\lambda)^{-1}$, see Sect. 5.3) The maximum power put out by bacteria in the process of dividing, and by animals of different body size during jumps per unit volume of their driving muscle, e.g., flea, grasshopper, locust, kangaroo rat and bush baby all coincide (Gorshkov, 1981, 1983b). This fact makes it possible to introduce the biochemical limit line, λ_{BCH} into Fig. 5.1.

The maximum existence rate, λ_{max}, must be significantly lower than the biochemical limit and be close to the optimal rate λ_{opt}. The rate λ_{max} in Fig. 5.1 is assumed to be equal to the maximum observed rate for eukaryotes, i.e. to the rate for infusoria of the smallest size (Gorshkov, 1981).

The observed body size of endothermic animals (mammals and birds with constant body temperature T_B) is limited by the condition of conservation of their body heat budget at environmental temperature T_0. For a given linear body size the lowest surface area is that of a sphere $s_B = 4\pi R^2$; its volume would be $(4/3)\pi R^3 = l^3$ (in agreement with the definition of l, Eq. (5.2.1), for average projection area $s = l^2$). Thus we have for a sphere $s_B \approx 5l^2$. For animals that would mean: $s_B \geq 5l^2$. The heat flux across the unit body surface area $j_B \equiv jl^2/s_B$ is equal to

$$j_B = h_B \nabla T = h_B \frac{\Delta T}{l_B}, \qquad \Delta T \equiv T_B - T_0, \qquad (5.2.4)$$

where h_B and l_B are the heat conductivity and thickness of the insulating layer (fur, fat, feathers). Apparently, $h_B \geq h_{min}$, ($h_{min} = 2.4 \times 10^{-2}$ W m^{-1}($^\circ$C)$^{-1}$) is a heat conductivity of air and of eiderdown (Childs, 1958) and $l_B \leq l$. As a result the minimum value of j for endothermic animals, $j_{e\,min}$ may be described by a relationship (Gorshkov, 1982a):

$$j_{e\,min} = 5 h_{min} \Delta T/l. \qquad (5.2.5)$$

At $T_0 = 0\,^\circ$C and $T_B \approx 40\,^\circ$C the dashed line for $j_{e\,min}$ in Fig. 5.1 crosses line 4 (mammals) near the actually observed minimal body size: $l = l_{min} \approx 1$ cm ($m_{min} \sim 1$ g), and line 3 (ectothermic ("cold-blooded") vertebrates) at $m_{min} \leq 1$ kg. Therefore large reptilia can be endothermic ("warm-blooded") (Bakker, 1975; Paladino et al., 1990).

The maximal value of $j_{e\,max}$ for endothermic animals is limited by the maximum possible heat release in terrestrial or aquatic conditions: $j_B < j_{e\,max}/5 = j_{Bcrit}$. E.g., at $T_0 \geq T_B$ in air the value j_{Bcrit} is given by possible available evaporation, which cannot exceed 200 W/m^2 at a relative humidity of 60%, i.e. $j_{e\,max} \approx 1000$ W/m^2 (presented by a dotted line in Fig. 5.1). Bird lungs feature a more advanced design that those of mammals (Schmidt-Nielsen, 1972). That is why the giant among passerine birds – the raven – compensates lack of sweat glands by the more effective (as compared to mammals) evaporation of water from the surface of its lungs. Lack of contact between the line for passerine birds and lines of biochemical limits is directly related to flying: energy expenditure during flight exceeds such expenditure during any other mode of locomotion (Gorshkov, 1984c).

5.3 Energetics and Body Size of Photosynthesizing Plants

The metabolic power of photosynthesizing plants is extracted from the absorbed solar radiation. If one assumes that, in the course of photoreactions, light is only used to synthesize organic compounds from inorganic ones, then the total power consumed by a green plant should be proportional to the import of inorganic substances needed for such synthesis. Knowing the respective calorific coefficients, one may determine the value of this metabolic power from measurements of matter exchange; it is then retrieved from the gross primary production of organic carbon. Its density per unit Earth's surface (gross primary productivity) may be denoted as P_0^+ and the respective power density as p_0^+, see Sect. 5.1 and Eq. (5.2.3). Were all the synthesized organic matter spent on ("autotrophic") respiration within a plant of a constant body mass, import and export of nutrients to the environment could be completely compensated. No such compensation occurs in the presently living plants, and if metabolism takes place, the mass of a plant always increases. The plant mass increment is its net primary production (this is the part consumed by heterotrophs), and we shall denote its density per unit Earth's surface (the net primary productivity) as P_1^+, and the respective power density as p_1^+.

The difference between the power of gross and net primary productions, i.e., the plant respiration (r_1^-) presents the metabolic power spent by plants to sustain their own life processes. Plants are immotile and may only consume the needed food from the environment via physical diffusion, similar to fungi and bacteria. It may be found empirically for photosynthesizing plants that the dependence of their metabolism (respiration) per unit projection area $(j \equiv r_1^-)$ and unit body volume $(\hat{\lambda}_1)$ on the vertical size l, coincides with the respective dependence for bacteria and fungi, see Fig. 5.1.

The law of conservation of energy and matter relates the rate of consumption P_n^- to respiration R_n, to production P_n^+ densities, and to velocity of biomass change $\dot{B}_n$ via the dependencies (Fig. 5.2):

$$P_n^- = R_n + P_n^+; \quad P_n^+ - \dot{B}_n = P_{n+1}^-; \quad n = 0, 1, 2; \tag{5.3.1}$$

$$p_0^- \equiv I, \quad P_2^+ = \dot{B}_2, \quad p_n^\pm \equiv K P_n^\pm, \quad r_n^- \equiv K R_n^-.$$

Here I is the solar radiation consumed by the biota; $P^\pm, R^-$ and $p^\pm, r^-$ are the variables in units of live mass and of energy, respectively, see Eq. (5.2.3) In steady state $\dot{B}_n = 0$ and $P_n^+ = P_{n+1}^-$, so that we have:

$$I = r_1^- + r_2^- + r_3^-, \quad p_0^+ = r_1^- + r_2^-. \tag{5.3.2}$$

Each box in Fig. 5.2 characterizes three independent variables P^-, P^+ and B. It is convenient to use the relative variables in each box in Fig. 5.2:

$$\Lambda \equiv \frac{P^-}{B}, \quad \alpha \equiv \frac{P^+}{P^-}, \quad \tau \equiv \frac{B}{P^+}, \tag{5.3.3}$$

$$\tau \equiv (\alpha \Lambda^-)^{-1}. \tag{5.3.4}$$

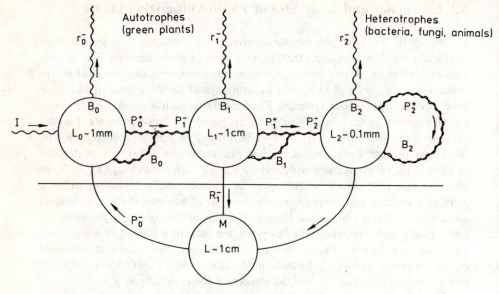

Fig. 5.2. Energy and matter fluxes in a local ecosystem. Solid lines – matter, wavy lines – energy fluxes. Combined solid and wavy lines – fluxes of organic matter. I – solar radiation, r_n^- – heat fluxes resulting from the destruction of the organic matter in the process of respiration; r_0 – light leaf respiration power flux (Govindjee, 1982; Lehninger, 1982). P_n^+ – production, P_n^- – consumption (destruction) densities of the organic matter. B_n – biomass, L_n – the organic matter layer thickness. $\dot{B}_n$ – the velocity of changing of biomass. M – inorganic matter resulting from destruction of the organic matter, L – its thickness; R_n^- – inorganic fluxes resulting from destruction of organic matter, P^- – total inorganic flux (total destructivity). Boxes in the scheme: $n = 0$ – photosynthesizing parts of plants, $n = 1$ – non-photosynthesizing parts of plants, $n = 2$ – heterotrophs. Laws of matter and energy conservation are satisfied in every box.

The relative variables Λ^-, α and τ remain meaningful for single individuals. The mass-specific consumption rate is $\Lambda^- = \eta\Lambda$, where $\Lambda = Q/m$ is mass-specific metabolic rate expressed in units of live mass, η is a digestibility. In most cases $\eta \geq 0.8$ (Sawby, 1973, Kendeigh, 1974) and we can approximately set $\Lambda^- \approx \Lambda \equiv Q/m \equiv \lambda g/K$ (Sects. 5.1 and 5.2). The coefficient α is the ecological efficiency of transforming the consumed product into body tissue (including meat and milk). For most locomotive animals of any body size $\alpha \approx 0.1$ (Whittaker and Likens, 1975). The time τ is the residence time of atoms in man's body tissue. This is an effective time scale for all life processes including the lifespan τ_L. The ratio $h \equiv \tau_L/\tau$ does not depend on body size and is a universal constant for large taxonomic groups (Brody, 1945). Therefore the lifespan τ_L is proportional to the inverse mass-specific metabolic rate Λ^{-1}:

$$\tau_L = c\,\Lambda^{-1}, \quad c \equiv \frac{h}{\alpha}. \tag{5.3.5}$$

For bacterial unicellular individuals $h \sim 1$, $\alpha > 0.5$ (Kendeigh, 1974; Whittaker, 1975) and the dimensionless coefficient c in (5.3.5) is of the order of unity. For most mammals the coefficient c is equal to about 100 (Brody, 1945). Man is the exception. For man the coefficient c is four times larger than for other mammals (Brody, 1945).

The law of conservation of energy and matter in steady state $\dot{B}_1 = \dot{B}_0 = 0$ relates the power of gross and net primary production to the power of plant respiration densities via the dependence:

$$p_0^+ = p_1^+ + r_1^-, \tag{5.3.6}$$

where the index "$+$" again denotes synthesis, see Fig. 5.2. Therefore, the level of respiration, r_1^-, is limited by the value of p_0^+. Plants, in contrast to animals, are not capable of increasing their energy consumption per unit projection area ($j = r_1^-$), independent of any possible morphological perfections. The vertical size of plants cannot be extended, except in the first taxonomic group. It is limited to the value of approximately 1 cm, (see Fig. 5.1). The biospheric average thickness, l, of the metabolically active layer of vegetation is of the order of 1 mm. In that sense the plants are dwarfs as compared to higher animals. The visible giant vertical size of plants, determined by their height, H_0, may only be reached because the volume of space, occupied by a plant, consists overwhelmingly of air and wood, and does not contain any live metabolically active tissue.

Solar energy may be transformed into the energy of organic matter at an efficiency level close to unity (see (5.1.3)). However the observed diurnal efficiency of photosynthesis never reaches 7%. Moreover, the observed annual average efficiency of photosynthesis for the whole biosphere constitutes about 0.3%, (Govindjee, 1982), see Table 5.1.

All the nutrients, except gaseous CO_2 and O_2, are consumed and transported by land plants along their bodily vessels as water solutions. The amount of water consumed by plants exceeds their net biochemical needs by many orders of magnitude. Therefore pure water must be constantly removed from plants. This occurs through transpiration – water evaporation by leaves. The amount of nutrients consumed by land plants, i.e., their net primary production, thus varies in proportion to transpiration. Due to the high leaf index of plants, i.e., to high effective evaporating surface and (particularly for trees), due to increase of the eddy diffusion in air at higher altitudes, transpiration may significantly exceed the level of regular evaporation from the open ground surface.

The estimates of net primary production and of plant biomass for various Earth ecosystems are given in Table 5.1.

The empirically measured dimensionless ratio of the annual average rate of transpired moisture to net primary production in live mass units is called the transpiration coefficient k_T, and is of the order of 100 (Larcher, 1976). Transpiration is proportional to total evaporation, which also includes evaporation by soil. The transpiration coefficient may be expressed as follows:

$$k_T = \frac{\alpha_T \rho E}{P_1^+}, \tag{5.3.7}$$

Table 5.1. The net primary production and biomass of the biosphere.

Ecosystem	S_e $10^{13}\,\mathrm{m}^2$	d_0	$\mathbf{P}_{1C}^+$ $\frac{\mathrm{GtC}}{\mathrm{year}}$	$\mathbf{B}_{1C}^+$ Gt C	P_{1C}^+ $\frac{\mathrm{tC/ha}}{\mathrm{year}}$	B_{1C}^+ $\frac{\mathrm{tC}}{\mathrm{ha}}$	τ year	τ_1 year	L_1 mm	β_2 %
Forests, bogs, swamps, marshes	5.1	8	40	750	8	150	19	2	16	5($<$ 1)
Grasslands, shrubs	3.3	4	13	50	4	17	4	1	4	10(1)
Cultivated (arable) lands	1.4	4	5	5	3	3	1	1	3	50(50)
Lakes, rivers	0.2	2	0.5	0.1	2	0.4	0.2	0.2	0.4	10(1)
Deserts, tundras	5	0.7	1	2	0.2	0.4	2	1	0.2	5(1)
Continents, total	15	4	60	800	4	50	13	1	4	7(1)
Open ocean (pelageal)	33	0.6	30	0.5	1	0.01	0.01	0.01	0.01	40(0)
Coastal waters (shelf)	3	2	8	1.5	3	0.1	0.2	0.2	0.6	30(0)
Ocean, total	36	0.8	40	2	1	0.06	0.05	0.05	0.05	40(0)
Earth, total	51	2	100	800	2	16	8	0.1	0.2	17($<$ 1)

- S_e is the area occupied by the ecosystem;
- d_0 is the leaf area index (the ratio of the leaf total surface area to their projection area upon the Earth's surface);
- $\mathbf{P}_{1C}^+$ is the net primary organic carbon production (Whittaker and Likens, 1975; Ajtay et al., 1979; Gorshkov, 1987a; Townshend et al., 1991; Townshend, 1992);
- $\mathbf{B}_{1C}^+$ is the total mass of organic carbon in living plants, including wood (Whittaker and Likens, 1975);
- P_{1C}^+ and B_{1C}^+ are the net primary productivities and the total biomass of organic carbon (Whittaker and Likens, 1975; Ajtay et al., 1979);
- $\tau = \mathbf{B}_{1C}^+/\mathbf{P}_{1C}^+ = B_{1C}^+/P_{1C}^+$ is the total biomass residence time; on average the net primary productivity of the metabolically active live mass P_1^+ is equal to $10P_{1C}^+$;
- τ_1 is the residence time for metabolically active biomass (Gorshkov, 1982b);
- $L_1 = P_1^+\tau_1/\rho$ is the layer thickness of metabolically active biomass;
- β_2 is the share of net primary production consumed alive by consumers (by vertebrates in brackets).
- Forests, bogs, marshes and swamps are joined because these ecosystems feature similar productivities and biomasses (Whittaker and Likens, 1975)

where α_T is the share of transpiration in total evaporation, ρE, from a unit soil area; E is the observed evaporation rate (m/year); P_1^+ is the net primary production in units of live mass (kg/(m^2 · year)). The share of the solar radiation power, η_T, spent on transpiration, is equal to:

$$\eta_T \equiv \frac{\alpha_T\,\rho E\,L_w}{I} \equiv \frac{\alpha_T\,E}{E_{\max}},$$

$$E_{\max} \equiv \frac{I}{\rho L_w} \approx 2\,\mathrm{m/year}, \tag{5.3.8}$$

where $L = 2.3\,\mathrm{kJ/(g\,H_2O)}$ is latent evaporation heat for water; $I \approx 150\,\mathrm{W/m^2}$ is the mean solar energy flux reaching the Earth's surface, see (2.2.3). Because of (5.3.7) the efficiency of net photosynthesis production, η_p, appears to be uniquely related to η_T, (5.3.8):

$$\eta_p \equiv \frac{p_1^+}{I} = \frac{K\eta_T}{L_w k_T} \equiv \frac{K}{L_w k_T}\alpha_T \frac{E}{E_{max}}, \quad (p_1^+ \equiv KP_1^+), \tag{5.3.9}$$

where p_1^+ is the power of net primary productivity in energy units; K is the energy content of living cells, (5.1.2). (The energy content of wood differs from that of metabolically active plant tissues. However, wood production constitutes no more than 10 % of the total plant production. Account of wood production would not change the results above.) The values of L_w, K and k_T are essentially physical and biophysical constants which cannot be changed by the biota. Therefore the efficiency of photosynthesis of land plants is completely determined by the rate of evaporation, E, which depends on the state of continental biota (Sect. 4.6).

In the most humid areas in the whole biosphere, such as tropical rain forests, evaporation occurs totally by way of transpiration, and more than 90 % of the available solar radiation power is spent on it (Larcher, 1976; Govindjee, 1982). This situation results in photosynthesis efficiency nearing its observed maximum in these areas (Larcher, 1976). Conversely, the efficiency of photosynthesis is sharply reduced in the areas of insufficient evaporation.

The amount of total land net primary production may be estimated from the known values of the average land evaporation rate $\bar{E}_b = 500$ mm/year, see Fig. 4.11, the land surface area (see Table 5.1), and the average annual value of the share of transpiration in total evaporation $\bar{\alpha}_T = 0.6$ (Gorshkov, 1980b). Using these values and Eqs. (5.1.1) and (5.1.2) in Eq. (5.3.9) we have the average annual photosynthesis efficiency $\bar{\eta}_p \approx 0.3\%$, the average power of net primary productivity $\bar{p}_1^+ \approx 0.5$ W/m^2 and the average land net primary productivity in carbon units $\bar{P}_{1C}^+ \approx 4$ t C/(ha·year) in accordance with the data of Table 5.1. The maximum evaporation rate is four times as large if all the available solar energy is spent on it (this follows from (5.3.8)). The maximum annually averaged values of η_p, p_1^+ and P_{1C}^+ are respectively $\eta_{max} \approx 1.2\%$, $p_1^+ \approx 2$ W/m^2 and $P_{1C}^+ \approx 16$ t C/(ha·year). The rate of evaporation from the ocean surface ($E_s \approx 1.3$ m/year) is more than twice as large as the contemporary evaporation rate from the land surface, see Fig. 4.11. The restoration of land surface vegetation coverage, mainly in the deserts, could significantly change the global evaporation regime and average land net primary productivity, increasing its severalfold. This would lead to reduction of heating of desert surfaces and to a change in the overall temperature regime of the planet (Henderson-Sellers and Cogley, 1982).

5.4 Fluctuations in Synthesis and Destruction of Organic Matter

Despite the extreme complexity of the overall structure and interspecies relationship within the local ecosystems there exist general laws which tie production and destruction to body size (more accurately, to average correlation radii of the individual). These apply to all the species active in both synthesizing and destroying organic matter. These laws follow from the conditions of matter cycle closure. To satisfy the conditions in (4.3.5) (see also (4.3.2) and (4.3.3)) the relative random fluctuations of P^+ and P^- have to remain below the value of steady state breach κ_0, see Sect. 4.3.

Only individuals from different species may interact in a correlated manner in a community. There is, first of all, a strict correlation between the species synthesizing and destroying the organic matter (i.e., between plants and animals), which is superimposed by correlations between carnivores and herbivores (their prey) in the animal kingdom. In the interest of natural selection the interaction of individuals within a species must be competitive. Since individuals of the same species are uncorrelated, there remains only one way to diminish the possible fluctuations of matter and energy fluxes. According to the well-known statistical law of large numbers, the relative fluctuation of a measurable variable in a non-correlated system is of the order of $1/\sqrt{N}$, where N is the number of mutually uncorrelated parts of the system (Sect. 2.3). Therefore, within a local ecosystem, organic matter should be synthesized and destroyed by $N \geq \kappa^{-2}$ uncorrelated elements. This condition may be realized through different mechanisms of synthesis and destruction.

Plants are immotile and form a continuous cover. The strongest synthesis fluxes usually flow through the largest plants in the community. But plants function as weakly internally correlated modular individuals (Begon et al., 1986). Let us denote the average correlation radius for plants (i.e., the average distance between the various parts of a plant functioning in a correlated mode) through r^+. Then, on account of the predominantly vertical stratification of correlated parts in plants, we obtain for the number of uncorrelated "patches" (columns) within a local ecosystem of size L_c (see Gorshkov, 1984a, 1985a):

$$N = \frac{L_c^2}{(r^+)^2} \geq \kappa^{-2} \quad \text{or} \quad r^+ \leq \kappa L_c. \tag{5.4.1}$$

We see that fluctuations in plant productivity are decreased by large plants which are actually formations with a loose inner correlation and which function in a mode similar to that of an equivalent colony of completely uncorrelated single cell algae. If there are n^+ plant species approximately equally represented in a local ecosystem which occupy different niches and, consequently, function in uncorrelated mode, then the number of such uncorrelated patches increases by the factor of n^+ and the expression for the average correlation radius transforms into:

$$r^+ \leq \kappa L_c \sqrt{n^+}. \tag{5.4.2}$$

We see that diversification of species in a community would increase the average correlation radius between plants without unbalancing the closed cycles of matter. The radius of a local ecosystem as a whole must be the same for plants (synthesizers) and for bacteria, fungi, and animals (destroyers) of the organic matter. Therefore the average correlation radius for plants (5.4.2) should be treated as a universal characteristic, which does not depend on the size of separate plants in the ecosystem. Irrespective of plants' size their parts follow similarly chaotic distributions, so that characteristic sizes of plants, forming the bulk mass of vegetation (i.e., the maximal distance between the various correlated parts of plants) have to be assessed from the height of their trunks and/or length of stems. Next, the relationship in (5.4.2) makes it possible to assess the size of the local ecosystem, L_c, from the average correlation radius of plants (r^+). Apparently, the vertical radius of correlation for plants r^+ in (5.4.2) cannot exceed the thickness of the metabolically active level of vegetation, l, (Sect. 5.3). Assuming that the latter is of the order of the thickness of a green leaf (i.e., $r^+ \sim (0.1–1)$ mm) we obtain: $L_c \sim (1–10)$ m.

Similarly, immotile fungi and bacteria also work to diminish fluctuations in the destruction of organic matter. Like higher plants, fungi have a small correlation radius, which is of the order of the thickness of their hyphas. In turn, bacteria present a non-correlated set of separate single-cell organisms. Thus ecological problems arise only after locomotive animals evolve and enter the ecosystems.

5.5 Immotile and Locomotive Organisms

Like any other macroscopic physical motions and processes, life is sustained by the free energy of solar radiation. The flux of solar radiative energy at the Earth's surface does not exceed 1 kW/m^2 at maximum (see (2.2.1)). Hence, no macroscopic process directly driven by the radiative solar energy should exceed this power density threshold.

The energy release during thunderstorms, hurricanes and tornadoes exceeds that value by a factor of several tens or even hundreds.[1] That may occur either due to concentration of the solar radiant power incident upon the larger area and transformed into mechanical energy, into a smaller surface area, or quickly releasing the potential energy previously stored over a long time period.

Concentration of solar energy from large territories into small areas only occurs when water is evaporated and precipitated. Residual precipitation, which failed to reevaporate, accumulates into rivers, and the resultant hydropower density significantly exceeds the radiative solar energy flux. But the global hydropower consists of a very small part of the total sunpower, see Table 2.1.

The absorbed solar energy always accumulates in the form of evaporation/melting latent heat. Slowly evaporating water vapor stores large amounts of energy, which may be released in a pulse by a tornado-like formation. Having spent within a second the energy previously stored in a given volume for several hours or even days, the tornado has to spatially move so as to consume energy

---

[1] The flux of wind energy is equal to the product of its velocity, u, with the density of wind energy $\rho u^2/2$, where ρ is air density. Dissipation of wind energy (its destructive power) is equal to $c\rho u^3/2$, where c is the coefficient of dissipation, practically independent of the velocity. The average global wind speed and the wind power flux are equal, respectively, to 7 m/s and 3 W/m^2 (Gustavson, 1979). When the wind speed close to the center of a typhoon climbs to 200 m/s, that is almost by a factor of 30, its power flux increases in proportion to u^3, that is by the factor of 3×10^4 reaching 100 kW/m^2. That power is clearly much higher at the very center of the cyclone.

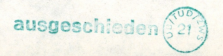

from the newly occupied volume, etc. The higher the tornado power, (i.e., its rate of energy release per unit volume), the quicker it has to move. Without movement the tornado would quickly break up and dissipate all its power.

The same goes for hurricanes too. The principal feature in using the potential energy accumulated in unit volume of the environment is that the object using that energy, whether a tornado or a hurricane, must move. If a mechanism were available to concentrate that energy from a large surface, local immovable tornadoes or hurricanes could appear which (like hydropower plants) would remain spatially stable (Jones, 1990), but this is not actually observed.

Fire presents a similar phenomenon. During a fire the energy from the organic matter synthesized for many previous years is spent almost instantly. Fire may only sustain itself if it spreads quickly. Similarly rock falls and avalanches release gravitational energy accumulated during the slow prolonged processes of snowfall and/or mountain formation. In all such cases high density power fluxes only become possible due to previous accumulation of potential energy in various forms.

Free energy of sunlight cannot be directly stored in the form of photons, since photons possess kinetic energy only and have no mass, see Sect. 2.6. Since plants live off absorbed solar radiation, they cannot produce power densities higher than that of incandescent light. Movement would have not helped plants to absorb more light. That is why they are immotile, weakly internally correlated modular individuals that form the continuous vegetation cover of the Earth's surface (Gorshkov, 1980b). This statement can be called *the law of plant's immotility*. Absorbing solar radiation, plants accumulate it in the form of potential energy of the organic matter they synthesize. The observed maximum power flux of organic matter producing photosynthesis is about $2.0\,W/m^2$. The average land surface power of net primary productivity is about $0.5\,W/m^2$ and, of the Earth as a whole, $0.25\,W/m^2$ (see Sect. 5.3 and Table 5.1).

Animals feed off the organic matter accumulated by plants. The power of the flux of organic matter consumed by an animal per unit (average) projection area may considerably exceed the respective plant productivity. For mammals and birds their consumption fluxes per unit average projection area exceed $1\,kW/m^2$ (Sect. 5.2), i.e., are above plant productivity by a factor of several thousand. Thus animal life may be sustained only through consumption of organic nutrients which are synthesized by plants at an area exceeding the animal's individual average projection area by the same factor. Passive consumption of organic matter synthesized at a large area bordering the surface of the animal's body would only be possible in a liquid environment. Such a feeding mode in combination with immotile existence is employed by several marine and fresh water animals (actinias, ascidias, some mollusks, and balanuses). In the absence of water-transported fluxes of organic matter an animal is capable of eating within an hour the organic matter synthesized in a whole year by all the plants around it. After that the animal has to move to a new area to be able to feed off the organic matter available there, etc. This movement is a necessary precondition of animal life. A moving animal inevitably destroys accumulated biomass. Its life would be impossible without previous accumulation of such mass.

The intensity of consumption flux is singularly connected with the animal's body size. Food enters the animal's body through its surface and is consumed within its volume. With increasing body size, l, the body surface grows as l^2, and its volume as l^3. Biochemical organization of life follows certain universal laws, which demand that energy release per unit volume of the animal's body, $\hat{\lambda}$, Eq. (5.2.2), stays close to an optimal level, see Sect. 5.2. For all the actively living organisms it amounts to about $10\,\mathrm{kW/m^3}$ (Fig. 5.1). Therefore, the power released per unit body surface, j, would increase with increasing body size and would linearly follow l ($j = \hat{\lambda}l$, see (5.2.2)). Such a dependence necessitates transition from diffuse absorption of nutrients by bacteria, protozoa and fungi to active mechanical feeding and development of specialized digestive and distribution systems in higher animals. In other words, an increase in body size is necessarily accompanied by an increase in animal complexity. Only microscopic or weakly internally correlated modulary individuals, for which the nutrient fluxes through their unit body surface area do not exceed the level of plant productivity, may remain immotile during their life span. It may be seen from Fig. 5.1 that only bacteria, protozoa, (except infusoria), and fungi with body size below $10^{-4}\,\mathrm{m}$ fall into this category (as for fungi, that characteristic size is determined as thickness of their hyphae). All other animals from infusoria to whale must move. As a consequence they must be strongly internally correlated unitary individuals (Begon et al., 1986). This condition would even hold for the case of one separate species which could consume the total plant production. When, as it were, this production has to be shared between many animal species, their feeding territories have to be widened, and the animals have to move faster, so as to be able to cover these territories. This statement can be called *the law of animal's immotility*.

The average correlation radius for locomotive animals is close to their body size: $r^- \sim l \equiv (m/\rho)^{1/3}$, where m is the animal's mass, and ρ is its body density, see Sect. 5.2. The area of correlated food consumption by an animal is of the same order of magnitude as its body projection area, $s = l^2$. The relative fluctuation of food consumption by an animal in the space region of the order of its body projection area is of the order of one. If a large animal of body size $l \sim L_c$ completely consumes production from a local ecosystem of size L_c, then its relative fluctuation, and, consequently, the local ecosystem breach, κ, would also be of the order of one. The only way for large animals to exist at all within closed matter cycles is to decrease their quota of consumption. An animal of body size $l \sim L_c$ should consume no more than $\kappa \sim 10^{-4}$ of the total primary production from a local ecosystem.

The more diverse the animal species in a given range of body sizes, the more weakly their consumption of plant production is correlated, and, hence, the lower are the overall fluctuations of that consumption. If a ceiling is set for possible fluctuations (a set value of the local ecosystem breach κ, Eq. (4.3.5), is adopted) and then increasing the species diversity makes it possible also to increase the total mass of animals in the given body size range. Let us introduce spectral densities per given body size of the consumption quota, β, and of the number of species, n (Gorshkov, 1981). Then, similar to (5.4.1) and (5.4.2), we obtain for that body size the number of non-correlated parts in a local ecosystem, $N = (L_c^2/l^2)n$, and the relative fluctuation of consumption (destruction) by animals of that body size, $\beta/\sqrt{N}$. The latter should not exceed the level of the local ecosystem breach, κ. As a result we have (Gorshkov, 1984b, 1985a):

$$\beta \le \left(\frac{\sqrt{n}}{l} \right) \kappa L_c. \tag{5.5.1}$$

In contrast to (5.4.2), where the condition of the cycles' closure dictates the internally uncorrelated structure of plant bodies, the relationship in (5.5.1) demands only that the destruction quota be specifically distributed as a function of the animals' body sizes. The strong internally correlated structure of animals' bodies is determined by their need to move. For large animals of body size in excess of $l = 10$ cm their consumption quota may be estimated from (5.5.1): if $\kappa \sim 10^{-4}$, $L_c < 10$ m, $n \sim 1$, then $\beta \sim 0.01$. Thus, the large animals' quota of consumption in the ecosystem must not exceed 1 %. This estimate agrees well with the empirical data available for all the ecosystems unperturbed by man, see Fig. 1.3 and Sect. 5.6.

Note, that the relationships in (5.4.2) and (5.5.1) entail that an increase in the species' diversity provides a way for more animals to exist among the more correlated higher plants without disrupting the closed matter cycles. To find a true dependence of β on l one has to know how the number of species n in (5.5.1) depends on l. That problem is analysed in Sect. 5.13.

Relationships in (5.4.2) and (5.5.1) describe the general structure of the local ecosystems. They demonstrate that the biosphere may, on the whole, be envisaged as a non-correlated set of live, internally correlated biosystems devoid of centralized control, averaging about 0.1–1 mm in size. This structure guarantees that the fluxes of organic matter synthesis and destruction do not fluctuate too strongly and remain within about 10^{-4} of each other. Large animals may exist within a stationary biosphere only on condition that their quota in consumption of organic matter produced in the biosphere does not exceed 1 %. In relation to large animals the existing biosphere is just an energy producing engine, working to support them, to provide them with food and oxygen and to stabilize their environment at an optimal level. However, this engine functions at an efficiency level of no more than 1 %. The other 99 % of energy fluxes must be consumed by the other species in the community, and that way they should be considered "added value", necessary to support the life of the larger animals.

The size distributions, Eqs. (5.4.2) and (5.5.1), which exclusively cover the data on correlation radii for differing species, play the role of the intensity characteristics of the natural biota, similar to energy distribution in thermodynamics.

5.6 Distribution of Consumption by Heterotrophs According to Their Body Size

Let us introduce the share, β_i, of net primary production consumed by an animal of a given body size, i.e., the ratio of consumption by that animal, P_i^-, to the net primary production, P^+: $\beta_i \equiv P_i^-/P^+$. It is a characteristic handy for comparing various ecosystems with differing net primary productions against each other. Summing up consumption by all the individuals within the body size interval from l to $l+\Delta l$, one may plot a distribution of the share of consumption with body size. However, the density of consumption per universal unit body size increment, Δl, has no sense within a wide range covering several orders of magnitude, since any function characterizing an individual can change within the characteristic range Δl of the order of the body size of that individual, l. (Consumption by bacteria having a body size of about $1\,\mu\text{m}$ changes noticeably while the body size is changed by $\Delta l \sim 1\,\mu\text{m}$. Consumption by large mammals of the body size of $l \sim 1$ m noticeably changes with the body size changing by $\Delta l \sim 1$ m, but does not change while that size changes by $\Delta l \sim 1\,\mu\text{m}$.) Therefore only a distribution function retrieved for a unit relative interval $\Delta x \sim \Delta l/l$, $\beta(x)$, is sensible, that is a dimensional size distribution or size spectrum, (Hutchinson and MacArthur, 1959; Sheldon et al., 1972), defined as follows:

$$\beta(x) \equiv \frac{1}{\Delta x} \sum_i \beta_i, \quad \Delta x \equiv 0.43 \frac{\Delta l}{l}, \quad \text{or } \beta(x) = 2.3\, l \left(\frac{1}{\Delta l} \sum_l^{l+\Delta l} \beta_i \right), (5.6.1)$$

$$\int_{x_{\min}}^{x_{\max}} \beta(x)\, dx = 1, \quad x \equiv \lg\left(\frac{l}{l_e}\right), \quad l_e = 1\,\text{cm}. \tag{5.6.2}$$

Summation here is conducted over all the species entering the body size range from l to $l+\Delta l$ and β_i is the i species' consumption share. Various age groups of individuals of the same species, strongly differing in their body size, are separated into different relative body size groups. The factor 0.43 accounts for decimal logarithms instead of natural ones. The function $\beta(x)$ is the relative body size spectrum, i.e., the density of the consumption share of the net primary production by individuals of a given body size, entering the unit range of relative size $\Delta x = 1$.

Figure 5.3 plots the distribution $\beta(x)$ based on published field studies from a large number of natural non-perturbed ecosystems. The histogram ranges in Fig. 5.3 correspond to: 1 – bacteria, protozoa and saprophito phagous; 2 – invertebrates; 3 – vertebrates. The solid line presents the average distribution over all the studied ecosystems (Gorshkov, 1981).

Histogram intervals are chosen to correspond to the groups 1–5 of individuals, presented in Fig. 5.1. The first interval, $10^{-6}\,\text{m} \le l \le 10^{-4}\,\text{m}$ is occupied by bacteria, protozoa and saprophito phagous (those destroying dead plants) and mycorrhiza (fungi in symbiosis with plant roots, Pankow et al., 1991). The fungi body size is assumed to be equal to that of hyphae, strings of mycelium composing the body of each fungi; they may be assumed to correlated weakly among themselves (Gorshkov, 1981, 1984b). In the second interval, $10^{-4}\,\text{m} \le l \le 10^{-2}\,\text{m}$,

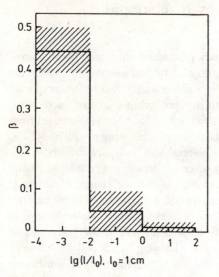

Fig. 5.3. Distribution of the organic matter destructivity vs the terrestrial heterotrophic body size (Gorshkov, 1981). $\beta = P_l^-(l)/P^+$, $P_l^-(l)$ – the spectral density of destruction produced by heterotrophic individuals (bacteria, fungi, animals) of a body size l, P^+ – net primary production (of terrestrial plants). Solid line – the universal distribution, observed in the natural non-perturbed ecosystems (Gorshkov, 1981). Area under the solid line is equal to unity. Numbers in per cent present the inputs from various parts of the histogram to the whole. The observed deviations from the mean distribution in some natural ecosystems are dashed.

consumption of net primary production is determined by invertebrates. Bacteria and fungi entering the second interval do not play any significant role there due to their low mass-specific consumption λ (Fig. 5.1), even though their biomass may exceed that of invertebrates. The third interval, $10^{-2}\,\text{m} \leq l \leq 1\,\text{m}$, is completely dominated by vertebrates, mainly mammals. The input from consumption by invertebrates to the third interval is insignificant. Scatter of the measured values in various ecosystems is shown by hatched areas.

As follows from Fig. 5.3, bacteria and saprophito phagous consume about 90 % of all the net primary production in natural ecosystems not perturbed by anthropogenic impact, invertebrates about 10 %, and vertebrates about 1 % of that production. Flowing waters, such as littoral, estuaries and rivers have to be excluded from this domain as having high influx of nutrients.

A distribution similar to that presented in Fig. 5.3 is also observed in shallow closed water ecosystems, where the principal part of primary production is controlled by large multicellular plants of high biomass (Kamenir and Khailov, 1987; Kamenir, 1991). In the open ocean and other deep waters where the total production is controlled by microscopic phytoplankton (its individual biomass is three to four orders of magnitude less than that of higher plants), there are no large herbivores, and all the net primary production is consumed by bacteria and zooplankton, which occupy the first part of the histogram in Fig. 5.3. A similar situation is observed for lichen.

Thus, with account of plant respiration, more than 95 % of the gross (total) primary production consumed by individuals in the community flows through immotile individuals. All the motile animals together comprise only a 5 % addition to the energy consumption structure of the community. However, being large animals with strongly slowed metabolism (Fig. 5.1) they may (as, for example, in the ocean) comprise a considerable (though metabolically not too active) part of the total community biomass.

Large vertebrates add the smallest part (less than 1 %) in the energy consumption structure of community. This part can have the largest relative fluctuation (larger than 100 times) during the shortest time interval without any apparent break in the community energy flow. That is why a high rate of reproduction of the so called r-selected species (Brain and McNab, 1980) and therefore high metabolic power and basal rate (Pianka, 1970) become advantageous in the presence of large fluctuations in population density. That is also the reason for the greater competitiveness of endothermic animals compared to ectothermic animals and of passerine birds compared to nonpasserine birds of equal body size.

The fact that practically all the energy flux goes through immotile individuals, and that the principal part of plant biomass is consumed after their natural death, together provide for closed cycles of nutrients, needing no horizontal transport of these nutrients, and also for highly effective absorption of solar energy in the community. The principal condition forced upon the immotile heterotrophs, is that the continuous layer into which they combine must not shade producers in the community from the Sun. Therefore immotile heterotrophs should find a place below the photosynthesizing parts of vegetation (either bacteria and fungi in the soil, or bacteria and zooplankton in oceanic depths).

The destructivity, $\beta_l P_1^+$ is distributed among all the individuals of a given body size positioned in the vertical layer of thickness L of their metabolically active biomass ($B = \rho L$), where β_l is the share of consumption by individuals of body size l averaged over all the species in the community. This consumption is equal to the product of consumption per unit volume of an individual, $\hat{\lambda} = j/l$, see (5.2.2), and thickness of the biomass layer L, i.e., $\hat{\lambda} L = \beta_l P_1^+$. Such a presentation makes it possible to determine the biomass layer thickness L from the equation $L = \beta_l(P_1^+/j)l$. The ratio $d \equiv L/l = \beta_l P_1^+/j$, which is equal to s/S (here s is the projection surface area of one individual; S is the effective consumption area (home range) per single individual: $sl = SL$) is equivalent to the leaf area index d_0, see Table 5.1, and may be called the projection area index for heterotrophs (Gorshkov, 1981, 1982a). The layer of biomass of bacteria and fungi in soil, of a thickness L, cannot be too thick: the bacteria size is $l \simeq 10^{-6}$ m, and the size of a fungus (its hyphae thickness) is $l \simeq 10^{-5}$ m, so that we have for bacteria: $L = ld \leq 5 \times 10^{-5}$ m, and for fungi: $L \leq 5 \times 10^{-4}$ m, since $d \doteq \beta_l P_1^+/j \leq 50$ ($P_1 \leq 2$ W/m^2, $j \geq 0.04$ W/m^2, hence $d \approx 5$–10 in reality, see Fig. 5.2).

Assuming the global average cover by bacteria both on land and at sea (Sieburth, 1976) to be equal to $L = 5 \times 10^{-5}$ m we obtain for the total live mass of all those bacteria (spread across the Earth's surface of 5.1×10^{14} m^2) a value of $M = 3 \times 10^9$ t. The average mass of a single bacteria is estimated at 10^{-18} t and their total number on Earth is given a figure of 3×10^{27}. That value may simultaneously give an estimate of the total number of living beings in the biosphere, since the number of individuals of all the other species together is several orders of magnitude lower. The number of species among the bacteria being estimated at 3×10^3 (Chislenko, 1981; Raven and Johnson, 1988), the number of bacteria within a single species is estimated at 10^{24}, and that fact has been covered in Sects. 3.15 and 3.16.

Note also a certain property of higher plants which makes possible the existence of large herbivores with a low share of consumption of primary production: while all the single-cell individuals and all motile (locomotive) animals function within the strict correlations between the separate parts of their individual bodies, and execute centralized control of that body as a whole, immotile multicellular individuals (higher plants and fungi) do not have any such control. They do not possess a head and consist of practically independent, weakly correlated parts of small sizes (e.g. leaves of a single plant). Moreover, these separate parts may compete among themselves for sunlight and nutrients. When one part of a plant perishes, that does not entail death of its other parts and of the whole, but stimulates development of those other parts. In that sense higher plants and fungi are more of a set of independent individuals (leaves, hyphae), which are partly correlated via a common woody trunk and the vessel system supplying nutrients, water and food from soil. Although weak, it is particularly this correlation which facilitates the high overall metabolically active mass of higher plants and fungi.

The motile herbivore animals are capable of eating only the metabolically active parts of plants which contain nutrients in the required proportions. Higher plants are noted for the maximum thickness of their metabolically active biomass layer and for lack of correlation between the separate parts of each individual. These features are particularly favorable for animals to feed off certain specific parts of plants, which may constitute only a small part of their metabolically active biomass. Meanwhile consumption of any small part of metabolically active mass of a rigidly correlated individual (particularly – of a single-cell one) is impossible, since it would lead to that individual's death.

Were all the large multicellular plants as rigidly internally correlated as the animals are, large animals would produce extremely high fluctuations in the natural distribution of vegetation, even with the share of consumption by those animals remaining quite small. (That, for example, is what happens when the vessel network in the cambium is damaged around the whole perimeter of the tree trunk.) That is why the appearance of mobile herbivores and of carnivores feeding off the former could only take place in the course of evolution after higher plants had appeared.

The share of consumption β_i by a species i, in the community may be used to estimate empirically the correlation radius of the community. Denoting the share of consumption of plant production by a heterotrophic species i, in the community as β_i^-, and using the normalization $\Sigma_i \beta_i^- = 1$ (summing is over all the heterotrophic species in the community) one may estimate that correlation radius for the community from the linear distance at which the sum is saturated reaching some value close enough to unity; for example, the distance at which $\Sigma_i \beta_i^- = 0.95$. It follows from the conducted analysis that the principal input to that sum is produced by a small number of bacteria and saprophyte fungi species. The same may be done for autotrophic plant species, understanding β_i^+ as the share of the solar energy or the share of inorganic nutrients consumed by the ith plant species in the community ($\Sigma_i \beta_i^+ = 1$). That approach indicates a significantly smaller size of the community (Gorshkov and Gorshkov, 1992) than the saturation length for the whole number of species, independent of their consumption share (Giller, 1984) which appears (in the case of non-perturbed ecosystems) to be close to estimates of the correlation radius of the community obtained in Sects. 5.4 and 5.5.

5.7 Daily Average Travelling Distance

Consider the movement of land surface animals. The total metabolic power of an animal moving at a speed u is usually estimated from the rate of its oxygen consumption. It may be written as (see (5.1.4)):

$$q(u) = [A(u) + 1] q_0. \tag{5.7.1}$$

Numerous experiments have demonstrated that the total activity $A(u)$ of an animal is linear with u up to the maximum speeds developed by that animal (Schmidt-Nielsen, 1972, 1984). This relationship holds for every species ever studied. Moreover, when the animal's speed of movement approaches zero, the value of $A(u)$ approaches a certain finite limit $A(0)$, i.e., the total power of movement does not smoothly taper out into the basal rate q_0 (Schmidt-Nielsen, 1972, 1984). It is natural to label the intercept $b \equiv A(0)$ "readiness" (for movement) (Gorshkov, 1983b, 1984c). The average value of b is close to unity (Fig. 5.4). Following the dimension condition (Sect. 2.6) the available empirical results may be presented as:

$$A(u) = a + b, \qquad a = \frac{u}{u_0}, \tag{5.7.2}$$

where the value of a is the net movement activity, and the fundamental dimensional constant u_0 has the meaning of the speed the animal develops when $a = 1$.

The speed u_0 determines the slope of the line presenting the dependence of the measured power, (5.7.1) and (5.7.2), on the speed of movement u. Experimental data from Fig. 5.4 show that u_0 is a universal characteristic of movement, independent of the animal body size within the given taxonomic group. The average value

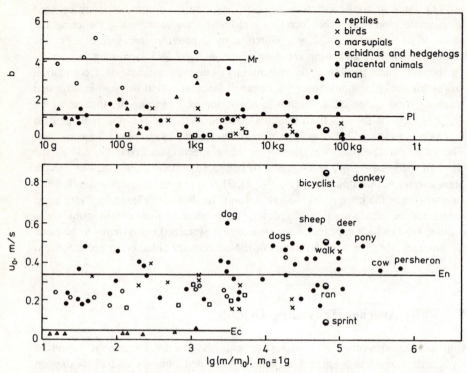

Fig. 5.4. The available speed and movement readiness (Schmidt-Nielsen, 1972, 1984; Gor-shkov, 1983b) Readiness b (intercept) presents the increment in metabolic power in units of the basal rate when going from the state of rest to movement at almost zero speeds. The achievable speed u_0 is the reverse total movement power-by-speed derivative (in units of the basal rate). Lines in the figure denote: En – average achievable speed for endothermic animals ($u_0 = 0.3$ m/s); Ec – same for ectothermic animals ($u_0 = 0.03$ m/s); Mr – average readiness for marsupials ($b = 4.2$); Pl – average readiness for all the other placental animals ($b = 1.0$); m – animal body mass. Man is a mediocre long-range runner, the worst sprinter among the endothermic animals, but one of the best walkers in the animal world. The absolute record-holder in energy parameters of movement among all the animals is the donkey.

is $u_0 = 0.3$ m/s $= 26$ km/day for all the "warm-blooded" (endothermic) animals. The record belongs to the donkey, for whom $u_0 = 0.8$ m/s.

Consider the meaning of speed u_0. The total diurnal activity $\bar{A}$ is limited by the existence rate q; according to empirical data available for most animals it is close to $\bar{A} \approx 1$. We denote the relative duration of the active state for an animal as $x_a = t_a/T$, where t_a is duration of the active interval, and $T = 24$ h. The total cumulative diurnal activity must coincide with its average value

$$\bar{A} = A x_a = \left(\frac{u}{u_0} + b \right) x_a,$$

from which we obtain:

$$x_a = \frac{\bar{A}}{u/u_0 + b}.$$ (5.7.3)

If $\bar{A} = 1$, $u = u_0$ and $b = 1$ we have $x_a = 1/2$, i.e., $t = 12$ h (a 12-hour working day). We further obtain from (5.7.3) for $A = 1$ and $b = 1$ that an animal cannot move at a speed different from zero for the whole 24 h in a day (if $x_a \to 1$, $u \to 0$). The distance L_T, travelled by an animal in a day is equal to $u\,t_a$, i.e., $x_a = L_T/u\,T$. We find from (5.7.3) that:

$$L_T = L_{T\ \max} \frac{u}{u + bu_0}, \qquad L_{T\ \max} = \bar{A}\,u_0\,T.$$ (5.7.4)

It follows from (5.7.4) that the maximum daily travelling distance is reached at speeds of movement $u \gg u_0$ because the readiness b differs from zero. Animals should move quickly but in short bursts. Note that $b \approx 1$ for untrained people, for athletes $b < 1$ (see Fig. 5.4). According to (5.7.4) the maximum distance walked in a day at the diurnal average activity of $\bar{A} = 1$ is about 26 km (for a donkey it amounts to 70 km/day). Finally, using (5.7.3), the average daily speed, $L_T/T = u\,x_a$, that the animal's metabolism may support (we may call it available speed, u_a) can be expressed as:

$$u_a = \bar{A}\,u_0 \left(1 - \frac{bx_a}{\bar{A}} \right).$$ (5.7.5)

At $\bar{A} = 1$ and $x_a \ll 1$ the speed u_0 is equal to available speed u_a.

5.8 The Maximum Speed of Movement for Animals

The speed u_0 however cannot be totally independent of animal body size. We shall demonstrate from the law of energy conservation that, starting from some critical body size, the speed u_0 must decrease for larger sizes l. Metabolic power is transformed into mechanical power at a certain efficiency level α which cannot be larger than the observed maximum efficiency of muscles. Within a living individual the latter does not exceed 25 % (Hill, 1960; Cavagna and Kaneko, 1977; Heglund et al., 1979). Therefore one may assume that $\alpha < 0.25$. The mechanical power put out at a constant speed u is spent to compensate for energy dissipated to ground and air friction. The law of energy conservation is then expressed as the equality between mechanical power and dissipative energy losses.

Energy dissipation during movement on soil is proportional to the product of body weight, mg, and the speed of movement u, and may be written as γmgu, where γ is the ground dissipation coefficient (it is similar to the coefficient of friction known from physics). The empirical data available on the animals' maximum velocities show that the value of γ depends neither on the speed of movement, nor on the body size (i.e. mass) of the animal, and is, on average, equal to 0.05 for most animals (Gorshkov, 1983b). Dissipation of energy to air friction is equal to c $l^2 \rho_c u^3 / 2$, where ρ_c is air density ($\rho_c = 1.2 \times 10^{-3} \rho$, $\rho = 1\,t/m^3$); $\rho_c u^3 / 2$ is the energy flux through a unit surface, equal to the product of energy density $\rho_c u^2 / 2$ and velocity u; cl^2 is the effective streamlined body surface. This value may be treated as the product of the resistance force $(c/2)\rho_c u^2 l^2$ and the velocity u. The air resistance coefficient c may be measured (see references in Gorshkov, 1983b, 1984c). It is equal to 0.5 for the majority of land surface animals. The body size l of mobile animals is related to their body mass by a relationship:

$$l \equiv \left(\frac{m}{\rho}\right)^{1/3}. \tag{5.8.1}$$

The mechanical power of movement is equal to $\alpha\, a\, q_0$. Equating it to cumulative dissipative losses we have:

$$\alpha\, a\, q_0 \;=\; \gamma_{tot} mgu \tag{5.8.2}$$

$$\gamma_{tot} \;=\; \gamma + \gamma_c \equiv \gamma\left(1 + \frac{Fr}{k^2}\right) \tag{5.8.3}$$

$$\frac{\gamma_c}{\gamma} \;=\; \frac{Fr}{k^2}, \quad Fr \equiv \frac{u^2}{gl}, \quad k^2 \equiv \frac{2\rho\gamma}{\rho_c c}. \tag{5.8.4}$$

Here γ_{tot} is the total dissipation coefficient, equal, by definition, to the ratio of resistance force to individual body weight mg; Fr is the Froude number, see Sect. 2.6; γ_c is the air dissipation coefficient, which is relatively small for $Fr/k^2 \ll 1$.

Using the expression for net activity a, Eq. (5.8.2), one may rewrite that expression (for $Fr/k^2 \ll 1$) in the form:

$$u_0 = \frac{\alpha}{\gamma}\lambda_0, \qquad \lambda_0 \equiv \frac{q_0}{mg}. \tag{5.8.5}$$

Since λ_0 drops for higher body sizes (Fig. 5.1) the observed constancy of u_0 for varying body size l means that either the efficiency α or the dissipation coefficient γ must change with body size l. Basing calculations on empirical data we shall demonstrate that the value of γ cannot change with body size. Consequently, the value of efficiency α must change.

The ratio

$$\varepsilon \equiv \frac{\lambda_0}{u_0} = \frac{\gamma}{\alpha} \tag{5.8.6}$$

presents the dimensionless energy cost of moving a unit weight along a unit distance (it is similar to automobile mileage); $\lambda_0/u_0 = E/mgL_d = aq_0/mgu$, where $E = aq_0 t$ is the net energy expenditure per distance travelled $L_d = ut$. The dependence of ε on body size l for animals is presented in Fig. 5.5. Due to constancy of u_0 the energy cost ε linearly falls off for larger body sizes as λ_0 and α^{-1}; this drop goes on until the efficiency α reaches its maximum possible level. Following that the value of ε must remain constant, independent of body size (Gorshkov, 1983b).

According to observational data, λ_0, u_0 and hence the ratio α/γ do not depend on the speed of movement. This means that animals move slowly enough that

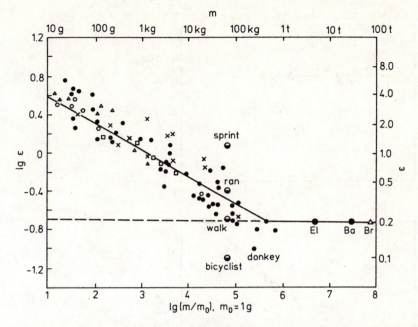

Fig. 5.5. Energy cost of movement vs the animal body size (mass). (Schmidt-Nielsen, 1972, 1984; Gorshkov, 1983b). The dimensionless energy cost of movement ε is equal to net expenditure of metabolic energy (the difference between the total metabolic energy and the metabolic energy output at the zero speed limit) per unit body mass per unit distance:

$$\varepsilon = [q(u) - q(0)]/(mgu);$$

$q(u)$ – the metabolic movement power at the speed of u; m – the animal body mass. For experimental points, see legend to Fig. 5.4. The solid line is the average value of ε. It does not depend on the absolute animal metabolic power and is identical for mammals, birds and reptiles of equal body size. Due to higher movement efficiency α the value of $\varepsilon = \gamma/\alpha$ decreases at higher body size as far as the maximum possible value of α and minimum value of ε. After achieving it, further decrease in ε for larger body sizes should stop. The solid line is numerically extended in the horizontal from the observed maximum efficiency α and the average dissipation coefficient γ for the mechanical movement energy (see Fig. 5.6). Ho – man; El – the maximum body mass for a presently living land animal, the African elephant (5 t); Ba – the maximum body mass for an extinct land mammal, Baludjiterium (30 t); Br – the maximum body mass for a dinosaur, the Brachiosaurus (80 t). For other notation see Fig. 5.4.

one may neglect air resistance (second term in (5.8.3)). Speeds of movement at which the resistance of air becomes equal to ground friction should be the top limit, because further energy expenditures (i.e., net activity a) would grow as u^3. Therefore the condition

$$\frac{1}{k^2}\frac{u_{\max}^2}{gl} = 1 \quad \text{or} \quad u_{\max} = k\sqrt{gl} \tag{5.8.7}$$

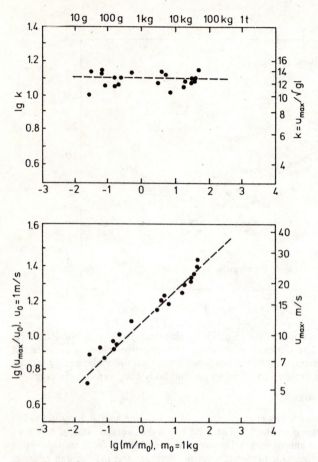

Fig. 5.6. Land animals maximum speeds of movement vs their body size (mass). The maximum speeds of animal movement correspond to a constant value of Froude's number $k^2 = u_{max}^2/g\,l$. Equating energy expenditures for overcoming ground and air resistance, Eq. (5.8.7), and accounting for the definition of ground resistance, Eq. (5.8.4), the ground resistance, γ, may be retrieved from a known air resistance coefficient $c = 0.5$. It averages $\gamma = 0.05$ (Gorshkov, 1983b, 1984b). At a movement efficiency of $a = 0.25$ we obtain a maximum energy cost of movement $\varepsilon = \gamma/\alpha \approx 0.2$, see (5.8.6) and Fig. 5.5.

must correspond to maximum speeds recorded for animals of body size l. Empirical data on these speeds (see Fig. 5.6) demonstrate that Froude's number $u_{max}^2/g\,l$ remains constant for any animal, i.e. depends neither on the speed u, nor on the size l. On that ground one may state that the dissipation coefficient γ is also constant; indeed, the constancy of the air resistance coefficient c had been repeatedly tested in independent experiments (see references in Gorshkov, 1983b, 1984c).

The above leaves the efficiency α as the only parameter to change with size l in the relationship (5.8.5); its changes should be such that the product $\alpha\lambda$ remains constant (Gorshkov, 1983b). Consequently the value α must increase with the body size l growing. But $\alpha \leq \alpha_{max} \approx 0.25$. Therefore $\varepsilon \geq \varepsilon_{min} = \gamma/\alpha_{max}$. One may see from the data available on u_0, γ and λ that this limit is reached for the animal mass of $m \approx 100$–300 kg, see Fig. 5.5. Direct measurements made for horse and man showed that their efficiencies are close to the top limit (Brody, 1945; Atkins and Nicholson, 1963). The value of α having reached its maximum, the speed u_0 (5.8.5) must start to decrease with λ_0 at even higher body size l.

The decrease in efficiency of locomotion α for lower body sizes is only observed when locomotion takes place in the regime of oxygen balance, and energy expenditure is compensated by oxygen consumed from the environment (Gorshkov, 1983b). All animals are capable of short bursts of locomotion in the regime of oxygen debt at maximum efficiency α, independent of their body size. That conclusion follows from the analysis of record jumps by animals of different body sizes (Gorshkov, 1983b, see Fig. 5.1).

The mechanical power per unit body mass, $\alpha\lambda$, necessary to support the animal's life, is observed to be independent of its body size. There is no physical property limiting the efficiency of locomotion α of small animals. Thus the decrease of α at smaller body size could be achieved by reducing the ratio of muscle mass to body mass at the same maximum efficiency of those muscles, which is not actually the case (Gorshkov, 1983b). Therefore we conclude that small animals only use their muscles at the maximum possible efficiency in extreme situations of oxygen debt. With the overwhelming part of their lives occurring in conditions of oxygen balance, the efficiency of muscles α drops for smaller body sizes, so that $\alpha\lambda$, the mass specific power of locomotion, remains the same for both the small and the large animals. That feature is apparently ecologically caused. It is only due to that feature that energy competitiveness of the large animals, controlled by their mechanical power, coincides with energy competitiveness of a congregation of small animals of an equal mass. The total competitiveness related to presence of inner correlation and to support of internal homeostasis (which is understood as building up a weakly fluctuating internal environment optimal for the functioning cells and organs of the body, that environment kept unchanged due to the controlling action of an "internal" Le Chatelier principle) increases for larger animals, so that there appears an energy supplied ecological niche for the existence of large animals surrounded by small ones.

However, with body size increasing, that property is only supported up to a certain critical size, at which the efficiency of locomotion reaches its maximum admissible value α, see Figs. 5.5 and 5.6. Large animals whose body size exceeds the critical value are forced to search for some exotic means of increasing their competitiveness and of gaining an ecological niche fit for their existence.

5.9 Maximum Permissible Share of Biomass Consumed by Mobile Animals

We denote the vegetation biomass B_1 per unit land surface as $B_1 \equiv \rho L_1$ where L_1 is the thickness of the metabolically active (edible) layer of plant biomass, see Table 5.1. Assume that moving across its feeding ground (home range) the animal eats part of the biomass equal to $B_L = \beta_L \rho L_1$, where β_L is the consumed fraction of vegetation biomass. The effective width of land band off which the animal eats vegetation is close to that animal body size l, Eq. (5.8.1). The vegetation mass consumed in unit time with the animal moving at an average daily speed of u is equal to $B_L l u = \beta_L \rho L_1 l u$.

The fodder assimilation coefficient (digestibility) for an animal may, for simplicity, be assumed equal to unity (for most animals it is actually equal to 0.8 (Gessaman, 1973; Kendeigh, 1974, see Sect. 5.3)). The energy contained in the fodder consumed during movement must be equal to the total existence rate: $q = (\bar{A} + 1)q_0$:

$$K\beta_L \rho L_1 l u = (\bar{A} + 1) q_0, \tag{5.9.1}$$

where K is the energy content of a unit live mass, Eq. (5.1.2). The relationship (5.9.1) determines the speed of movement needed to support the animal's existence. It may be called the ecologically necessary speed u_n:

$$u_n = \frac{(\bar{A} + 1)q_0}{K\beta_L \rho L_1 l}. \tag{5.9.2}$$

The animal may only survive if its available speed u_a, Eq. (5.7.5), is larger than or equal to u_n. Using (5.7.5), (5.7.2), (5.8.5) and (5.8.6) this inequality may be rewritten as a limitation upon the consumed share of vegetation biomass β_L (Gorshkov, 1982a, b):

$$\beta_L \geq \beta_{L\,min} \equiv \frac{\bar{A}+1}{\bar{A}} \frac{g}{KL_1} \frac{1}{(1 - bx_a/\bar{A})} \varepsilon l^2, \quad \varepsilon \equiv \frac{\lambda_0}{u_0} = \frac{\gamma}{\alpha}, \tag{5.9.3}$$

or as a limitation upon the consumed biomass:

$$B_L \geq B_{L\,min} \equiv \frac{\bar{A}+1}{\bar{A}} \frac{g\rho}{K} \frac{1}{(1 - bx_a/\bar{A})} \varepsilon l^2, \quad (B_L = \beta_L \rho L_1). \tag{5.9.4}$$

All the variables entering the righthand part of (5.9.3) and (5.9.4) are wellknown. The thickness of the metabolically active biomass L_1 is estimated in Table 5.1. The energy cost, ε, is determined by the dissipation coefficient, γ, and the efficiency, α, and hence it cannot depend on the taxonomic group the animal belongs to, see Fig. 5.1. Therefore the limitations in (5.9.3) and (5.9.4) are equally justified for all the land surface animals: insects, larvae, amphibia, reptiles, mammals and birds. (A pole at $x_a = \bar{A}/b$ is produced by the zero available speed, Eq. (5.7.5), at such a value of x_a.)

5.10 Settled and Nomadic Lifestyles for Locomotive Animals

The relationship (5.9.1) determining the animal's necessary speed of movement u_n may be presented and interpreted in various ways. The metabolically active biomass of vegetation $B_1 = \rho L_1$ may be expressed as $P_1^+ \tau_1$, where τ_1 is the turnover time for the metabolically active (short lived, see Table 5.1) biomass; P_1^+ is the net primary productivity in units of live biomass (kg m^{-2} year^{-1}). The area of feeding ground for an animal (approximately equal to "home range" (Harestad and Bunnell, 1979; Damuth, 1981a, b)) may be expressed as S ($S \equiv N^{-1}$, N is the population density number). The distance travelled by an animal across this territory is equal to S/l. Denote the time in which the animal makes a round of this whole territory as τ_S. (The band of width l must scan the whole territory in time τ_S.) Then the speed u_n must be equal to $(S/l)/\tau_S$.

The rate of fodder consumption by an animal $Q \equiv (\bar{A} + 1)q_0/K$ equals the consumed fraction of plant production over the total feeding ground $\beta_l P_1^+ S = Q$, where β_l is the species consumption share of the net primary production. Substituting these values into (5.9.1) and cancelling identical terms in both parts of the equality we obtain the relationship between the species consumption share of vegetation biomass β_L and the species consumption share of the net primary production β_l:

$$\beta_L = \beta_l \tau_S / \tau_1. \tag{5.10.1}$$

The species consumption share $\beta_l = Q/(P_1^+ S)$ may be expressed via the animals's biomass $B = \rho L$ (L is the layer thickness for such a biomass). The consumption territory S is related to biomass B by relationship: $SB = m$, ($SL = l^3$, $m = \rho l^3$). We obtain for species consumption share:

$$\beta_l = \frac{\Lambda L}{P_1^+}, \tag{5.10.2}$$

where $\Lambda = Q/l^3$ is the rate of fodder consumption per unit volume of the animals's body, see Sect. 5.1.

The relationship in (5.10.1) makes possible quantitative differentiation between settled and nomadic life styles. If an animal rounds its feeding ground in time τ_S equal to vegetation reproduction period τ_1, it would appear at a given area within its feeding ground in exactly the time needed for the vegetation to reproduce the part of biomass eaten by that animal before, during its preceding visit. In that case the share of consumed biomass and the plant production would coincide with each other: $\beta_L = \beta_l$.

In reality most small-sized animals round their feeding grounds in a shorter time ($\tau_S \ll \tau_1$), each time eating away an amount of biomass significantly smaller than their permissible share ($\beta_L \ll \beta_l$). Such a situation permits the animal to visit any part of its feeding ground at practically any time, and thus reduces fluctuations of biomass of vegetation due to its consumption by an animal. Small-sized animals may therefore exist in conditions of abundance of food and metabolic energy. Fluctuations of vegetation biomass due to its consumption by an animal

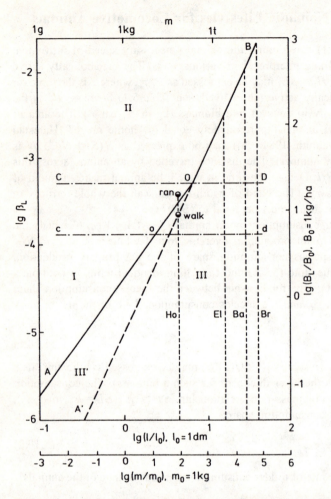

Fig. 5.7. The share of vegetation consumption by herbivores vs their body size (mass). The solid line shows the minimal consumed biomass $B_{L\,min}$, Eq. (5.9.4) (righthand scale) and consumption share of the total plant biomass β_L, Eq. (5.9.3) at $L_1 = 4\,mm$ (lefthand scale), which, when consumed, provides the energy of animal movement across their feeding ground ($\bar{A} = 0.5$; $x_a = 0.25$). The solid line breaking point corresponds to such a point in Fig. 5.5. Movement efficiency is at maximum to the right of point O. Dashed extension of the line A′OB corresponds to the absolute maximum movement efficiency, independent of the animal body size. Line AO corresponds to the observed decrease in efficiency for lower body sizes, see Figs. 5.4 and 5.5. Dash-dots in CD present the observed average consumption share of vegetation products by mammals in the natural land ecosystems (Damuth, 1981a, b) β_l, Eq. (5.10.2), computed from the average forest, savanna and steppe productivity ($p_1^+ = 1\,W/m^2$, $P_{1C}^+ = 0.8\,kg\,C/(m^2\,year)$), see Table 5.1. The observed animal biomass $B = \rho L$ increases with body size as inverse mass specific metabolic rate, Λ^{-1}, (Damuth, 1981a), so that β_l remains independent of the latter, see (5.10.1). The dotted extension of line CD is an extrapolation to body sizes of extinct animals, see Fig. 5.5. Line COD crosses line AOB at the latter's breaking point (Gorshkov, 1982a, b). Line cod gives an admissible share of vegetation consumption by foragers-collectors (four times less

do not exceed the natural fluctuations of that biomass in the absence of animals. The presence of animals does not leave any noticeable trace and does not change distribution of the vegetation.

A large animal is forced to consume an excessive part of vegetation biomass ($\beta_L \gg \beta_l$). The vegetation and the whole community around it are then destroyed, and the closed matter cycle in a local range where consumption took place is disrupted. Then the animal leaves the destroyed area and returns to it only after a time τ_S, when steady state vegetation, community, and the closed character of matter cycles are restored. During that succession time (which is much longer than the vegetation reproduction period $\tau_S \gg \tau_l$) the net primary production is consumed by other "repairing" species which act to close the matter cycle again. As a result the effective share of net primary production consumed by large animals remains within the ecologically admissible norm, see Fig. 5.3. However, such an animal leaves a noticeable trace in the observable distribution of vegetation, visible e.g. from on board an aircraft. At any given instant only a tiny part of the enormous feeding ground appears to be fit for life for a large animal. This part is equal to the ratio $\tau_l/\tau_S = \beta_l/\beta_L$, see (5.10.1). All the rest of the territory must be closely guarded against the intervention of competitors. A large animal constantly remains in a state of food and energy deficit (see Fig. 5.7).

The strategy of existence in which the round of the feeding ground is completed during a time shorter than that of reproduction of vegetation, so that this round does not leave any traces in the natural distribution of vegetation, corresponds to settled lifestyle. The strategy in which such a round takes more time than the reproduction period for vegetation, and leaves a noticeable trace in the natural distribution of vegetation, corresponds to the nomadic lifestyle (Gorshkov, 1982a,b).

If the consumption share of vegetation production β_l is fixed, all the large animals having $\beta_{L\,max} > \beta_l$, may only exist in the nomadic regime, Fig. 5.7. With an anomalously low species-specific value β_l even small animals featuring $\beta_{L\,min} > \beta_l$ fall into an obligatory nomadic lifestyle. Small animals may also turn sporadically to a nomadic lifestyle if they reach extremely high population density and consume an extremely high share of vegetation biomass, while the relationship $\beta_L > \beta_l > \beta_{L\,min}$ holds, Fig. 5.7. Such facultative nomadic behavior apparently arises in communities perturbed by man (invasions of locusts, forest "damagers", etc.).

---

than the herbivores' share (Gorshkov, 1982b, 1984b)). Range III to the right of line A'OB is prohibited energetically. Range III', limited by lines A'OA, is prohibited physiologically. Within that range animals would not be capable of moving across their territories by eating the available vegetation. Range I, limited by lines AOC for herbivores (Aoc – for foragers-collectors) is open for them in a settled regime $\beta_L/\beta_l < 1$. Range II, limited by lines COB (coOB – for foragers-collectors) is open for nomadic herbivores: $\beta_L/\beta_l > 1$. The existence of animals of body size falling to the right of point O for herbivores (and to right of point o for foragers-collectors) is possible only in a nomadic regime. For other notation see Figs. 5.4 and 5.5.

In a settled regime any animal in its natural community eats less than 20 % of all the edible biomass in any given spot of its feeding ground (Golley, 1973), which guarantees sustained stability of the whole of the community under any fluctuations.

In a nomadic regime the share of biomass consumption may even reach unity, (all the biomass is completely destroyed when it is "edible"), and, consequently, the whole community perishes. Following that a long restoration period is needed during which the biomass and the community as a whole are generated anew and then proceed at their most competitive steady state. Such extremely rare cases of nomadic behavior are only encountered in the human population (slash-and-burn agriculture and modern wood clearing) and also in certain insects in communities perturbed by man (Holing, 1978; Finegan, 1984; Isaev et al., 1984). Nowadays such communities are permanently destroyed every few tens of years ($\tau_S/\tau_1 \approx 10$), so that they are never able to reach their steady state. They might only be restored if such destruction was repeated every few hundred years, i.e. if perturbations were reduced by several orders of magnitude.

5.11 Carnivores

Biotic and environmental stability only depend on the interaction between autotrophic plants and heterotrophic herbivores, see Fig. 5.2. Dividing the heterotrophic block of the biosphere into herbivores and carnivores is equivalent to undoing the structure of correlations within the heterotrophic block. Consider specific features of carnivores.

Biomass production by herbivores is ten times less than the production of vegetation they consume, i.e., it is less by much more than an order of magnitude than the net primary production. Therefore all the carnivores must be mobile animals. Their feeding ground must be ten times larger than the feeding territory of their prey and their population density should correspondingly be ten times less (at a metabolism level similar to that of their prey).

Predators should not only be mobile animals themselves, but may only feed off mobile prey. Production by motile prey is concentrated into their projection area and presents a "source" of a productivity density exceeding net primary productivity by several orders of magnitude. In contrast to a herbivore, a carnivore does not need to collect the evenly spread products from its whole feeding ground; it is enough for such an animal to move from one "source" to another or to keep attached to the "source" itself (the phenomenon of parasitism). All the carnivores, despite the enormous feeding ground they cover, remain in the state of complete energy abundance (Gorshkov, 1982a, b).

In contrast to herbivores, whose mean share of vegetation consumption is much less than the net primary production, predators consume the main part of the production of their prey. Under natural conditions they cannot increase their number if the number of their prey remains constant. Therefore natural predators of any individual size are incapable of disrupting ecological equilibrium in the community. (However, dogs and cats living off man in suburban areas may completely extinguish their natural prey.)

The role of predators in the community is to eliminate decay individuals from the prey species of the same community. In strongly perturbed external conditions the decay polymorphism sharply increases. This causes a sharp increase of the population number of the respective predator species. If, in contrast, decay polymorphism of the prey species were to reduce to zero, the predator species would not be needed and would become absent in the community. The same reasoning is valid for the correlation between plants and herbivore consumers, mainly insects. The sharp increase of the decay polymorphism in plants precepitates a corresponding sharp increase in the population of herbivore insects. Such processes are observed after fires, forest clear cutting and other strong perturbations of natural communities (Holing, 1978; Isaev et al., 1984; Morneau and Payette, 1989). Were the decay polymorphism to vanish in all the species, all the consumer species would disappear from the community and only dead bodies would be destroyed by reducers.

As noted in Sect. 5.3 the lifespan of humans is about four times as long as that of other mammals of the same body size. Humans have the lowest productivity, τ_L^{-1}, and ecological efficiency α among mammals, see (5.3.5). We have for humans $\alpha \sim 0.025$ instead $\alpha \sim 0.1$ for other mammals. Obviously the limit $\alpha \to 0$ and $\tau_L \to \infty$ ("immortal" individuals) would entail that the prey has zero productivity, so that the consumption of prey by predators becomes impossible. There should be some low but finite critical value of the ecological efficiency of prey, α_{min}, at which its consumption by predators ceases to be energetically advantageous. Apparently humans have reached such a critical minimal value of α. Indeed, there is no predator now and evidently has never been in the past which specialized in consuming humans (Blumenschine and Cavallo, 1992). That is why man has always been forced to eliminate decay individuals from his own population himself.

5.12 Diffusion of Excreta

There is one more limitation on consumption by locomotive animals. Recall that the fall-off of dying vegetation provides for stability of concentration of nutrients in a local ecosystem; these nutrients, randomly distributed in the fall-off, only have to diffuse quickly in their initial position. This may happen in two ways: separate leaves falling off are small enough to be distributed evenly, while large tree trunks slowly grow and just as slowly decompose after falling. Insignificant fluctuations of nutrient concentrations within the local ecosystem may also be compensated because of the Le Chatelier principle acting in the community.

Moving herbivores collecting nutrients from their feeding grounds transport biogenic elements within their bodies and concentrate them in their excreta, of which 80% fall to urine and 20% to feces (Kleiber, 1961; Kendeigh, 1974). As follows from the data presented in Fig. 5.3, small mobile animals (like dungbeetles) feeding off the feces consume no more than 10% of them. The principal part of this product is destroyed by bacteria and fungi. Therefore a stationary state is only possible when the nutrients, transported and concentrated in the excreta, undergo diffusion and/or are transported with the external matter fluxes across the territory they had been concentrated from; this process should not take longer than the period of vegetation reproduction τ_1.

Let the average distance between separate animals' excreta be L_{ex}. The average amount of excreta, proportional to the animals' body size, may be denoted as δl^3, where $\delta \approx 10^{-3}$ (Kleiber, 1961). Moving along the distance L_{ex} the animal eats the amount (volume) of vegetation of $\beta_L L_{ex} l L_1$. The "excretion distance" L_{ex} is determined by the equality $\beta_L L_{ex} l L_1 = \delta l^3$, i.e.

$$L_{ex} = \frac{\delta l^3}{l L_1 \beta_L} = l^2 \left(\frac{\delta}{L_1 \beta_L} \right).$$

The time excreted nutrients take to diffuse the distance from which they had been concentrated is the order of:

$$\tau_D = \frac{L_{ex}^2}{D} = \frac{\delta^2}{\beta_L^2 D L_1^2} l^4, \tag{5.12.1}$$

where D is the diffusion coefficient with dimension cm^2/s (that is why the term L_{ex}^2/D has the dimension of time). When dissolved in water excreta mainly diffuse via molecular diffusion in water (including molecular diffusion in vegetation roots). The molecular diffusion coefficient in water is of the order of magnitude $D \approx 10^{-5}$ cm^2/s $= 10^{-2}$ m^2/year. The condition $\tau_D \leq \tau_1 \approx 1$ year limits the value of l:

$$l \leq l_D \equiv (\tau_1 D)^{1/4} \left(\frac{L_1 \beta_L}{\delta} \right)^{1/2}. \tag{5.12.2}$$

Assuming the average thickness of the metabolically active biomass layer of vegetation $L_1 \approx 4$ mm (see Table 5.1), $\delta \approx 10^{-3}$, $\beta_L \approx 10^{-3}$, $\tau_1 \approx 1$ year, $D \approx 10^{-2}$ m^{-2}/year, we obtain $l_D \approx 1$ cm. As seen from (5.12.2) this value is hardly sensitive to even significant variations in any of the input variables.

Therefore, there is no problem of the excreta spread for individuals of $l \leq l_D$; this spread, even by means of the slowest process of them all, molecular diffusion in liquid, takes less time than reproduction of vegetation. On the other hand, for animals of sizes $l > l_D$ the time of diffusional spread τ_D quickly increases, see (5.12.1). The τ_D increases by four orders of magnitude, while l increases by only one. At $l \approx 10^{-1}$ m the time interval $\tau_D \approx 10^4$ years; at $l \approx 1$ m we have $\tau_D \approx 10^8$ years. These estimates do not change, in principle, even if the diffusion coefficient changes by a few orders of magnitude. Therefore, nutrients excreted from the bodies of large animals cannot be returned to those places from which they had been collected by the process of diffusion.

Stable ecosystems containing large animals may only exist because of the external natural fluxes of matter, which mix and transport the animals' excreta across the land surface. The principal role in mixing the excreta of large animals is played by the surface runoff of precipitated water. The amount of nutrients mixed by surface water runoff may be assessed from the level of ionic runoff of carbon, which amounts to about 10^{-3} of the organic carbon production (Watts, 1982; Schlesinger, 1990). In a stationary case the amount of nutrients concentrated in the excreta of large animals must not exceed the amount of nutrients returned to their initial state by the surface ionic runoff. Consequently the global average share of consumption by all the large animals must not exceed several tenths of a percent of net primary production, which corresponds to the distribution presented in Fig. 5.3. In areas of low surface runoff, large animals may comparatively quickly desertify the land surface (Gorshkov, 1981, 1982a).

In coastal areas, estuaries, river floodlands and also in rivers and lakes themselves, where the ionic runoff locally approaches the level of net primary production, the share of consumption by large animals may be significantly larger than their average global consumption share.

Following the destruction of an ecosystem (including the destruction of soil cover and of the natural homogeneous distribution of nutrients) locomotive animals may play a significant role as "repairing" species in spreading nutrients across the territory, further to be evenly distributed due to diffusion processes. Therefore the structure of fresh vegetation during the period of successions suggests a larger share of consumption of its production by locomotive animals than in a stationary case.

5.13 Detailed Distribution of Destructiveness with Body Size

Theoretically treating fluctuations of destructiveness and demanding that these are kept small we arrived, using the law of large numbers, at the formula given in (5.5.1) which describes the dependence of share of consumption upon the body size. It follows from that formula that the dependence of the share of consumption β by animals of a given body size l of all species in the community is defined by the behavior of the density of the number of species n vs l.

The share of consumption β in the community by species entering the prescribed interval of body sizes is related to the average share of consumption by a single species β_l (falling into the same body size interval) by the obvious expression:

$$\beta_l = \frac{\beta}{n}. \tag{5.13.1}$$

We find for β_l from (5.5.1):

$$\beta_l \sim \frac{1}{l\sqrt{n}} \kappa L_c. \tag{5.13.2}$$

The dependence of density of the number of species and of consumption shares β and β_l on body size l may be presented in power (allometric, see Sect. 2.6) form $n = n_0 (l/l_0)^{n'}$, $\beta = \beta_0 (l/l_0)^{\beta'}$, $\beta_l = \beta_{l0} (l/l_0)^{\beta'_l}$. The slopes, β', β'_l will change in accordance with (5.5.1) and (5.13.2), so that they are related to each other via:

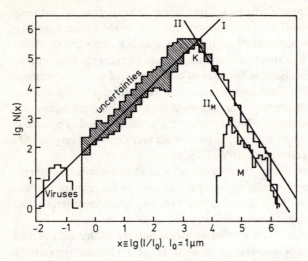

Fig. 5.8. Size spectrum of the world's herbivore species. $N(x)$ is the number of species per unit of the relative body size interval, Δx; $x = \lg(l/l_0)$, $l \equiv (m/\rho)^{1/3}$, where l, m and ρ are the size, mass and density of the body, respectively. The histogram K is the distribution of the total land herbivore species including reducers (Grant, 1977; Chislenko, 1981; Gorshkov, 1985a, b; Wilson, 1988; Thomas, 1990; May, 1990, 1992). The uncertainty is shown dashed. The histogram M is the distribution of mammals (Chislenko, 1981; Eisenberg, 1981). I, II, II_M are the scaling approximations. The slopes of lines are $N' = 0.96$ for I, $N' = -1.6$ for II and II_M.

$$\beta' = \frac{1}{2}\,n' - 1, \qquad \beta_l' = -\frac{1}{2}\,n' - 1. \qquad\qquad (5.13.3)$$

When $n' = 0$ we have $\beta' = \beta_l' = -1$ and β and β_l decrease in proportional to l^{-1} for higher body size l. If we have $n' > 0$ for the constant slope n', the drop off in β will slow down for higher body sizes l, while the drop off in β_l will, inversely, speed up. When $n' < 0$ the tendencies will be opposite. In particular, at $n' = -2$ the fall-off in β_l may be stopped for larger body sizes, see Fig. 5.7.

The empirical data accumulated indicates that the distributions n are close to each other for various land ecosystems (Chislenko, 1981). Thus it is natural to consider the task of finding the distributions of β and n for a globally averaged local land ecosystem. Distributions for β and β_l may be found that way and compared to the available empirical data.

The distribution n averaged over all the ecosystems may be found from the distribution N, similar to it and available for all the continental herbivore species in both fauna and flora, Fig. 5.8 (Gorshkov, 1984b, 1985a; May, 1990, 1992).

It follows from Fig. 5.8 that the density of the number of species, N, grows for $l < l_m \sim 1$ mm ($m < 1$ mg) at a slope $N' \approx 0.96$. Then that density N falls off at a slope $N' \approx -1.6$. Substituting those data into (5.13.3) we find the slopes β' and β_l' for respective size intervals. The absolute value of distribution β may be retrieved from the condition of normalization: the sum of values of β over all the

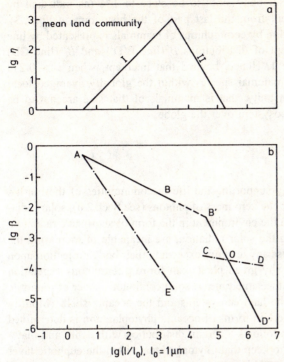

Fig. 5.9a,b The size spectrum of the mean World destructivity: (**a**) the size spectrum for the number of species in the mean land local ecosystem; the straight lines I and II are the scaling approximation, see Fig. 5.8; (**b**) the size spectrum for the shares of consumption by a community β (line ABB'D') and by a single species β_l (lines AE and COD), see text for details.

size intervals should be equal to unity (that is all the primary production should be destroyed). The absolute value of β_l is defined by (5.13.1). That approach opens the possibility of finding details of the distribution in the first, most important part of the histogram in Fig. 5.3. The part of the distribution thus obtained – that is line AB in Fig. 5.9 – agrees quite well with the data for communities of soil species in the range $l < l_m$ (Gorshkov, 1984b, 1986a; Tseitlin, 1985; Tseitlin et al., 1986).

Data are also available for the dependence of the share of consumption of β_l, a single species of mammals, on their body size (Damuth, 1981a). The slope β_l', retrieved from the value of n', Eq. (5.13.3), for mammals (see Fig. 5.9) agrees quite well with those data (Gorshkov, 1984b, 1986a). The contribution of consumption by mammals to general consumption by the community is small and cannot be retrieved from the general condition of normalization for β within the empirical error level. The absolute values of share of consumption by a single species β_l for mammals the world over agree with the observed value of β_l (line CD, see also Fig. 5.7), if one assumes the cumulative share of consumption by the whole community of mammals of all body sizes to be close to 1% (as indicated by the empirically available input from the last part of the histogram in Fig. 5.3). The dependence of consumption by communities of mammals is presented by line B′D′ in Fig. 5.9. The intercept of distributions β (line B′D′) and β_l (line CD) follows Eq. (5.13.1) for $n = 1$. Hence, beyond that intercept, when $l > 0.2$ m ($m > 8$ kg), the number of mammal species within the globally averaged local ecosystem becomes less than unity, that is mammals of that size are not to be encountered in every local ecosystem over the globe.

5.14 Brief Conclusions

The source of external energy supporting the life of communities of the Earth's biota is solar radiation. Due to the zero mass of photons (see Sect. 2.6), solar radiation cannot be accumulated in the environment in the form of shortwave radiation. The Earth's plants, absorbing the solar radiation, are incapable of increasing the absorbed flux by moving across any territory exceeding their body projection upon the Earth's surface. That is why green plants can form a continuous vegetation cover, remaining immotile at the same time. A solid continuous cover of immotile vegetation is typical for all the land ecosystems and the oceanic shelf. (Motility of single-cell individuals in certain forms of oceanic phytoplankton is determined by the fact that their biomass follows a certain distribution with depth and that a vertical movement is needed to keep that phytoplankton within the euphotic layer (Sieburth, 1976; Gorshkov, 1980b).)

Immotility of green plants results in the possibility of loosely correlated (modular) multicellular plant individuals. The mode of functioning of such individuals is close to that of the completely uncorrelated single-cell individuals of equal metabolically active mass. That feature lowers the fluctuations of photosynthesis of organic matter within the local ecosystem, as based on the action of the law of large numbers (see Sects. 2.3 and 3.2).

The destruction of photosynthesizing matter in the community is also performed by the immotile, weakly correlated individuals – bacteria and fungi. (Motility of certain forms of bacteria, similar to that of certain forms of phytoplankton, pursues the aim of vertical movement through soil layers.) Taking account of the body size distribution of destructivity, Fig. 5.3, immotile individuals destroy more than 95% of the photosynthesized organic matter (see Sect. 5.6). Similar to the synthesis of organic matter, this makes it possible to reduce fluctuations in the destruction of that matter within the local ecosystem, as based on the action of the law of large numbers.

Organization of the community on the basis of a large number of non-correlated or modular, weakly correlated parts, makes it possible to control both the rate of synthesis and of destruction of organic matter to a high degree of accuracy. That, in its turn, makes it possible to keep the matter cycles strictly closed, and the environment steady provided there are no external perturbations, as well as enabling an adequate reaction of the community towards compensation of any external perturbation of the environment. There are indeed organized communities of immotile individuals alone, such as epilythic lichen, see Fig. 4.1a,b.

The existence of a universal minimum admissible value of energy consumption per unit volume (or mass) in all the living beings results in a strict limitation upon the admissible vertical size of an individual, provided the flux of energy incident upon the single projection area of that individual upon the Earth's surface is constant. That size is controlled by the flux of solar radiation and by photosynthesis efficiency. For the biosphere, on average, the solid cover of the metabolically active biomass for both the photosynthesizers of the organic matter (green plants), and its reducers, heterotrophs (bacteria and fungi), may reach a depth of no more than 3 mm. The observed extremely large body size of woody plants is explained by the fact that the overwhelming part of space occupied by that plant is empty, while most of the biomass of such plants is metabolically inactive (actually it is dead).

To support life of large individuals with a metabolically active layer much thicker than that formed by plants and other immotile organisms, one needs to employ energy fluxes which by far exceed the flux of solar energy, even when the efficiency of that solar energy consumption (the efficiency of photosynthesis) is equal to unity. Hence, large individuals cannot form a solid continuous cover (the "stationary crowd"). The feeding energy for these individuals should be collected from a large surface, significantly exceeding the individual's projection upon the Earth's surface. Since, apart the solar radiation, there are no other forms of primary energy available, and solar radiation does not accumulate, such individuals cannot feed off the solar energy immediately. Hence large individuals may only feed off the secondary energy of synthesized organic matter, which feature the property of mass and can be accumulated locally. In other words, large individuals may only be heterotrophic, and can only participate in destroying organic matter. Feeding off the locally accumulated plant biomass is only possible via movement of large individuals over their feeding ground. Movement, on the other hand, demands that the body of a large individual is a rigidly correlated unitary body of a motile (locomotive) animal.

The community consisting of immotile, and, hence, of small vertical size modular individuals may only exist on condition of strict equality between the synthesis and destruction over any arbitrarily small time interval, hence of strict constancy of the organic and inorganic mass in each local ecosystem, that is, in the environment. Introduction of mobile animals into the community results in a total change of functioning mode for that community. Mobile animals feeding off the accumulated biomass inevitably precipitate oscillations of that biomass in any local area of the community, since the animal very quickly eats that biomass away, and then it is recovered very slowly by way of production, see Fig. 5.10a. That, in its turn, results in oscillations of inorganic matter introduced by the animal into the environment after it consumes that organic matter. Hence, the state of the environment ceases also to be stationary, and suffers significant oscillations. Stationariness of the environment may only be reached after averaging over a long enough time

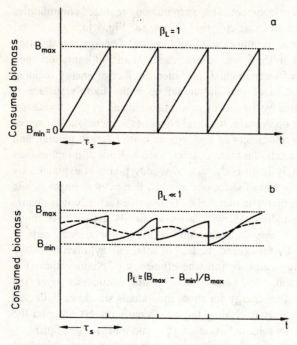

Fig. 5.10a,b Oscillations of the community biomass in the presence of large animals: (**a**) change of the plant biomass, B, with time, t, within a local area when large animals consume the total biomass, $\beta_L = 1$ (the case of cultivated land); (**b**) changes in plant biomass with time when large animals consume only their admissible quota of plant biomass, which does not exceed the natural fluctuations of vegetation. The dashed line indicates the natural fluctuations of plant biomass; the solid line shows oscillations of biomass with large animals present, β_L is the consumed share of vegetation biomass, τ_S is the time in which the animal rounds of its whole territory, see Sects. 5.9 and 5.10.

period. That result imposes strict limitations upon the possible species composition and the behavior of the animals entering that community.

When random oscillations of biomass and of destruction rate of organic matter in a community are strong, it becomes impossible to close matter cycles and to satisfy the Le Chatelier principle. Therefore the average consumption quota of plant products by mobile animals should not exceed the natural fluctuations of plant production. When that condition is met, the presence of animals in the community does not leave any apparent traces in plant biomass (Fig. 5.10b). Biomass oscillations grow with the body size of those animals. Hence the quota of consumption of plant production by those animals should drop for larger body size of the consumers. That conclusion agrees with the observed distribution of plant production with consumers' body size, Fig. 5.3. Reducing the number of species of large animals slows the rate at which that consumption quota drops for a separate species with their body size increasing.

Energy spent by an animal for making the rounds of its feeding ground quickly increases with the animal's body size for purely physical reasons (see Sect. 5.8). The life of an animal is physically possible when the energy it spends to round that territory is covered by the energy of food it consumes. According to the ecological reasons outlined above, the energy of food consumed by the animal should, conversely, reduce with that animal's body size (see Sect. 5.9). The last ecological condition is only met for small enough animals, their size not exceeding a certain critical value (Sect. 5.10). The body size of man coincides with that critical body size in its order of magnitude. With the body size exceeding that critical limit, the share of plant food it consumes inevitably grows. To support ecological equilibrium such animals may only exist in nomadic mode, at a very low average density of their population, while at the same time defending an enormous feeding ground against intervention of competitors.

Maintaining the density of the population of large animals is quite a difficult ecological problem, solved within a whole ecosystem, that is within a hyperpopulation of competitively interacting communities. That necessity results in very strict limitations on both the presently existing and formerly existing species of large herbivore animals, and to limitations upon the relative lifespans of such species, as measured in lifespan units of a single generation, in other words, in their relatively quick evolutionary sequence. (According to paleodata, the absolute life duration for a species does not depend on body size (Simpson, 1944), while the lifespan of a separate generation increases in proportion to body size (Gorshkov, 1982a), so that the number of generations fitting into the lifespan of a species reduces with increasing body size.)

The overall spreading of the locomotive animals means that communities including such animals are more stable. Apparently the locomotive animals are the main repairing species that increase the relaxation rate of biota and environment to the normal state after its external perturbation. This conclusion follows from the observable fact that the population of the most locomotive animals increases during succession processes in the ecosystems after such events as fires, wood cleaning and other destruction of the natural biota.

Apparently more than 90% of all the terrestrial species of the biosphere (including the majority of plant and insect species) are repairing species. The species diversity usually reaches a maximum about several tens years after a strong external perturbation (fire, volcanic and nuclear eruptions, etc.) and then drops and stabilizes at a low value (Morneau and Payette, 1989; Gorshkov and Gorshkov, 1992). The genome of all the repairing species should contain the information about population density and behavior of individuals that is needed for the rapid restoration of the ecosystem after its external perturbation. Such genetic information can be realized only in the perturbed external condition and should decay in normal ones. The external perturbations of the environment and the biota are random and irregular. The genetic program of repairing species may decay and they may lose their capacity to restore the perturbed ecosystem during occasionally very long periods of concentration of the natural (unperturbed) conditions.

Then the biota should contain the internal mechanisms of regular perturbation of the ecosystem. It may be produced by the largest animals (including man) living nomadic life styles (see Sect. 5.10).

It follows from the estimates on the size of local ecosystems which are capable of closing the matter cycles, thus meeting the Le Chatelier principle with respect to external perturbations, that this size is significantly smaller than the feeding ground (home range) of a large animal. That situation is similar to that occurring with biological regulation of globally accumulated substances, see Sect. 4.6. It follows from that reasoning that the large animals cannot control the community. Violation of that rule results in the breaking up of whole hyperpopulation of the communities and in extinction of the large animals. Significant changes that the communities suffer after forceful extinction of large animals do not contradict the last rule. Communities should change in exactly the same way as a result of extended perturbation of the environment. However all of these changes should comply with the Le Chatelier principle with short-term perturbations of the environment. If there are some slight changes in one of the communities, such that the excessive share of consumption by the larger animals is reduced as a result (for example the share of plants with thorns increases), that community gains some edge over the other ones, and gradually ousts the other communities. Reductions in the population of larger animals should bring about such changes in the community which would stimulate an increase in those numbers and vice versa.

The population density for all the larger animals in natural communities is determined by the necessity to have a stable closed cycle of matter in these communities, and not by the available amount of food (the latter always exceeds the animal's needs, see Sect. 5.10). The information about optimal population density is written into the normal genome of the animal, the same way the rules for interaction with all the other species in the community are. The principal threat to the community integrity consists in the possible increase of the density of population of larger animals above that optimum. Therefore, most behavioral traits are aimed at preventing that excessive growth in density of population, rather then increasing that density to the limit the food base can stand (Maynard Smith, 1964). That aim is attained via strict control of the size of the feeding ground per single individual (McNab, 1983). That control is executed by way of diverse forms of competitive interaction between the individuals at every level in the community (sound signals of neighbors, migration of animals getting above that optimal density (McFarland, 1985), parasites and carnivores included). Expansion of large animals into new territories goes on with all those traits remaining intact. All such diverse interactions between the different species in the community are aimed at supporting the highest competitiveness of the community as a whole. It is not the species that survive, but the communities which are most efficient in controlling the optimal environmental life conditions. Species devoid of such altruistic traits increase their numbers outside that limit, disrupt the correlation in the community, perturb the environment and die out together with the community in which they originated.

It may be said that all the large motile animals comprise a certain component of the environment, which is kept, together with concentrations of the biochemically active components (global biologically accumulated nutrients), at a certain level by the population of communities consisting of plants and microorganisms (see Sects. 4.6 and 4.8). (Note that it is erroneously assumed sometimes that the community should include whole populations of all the species of large animals entering that community. In that case the size of the community could not be much less than the largest territory occupied by a population of large animals, and there would be no hyperpopulations of communities possible at all, see Sect. 3.2.)

Biological regulation of the environment is determined purely by the relation between the synthesis and destruction of organic matter. The possible forms of such a relation are limited by the above enumerated strict laws of nature. Within the limitations set by those laws the biological relations may assume any forms, however complex. One of those forms is the trophic structure of the destruction of organic matter, that is the way the heterotrophs are divided into reducers, destroying dead organic matter, and the consumers, who devour live individuals. Herbivores, carnivores of the first order, eating away the herbivores, carnivores of the second order, who feed off carnivores of the first order, etc. are identified. Such a division into different levels forms a well-known ecological pyramid of energy fluxes, which is often envisaged as the basis of ecology (Odum, 1983). It only makes sense on condition of a low ratio of production to consumption in the population of each species, and loses sense for the reducers, in which that ratio is not low (Gorshkov and Dolnik, 1980; Gorshkov, 1982a). Carnivores also feature certain peculiarities, enumerated in Sect. 5.11, and based on the general physical laws of nature.

However, details of the interaction between carnivores and their prey are controlled by the correlated nature of interaction between all the species in a natural community, which, in principle, is a different form of symbiotic interaction. Dividing the interaction between the species in the community, such as commensalism, amensalism, predation, parasitism, symbiosis, etc. (Begon et al., 1986) is quite artificial, and in no way defines the actual sense and diversity of these interactions. All such interactions are but different forms of correlations between the species in a natural community and are similar to correlations between the different organs in a body or organelles and biological macromolecules in a cell.

The enormous powers of information fluxes processed by the molecular structures of living organisms in a natural community, which are incomparably higher than the maximally achievable fluxes of information flowing through all the computers of modern society, indicate that it is hopeless to try to construct any mathematical models pretending to describe the actual processes within the natural communities (Sect. 2.8). These processes are many orders of magnitude more complex than the processes taking place within a separate living individual, in particular those evolving within the brains of large animals and man, and will apparently never become amenable to detailed modelling. (That comment does not refer to artificial communities, devoid of a program of stabilization of the environment, the only aim of their construction being to provide enough food for man.) At the same time studying the physical limitations upon the processes taking place in the community brings some clear results opening the way to unequivocal conclusions.

6. The Ecology of Man

Before proceeding to treat the ecology of modern civilized man, we consider behavioral traits common to man and other mobile animals, based on their genetic programs, which remain intact even in conditions of civilization.

6.1 Behavioral Strategy of Mobile Animals

All the forms of interaction with the environment necessary for immotile multi-cellular individuals, such as photosynthesizing plants and fungi, are rigidly programmed at their genetic base level. Any external forcing of those individuals always produces a strictly determined biochemical reaction. Partial correlation in plants allows a certain reaction in some parts of those plants when other parts are affected (such as the reaction to light, to obstacles, etc. (Raven and Johnson, 1988)). These individuals do not need any program of selection between several alternative behavioral patterns. Neither do they need a nervous system to execute a centralized control of the whole individual.

Mobile animals must first of all command the locomotion capability for the individual as a whole. That calls for a rigid correlation between all the parts of the individual body, for the presence of measuring organs (those capable of sight, sound, smell, taste, and feel), and for a central nervous system. When moving, the animal faces some particular new environmental situation each time, one that its parents might never have encountered during their lifespan. Only the average characteristics of the animal's ecological niche (the set of natural stimuli) remain intact.

Since the amount of information coming from the environment considerably exceeds that contained in the genome of any individual (see Sect. 2.8), it is impossible to program correct reactions to any external forcing an animal might face into the genome (such that they would guarantees a stable life support). The animal appears to face an unavoidable choice between the differing tactical opportunities which are alternatives to each other. Only a correct strategic line of behavior may be programmed into the genome, based, as it were, on the permanency of the averaged characteristics of the animal's ecological niche. The situation is similar in statistics, when no individual movements of each separate molecule can be traced, and the characteristics of state are only the average ones of the type temperature and pressure.

The operation of that program is supported by the system of genetically fixed positive and negative emotions. Positive emotions (desires, appetites) stimulate actions in the "right" direction which work to preserve the species securely. Negative emotions prevent the actions directed towards destroying that stability. Positive and negative emotions are values measurable from the actions the animal performs. An animal tries to act in such a way that is associated with positive emotions, and tries to evade actions associated with the negative ones (Lorenz, 1981; Livesey, 1986). Finding the correlations between various actions by the animal and the biochemical reactions or bodily movements (motor patterns) accompanying them makes it possible to measure the intensity of, and retrieve the dimension of, various complex emotions, as described in Sect. 2.6. Similarly the observed correlation between the volume of some liquid and temperature is used for the measurement of temperature. If two emotions seem to be identical (such as love and sexuality), but have different dimensions, that means they are two different emotions and vice versa. (Everybody knows that tail wagging is associated with actions producing positive emotions in a dog. However the dog could not indicate it to the man in any direct way. Hence that correlation had been measured by the method described above.)

Emotions are usually considered as a characteristic of human behavior. The instincts (species-characteristic drive) are generally investigated in animals. Both emotions and instincts may be measured only during the respective actions performed by the individual. Thus the dimensions of emotion and corresponding instinct are the same and, hence, they should be regarded as identical characteristics (see Sect. 2.6).

The program of emotions controlling the behavioral strategy of animals may be quite complicated, but anyhow it is genetically fixed, singular, and unchangeable for each species (each normal genome). It cannot be subjected to any correction or upbringing as conditions vary, the same as the morphology of the animal body (Lorenz, 1981). As with any information written into the genome, this program may suffer decay, that is be perturbed and distorted in decay individuals. The distortion of the program of emotions results in erroneous behavior, which is perceived as pathology of the psyche in man (Gershon and Rieder, 1992). Pathological behavior almost inevitably leads to the death of the individual. That is why decay mutations leading to behavioral and psychic distortions are the most serious deleterious decay changes of the genome in mobile animals. Under natural conditions normal individuals should feature the highest frequency of occurrence, which makes it possible to empirically find the natural system of positive and negative emotions in each species, not distorted by pathologies.

The program of correct actions cannot be based on positive emotions alone. The positive emotion should be saturated (there should be action-specific exhaustion) if the corresponding action has been performed by an animal (Lorenz, 1981). Introduction into the genetic program of stationary negative emotions which prevent actions directed towards destroying the individual, population and community is also necessary. Neutral actions, not associated with any emotions, are ecologically senseless in natural conditions, and are thus wasteful from the point of view of energy expenditure. However, extreme diversity of the external conditions inevitably results in overlapping of actions associated with positive and negative emotions. Correct actions towards positive emotions may happen to lie beyond a penetrable barrier of negative emotions. A specific direction of actions may arise within the lifespan of one individual and remain absent from that of another one. The information on the existence of such a direction of correct actions should be available to an individual but cannot be included in its hereditarily information fund. That is where the necessity for extragenetic memory (of learning) in animals appears from, such that the information is kept in it during the lifespan of an individual and is not be transmitted to the following generations. Differences in learning result in tactical behavioral differences of individuals with the same inherited program of emotions, that is with identical behavioral strategy (Lorenz, 1981).

All the mobile animals possess such a memory. It includes such elements as conditioned reflexes and imprinting (McFarland, 1985), covering the information imprinted into the memory for a long time period or for life at an early age. Particular cases of imprinting include the formation of urbanized populations of wild species, memorizing the coordinates of birthplace (philopatry) by migrating birds (Dolnik, 1982; Sokolov, 1991), and speech in man. In the absence of emotions (of consciousness) no information may be introduced into the extragenetic memory of the individual. Consciousness is thus metabolically active state of the individual's life in which correct perception and processing of information coming from the environment are possible on the basis of the program of positive and negative emotions (Edelman, 1990; Crick and Koch, 1992). The unconscious state means that either perception of information or its processing is lacking. In that sense, consciousness is a measurable characteristic, singularly associated with the organs of perception and emotions, see Sect. 2.6. Hence consciousness is a property common for all the moving animals, not just man alone (Goldman-Rakic, 1992; Zeki, 1992).

The observed assimilation times for the information that the animal perceives from its environment are much shorter than the characteristic times of cell division and transformation. It follows that the information of the long-term (associative) extragenetic memory is perceived and localized in memory cells of molecular, instead of macroscopic size, see Sect. 3.3. Such molecular memory cells should reside in neural cells, the neurons (Fischbach, 1992; Kandel and Hawkins, 1992; Stevens, 1993). Apart from DNA, there are no polymer molecules in cells that are capable of duplication, that is of copying the information they contain. That is why the neurons containing long-term extragenetic memory are incapable of division, since otherwise that information would be lost. Therefore the time interval during which the information is preserved in the long-term extragenetic memory should coincide with the average lifespan (the decay time) of a neuron, τ_n.

An animal or a human exists itself for as long as its brain retains memory. Therefore the lifespan of an animal, τ_L, should coincide with the average lifespan of a neuron containing information of the long-term memory, τ_n. The biochemical organization of the brain is identical in all the mammals (Hubel, 1979). Hence, the average lifespan of the neurons should be the same for all the mammals with similar body size and metabolic rate (Sect. 5.2). One could thus conclude an equal lifespan for all the mammal species of equal body size. That is indeed the case except for man (Brody, 1945). Man enjoys a lifespan of about four times as long as any mammal of the same body size (Brody, 1945), see also Sects. 5.3 and 5.11. It is enough to cite the example of a dog of body size equal to that of man. The average lifespan of a dog is about 15 years, while man's average exceeds 60 years. There exists an apparently unique possibility to practically unlimitedly extend the individual's lifespan, τ_L, retaining its extragenetic memory accumulated in the brain, while the average lifespan of the neurons, τ_n, remains fixed (Gorshkov, 1982a). It would be sufficient to repeatedly copy all the information contained in the memory into different areas of the brain weakly correlated to each other. We denote the minimal number of rigidly correlated neurons capable of retaining all the information from the extragenetic memory as N_{min}. We shall call that combination of N_{min} neurons a "memory block". The storage time for information in a single memory block coincides with the average lifespan of the neurons, τ_n.

If a larger number of weakly correlated autonomous memory blocks carrying the same information exist at the initial time moment, the law of the decay of information in such a set of memory blocks will coincide with the common law for the decay of radioactive substances. Let the initial number of neurons containing memory information and accumulated over the whole period of body growth be $N_0 \gg N_{min}$. The number of independent memory blocks will then be N_0/N_{min}. The law of decay of the neurons and of the memory blocks they form with time t elapsed after the body ceased to grow will have the form:

$$N = N_0 e^{-t/\tau_n}. \tag{6.1.1}$$

A human does not lose either its memory or identity so long as there is still at least one memory block undecayed in its brain. After the last memory block decays serious memory lapses and senility set in (Selkoe, 1992). The time, t, after which all the memory blocks have decayed, coincides with the average lifespan for the human species, τ_L, and may be retrieved from the equation:

$$N_{min} = N_0 e^{-\tau_L/\tau_n}, \quad \text{or} \quad \tau_L = \tau_n \ln(N_0/N_{min}). \tag{6.1.2}$$

Assuming $\tau_L/\tau_n \approx 4$, we find that $N_0/N_{min} \approx 50$. Hence, the brain of a young human should contain 50 times as many neurons as that of a dog carrying the same memory information load. The dog's brain, however, is only several times as small as that of a human. It follows then that memory information must be contained in just a small share of brain neurons. Simple estimates (Sects. 2.8 and 6.4) show that the amount of extragenetic memory accumulated by a human in the course of his/her lifespan coincides in its order of magnitude with that genetically contained in the human genome. Since both types of information are written into the memory cells of molecular size, all the extragenetic memory should be localized in a volume of the order of volume of DNA from a single cell. That is why all the network of human memory blocks may occupy only a tiny part of the brain volume, which clearly strongly complicates its experimental localization.

Every autonomous memory block should necessarily contain the complete information that an individual assimilates from its environment. That is why after quick assimilation of new information during immediate contact of a human individual with the environment the newly obtained information has to be accurately spread throughout all the memory blocks. The latter metabolically active process in the brain should happen slowly and continuously, without any contact with the environment (Goldman-Rakic, 1992; Kandel and Hawkins, 1992). It may be accompanied by discovering correlations existing between the various elements of the newly acquired information. That, apparently, constitutes the essence of thinking, which would thus be either completely absent from or remain rudimentary in other animals.

Recollection of a correct action resulting in positive emotions may weaken the negative emotions preventing that action in the given individual; however such emotions should be conserved in the genome. It is only when action associated with positive emotions repeatedly and forcefully meets the same barrier of negative emotions for many generations to come, over the period of evolution of the order of several million years, that these negative emotions may cease to reflect the actual environmental conditions and vanish from the species genome.

The possibility of action towards negative emotions, based on the memory of gratification associated with that action (that is, will) should also be written into the genome. Animal training is based on that property of the genome. Repeated food gratification helps to teach an animal to perform actions unnatural for that species, which it never performs under natural conditions, and which should, by definition, produce some penetrable but certainly negative emotions in that animal (Gould and Marler, 1987).

A given individual might never encounter the possibility of actions precipitating certain emotions programmed into its genome during its lifespan. Leaving the natural ecological niche and meeting with some unnatural conditions, the genetic system of emotions may fail to meet the condition of supporting the species stability (as, for example, is the case with man's narcotic addiction).

The strategic program of the basic positive and negative emotions is identical in all the mobile animals. Freedom of movement should provide for animal feeding needs. These actions should be included in the program of positive emotions. However, the principal positive emotions should be associated with preservation of the population. These are positive emotions supporting competitive interaction and reproduction. Negative emotions (such as pain, fear, etc.) support the life of an individual.

6.2 Herd Animals

Competitive interaction among mobile animals may be implemented following a mode much more advanced than in immotile individuals. The principal task of competitive interaction is to determine rank. Ranking immotile individuals according to their level of competitiveness may only be simultaneously conducted for immediate neighbors. The relative level of competitiveness of the spatially separated immotile individuals may only be clarified for their offspring after a long time. Mobile individuals acquire a unique ability for simultaneous rating of their competitiveness among a large number of individuals, banding into herds, the partially correlated flocks of individuals.

A herd makes it possible to organize a hierarchical structure. The most advanced form of hierarchical structure is linear (similar to ranking among sportsmen): the individual of first rank (called elite male below) dominates all the rest, the individual second in its rank dominates everybody but the first, and so on (Panov, 1983; McFarland, 1985). With decreasing rank the advantages enjoyed by the individual in feeding and breeding decrease. Such a structure demands high energy expenditures on competition during the initial period of herd formation only. Later on competitive interaction takes place among the two immediate neighbors in the hierarchical structure. The new competitive individual may always move up the hierarchical ladder up to the place corresponding to its potential without disrupting the general structure of the herd. However all the fully-fledged members of the herd bear a constant psychological burden of daily demonstrating (without undue conflict, as a rule) the level of their competitiveness to all the other members of that herd. The principal positive emotion, boosting competitive interaction among the herd animals to the highest possible level of efficiency, is related to the drive for higher rank (rating, prestige) on the hierarchical ladder.

Clear rank is most important at the top of the hierarchical structure, since the genome of individuals residing there is closest to the normal one. It is particularly that genome which should be transferred to the following generations. The lower part of the hierarchical ladder does not need any ranking. The rating of all individuals residing there is practically the same.

The popular notion that the herd or the pack forms either to provide defence against the beasts of prey or for a more efficient use of energy of movement, or of food resources has no sound foundation. When animals join into herds, all the energy characteristics of their movement and feeding remain exactly the same as for animals separated into individual feeding groups (Gorshkov, 1982b). The phenomena of correlated behavior that herd individuals demonstrate during predators' assaults are secondary in nature. The predatory mode of living does not vanish after herds form. Herd animals have as many predators as individual ones. Moreover, feeding problems are simplified for predators when their prey join into herds. The rate of movement of a grazing herd is much slower than the individual speeds of movement of separate animals feeding off that ground (Gorshkov, 1982a,b). These speeds only even out for long-range migrations. Therefore, a predator who has found a herd can save energy needed for hunting the prey and be satisfied with following the herd, spending much less energy on movement than its prey (Gorshkov, 1982a,b). Besides, all the predators have a genetic program preventing extermination of the prey which would entail the perishing of the predator itself.

Finally, many species, such as elephants, to give an example, follow a herd life mode while having no predators at all. The reason for the formation of a herd may only be explained by the unique possibilities of increasing the efficiency of competitive interaction.

The hierarchical structure of a herd, in which every individual is capable, at least in principle, of occupying any position, should not be confused with rigidly correlated organizations known, for example, in social insects. Specialization of various groups of individuals in those creatures is hereditarily fixed (written into the normal genome) and cannot be changed. Competition between the different groups is impossible, as it is impossible between the different organs in a single body. Stratifying into hereditary specialization in herds is only present in the form of division into different sexes and into adults and juveniles, prepuberal individuals. Competition for childbearing between the male and the female is just as impossible as competition between a juvenile and an adult individual (Gorshkov, 1982a). Adults and juveniles either occupy different ecological niches (such as nymphs and imagos in insect species or fry and adult fishes in fish species), or are correlated via parental care (as in bird and mammal species).

The degree of competitiveness of an individual should be tested in all the life situations encountered, so the everyday herd existence is most favorable for adequate identification of the hierarchical structure. Joining into herds takes place every time it is permitted by the ecological niche. When the ecological niche does not permit everyday existence in a herd, short-term banding into herds takes place, so that the hierarchical structure is identified in some vital criteria only (this is the essence of bird mating calls, of long-range seasonal migration in bird, fish and mammal species, of walrus and seal rookeries during the breeding season, etc.).

The lowest steps in the herd's hierarchical ladder are occupied by noncompetitive decay individuals. The low prestige (rating) in a herd may drive the animal into an extended state of negative emotions (into distress). That state results in certain genetically programmed physiological reactions of organ destruction, so that the animal perishes as a result (Selye, 1974; Manning, 1979). In cases of overpopulation a whole lower strata of the hierarchical ladder is cut off, while the top levels of that ladder still reside in conditions of food abundance. That is how the death rate is regulated for decay individuals (Sect. 3.11).

Formation of a herd with a hierarchical structure provides not only for efficient stabilization of the existing level of species organization, but for a quick fixation of newly appearing favorable evolutionary traits in all the members of the herd in just a few generations. As a result the evolution of mobile animals is accelerated, and the rate of species formation in them significantly exceeds the rate of such formation in immotile individuals. That conclusion is substantiated particularly by comparing the number of contemporary species in plants and animals: there are about two hundred thousand of the former, and over several millions of the latter (Chislenko, 1981; Wilson, 1988; Thomas, 1990).

Support of the herd as a correlated formation of a group of individuals may only result from competitive interaction between the different herds. (Joining of various herds into a single macroherd during long-range migrations only works to intensify competitive interaction between the separate individuals.) The presence of sexual dimorphism and polygamy in herds works to regulate, at a high efficiency, the birth rate of decay individuals (Sect. 3.11).

Most ectothermic (cold-blooded) species typically lay an enormous number of eggs (e.g. fish) without further bothering with their progeny. The share of individuals reaching the reproductive age is kept strictly constant through the working of the law of large numbers (Sect. 2.3). In that case a correlated interaction between the sexes, including the search for a sexual partner and fertilization, are completely within the scope of positive emotions of the type of sexuality. Reproducing a large number of offspring is impossible in any endothermic (warm-blooded) species, since endothermicity features a minimum body size (Sect. 5.2). Thus endothermic animals, birds and mammals, are forced to help their young to survive, channelling some metabolic energy of the parents into childcare.

That effect results in a need for a new positive emotion–parental love, maternal love in particular, in mammals. Channelling metabolic energy of one individual to support another contradicts the principal basis of competitive interaction between independent individuals within the population. That is a manifestation of correlated interaction which may be supported by competitive interaction between different families, consisting of mothers and their young. Motherly love is not correlated with sexuality (*libido*). That is why sexuality, as a positive emotion of sexual interaction, and love, as capacity to provide other individuals with care (i.e. to spend the metabolic power of the individual in the direction of maintaining the life of other individuals), have differing dimensions (Sect. 2.6), that is they have nothing in common. The necessity to care for the young during the period of reproduction switches mammal females out of competitive interaction, which is then carried on during that period by males only, who do not participate in childcare, and who band into herds and packs.

In the herd lifestyle with its fixed hierarchical structure, the behavior most advantageous for the species is for the females to mate with the bearers of the best genes, that is with elite males from the top of the hierarchical structure.

When the mammal females are capable of raising their young by themselves, they group around the elite male, forming a harem. The rest of the males then band into herds for the period of reproduction and identify the contender for the role of the new elite male among themselves, competitively interacting with each other.

Interesting features may arise in herd animals when the female herself is incapable of raising her young (Gorshkov, 1982a). A single elite male cannot provide help in metabolic energy to all the breeding females. Most of those are busy breeding. The only individuals left free of reproductive burden appear to be the males from the lower part of the hierarchical ladder. The only way out, making the existence of such species possible, is the appearance of a new positive emotion in those males, that is fatherly love to both the young and the female (if she is tied to her young by lactation, as is the case with mammals). That emotion is of the same dimension as motherly love, and it has nothing in common with elite male sexuality. It is related, as in the mother, to selfless drive of this male helper to help the young, passing to them part of his metabolic energy. The elite male should be completely free of that quality, since he has completely different functions within the species. Both types of behavior are written into the normal genome and are inherited from the elite male. If the elite male perishes, one of the non-elite male helpers takes his place, and his behavior goes through a complete transformation in accordance with the program of the normal genome.

The absence of sharp genetic differences between the elite male and the weakly decay males in the middle part of the hierarchical structure brings into conflict emotions driving the male to higher rank with those stimulating him to pass a part of his metabolic energy to the young. To smooth those, females in certain species employ continuous sexual gratification (by analogy with food gratification) of the male helpers (Gorshkov, 1982a; Andelman, 1987). Since bringing up the young takes much time, the female should be capable of manifesting capacity for being sexually receptive during most or the whole of that period. It may be achieved by means of transition from estrus to menstrual cycles (Lovejoy, 1981, 1988; Austin and Short, 1984; Andelman, 1987).

With this sexual gratification the female should have some physiological mechanism of preventing possible egg fertilization by the sperm of the male-helper (like blocking the ovulation during lactation, by weakening of the female sexual excitation during copulation with the male helper, by conservation of the elite male sperm in the female body during long periods of time, etc. (Shugart 1988; Maksudov et al., 1988)). The number of copulations between the female and the male helper significantly exceeds the number of copulations with the elite male resulting in delivery of the young. Such a reproductive strategy is thus envisaged as monogamy accompanied by rare infidelities. The latter may be erroneously treated as either deviation from the normal sexual behavior or as manifestations of polyandry. Real polyandry takes place only in birds when young are raised by the male. The reproductive strategy based on true monogamy or on promiscuity, that is on chaotic sexual contacts (Lovejoy, 1981), inevitably means refusing to regulate the birth rate and falling back to regulating the death rate of decay individuals, that is to high death rate at infancy.

The female cannot be unfaithful to the elite male during the whole period of her relationship with him. Such an infidelity on her part means that the female has lost her faith in the elite male, that is, she has stopped considering him as such. Adequate relations between the sexes are adjusted by the negative emotions of jealousy. The elite male should be jealous towards all the other males during his cohabitation with the female. The male helper should not be jealous of the female, letting her mate with the elite male at any time. The female, on her part, cannot be jealous of the elite male, since his functions include mating with as many normal females as possible. At the same time the female is jealous of her male helper, because his energy is necessary for her reproductive success. Female manifestations of jealousy towards a male definitely indicate that she regards him as a male of the lower rank and is ready to cuckold him at the first opportunity.

These peculiarities of sexual behavior are the reason for the intimate character of copulation of sexual partners which they conceal from other individuals of the population. Collective sexual contacts (excluding elite male contacts with many females) should be accompanied by a negative emotional load. It is an unnatural behavior in individuals of species with sexual gratification.

The interaction between the elite male and the female is not energy correlated. The elite male does not need any help and cannot give such help to his females. The female and the male helper should combine into an energy correlated couple – family, working to provide for the well-being of the young. As in the case of true monogamy, that correlation should be supported via competitive interaction between different families, or that correlation will inevitably decay. The female is interested in the good health of her male helper, who is weaker than the elite male. She should support him in case of need, the same as her own young, that is she should feel true love towards him.

All these genetically programmed behavioral features typical for individuals in a herd characterize the internal correlation in it, and are kept from disintegration by competitive interaction and selection among different herds (Wrangham, 1977; Harvey, 1985; Foley, 1987).

The strategy of regulating the birth rate based on polygyny of the elite males, with their females employing concealed ovulation and sexual gratification of the male helpers, is apparently present in rudimentary form in vervet monkeys (Andelman, 1987). However, it has found its most pronounced development in the human species. Significant morphological differences between men and women, that is the noticeable sexual dimorphism, indicate the presence of polygamy in man as in most primates (Lovejoy, 1981).

The development of the brain and the necessity for mastering the hereditary cultural information both resulted in extension of childhood (Brody, 1945; Foley, 1987), which increased energy demands of childcare. The mother appeared incapable of bringing up her children alone. That development resulted in the formation of the family based on the genetically fixed male love and kindness, that is on the tendency of men to care for mothers and for their children. The correlation between the spouses is also supported by the genetically fixed possibility for continuous intimate sexual life, a feature absolutely unique in the animal world (Lovejoy, 1981; Andelman, 1987). On the other hand the phenomena of feminine prostitution and homosexuality (Lesbian love) are consequences of the normal feminine behavior based on the genetically fixed capability of sexual gratification. However male prostitution and homosexuality are always evidence of genetically abnormal (decay) behavior.

As noted above the behavioral strategy, as well as morphology of individuals of the species, cannot be arbitrarily changed and fitted to any unfavorable conditions. So humans following polygamy and sexual gratification cannot discard such strategy and turn to monogamy under the pressure of the AIDS pandemic.

6.3 Territorial Animals

Immotile heterotrophic fungi and bacteria may exist even though the production of plants maintains an absolutely unchanging biomass of a community. The stability of that community with immotile heterotrophs present is supported by keeping a balance between the synthesis and destruction of organic matter.

All the mobile animals inevitably perturb the community biomass within their feeding ground, which is many orders of magnitude larger than their body size. They should provide not only for the stability of their own species, but for that of the community to which they belong, as a whole. The long time periods needed to restore the destroyed part of the community biomass result in rigid limitations upon the number of mobile animals. The principal feature of their hereditary program is keeping their population numbers far below the threshold which the food base permits.

Apparently the most rational means of controlling the animal population numbers is animal territorialism. With this the whole area fit for the existence of the population is separated into individual territories. Each such territory belongs to only one self-reproducing individual, who guards it against all potential competitors. The size of that territory is genetically fixed. The admissible correlation between the size of that territory and the possible variations of the external conditions, such as the value of primary production, to give an example, is also genetically fixed (Wynne-Edwards, 1962). To control the numbers of the species it is sufficient to support such territorialism during the reproductive period only. Outside that period the animals may band into herds, losing their territorial behavior. This behavioral mode is typical for many birds and mammals. Animals guard their territories by direct contact with their neighbors at the border, by leaving smelly spots and by uttering sound signals (Tinbergen, 1968; Hinde, 1970; Manning, 1979; McFarland, 1985). Singing birds spend a considerable part of their time singing (Dolnik, 1982). However, after the end of the reproductive period, by midsummer in the temperate zone, birds stop singing, lose their territorialism, and band into flocks (Hinde, 1970).

Lack of territorialism during the reproductive period makes senseless its support outside that period, since then control of the population numbers is inevitably lost. However, supporting territorialism during the reproductive period strongly hampers or renders completely impossible regulation of the birth rate of decay individuals, based on sexual dimorphism and polygamy (Sect. 3.11). Polygamy in territorial animals may only be preserved by way of organizing display (of the type of heathcock mating-place), when owners of individual territories come to a certain place from afar for the purpose of polygamous mating (McFarland, 1985). In every other case territorialism combined with sexual dimorphism inevitably means monogamy (Hinde, 1970). An elite male may at best mate with his closest neighbor females. Competitive interaction and breeding of territorial animals becomes similar to that found in immotile plants. Sexual dimorphism then makes it possible (if needed) to raise the young by two parents in bird and mammal species. Due to the impossibility of promiscuity the territorial couple often forms a lifelong unit with elements of mutual help and support. The genetically fixed fidelity and mutual love appear to be correlated emotions in that case, that is notions identical to each other (see Sect. 2.6; Gorshkov, 1982a; Austin and Short, 1984). All the other advantages of sexual dimorphism vanish then and regulation of breeding decay individuals becomes impossible. All the competitive interaction changes to being based on regulating the death rate in decay individuals (Coleman, 1972; Freed, 1987; Hofshi et al., 1987), and the latter becomes most efficient during the period of loss of territorialism and of formation of herds and packs. This in particular explains the appearance of large accumulations of migrating animals, and also of the formations of male stocks during the reproductive period, who take no part in breeding and raising of young.

Thus lack of territorialism and herd formation combine to open the possibility of extremely efficient stabilization of the species, as compared to that executed in territorial animals. However, the problem of preserving the community and of keeping the environment from disintegration is heavily aggravated for herd animals. The control of their population numbers may be realized by fixing a given territory as property of a given herd, envisaged as a correlated group of individuals, so that competitive interaction goes on between the different herds (Clutton-Brock, 1974). In that case each individual in the herd should be marked according to its belonging to that particular group. The normal genome should be identical for every herd. The normal genotypes of individuals from the same group should be similar. But the normal genotypes of individuals from the different groups can show discernible variation within the range of normal polymorphism of the species (Sect. 3.8). Thus individuals from the different groups can be genetically marked. The individual marking may also result from protracted contact between the individuals, and from the knack of separating the individuals into friends and aliens, based on extragenetic memory. The possibility of such marking should also be genetically fixed.

However, a transfer to a nomadic life mode is inevitable for large animals, and they have to protect an enormous territory occupied by communities in the process of regeneration. This heavily complicates the task of controlling the population numbers in herd animals. Large herd animals appear to be the principal potential destroyers of the environment. The admissible share of their consumption of 1 % of the total energy flux in the community (Sect. 5.6, Fig. 5.3), which is in agreement with the law of conservation of energy, may fluctuate, increasing by two orders of magnitude and reaching 100 % . Meanwhile invertebrates (mainly insects), consuming 10 % of the total flux, may only increase that consumption by one order of magnitude, while bacteria and fungi, their normal share of consumption exceeding 90 % , are only capable of bringing that share up 10 % . Large fluctuations of consumption are hardly probable in large territorial animals. It should all result in species instability and higher probability of extinction of large herd animals, as compared to territorial species. Together with quick fixation of new evolutionary traits, that feature may be interpreted as a tendency for quick evolution of large animals (Erlich and Holm, 1963).

6.4 Genetic and Cultural Heritage

Radical new "discoveries" resulting in the appearance of new species, essentially different from all the preceding ones, have taken place several times in the process of evolution. This is how multicellular species appeared, then vertebrates, endothermic animals with constant body temperature (birds and mammals). Such "discoveries" have happened only extremely rarely. The coincidence of two or more such fundamental discoveries in time is quite an improbable event. That is why the appearance of all the new large taxa resulted from monophyletic processes, that is from evolutionary divergence of a single predecessor species, a major progressive restructuring taking place in its genome. The appearance of man is also related to a fundamental, genetically fixed "discovery", which had placed man into an exceptional position in the whole animal world. As in every other case that was a single momentary happening, all the other features and traits of man being its consequences.

All the species known, except man, contain all the information they need on the environment, necessary for their existence, in their genome. That information is safely preserved and cannot be lost, as long as the number of individuals available is sufficient for reproduction of the species. Fluctuations leading to sharp drops in the number of those individuals are not catastrophic. The species may be saved even if its individuals are kept for many generations only in zoos, outside their natural environment, provided their number is sufficient for reproduction. At some later stage the species may be transferred back to its natural environment, and keep on existing, as it would after an extended perturbation of the external environment (Sect. 3.9).

Mobile animals are capable of training and learning (Gould and Marler, 1987). However, everything the animal should learn in its natural environment is written into its genome. The animal should be capable of taking and memorizing the coordinates of the locality it had been born in, of fixing the size of its feeding ground. If the program envisages parental childcare, a hereditary program is possible for the young to be taught by their parents. An animal artificially brought up without such training will nevertheless teach its own young in exactly the same way its own parents would have. No animal ever transfers its teachings obtained from its training, to its offspring. All the information in extragenetic memory is only preserved for the duration of the individual lifespan. This prevents the likelihood of animals transferring to the following generations some erroneous or unnecessary information from the point of view of the given species. Many animals use tools in their daily activities. The Egyptian vulture breaks eggs with stones. The Darwin finch in the Galapagos Islands uses horns to extract insects from tree slits. Chimpanzees use sticks (Raven and Johnson, 1988). It has been proven by raising the young without any connection to their parents that the skills of using tools are hereditary, that is the information on such use is contained in the normal genome.

Examples of "biological cultural heritage", not related to memorizing the trained skills, but significantly improving competitiveness of the animals, are known from the animal world. That is the bacterial stomach flora of ruminant mammals and white ants. That flora gives these animals the ability to digest vegetation which is not consumable by other animals. It is proved that a calf raised in sterile conditions does not receive that kind of flora and becomes incapable of digesting fodder common to that species. The behavioral traits, driving the young to borrow such bacterial flora from parents, is genetically fixed.

In social structures a transfer is possible of information accumulated during the lifespan of a single individual to other individuals in the group. For example, having found a source of food, honeybees transmit the coordinates of that source to other bees in the beehive (Frisch, 1977). Having learned a new way to get food from anthropogenic sources, birds may demonstrate that technique to other members of the flock, thus cutting the time needed for independent mastering of that technique (e.g., they learn how to open milk bottles, Foley, 1987). Monkeys in a pack may start to wash sand off fruits when the source of food is polluted (Kawai, 1965). Heathcock and woodcock mating places are transferred from generation to generation. Such behavioral patterns demonstrated by animals are not elements of culture. They only demonstrate the genetically programmed limits of acquiring and processing information in extragenetic memory of a social structure (a hyperindividual, see Sect. 3.2). The loss of that information does not endanger survival of the species. Moreover the animals should discard that information as unnecessary whenever their environmental conditions change. However, if placed again into similar conditions, the animals will again in due time acquire the know-how on broadcasting the position of sources of food, on opening milk bottles, and on washing fruits.

The formation of culture and civilization, accumulated and transferred from generation to generation in the process of teaching, and which is not contained in the genetic program, is a property unique to man. The cultural heritage is based on the genetically fixed behavior. But it is only man who has learned to use his scientific, technical, and cultural heritage to increase his competitiveness and change his environmental situation. Discovering the ability to accumulate cultural information in addition to genetic infortmation has led to evolution of the genome and of the morphological structure of man towards better use of that ability. First of all, brain capacity further increased to produce a bigger buffer in which to store that cultural information, and, second, speech developed as a means to transmit the information accumulated. The direct consequence of the evolution of culture is the material culture of man, that is his use of material, tools and fire (Lovejoy, 1981; Foley, 1987).

Intense competition had taken place in the process of the formation of man's genome between related species with differing genetic programs and it went on until the rates of accumulating genetic and cultural information became comparable to each other, that is until both the rate of acquiring the new morphological changes and of accumulating cultural know-how worked together to increase competitiveness of the respective species (Foley, 1987). As soon as the rate of progress (that is of accumulation of cultural information) exceeded the rate of evolution (that is of accumulation of genetic information) in a certain species, it appeared unreachable for all of its competitors.

Prior to development of speech, all the cultural information had to be stored in every separate man's brain. That resulted in quick evolution towards the increase of brain volume and capacity. The volume of brain had reached its maximum in Neanderthal Man (*Homo sapiens neanderthalensis*), who lived from 2×10^5 to 4×10^4 years ago (Johanson and Edey, 1981; Elinek, 1982; Rucang and Shenglong, 1983; Foley, 1987). The accumulated cultural information had to be transmitted from generation to generation without losses, by means of the language of mimics and gestures, still present in modern man (a sizeable part of brain core in man has the single function of identifying human faces (Geschwind, 1979; Fischbach, 1992)). It resulted in the teaching process becoming exceptionally important, so that the relations between the generations were drastically altered in the human species, as compared to all the other animals.

The appearance of modern man (*Homo sapiens sapiens*) is related to another major change in the genome – the development of speech, that is the capacity to take in and transfer to following generations the cultural language of sound signals, which differ from the genetically fixed sound signals used by other animals. Any specialization in the social structures of animals is genetically fixed (Frisch, 1977; Brian, 1983). With speech developing it became possible for different people to accumulate specialized cultural information. In its turn such a development resulted in the need for society to develop, i.e. a new internally correlated social structure based on cultural specialization, with the inevitable elements of altruistic interaction between individuals not kin to each other (Simon, 1980). Now all the cultural information could be stored in several brains, instead of just one, these brains belonging to different members of the society. Further progress of the civilization of modern man occurred on the basis of competitive interaction of, and selection among, the new hyperindividuals (Sect. 3.1), societies with optimal culture (nationalities).

The appearance of cultural specialization made it possible for the brain of a single man, the most vulnerable part of the human body, to stop growing and even to shrink somewhat. Apparently, it was particularly the formation of society based on advanced speech (resulting from the formation of chin, the reduction of mass and increase in mobility of the lower jaw) which gave the decisive advantage to modern man, having formed about $(4-10) \times 10^4$ years ago (Elinek, 1982; Rucang and Shenglong, 1983; Foley, 1987) and which enabled him to quickly force out Neanderthal Man completely.

The genetically fixed specialization in social structures of animals does not have any centralized control. The appearance of cultural specialization in man demanded that law and moral norms of correlated interaction between society members be developed without fixing them in the genome. These norms inevitably change with developing culture and need the formation of state organs for centralized control and steering of society. Aesthetic perception of man is basically formed via imprinting (Sect. 6.1). That is what makes the young generation so receptive to any new lifestyle while people of riper age, having grown up in different conditions, often appear not to accept it.

However all the actions of man are still dictated by the genetically programmed system of positive and negative emotions, which do not depend on the acquired cultural heritage and cannot be changed via upbringing. The basis for competitive interaction remains without changes the one preventing the decay of the genome in the human population as in any other population of bi-sexual species. It is based on regulating the birth rate (Sects. 3.6, 3.11, and 6.2) and on preserving the lives of most of the newborn members of society. The existing hierarchical structure at all levels of cultural specialization is supported by the drive to raise the prestige (the rating) of members of all such structures. The creativity drive is apparently written into the normal genome of man. However, that genetic property may only be saved from decay if man may demonstrate the results obtained, that is if he can raise his rank in society as a result.

In animal world, it is only the genetically fixed information content of the normal genome which is transmitted to generations to follow, the one determining the highest competitiveness of the individual. In contrast to animals, any information may be transmitted down the generations in modern man, thus forming the basis for the existence of pure mathematics, of humanitarian sciences, of art, and sports and games, and astrology and other anti-sciences. The development of those branches of culture is possible in highly developed and competitive society and, in contrast to accumulation of knowledge in natural science and technology, which develop in the direction of higher competitiveness of the society, can go any arbitrary way, increasing the level of professionalism and raising higher the scientific prestige of its participants, as forced by competitive interaction of experts working in these fields. Quite possibly that development is similar to development of non-adaptive handicap characteristics, which work to increase competitiveness of individuals, such as bright feathering in birds or giant antlers in deer's, in the natural biota (Zahavi, 1975.)

Actions promoting the maximum prestige depend on the state of culture in the society and may, for example, differ from the totalitarian to democratic societies. Disinformation based on genetic heritage within a single population is absolutely impossible. The genetically programmed disinformation is only employed during interaction between the different species (such as mimicry (Hinde, 1970; Raven and Johnson, 1988)). Culture makes it possible to use disinformation within the society to raise the prestige of a separate member of that society. Actions increasing the level of prestige are demonstrated to all the members of the society. Conversely, actions lowering the prestige are painstakingly masked from everybody. Supporting the prestige of a separate individual may alternatively go by way of artificially lowering the level of prestige of those around the individual (egoism, see Simon, 1980). Such tendencies in society are only limited by the loss of competitiveness of the whole society inevitably accompanying them.

There is no analog of a normal genome with respect to cultural heritage. Therefore, there is no stabilization of cultural heritage by means of relaxation to the normal state (Sect. 3.9). The presence of the relaxation to the normal state in the genetic heritage and the absence of such relaxation in the cultural heritage should be taken into account in all investigations of human evolutionary history (Cann et al., 1987; Wilson and Cann, 1992; Thorne and Wolpoff, 1992). In contrast to genetic heritage, cultural heritage may be lost during the lifespan of the species. It is a process partially going on through the process of accumulation and evolution of cultural information in exactly the same way happens to genetic information in the process of evolution of the species. The amount of cultural information accumulated does not lack as much as that in the human genome. The information content of human DNA is about 10^{10} bit (Sects. 2.8 and 3.4). The human brain is capable of assimilating information at a rate of no more than 100 bit/s, that is of accumulating no more than 10^{10} bit during the whole of a man's life. Recalling the inevitable repetitions during that lifetime, as well as repetitions in the genome, the unique component of both information sets is reduced by several orders of magnitude (apparently down to 10^8 bit). The cultural information of the whole of mankind (the information contained in the artificial environment surrounding man) is composed of non-overlapping parts of memory contents of each individual man. Information written into books and computers is only alive when it is contained in the memories of the living individuals of society. The upper level of cultural information commanded by mankind may be estimated as a product of the human population (5×10^9 persons) by the information content of a separate individual (10^{10} bit/man), that is about 10^{20} bit. Accounting for the process of accumulation of information during teaching and for social sciences the overall cultural information possessed by mankind should be reduced by two to three orders of magnitude, that is down to 10^{17} bit. The hereditary information contained in all the species of the biosphere is of the same order of magnitude, see Sect. 2.8.

The amount of memory accumulated during the lifespan of an animal does not change from generation to generation. This amount is necessary and sufficient for maintaining the steady state population number of individuals and their natural environment. The cultural heritage of modern man increases continuously. The human population growth is the consequence of such increase. The sustainable development of human civilization without destroying its environment would be possible if the inevitable increase of cultural heritage were not accompanied by the growth in the human population, which should be less than the definite threshold number depending inversely on the level of development. The value of this threshold and possible mechanisms of preventing the human population growth should be found and included in human culture.

Culture and civilization are absolutely necessary for man's life in exactly the same way as is his genetic program. Destroying the existing culture would render man incapable of existence. It may be said that modern man bears a "part of his genome", necessary for his existence, in the vulnerable form of his cultural heritage. Changing his environment, man changes his own culture too. If it is found that such changes do not support man's survival, then man, having already progressed beyond the present civilization, will be incapable of returning to his former existence without that culture, which is completely opposite to what happens with animals released from the zoo.

The natural biota consists of widely diverse species of equal competitiveness. The amazingly quick rate of change of civilization results in a single lifestyle having the highest competitiveness at any given time, and the whole of mankind must inevitably follow this. That is the scientific-technical revolution of the present day, and no other modes of man's existence may compete with it.

6.5 The Ecological Niches of Man

Paleontological data (Johanson and Edey, 1981; Elinek, 1982; Foley, 1987) demonstrate that the ancestors of modern man occupied the niche of the forager, a species with a wide spectrum of consumption of vegetation food, with flesh food approximately ten times scarcer. Assuming the daily average speed of movement of a foraging man over his feeding ground to be $u = 15$ km/day, see Sect. 5.9, the foraging bandwidth for one man to be $l \approx 1$ m/person, the time of reproduction of food products $\tau_1 \approx 1$ year, we obtain for the extent of feeding ground $S = lu\tau_1 \approx 550$ ha/person, see Sect. 5.10. If we assume the total area of the primeval foragers to be of the order of 10^9 ha (which is close to the total area of today's arable lands, see Table 5.1), we find that the primeval human population of Earth did not exceed two million people. The discovery of fire about a million years ago (Johanson and Edey, 1981; Rucang and Shenglong, 1983) permitted man with his new niche of the hunter to populate vast areas of temperate climate, where life by foraging is impossible. The population of Earth did not noticeably increase as a result, because the consumption territory of a hunter is larger than that of a forager (Gorshkov, 1980a, 1984b; Bromley et al., 1983, Foley, 1987).

Man's body is large and devoid of hair cover. Mammals' hair forms a thermo-insulating layer, supporting constant body temperature. The loss of hair by man points to the fact that under natural conditions his body was constantly overheated (Gorshkov and Dolnik, 1980; Foley, 1987). Man must have spent more energy on moving across his feeding ground than other animals of equal body size. Man is capable of walking 40 km a day and more, which exceeds the average daily running distance of other mammals by about a factor of two (Sect. 5.5). That is only possible at twice as high average daily activities ($\bar{A} \approx 2$, instead of $\bar{A} \approx 1$). It all indicates that man must have been permanently in a state of energy deficiency, leading a nomadic life and being forced to protect an enormous feeding ground (Sect. 5.10). Man's exclusive position in his energy demands was the factor determining his evolution towards higher cognitive powers.

The discovery of agriculture opened the way for man to increase his share of consumption of vegetation food products from arable lands to values comparable to the total net primary production, via growing edible monocultures and forcing most competing consumers out. Simultaneously the surface area necessary for a single man's consumption reduced to just several hectares per person. The energy formerly spent on making the rounds of the foraging territory was now to be spent on land cultivation.

Agriculture meant transition from the large nomadic groups of people to a settled life mode. Minimal energy expenditures were provided by land toilers separating into individual land patches in which either farms or small villages formed, so that the life mode became similar to that of territorial animals. Meanwhile the genetically fixed strategy of competitive interaction and reproduction of human beings remained the same, that is corresponding to formation of large civil groups, see Sects. 3.11 and 6.2. The stability of the population could thus only be provided by the appearance, simultaneously with agriculture, of cities, of large settled groups of people, feeding off the product grown by the agricultural population. Apparently, the cities must have indeed appeared simultaneously with the invention of agriculture.

Constant exchange of people should have taken place between the village and the city, so that the state appeared as a result. Keeping the state internally correlated was made possible by competitive interaction between the different states. City population had accepted upon itself the principal functions of competitive interaction, including that of the defence of the state.

The farmer was now already unable to acquire the necessary amount of animal products from the new consumption area reduced by a factor of several hundred. Thus farming over large territories could emerge only together with animal husbandry pastures. Since production by livestock is ten times lower than its fodder, to produce a tenth of his food in the form of animal products, man was forced to have the total animal biomass of the same order as that of the human population itself, and the pasture land areas as large as that of the arable lands. Using such arable lands man already consumes such a share of the overall biomass produced, that its natural reproduction is no longer possible. Man is thus forced to take the function of that reproduction upon himself, annually ploughing, fertilizing, and seeding arable lands. Agriculture and animal husbandry gave man a way to manage significant new areas in the temperate climatic zone, increasing the overall human population of Earth by a factor of about 20, as compared to that of the foragers.

About 200 years ago the energy of fossil fuel started to be used for transportation of people and food and for processing arable lands. That development made it possible to increase the share of consumption from such lands to that maximally possible, and to introduce many new lands, not fit for manual tilling, into the cultivation cycle, which resulted in a quick population growth. Earth's population had been slowly growing from the times of discovery of agriculture up to the very start of industrialization, increasing by a factor of about ten in ten thousand years (Bogue, 1969; Meadows et al.,1992). The last 200 years of additional energy input resulted in a new increase of the Earth population by another factor of five, now reaching 5×10^9 people.

The observed relative rate of the world human population growth, $r \equiv (dN/dt)/N$, has changed proportionally to the overall human population N,

$r = N/N_{cr}$, $N_{cr} = $ const, across the whole interval of the existence of mankind (Shklowsky, 1987; Gorshkov and Dolnik, 1980; Gorshkov, 1980b, 1984b). Thus the growth of world human population was hyperbolic, instead of exponential, see Fig. 6.1:

$$\frac{dN}{dt} = \frac{1}{N_{cr}} N^2, \quad N = \frac{N_{cr}}{t_{cr} - t}; \tag{6.5.1}$$

$$N_{cr} = (2.0 \pm 0.2) \times 10^{11} \text{ peoples} \cdot \text{years}, \quad t_{cr\,A.D.} = 2025 \pm 5. \tag{6.5.2}$$

The dimensional constants, Eq. (6.5.2), were found from empirical data (Urlanis, 1978; Starke, 1987, 1990) by the least mean square deviations technique. The presence of a pole singularity in (6.5.1) means that the character of growth must change as the singularity is approached, see Fig. 6.1. However, no appreciable deviation from hyperbolic growth has been observed up to now.

As a result the existence of people on both the newly managed territories and the territories traditionally inhabited by man appeared impossible without additional energy expenditure. Despite the fact that transportation consumes about one third of the total energy used by society (Cook, 1971; Davis, 1990), it was particularly the discovery of mechanized movement and its further development, which was the cause of the scientific-technological progress going on now. Modern civilization and the environmental overburden it produces (Sect. 4.12) would have been unthinkable otherwise. The process of overpopulation of the planet and the crisis of the environment had started with the discovery of mechanical movement across the water and air routes, and with constructing a modern network of highways and railroads, and not with the development of modern industry, power stations, or nuclear industry.

Contemporary consumption of energy by man is based on non-renewable stores of fossil fuel (carbon, oil, and gas), and is equal to 10 TW (2 kW/person), which is approximately one order of magnitude higher than the power of renewable energy sources available to man (such as solar, wind, geothermal, tide, river hydropower, and wood growth, see Table 2.1). Consumption of biospheric organic production by man (food for man and livestock, wood consumption) rises in proportion with the human population and is now equal to about 5 TW (1 kW/person) in energy units (Sect. 5.1) (Whittaker and Likens, 1975; Gorshkov, 1980b, Vitousek et al., 1986).

Each alternative means used to extract food reserves, sufficient to support the population for an extended time period, may be treated as a separate ecological niche. Figure 6.2 presents a comparative estimate of energetics of different ecological niches of man (Gorshkov, 1980a; Gorshkov and Dolnik, 1980), see Appendix C.

The required amount of food, 280 kg/year of calorie-equivalent grain per person, i.e. 134 W/person, is obtained from the amount of food required for a balanced diet of a single person (12 % animal food): 500 kg/year of calorie-equivalent grain, half of which is consumed by man and another half by domestic animals who transform it into 33 kg of animal production (in terms of calorie-equivalent grain). In

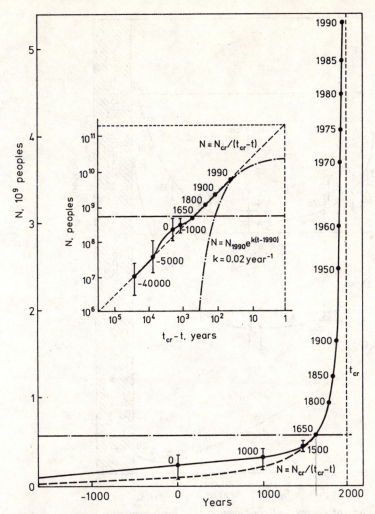

Fig. 6.1. World human population growth. Crosses and solid lines describe the observed growth of world human population. The dashed line is the hyperbolic growth, see (6.5.1). Vertical and horizontal dashed lines are dimensional constants, see (6.5.2). Inner figure is the same on the doubly logarithmic scale; dash-dotted curve is the exponential population growth at a constant $k \equiv (dN/dt)/N = 0.02\,\text{year}^{-1}$, that equal to the observed average growth of world human population in 1970–1990. Dash-dotted horizontal lines are the ecologically permissible limit for the world human population, see Figs. 1.4 and 4.10.

case of livestock grazing, fishing, and hunting, when no energy is expended on feeding animals and humans themselves only consume the animal products, the given quantity of food equals 280 kg/year in terms of calorie-equivalent grain.

The area utilized is computed as the territory from which the amount of food products indicated above is retrieved using the given technique. We find a definite

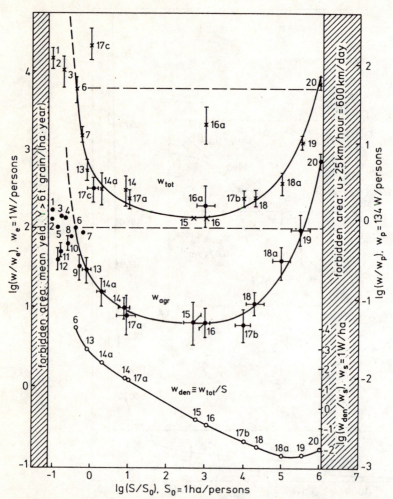

Fig. 6.2. Expenditure of energy and consumption area for a man with a normal diet in different niches. The vertical axis corresponds to energy consumption, w, in W/person and the horizontal axis corresponds to consumption area, S, in ha/person. The dots and the curve, w_{agr}, correspond to net energy expenditure for the consumption area for all forms of activity related to gathering food for a consumption norm (see text). The crosses and curve, w_{tot}, correspond to the total energy expenditure for production of the same quantity of food (including the energy expended on food for humans and domestic animals, household heating, food preparation, industry and transportation). The circles and curve, $w_{den} \equiv w_{tot}/S$, correspond to the density of the energy expenditure per unit area (additional scale on the right in W/m²).

Data: 1–12 denote various countries in the world. 1 – Japan, 2 – England, 3 – USA, 4 – Israel, 5 – Western Europe, 6 – World average, 7 – Asia and India, 8 – Oceania, 9 – Africa, 10 – Latin America, 11 – Taiwan, 12 – United Arab Republic, 13 – traditional agriculture, 14 – slash-and-burn agriculture, 14a – Tsembago, 15 – foraging, 16 – fishing, 16a – modern fishing, 17 – animal husbandry: a) pasture, b) primitive, c) in stalls; hunting: 18 – primitive, 18a – modern hunting by Eskimos, 19 – on horseback, 20 – motorized.

relationship between the area used and the power expended from Fig. 6.2, where the area used is shown along the abscissa while the ordinate gives the power expended in application of various methods of food extraction. Regions I and II are forbidden: region I corresponds to the average crop yield $\bar{Y} > 6$ t/(ha year) of grain (Revelle, 1976), while region II corresponds to speeds of motion $u > 25$ km/h = 600 km/day. The dashed line shows the "profitability" for an energy input which corresponds to the present global average input of energy into products obtained from cultivated fields (Rodin et al., 1974). Points above the dashed lines correspond to unprofitable input of energy. Niches that correspond to points located between the dashed lines and the main curve are energetically profitable but unstable: prolonged input of excessive energy results in exceeding permissible norms for consumption, and either the surrounding environment degrades, which is accompanied by a drop in productivity and a transition to the right side of the curve, or the productivity increases as a result of land cultivation and there follows a transition to the left side of the curve. For that reason, if the constant energy input is sufficiently prolonged, the niches around points at which the curves intersect a given level of energy input appear stable (compare niches 16a and 17c with other niches).

With the per capita energy input w_{tot} remaining prescribed, the left-hand stable niche is characterized by high density of energy input per unit surface area, w_{den}, (see lower curve in Fig. 6.2 and the right-hand complementary scale) and by higher population density, S^{-1}. That is why it is more competitive and forces the right stable niche out. The latter may only exist in the ranges where the formation of the left stable niche is impossible. Because of that, with energy consumption per single person growing, the basic mass of humanity shifts to the left along the curves, which results in a growth of population and in an even quicker growth of energy consumption of all mankind, including the anthropogenic share of biospheric production consumed.

Modern civilization has also brought the genetic program of man into conflict with the ecological niche he occupies presently. The growth of the amount of energy available per person has given woman the ability to raise her offspring alone. There appears to be no more need for male helpers anymore. That is why the number of divorces has grown on women's demand. The genetically imprinted need to have contact with women and to cater for family and offspring in most men has simultaneously been frustrated, loading to crime, prostitution, alcoholism, narcotic addiction and obscene language.

As for the animal world, with the metabolism increasing when one proceeds from invertebrates to vertebrates and from ectothermic to endothermic mammals and birds (Gorshkov, 1984b), the feeding territory increases, while the share of

---

Dashed horizontal lines indicate the average world-wide levels of energy expenditure. The horizontal and vertical short lines accompanying the dots and crosses indicate the possible scatter in the corresponding values. The computational methods and the initial data are discussed in Appendix C.

consumption by the given species, β_l, decreases, so that it corresponds to a shift towards the right-hand stable branch of the curve (see Fig. 6.2). That is related to the share of consumption by an animal being fixed according to the condition (5.5.3), provided that the animal body size is limited, and that condition does not depend on the animal's level of metabolic rate. Thus with metabolic rate, q, of the animal increasing, its consumption ground area (home range), S, should increase, while the density of the population S^{-1} and consequently the consumption share of the species, β_l, should drop off. Animals violating that condition tended to destroy their community, to wear out their feeding base, and to die out.

Mankind had existed for 2×10^5 years in niches 15 and 16 with a minimal biological energy consumption, while occupying niches 14, 17, and 18 for 10^4 years, (doubled energy consumption), niche 13 for 1000 years (five times higher energy consumption), and spending 100 years in niche 6 (20 times as high energy consumption).

As demonstrated in Sect. 4.12, modern civilization has resulted in the violation of the Le Chatelier principle in land biota. To recover both environmental and biotic stability, land areas not perturbed by man should be significantly expanded. That may only be achieved by stopping energy consumption and land use in these territories with simultaneous cessation of industrial activities and energy input in them, by removing roads carrying motor vehicles within these territories, and by banning mechanical transportation on the respective rivers and lakes. People might be admitted into those territories for recreational purposes, provided they use muscle driven transportation only. In other words, it seems to be enough to form sufficiently large national parks completely free of industrial activities, also prohibiting all motorized movement within their borders.

6.6 Climatological, Biological, and Ecological Limits of Energy Consumption by Man

The average characteristics of the Earth's climate, in particular its annual average temperature, are characterized by relative constancy. The species composition of the biosphere is adapted to the existing climate and to its observed fluctuations. Therefore, to preserve the existing biosphere no forcing of climate driving it outside the naturally admissible fluctuations should be tolerated.

The observed trend of fluctuations in the average climatic temperatures is presented in Fig. 6.3, and shows that temperature oscillations did not exceed $10\,°C$ in 10^4 years, making it $1\,°C$ in 10^3 years, and shrinking to several tenths of a degree in about 100 years. In accordance with the Stefan-Boltzmann law (2.2.4), a change of temperature by $0.1\,K$ corresponds to a change of radiation flux of $0.1\,\%$. Since the solar radiation incident upon the Earth's surface is of the order of $10^5\,TW$, see Table 2.1, the change in that flux over several tens of years, harmless for both the existing climate and the living beings, may reach about $100\,TW$. That change may be produced by both the anthropogenic change in the greenhouse effect and the change in albedo (Sect. 2.7). The same effect might also

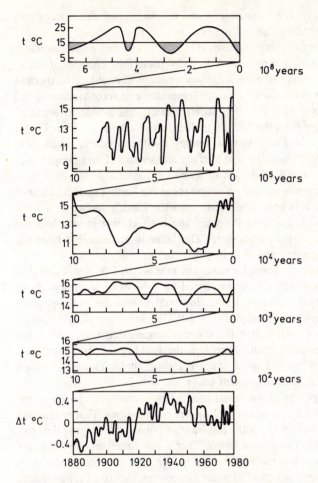

Fig. 6.3. Time variations of the Earth's surface temperature. Solid lines are the observable temperature variations in the different scales (Watts, 1982). The glacial eras in the upper figure (Berggren and Van Couvering, 1984) are shaded.

be produced by using sources of energy complementary to the solar one (such as combustive fossil fuel, using nuclear power, irradiating the Earth's surface by solar reflectors placed in outer space (Summers, 1971), or by initiating additional absorption of the incident solar energy (used to melt ice for fresh water), by heating the oceanic depths through extraction of energy from surface to abyssal water temperature difference (Meadows et al., 1974; Mesarovic and Pestel, 1974; Gorshkov and Dolnik, 1980; Penney and Bharathan, 1987). Spatial redistribution and restructuring of the surface budget of solar radiation against that naturally formed to the extent of more than 100 TW is also inadmissible. The latter limitation refers to using the solar energy from deserts and to transporting that energy into the areas of maximum concentration of population.

Use of external sources of energy by man at the Earth's surface means its transformation into thermal energy along some initially prescribed channel of decay of that external (free) energy, see Sect. 2.2. Generation of that additional thermal energy inevitably increases the Earth's surface temperature in accordance with the Stefan-Boltzmann law, see Sect. 2.7. It is fundamentally impossible to evacuate used waste thermal energy from the Earth's surface without some additional heating of that surface. Only the free (external) energy itself may be evacuated from the Earth's surface without changing that surface temperature. For example, part of the solar energy may be reflected back to space via increasing the albedo, see Sect. 2.7. Then that energy will initiate no processes at the Earth's surface, i.e. will not be used in any way. It is only possible to cool the Earth's surface at a fixed level of heat production via reducing the greenhouse effect, that is via changing the existing composition of the atmosphere. The latter is inadmissible from the point of view of life in general and man in particular.

Present-day energy consumption by mankind reaches 10 TW, see Table 2.1, hence energy consumption may still be increased by a factor of about ten above the present level. That is the climatic limit. However present-day anthropogenic change in the greenhouse effect amounts to 10^3 TW, see Table 2.1, Sect. 2.7, which is a hundred times higher than the energy consumption level and is ten times higher than the climatic limit. Therefore the build-up of the greenhouse effect is the development causing most concern among climatologists, to whom the politicians have finally started to listen lately.

The total biospheric power of the initial production is controlled by the moisture regime on land and by the structure of deep-sea communities. That production uses 100 TW of solar power and is at the top limit of power still keeping the temperature fluctuations within the natural limits. That is not a random coincidence – the power of the biosphere has reached the top power limit still compatible with climate stability. The energy structure of plant photosynthesis makes it possible to increase biotic power by at least a further order of magnitude, e.g., substituting the common C_3 plants by the C_4 ones, that is by such plants as corn and sugar cane (Govindjee, 1982). If man could only raise the average power of photosynthesis by an order of magnitude (a target for which researchers are incessantly striving), that would mean a catastrophic restructuring of the solar radiation budget. Such a tendency is as dangerous as excessive consumption of energy. That would correspond to breaking outside the climatic limit. Therefore, within the present-day climate, the total biospheric power of the biota cannot be increased.

According to the law of energy conservation, no more than the total power of the global biota, that is of 100 TW, may be transferred into the anthropogenic channel. That corresponds to increasing the share of anthropogenic consumption, that is of human food, cattle fodder, and wood by about an order of magnitude above the present level. That is the biological limit.

The increase of the anthropogenic share of consumption of biospheric production goes via increasing the total energy consumption by man. Presently the latter is far ahead of the former, see Fig. 1.4 and (4.12.6). That shows how strongly the biota resists destructive forcing by man. The increase in the greenhouse effect is produced by the increase of concentration of atmospheric CO_2. The latter effect is traditionally related to the combustion of fossil fuel. As a result of anthropogenic perturbation of the greenhouse effect, the climatic limit has already been exceeded by ten times. That is why both climatologists and politicians see the main thrust in their struggle for preservation of the global environment as reducing emissions of fossil carbon and in transferring to alternative "ecologically pure" sources of energy. After implementing such a transition and stopping emissions of fossil fuel into the atmosphere, in pursuit of the regime of energy saving, one might expect to return below the climatic limit and to reach the biological limit earlier than the climatic one during the subsequent economic growth, see Fig. 1.4 (Lovins et al., 1981; Hafele et al., 1986).

However, neither of these limits, repeatedly discussed in various publications (Duvigneaud, 1974; Meadows et al., 1974, 1992; Mesarovic and Pestel, 1974; Govindjee, 1982) have any relation whatsoever to reality. The actually existing limit to mankind's growth is the ecological one. It is related to supporting the stability of the environment, and to the action of Le Chatelier's principle in the natural biota, see Figs. 1.3 and 1.4. This limit is determined by the energy consumption level, independent of the source of energy consumption. As demonstrated in the present monograph there are ample grounds for believing that this limit has already been exceeded by an order of magnitude. It is particularly the high level of energy consumption, rather than CO_2 release in the fossil fuel combustion, that causes all the global changes including the build-up of the greenhouse effect and the exceeding of the climatic limit by an order of magnitude.

Were the anthropogenic perturbation of land biota to remain far below the threshold of its disintegration, the present-day emissions of fossil carbon would have been completely compensated by its absorption from the atmosphere by the non-perturbed biota both on land and at sea (Sect. 4.12). There would have been no increase of atmospheric CO_2 observed then. The transition to the so-called ecologically pure energy sources would not have prevented anthropogenic perturbation of the global biota, because it is determined by the level of energy consumption instead of the source of that energy. Therefore the rate of global destruction of the environment cannot be reduced by mere substitution of one energy source for another, while the power of that source either remains unchanged or even increases. The improvement of the ecological situation may only result from a reduction of power consumed down to its ecological limit, Fig. 1.4.

Going beyond the ecological limit results in disintegration of the natural communities in the biota, in cessation of the compensating action of the Le Chatelier principle, and in a violation of stability of the environment. Alterations in the part of the environment controlled by the biota bring about changes in the greenhouse gases and in moisture and temperature regimes of the planet. That, in its turn, breaks up climatic stability, affecting life conditions of both the biota in general and man in particular. Both the climatic and biological limits are then automatically violated.

6.7 Science and Religion

Restructuring the biosphere on the basis of scientific-technological progress is based on studies of objects that are capable of affecting the biota. The spatial sizes of such targets span the dimension range from that of the proton (10^{-15} m) to that of the planet Earth (10^7 m). Scientific discoveries in the areas of the micro- and macrocosm (astrophysics), made outside that scope of size ranges, cannot instigate a disintegration of the environment and the biota (Ginsburg, 1980). Up to the present times all the achievements of scientific and technological progress and the level of prestige of all scientific discoveries is actually estimated from the viewpoint of their efficiency in forcing the natural biota out of the environment and in further increasing the human population.

It was religion which was meanwhile formulating the rules of human behavior in man's interrelation with the environment and inside society. The cultural moral was formed on the basis of the genetically founded program of sustaining and raising the person's prestige in society. Actions motivated by some of the natural drives of man were prohibited: they violated moral standards and resulted in lowering of the person's prestige. Religion unified people into a community following one and the same moral. Competitive interaction between the various societies resulted in selection among the different religions and moral systems which provided for the most stable state of society and of its environment. The destruction of natural biota is forbidden in most religions. Presently the moral proclaiming a refusal to regulate the human population has failed to provide for further stability of either mankind or his environment. The present-day behavioral strategy should be formed taking account of the whole set of scientific data available. However, selection of an adequate model of behavior and of morals may only result from comparison (from competitive interaction of) of the results of activities of different societies with differing civilizations and cultures.

Religious dogmas, during the middle ages, hampered scientific-technological progress. As a result man did not exceed the admissible share of consumption of biological production of the biosphere as late as the eighteenth century. With the start of the industrial revolution, the developed countries quickly reached a high standard of living of their population through the development of their economies in the conditions of free market economy, while the environment was strongly perturbed locally. Locally emitted pollution was dissipated through the whole of the biosphere. However the biota of the "developing" countries, still non-perturbed by civilization, kept compensating for anthropogenic perturbations on the global scale. Thus the environment of the biosphere had hardly changed on average, until the beginning of the present century.

Therefore it may be stated that the economic growth of most of the developed countries, based on scientific-technological progress and taking place in environmental conditions acceptable for life on the whole, was achieved because of the lack of such progress and economic growth in the "developing" countries, so that the latter could preserve their natural biota. Were there no "underdeveloped" countries, living according to the moral prescriptions of their various religions, and no natural environment of those, the developed countries would have to spend up to 99 % of their national income to support the natural environment in its non-perturbed state. There could then be no scientific-technological progress, and the developed countries would have remained "undeveloped".

Instead of the direct pollution of the environment, Man's impact upon the biosphere consists in disrupting its natural biotic control. During the present century anthropogenic perturbation of the natural communities has exceeded the admissible threshold on the global scale, and the environment has started to deteriorate for the biosphere as a whole. The only solution now lies in reducing the anthropogenic perturbation of natural biota and recovering the areas occupied by the non-perturbed biota. To do that one has first of all to stop the progressive destruction of the wildness area in the developing countries, because the virgin nature of the developed countries is practically not preserved anywhere (Sect. 1.10). There appears to be no other way to preserve modern culture.

7. Conclusion

The principal statements of this monograph may be summarized as follows. All living things are organized on the basis of most complex internal correlations. All the types of biological correlation are unstable and are subject to constant decay. Both statements have been empirically tested at every level, from genetic to social. Any and all forms of correlation in biology, from cellular to communities, are supported via competitive interaction of individuals in the population, and via the stabilizing selection. (That latter statement has only been tested for some organisms and for some of the simplest communities.) No other means of compensation of continuously occurring decay are known.

Stability of the environment may only be explained as based on biological compensation of all the fluctuations and the directional abiogenic changes in it. This statement is testified to by extensive empirical data. The capability of the communities to keep the matter cycles closed and to extinguish external fluctuations of the environment cannot be supported by the competitive interaction between the individuals in each species comprising the community. The competitive interaction within the species is only capable of supporting the paired correlations between the species, such a correlation containing no information on the necessary interaction of the community as a whole with its environment. That information, contained in the genome of each natural species of the community, may be withheld from decay only via competitive interaction between the different communities. It follows then that all the communities may only exist in populations of competitively interacting communities, similarly to all individuals. The last statement does not contradict any of the empirical data so far known, and enjoys diverse proxy support. The measurements available for the size of communities and for the numbers of their populations are as yet indirect (Gorshkov and Gorshkov, 1992).

Communities are the most complex forms of biological correlation. The formation of the community is only related to the necessity to keep the cycle of matter closed, and to stabilize the environment. There exist many examples of stable existence of populations of separate species outside their natural communities where the cycles of matter are open. There are no grounds to believe that artificial communities may be constructed, which could stabilize the environment at the same level of accuracy that natural communities are capable of providing. Therefore, reducing the natural biota to within a volume smaller than some threshold value robs the environment of its stability, which cannot then be restored by building new cleaning complexes, by proceeding to no-waste industrial cycles, or by using ecologically pure sources of energy.

The level of that threshold was found from certain independent empirical results. It is demonstrated that the share of consumption by large animals in all the known natural communities does not exceed 1 % of the natural biological production. Starting from the analysis of the data on the carbon cycle, it is demonstrated that stabilization of the environment by land biota first failed after the start of the industrial revolution, when the anthropogenic share of consumption of the production from biosphere exceeded 1 %. For all of the several thousand years prior to those times, that part of the biosphere which had remained so far non-perturbed, could compensate for all the perturbations introduced by man's activities, man having already transformed practically all the natural communities of Europe and most of Asia.

The biosphere, consisting of the natural biota formed in the process of natural evolution and interacting with the external and immediate environment, is, by all appearances, the only system capable of supporting the stability of the habitable environment under any perturbations likely to happen.

Referring back to past catastrophes in the history of Earth is of little use. There is still no empirical proof available to show these to have been accompanied by a loss of biological control over the environment on a global scale. The information on such catastrophes has mainly been obtained from paleontological data on the large mobile animals, which have been shown to comprise only a fine superstructure of the natural biota. Extinction of such animals hardly perturbed the normal functioning of the biota in stabilizing the environment.

Let one assume that catastrophes destroying the overall correlation in the biota are still possible. Then, upon the imagined complete destruction of all the communities in the biota, following the single catastrophic event, and the ensuing loss of biological control of the environment on a global scale, two mutually independent processes should start: the process of restoration of the natural biota, and the process of the directional abiotic change of the environment no longer controlled by the biota. Whether life will be preserved after that or not depends on the relative rates of these two processes. The available data apparently indicate these two rates to be of the same order of magnitude. In other words, the perturbed biota, having lost its control of the environment, might have had time enough to regenerate evolutionarily and resume such a control within the time of abiotic changes of the environment to a state unfit for life. The very fact of the evolution of life and of the biological control of the environment testifies to that.

If one assumes that the present anthropogenic perturbation is similar to such a catastrophe destroying the biological stability of the biosphere, then, after the complete loss of correlation in contemporary biota, the stable environment fit for life and its biological control will be regained only after several hundred thousand years. However, during that period of regeneration the environment and the biota may well be in a state unfit for the existence of any mobile animals, man included, and, possibly, multicellular life forms in general. The newly regenerated stable biota might contain no ecological niches fit for multicellular individuals at all. Thus all those species would irreversibly vanish from the face of the Earth, so in that sense such a catastrophe would not in any way differ from a complete extinction of life for mobile animals and man.

Therefore preserving the natural communities and the existing species of living beings to the extent necessary to satisfy the Le Chatelier principle with respect to global perturbations of the environment, is the principal condition for further life on the planet. To do that it is necessary to preserve the virgin nature of most of the territory of the planet Earth, rather than conserving the biodiversity in gene banks, reservations, and zoos of negligible surface area (Riviere and Marton-Lefevre, 1992). It is necessary to raise the questions of organizing whole reserved continents and oceans. The first step in that direction might be preserving the continent of Antarctica intact, as is being widely discussed all over the world.

Appendix A
Details of Calculations in Sect. 4.11

Consider in detail the task of calculating the increment in production of the dissolved organic carbon (Gorshkov, 1991b, 1993a). Concentrations of radiocarbon vary at an approximately constant gradient from the surface (s) to depth L, less than 1 km, and then at deeper levels (d) remain approximately constant down to the very seabed at depth H. We denote all the surface preindustrial values by the additional subscript "0". Denoting the concentration of isotope $^\nu C$ by the same symbol in italics (and indicating additionally its localization in brackets in either the organic (+) or inorganic (−) reservoir, e.g. $^\nu C(s_0^+)$ or $^\nu C(d^-)$), we arrive at the following equation of mass budget for carbon (either "+" or " − ") in the oceanic column of unit area and depth H:

$$H \frac{d\,^\nu C(d)}{dt} = {}^\nu F - \frac{^\nu C(d)H}{^\nu T}, \tag{A.1}$$

where $^\nu F$ is the influx to that reservoir column, $^\nu T$ is the residence time for atoms of carbon isotope $^\nu C$ in the reservoir. The mass of carbon in the oceanic column is assumed equal to $^\nu C(d)H$. Deviation of preindustrial concentration in the surface layer from its value at depths influences the total mass of carbon by only several per cent, see Fig. 4.4.

The influx channel to reservoirs of both organic and inorganic carbon is the same for both ^{12}C and ^{14}C. However, ^{14}C has an additional escape channel from each reservoir, the decay channel. The last term in Eq. (A.1) for ^{14}C actually is a sum of two terms:

$$^{14}C(d)H(^{12}T^{-1} + T_c^{-1}),$$

and the residence time for ^{14}C in the reservoir is determined by the well-known relationship for any two parallel channels:

$$\tau^{-1} = T^{-1} + 1, \quad \tau \equiv {}^{14}T/T_c, \quad T \equiv {}^{12}T/T_c, \tag{A.2}$$

where T_c = 8267 years is the average lifetime of ^{14}C (Degens et al., 1984).

The influx $^\nu F$ in both organic and inorganic reservoirs is proportional to surface water concentration of inorganic radiocarbon $^\nu C(s^-)$. The equation $d\,^\nu C/dt = 0$ had held for the stationary preindustrial steady state, and the influxes $^\nu F_0$ into the reservoir coincided with the escape fluxes from the reservoir:

$$^\nu F_0 = {}^\nu C(s_0^-)\,^\nu v, \tag{A.3}$$

$$^{\nu}F_0 = {}^{\nu}C(d)H/{}^{\nu}T_0.\tag{A.4}$$

Here $^{\nu}v$ is the proportionality coefficient. The flux ratio, $^{14}F_0^{\pm}/{}^{12}F_0^{\pm}$ is equal to the concentration ratio, $^{14}C/{}^{12}C = {}^{14}R(s_0^-)$ in the "s_0^-" range with the accuracy of isotopic fraction corrections of the order of several percent ($^{14}v = {}^{12}v$). Certain chemical reactions take place there, so that carbon is channelled to both the organic and inorganic reservoirs from the dissolved gas (CO_2). We have from (A.2)–(A.4) for both the " + " and " − " reservoirs:

$$\frac{T_0}{T_0} = \frac{{}^{14}R(d)}{{}^{14}R(s_0^-)} = \frac{\Delta^{14}C(d) + 1}{\Delta^{14}C(s_0^-) + 1},\tag{A.5}$$

$$\Delta^{14}C(x) \equiv \frac{{}^{14}R(x)}{{}^{14}R(a_0)} - 1,\tag{A.6}$$

where $^{14}R(x)$ and $^{14}R(a_0)$ are the $^{14}C/{}^{12}C$ ratios for a single reservoir (+ or −) in the observed region, x, and at the initial time moment, a_0, respectively. At that moment the reservoir was in equilibrium with the preindustrial atmosphere. The value of $\Delta^{14}C$, Eq. (A.6), does not depend on the nature of the reservoir, and is exclusively determined by the age of radiocarbon:

$$\Delta^{14}C = \exp\left(-\frac{t}{T_c}\right) - 1 \quad \text{or} \quad \frac{t}{T_c} = -\ln(1 + \Delta^{14}C).\tag{A.7}$$

The ratio ^{14}R in any given sample is usually compared to the same ratio $^{14}R^A$ in a certain standard (a standard reservoir). Using that symbol:

$$\delta^{14}C(x) = \frac{{}^{14}R(x)}{{}^{14}R^A} - 1\tag{A.8}$$

we retrieve the following expression from (A.5) and (A.6) (see Stuiver and Pollach, 1977):

$$\begin{aligned}
\Delta^{14}C(x) &= \frac{1 + \delta^{14}C(x)}{1 + \delta^{14}C(a_0)} - 1 \\
&= \delta^{14}C(x) - 2\left(\delta^{13}C(x) - \delta^{13}C^A\right)\left(1 + \delta^{14}C(x)\right);
\end{aligned}\tag{A.9}$$

$$\delta^{14}C(a_0) = 2\left(\delta^{13}C(x) - \delta^{13}C^A\right), \qquad \delta^{13}C(x) = \frac{{}^{13}R(x)}{{}^{13}R^S} - 1.\tag{A.10}$$

It is assumed here that isotopic fractionation is controlled by the difference in isotope masses. Then the value of $\delta^{14}C(a_0)$ is twice as large as that of $\delta^{13}C(a_0)$. The isotope ^{13}C is stable, so that $\delta^{13}C(a_0) = \delta^{13}C(x)$. The standard samples A and S for isotopes ^{14}C and ^{13}C differ from each other. That is why $\delta^{13}C^A$ is subtracted from $\delta^{13}C$. Equation (A.9) is true to the accuracy of terms quadratic in $\delta^{14}C(a_0)$ and $\delta^{13}C(x)$. (The value of $\delta^{14}C(x)$ may be close to -1.) To simplify our expressions we use the following notation below:

$$\Delta^{14}C(x) \equiv \Delta(x).\tag{A.11}$$

The values $\Delta(s^\pm)$ and $\Delta(d^\pm)$ are borrowed from Druffel and Williams (1990) and $\Delta(s_0^-)$ from Druffel and Suess (1983), and Gorshkov et al. (1990). Generating the ratio $^{14}F_0/^{12}F_0$ in (A.4) and using (A.2), (A.5), (A.6), and (A.11) we obtain:

$$\tau_0^\pm \equiv \frac{^{14}T^\pm}{T_c} = \frac{\Delta(s_0^-) - \Delta(d^\pm)}{1 + \Delta(s_0^-)}; \quad T^\pm = \frac{^{12}T^\pm}{T_c} = \frac{\Delta(s_0^-) - \Delta(d^\pm)}{1 + \Delta(d^\pm)}. \tag{A.12}$$

Using (A.11) and (A.12) we have:

$$\Delta(s_0^-) = -0.05, \quad \Delta(d^-) = -0.23, \quad \Delta(s^-) = 0.13, \quad \Delta(d^+) = -0.53, \tag{A.13}$$

$$\Delta(s^+) = -0.18; \quad \tau^+ = 0.51, \quad T^+ = 1.02, \quad \tau^- = 0.19, \quad T^- = 0.23.$$

Note that the residence time T coincides with the age t at low $\Delta(d) \ll 1$, and $\Delta(s) \ll \Delta(d)$ only. The value of $\Delta(s_0^+)$ may be calculated from the condition that the flux of carbon to oceanic depths due to eddy diffusion was equal to influxes and escape fluxes from the reservoir, Eq. (A.4), during the preindustrial era:

$$^{14}F_0^\pm = \frac{D}{L}\left[^{14}C(s_0^\pm) - ^{14}C(d^\pm)\right] = \frac{^{14}C(d^\pm)H}{^{14}T^\pm}. \tag{A.14}$$

Here D is eddy diffusivity and L is the depth above which the ^{14}C concentration gradient is observed. The values D and L remain the same for both organic and inorganic carbon. We have from (A.11) and (A.14):

$$\frac{\Delta(s_0^+) - \Delta(d^+)}{1 + \Delta(d^+)}\tau^+ = \frac{\Delta(s_0^-) - \Delta(d^-)}{1 + \Delta(d^-)}\tau^- \tag{A.15}$$

and from (A.13) and (A.15):

$$\Delta(s_0^+) = -0.49. \tag{A.16}$$

The present-day influxes of radiocarbon to organic and inorganic reservoirs ($^{14}F^\pm$) far exceed their escape fluxes, see (A.1) and are equal to the rate at which the masses of radiocarbon accumulated have kept increasing over the period elapsed since the beginning of surface nuclear tests in 1955 (date of minimum atmospheric radiocarbon; Druffel and Suess, 1983). Such masses are proportional to the areas of the triangles ($d^\pm$, $s^\pm$, $s_1^\pm$) cut out by the measured at 1986 (Druffel and Williams, 1990) and the prebomb at 1955 profiles of concentration of radiocarbon, see Fig. 4.4:

$$^{14}\bar{F}^\pm = \frac{^{14}C(s^\pm) - ^{14}C(s_1^\pm)}{2\,\Delta t}L. \tag{A.17}$$

Here $^{14}\bar{F}^\pm$ are the radiocarbon fluxes averaged for 1955–1986, $C(s^\pm)$ and $C(s_1^\pm)$ designate the oceanic surface radiocarbon concentrations at 1986 and 1955 respectively, $\Delta t = 1986 - 1955 = 31$ years.

The value $\Delta(s_1^+)$ is unknown. This value can be found as follow. The rate of change of DOC mass, $\dot{m}_s^+$, is proportional to the known atmospheric increment of carbon mass, m_a: $\dot{m}_s^+ = k_s^+ m_a$, see (4.4.1), (4.4.2) and (4.12.2) in Sects. 4.4 and 4.12. Integrating this equation over time at constant k_s^+ we find that 43% of total increment of DOC mass, m_s^+, have been accumulated between 1955 and 1986; (Staffelbach et al., 1991), see Fig. 1.2: Thus using (A.5) and (A.10) we have:

$$[\Delta(s^+) - \Delta(s_1^+)]/[\Delta(s^+) - \Delta(s_0^+)] = 0.43.$$

From the last equation using (A.13) and (A.16) we have:

$$\Delta(s_1^+) = -0.31.$$

The value $\Delta(s_1^-)$ is known from the direct measurements (Druffel and Suess, 1983):

$$\Delta(s_1^-) = -0.06.$$

Recalling that the values of L and Δt are identical for both organic and inorganic carbon, we find from (A.4) and (A.11)–(A.17):

$$\frac{^{14}\bar{F}^+/^{14}F_0^+}{^{14}\bar{F}^-/^{14}F_0^-} = \frac{[\Delta(s^+) - \Delta(s_1^+)][1 + \Delta(d^-)]\tau^+}{[\Delta(s^-) - \Delta(s_1^-)][1 + \Delta(d^+)]\tau^-} = 3.1. \tag{A.18}$$

The ratio $^{14}F^-/^{14}F_0^-$ may be calculated from the total influx of radiocarbon into the ocean: $^{14}F =^{14}F^- +^{14}F^+$. The ratio $^{14}F^-/^{14}F^+$ from (A.4), (A.13) and (A.14) is equal to $^{14}C(d^-)\tau^+/^{14}C(d^+)\tau^- \approx 54$. Indeed, the ratio $^{14}C(d^-)/^{14}C(d^+)$ is equal to the mass ratio of the oceanic dissolved inorganic and organic carbon, which is of the order of 20, see Sect. 4.11. We further obtain from (A.18) that $^{14}F^-/^{14}F^+$ has decreased by a factor of 3, so that now it approximates to about 18. The ratio $^{14}F/^{14}F_0$ may be calculated using the well-known expressions (see, for instance, Gorshkov (1987a)):

$$^{14}F = \frac{b\,^{14}C(a) - ^{14}C(s)}{R_{as}}; \qquad ^{14}F_0 = \frac{b\,^{14}C(a_0) - ^{14}C(s_0)}{R_{as}}, \tag{A.19}$$

where $^{14}C(a)$ and $^{14}C(s)$ are concentrations of $^{14}CO_2$ in the atmosphere (a) and in the surface ocean (s), R_{as} is the air-sea interface resistance (Gorshkov, 1987a), b is the CO_2 solubility. Recalling that the ^{12}C concentration is about at equilibrium: $b\,^{12}C(a) = ^{12}C(s)$, dividing the right hand sides of (A.19) by $^{12}C(s)$ and $^{12}C(s_0)$ respectively, and averaging over time elapsed since land surface nuclear tests ceased (1963–1986) (Druffel and Williams, 1990), we obtain:

$$\frac{^{14}\bar{F}}{^{14}F_0} = \frac{\bar{\Delta}(a) - \bar{\Delta}(s^-)}{\Delta(a_0) - \Delta(s_0^-)} \approx 7.0, \tag{A.20}$$

$$\frac{^{14}\bar{F}^-}{^{14}F_0^-} \approx 6.8 \tag{A.21}$$

where $\Delta(a)$ and $\Delta(a_0)$ are taken from publications (see Gorshkov et al., 1990; Druffel and Suess, 1983). As a result we find from (A.17) and (A.19):

$$\frac{^{14}\bar{F}^+}{^{14}F_0^+} \approx 3.1 \cdot 6.8 \approx 21. \tag{A.22}$$

Taking (A.6) into account we have:

$$\frac{^{14}F^+/^{14}F_0^+}{^{12}F^+/^{12}F_0^+} = \frac{^{14}R(s^-)}{^{14}R(s_0^-)} = \frac{\Delta(s^-)+1}{\Delta(s_0^-)+1} = 1.2. \tag{A.23}$$

Finally, we have:

$$\frac{^{12}\bar{F}^+}{^{12}F_0^+} = \frac{21}{1.2} \approx 18. \tag{A.24}$$

Equations (A.18) and (A.20) are obtained assuming a constant concentration of ^{12}C. In reality the latter has increased in both the ocean surface and the atmosphere by approximately 12–25 % (Gorshkov, 1987a; Gorshkov et al., 1990). That effect results in the appearance of factors of the order of $1.12 - 1.25$ in $\bar{\Delta}(a)$ and $\bar{\Delta}(s^\pm)$. However, such adjustments are practically completely compensated for in the final result, (A.22).

The values entering (A.17) are approximately the same for the various regions of the world ocean (Williams and Druffel, 1987; Druffel and Williams, 1990). Only the depths L and H differ, the final result, (A.22) remaining independent of them, however. Therefore, one may assume that the ratio in (A.22) remains typical for the world ocean as a whole. We may retrieve the absolute values of DOC production P^{+DOC} and P_0^{+DOC} if we use the relations:

$$P^{+DOC}/P_0^{+DOC} = {}^{12}F^+/{}^{12}F_0^+; \quad P_0^{+DOC} = M_0^{DOC}/{}^{12}T^+,$$

where M_0^{DOC} is the total preindustrial mass of DOC. The modern estimation of DOC mass is, $M^{DOC} \approx 2000$ Gt C (Sugimura and Suzuki, 1988; Ogawa and Ogura, 1992; Martin and Fitzwater, 1992). The total DOC mass increment is about 15–20 % of M^{DOC} that is less than the uncertainties of the value of M^{DOC}. So we can put $M_0^{DOC} \approx M^{DOC}$. The average residence time for ^{12}C in its dissolved organic form is $^{12}T^+ = 8400$ years, see (A.13). Thus we obtain:

$$P_0^{+DOC} = P_0^{-DOC} = 0.24 \text{ Gt C/year}, \qquad P^{+DOC} = 4.2 \text{ Gt C/year} \tag{A.25}$$

For the rate of DOC accumulation, $\dot{m}_s^+$, we have:

$$\bar{\dot{m}}_s^+ = \bar{P}^{+DOC} - \bar{P}^{-DOC} = 4.0 \text{ Gt C/year}, \tag{A.26}$$

where the variable $\bar{P}^{+DOC}$ corresponds to the average production of the dissolved organic carbon (DOC) over the period 1955–1986, and $P^{-DOC} = P_0^{-DOC}$. The uncertainties of the result in (A.24) and (A.25) are less than 20 %. They are determined mainly by the uncertainty in the accepted mean value M_0^{DOC}.

The total mass of particulate organic carbon (POC) is of the order of several per cent of the total DOC mass (Mopper and Degens, 1979; Druffel and Williams, 1990). The possible rate of POC mass change due to change of POC production, sinking or destruction is, in any case, negligibly small as compared with the obtained DOC mass change (A.25).

Appendix B
Details of Calculations in Sect. 4.12

The carbon rates of change $\dot{m}_s^+$ and $\dot{m}_s^-$ and the coefficients k_s^+ and k_s^-, Eq. (4.12.2), may be directly retrieved from the observable changes of distributions of ^{13}C and ^{14}C in the DOC and DIC (see Appendix A) within the world ocean without using the unreliable value of global average air-to-sea exchange coefficient, see (Broecker et al., 1986; Gorshkov, 1987a, 1993b; Etcheto et al., 1991).

The value of k_s^+ may be retrieved from (4.12.2) and (A.26) taking the average for the years of 1955–1986 at $\dot{m}_s^+ = 4.0$ Gt C/year, $m_a \approx 106$ Gt C (Trivett, 1989; Gorshkov et al., 1990):

$$k_s^+ = \frac{\dot{m}_s^+}{m_a} = 0.038 \text{ year}^{-1}. \tag{B.1}$$

To obtain the k_s^- coefficient we may use the data on the distribution of ^{13}C in the world ocean (Quay et al., 1992). Equation (4.12.1) may be used for two carbon isotopes ^{12}C and ^{13}C. The rate of change for $^{13}\dot{m}_i$ may be written in the form:

$$^{13}\dot{m}_i \equiv \frac{d}{dt}(^{13}M) = \frac{d}{dt}(M_i\,^{13}R_i) = \dot{m}_i\,^{13}R_i + M_i\,^{13}\dot{R}_i, \tag{B.2}$$

$$M_i \equiv\ ^{12}M_i, \quad \dot{m}_i \equiv \frac{d}{dt}M_i, \quad ^{13}R_i \equiv \frac{^{13}M_i}{^{12}M_i}. \tag{B.3}$$

The land and oceanic biomasses have approximately equal ratios $^{13}R\colon\ ^{13}R_b \approx\ ^{13}R_s^+$ (Degens at al., 1968, 1984; Gorshkov, 1987a). The total organic mass of the land + oceanic biota is $M_B \equiv M_b + M_s^+$ and their increment is $m_B \equiv m_b + m_s^+$. Equation (4.12.1) for ^{12}C and ^{13}C have the form:

$$\dot{m}_a + \dot{m}_f + \dot{m}_s^- + \dot{m}_B = 0, \tag{B.4}$$

$$\dot{m}_a\,^{13}R_a + \dot{m}_f\,^{13}R_f + \dot{m}_s^-\,^{13}R_s^- + \dot{m}_B\,^{13}R_B +$$
$$M_a\,^{13}\dot{R}_a + M_s^-\,^{13}\dot{R}_s^- + M_B\,^{13}\dot{R}_B = 0; \quad (^{13}\dot{R}_f = 0). \tag{B.5}$$

Using the notation (see (A.10)):

$$\delta_i \equiv \delta\,^{13}C_i \equiv (^{13}R_i/^{13}R^S) - 1 \tag{B.6}$$

we obtain from (B.2) and (B.3):

$$\dot{m}_s^- = \quad -\frac{\delta_a - \delta_B}{\delta_s^- - \delta_B}\dot{m}_a \quad -\frac{\delta_f - \delta_B}{\delta_s^- - \delta_B}\dot{m}_f \quad -\frac{\delta_a M_a}{\delta_s^- - \delta_B} \quad -\frac{\delta_s^- M_s^-}{\delta_s^- - \delta_B} \quad -\frac{\delta_B M_B}{\delta_s^- - \delta_B},$$

$$2.1 = \qquad\quad -1.8 \qquad\qquad -0.38 \qquad\qquad -0.59 \qquad\quad +3.7 \qquad\quad -0.03$$

(B.7)

$$\dot{m}_B = \quad -\dot{m}_a \quad -\dot{m}_f \quad -\dot{m}_s^- .$$

$$0.1 = \quad -2.9 \quad +5.1 \quad -2.1$$

(B.8)

The figures below respective terms give their observed values in Gt C /year for the period 1970–1990. The leading term, $\delta_s^- M_s^-$, on the right hand side of (B.7) within the world ocean is obtained by Quay et al. (1992). Note that the rate of change of the total biomass $\dot{m}_B = \dot{m}_s^+ + \dot{m}_b$ is approximately equal to zero, i.e. $\dot{m}_s^+ \approx -\dot{m}_b$. Therefore the observed changes of global oxygen stores and fluxes (Keeling and Shertz, 1992) cannot provide evidence of rates of biomass change. The value of k_s^- may be retrieved from (B.7) and (4.12.2) taking the average for years 1970–1990 at $\dot{m}_s^- = 2.1$ Gt C/year, $m_a \approx 130$ Gt C (Trivett, 1989):

$$k_s^- = 0.016 \text{ year}^{-1}.$$

(B.9)

Finally, we obtain for k_s (see (B.1)):

$$k_s = k_s^+ + k_s^- = 0.054 \text{ year}^{-1}, \qquad \frac{k_s^+}{k_s^-} = 2.4.$$

(B.10)

The solution of (4.12.1) and (4.12.2) at constant k_s is as follows:

$$M_a(t) - M_a(t_0) = \int_{t_0}^{t} G(t - t')\dot{m}_A(t')at$$

(B.11)

$$G(t - t') = e^{k_s(t - t')}, \qquad \dot{m}_A(t) \equiv \dot{m}_f(t) + \dot{m}_b(t).$$

The solution (B.11) has analytical form in the case of logistic behavior of the total anthropogenic perturbation $\dot{m}_A(t)$ (Gorshkov, 1982c). If $\dot{m}_A(t)$ is constant in the future ($\dot{m}_A(t) = \dot{m}_A(t_0)$, $t_0 = 1990$ years) the solution (B.11) has a simple form:

$$M_a(t) - M_a(t_0) = \frac{\dot{m}_A(t_0)}{k_s}\left[1 - e^{-k_s(t - t_0)}\right].$$

(B.12)

Taking into account that a carbon mass of 2.1 Gt C corresponds to a carbon concentration 1 ppmv in the atmosphere (Watts, 1982) and using the numerical values, see Figs. 4.5–10, we obtain that asymptotic atmospheric concentration will not be larger than 460 ppmv:

$$[CO_2]_a = \{350 + 110[1 - e^{-0.054(t_{A.D.} - 1990)}]\} \text{ ppmv}.$$

(B.13)

However the real behavior of $\dot{m}_A(t)$ is not known and the coefficient k_s may not be constant if the perturbation $\dot{m}_A(t)$ should increase in the future, see Sect. 4.12.

Appendix C
Details of Calculations of the Results in Fig. 6.2

In Fig. 6.2, points 1–12 denote the average expenditures of energy on cultivated fields in 1964–1965 in different countries (Meadows et al., 1974). Manual labor corresponding to 10 W/person is added to points 9–12; the data of Starr (1971) and Hubbert (1971) correspond to the lower limit of the error cited. The crosses 1–6 were computed from data on total energy consumption (including consumption of the products of the biosphere) and grain production in the entire country. The deviation of the points from the curve is related to the difference between the value of the productivity and the world-average value. The points showing high productivity to the left of the curve are balanced by point 7, corresponding to half of the population on Earth.

Remaining data:

Point 13 – traditional agriculture (Russian, 1897) using working livestock. Computations from the data: average productivity, 0.6 t/(ha year) of grain (World Food Problem, 1967; Meadows et al., 1974); 1 horse per 4 ha of plowed field (Yuzhakov, 1904), average mass of a horse, 400 kg; grain equivalent: of consumption by a horse, five times its mass per year or 2000 kg/year or 1000 W (Brody, 1945) developed in the meadows and pasture-land; average consumption power by horse in the fields, 250 W/ha or 210 W/person (for production of 500 kg/year of grain); average working power of a horse, 125 W (one-eighth of the consumption (Brody, 1945)), average working power of a horse in the fields, 31 W/ha or 26 W/person (for 500 kg/year of grain); average power of manual labor in the fields 5 W/person (plowman with an average power of 15 W, feeding three people, including himself), i.e. $S = 0.83$ ha/person, $w_{agr} = 31$ W/person, $w_{tot} = 540$ W/person (134 W/person for food, 200 W (about 1.5 times the food power) for fire, 210 W for the horse).

Point 14 – slash-and-burn agriculture using manual labor with an average power $w_{agr} = 10$ W/person with productivity of 0.6 t/(ha year) during the cultivation periods and a regenerating period equal to ten of the cultivation periods: $S = 8.3$ ha/person, $w_{tot} = 300$ W/person (134 W for man food and 170 W for the fire used).

Point 14a – present tropical slash-and-burn agriculture practiced by the people of Tsembaga (Rappaport, 1971); the productivity during the periods of cultivation, 6.3 t/(ha year) of grain; regeneration time, 25 years; $S = 2$ ha/person; ratio of the energy in the harvest to the energy expended equals 16; $w_{agr} = 15$ W/person (per 500 kg of grain), $w_{tot} = w_{tot}^{(14)} = 300$ W/person.

Point 15 – primitive foraging without the use of fire; $S = 500$ ha/person; $w_{agr} = 6.6$ W/person; $w_{tot} = 134$ W/person; the quantities are computed on the basis of $S = 3 \times 10^7 \cdot l^2$ (territory intermediate between that of an herbivorous mammal, $10^7 \cdot l^2$, and that of a predator, $10^8 \cdot l^2$ (Calder, 1974; King, 1974), where l is the linear size (for man $l = 0.4$ m) and the motive power $w_{agr} = Fu$ for moving about the territory with an average speed $u = S/(l_{eff}\tau) \sim 0.17$ m/s $= 14$ km/day; it is assumed that in moving about a man forages over a strip of width $l_{eff} = 1$ m, where $\tau = 1$ year, the time for producing the food required for one year, $F = \gamma_a$ mg is the force, proportional to the weight, $\gamma_a = 6 \times 10^{-2}$ (Brody, 1945), see Fig. 5.6.

Point 16 – primitive fishing; $S = 10^4$ ha/person, computed from the average catch of 1–2 kg/(ha year) of live mass; the energy expenditure of the fisherman and the forager are taken as equal.

Point 16a – present-day marine fishing; computed from data on present-day catch of 7×10^7 t per year of live mass from an ocean area of 3.6×10^{10} ha; over-all power of world fishing fleet estimated at 1.5 times the calorific value of the fish caught (Meadows et al., 1972, 1974; Mesarovic and Pestel, 1974; Odum, 1983).

Point 17a – traditional animal husbandry using pastures, providing a consumption of 280 kg/year person of animal production calorie-equivalent to grain with a coefficient of transformation of vegetative energy into the animal production equal to 14 (twice as great as for the transformation of grain into meat (Meadows et al., 1974)), with average primary productivity of pasture land, 3 t (dry mass)/(ha year) or 1.4 t C/(ha year) or 1.8 W (ha year) (Brody, 1945; Whittaker and Likens, 1975; Odum, 1983) and with the present-day world-average grazing standards (20 % of the total primary production of pastures is consumed); $w_{agr} = 8$ W/person, determined mainly by expenditures of energy on maintaining pastures, taken as equal to one-quarter (present ratio of the expenditures of energy on pastures and on plowed fields (Burwell, 1978; Odum, 1983)) of the average expenditures of energy on pastures in niche 13; $S = 8.4$ ha/person; $w_{tot} = 240$ W/person (134 W as food for man, 80 W as cooking fire (60 % of the production from livestock (milk) is eaten in its raw form), 40 W as food for dogs) (Whittaker and Likens, 1975; Harlan, 1976; Janick et al., 1976; Schrimshaw and Young, 1976; Wortman, 1976);

Point 17b – primitive animal husbandry using pastures with 0.02 % of the production of pastures consumed at a rate 1000 times less than in 17a (two times greater than the consumption by corresponding wild animals)(McNeill and Lawton, 1970; Calder, 1974; King, 1974); $S = 10^4$ ha/person. As in 15, energy expenditures are determined by the movement of the herder over the pasture with $l_{eff} = 30$ m (average distance separating the sheep and the sheep herder); the herder eats eight times his weight per year, i.e., about 10 sheep, with a reproduction time for the sheep of the order of three years. Correspondingly, the herder must own a herd of 30 head; $w_{agr} = S/(l_{eff}\tau_1) = 6$ W/person ($\tau_1 \sim 1$ year, the regenerating time of vegetation); $w_{tot} = w_{tot}^{(17a)} = 250$ W/person.

Niches 17a,b corresponding to animal husbandry in pastures are most energy self-sufficient.

Point 17c – present-day animal husbandry in stalls using the production of pastures with a coefficient for transformation of energy from grain into energy of animal production equal to $\alpha_2 = 1/7$ (Meadows et al., 1974) and consumption of $7 \cdot 280$ kg/(year·person) = 2000 kg/(year·person) of grain is four times greater than that given in niche 6;

$$S = 4S^{(6)} = 1.6 \text{ ha/person}; \quad w_{agr} = 4w_{agr}^{(6)} = 400 \text{ W/person};$$

$$w_{tot} = 4w_{tot}^{(6)} = 24 \text{ kW/person}.$$

The niches 17c and 16a are territory and energy consuming. They can be used only when production exchange with other niches is available.

Point 18 – hunting on foot with one dog per person; $w_{agr} = 12$ W/person; $S = 2 \times 10^4$ ha/person; $w_{tot} = 240$ W/person = $w_{tot}^{(16)}$. The territory is estimated by postulating existence supported by a single species of game with a normal average biomass density of 210 g/ha of live weight (~ 52 g/ha of dry mass (Calder, 1974; King, 1974; Andrijanov, 1978). (In Andrijanov, 1978 the territory of a hunter in Siberia is estimated as $(2–3) \times 10^4$ ha/person), a regeneration time τ of the order of 1 year and harvesting of 25 % of the production of game. The power developed by the hunter corresponds to movement over the territory with an average speed of $u = 0.2$ m/s = 20 km/day (see niche 15), $l_{eff} = 30$ m, corresponding to an armed hunter making a kill at a distance of 15 m. The power involved in stalking and making a kill is taken as equal to one-quarter of the motive power involved in stalking. The motive power associated with a dog equals one-quarter of the motive power of a human.

Point 18a – present-day hunting by Eskimos (Kemp, 1971) (Canada, Baffin Island). The territory is estimated from the attached map as $S = 10^5$ ha/person (2.3×10^6 ha per 26 persons); $w_{agr} = 40$ W/person (30 W/person for gasoline engines, 10 W as the motive power of a man and a dog), $w_{tot} = 400$ W/person (170 W/person for gasoline, 50 W/person for kerosine or seal oil for heating a dwelling, 134 W/person for food for people, 40 W/person for dog food), the efficiency of the engines is assumed equal to 20 % (Summers, 1971).

Point 19 – hunting on horseback for large animals (bison, regenerating time $\tau \sim 3$ years) with one horse per person. The motive power of a horse $w_{agr} = 100$ W $= \gamma_h mgu$; $\gamma_h = 0.04$ (Schneider, 1976), $u = 0.63$ m/s = 54 km/day = $S/(l_{eff}\tau)$, $l_{eff} = 30$ m, $\tau = 3$ years, $S = u\tau l_{eff} = 3 \times 10^5$ ha/person, $w_{tot} = 1300$ W/person (1000 W for the horse, 134 W for the man, 150 W for fire).

Point 20 – motorized hunting; $l_{eff} = 50$ m, $S = 10^6$ ha/person, $u = 6.4$ m/s $= 550$ km/day, $\tau = 1$ year, $w_{agr} = \gamma_M mgu = 800$ W/person = 1 hp/person, $\gamma_M = 0.04$, m = 300 kg (mass of the machine including the person), $w_{tot} \sim 7000$ W/person; the efficiency of the engine is 20 % (Summers, 1971), the power for manufacturing the engines (fraction of the total energy used by our civilization) is taken as equal to the power of the engine (Cook, 1971).

In niches 19 and 20, existence supported by hunting is possible with game having a biomass density less than the average normal value (niche 18) by a factor of 15 and 50, respectively.

Estimates of the errors in the values of w and S for the average productivity of land ($0.5 \, W/m^2$) are shown on the graph.

Appendix D
List of Frequently Used Symbols

Symbol	Definition and Units	First Use
	Chapter 2	
T_S	absolute temperature of the Sun's surface, K	Sect. 2.2
T_o	absolute temperature of the Earth's surface, K	Sect. 2.2
η	maximum radiation efficiency, dimensionless	Sect. 2.2
I_S	solar constant, W/m^2	Eq. (2.2.1)
I	average relative flux of solar radiation per unit area of the Earth's surface, W/m^2	Eq. (2.2.1)
I_e	average absorbed flux of solar radiation per unit area of the Earth's surface, W/m^2	Eq. (2.2.2)
A	Earth's planetary albedo, dimensionless	Eq. (2.2.2)
I_o	average flux of solar radiation absorbed by the surface of the Earth, W/m^2	Eq. (2.2.3)
k_B	Boltzmann's constant, JK^{-1}molecule^{-1}	Sect. 2.3
T	absolute temperature, K	Sect. 2.3
$t\,^\circ C$	temperature, degrees Centigrade	Sect. 2.3
N_A	Avogadro's number, molecule/mole	Sect. 2.3
n_E	number of moles of matter	Eq. (2.3.1)
E	energy of mole of matter, J/mole	Eq. (2.3.1)
R	gas constant, JK^{-1}mole^{-1}	Eq. (2.3.1)
N	number of molecules or of particles	Sect. 2.3,
$z(t)$	measurable, time-dependent variable	Eq. (2.6.1)
$\dot{z}(t)$	time derivative of $z(t)$	Eq. (2.6.1)

Symbol	Definition and Units	First Use
$k(t)$	relative temporal rate	Eq. (2.6.1)
l	length, m	Eq. (2.6.2)
g	acceleration of free fall, m/s^2	Eq. (2.6.2)
u	speed, m/s	Eq. (2.6.2)
Fr	Froude number, dimensionless	Eq. (2.6.3)
z	measurable variable of a given dimension	Eq. (2.6.4)
β	dimensionless coefficient of proportionality between the relative changes of two variables of differing dimension	Eq. (2.6.4)
l_e	arbitrary unit of length	Eq. (2.6.7)
x	logarithm of length l measured in units l_e	Eq. (2.6.7)
z_e	arbitrary unit of measurable variable z	Eq. (2.6.7)
y	logarithm of z measured in units z_e	Eq. (2.6.7)
z'	slope of scale invariance x-dependence of y	Eq. (2.6.8)
q_e	flux of effective thermal radiation emitted by planet into outer space, W/m^2	Eq. (2.7.1)
c	thermal heat capacity, $JK^{-1}m^{-3}$	Eq. (2.7.2)
$q_{e0}; I_{e0}; A_0$	equilibrium values of $q_e; T_e; A$	Eq. (2.7.2)
σ	Stephan-Boltzmann constant, $Wm^{-2}K^{-4}$	Eq. (2.7.3)
q_R	thermal radiation flux of the planet at zero albedo, W/m^2	Table 2.7
T_R	temperature of planet surface at zero albedo and greenhouse effect, K	Table 2.7
T_e	effective temperature of planetary thermal emission, K	Table 2.7
q	planetary surface thermal emission, W/m^2	Eq. (2.7.4)
q_0	equilibrium value of q, W/m^2	Table 2.7
$\alpha; \alpha_0$	normalized greenhouse effect; its equilibrium value	Eq. (2.7.4)
z	relative change of temperature	Eq. (2.7.9)

Symbol	Definition and Units	First Use
k_0	coefficient of stability , year^{-1}	Eq. (2.7.9)
c_0	equilibrium heat capacity , $JK^{-1}m^{-3}$	Eq. (2.7.9)
λ_0	sensitivity of climate , $Wm^{-2}K^{-1}$	Eq. (2.7.9)
$A_0'; \alpha_0'$	derivatives over temperature of $A_0; \alpha_0$	Eq. (2.7.10)
N_e	flux of Earth's long-wave photons into space, photons $m^{-2}s^{-1}$	Eq. (2.8.1)
N_s	flux of short-wave solar photons absorbed by the Earth, photons $m^{-2}s^{-1}$	Eq. (2.8.2)
η_e	efficiency for solar energy, dimensionless	Eq. (2.8.3)
n_e	average number of long-wave terrestrial photons into which a single short-wave solar photon decays	Eq. (2.8.4)
q_{min}	minimal possible flux of Earth's thermal radiation, W/m^2	Eq. (2.8.5)
Chapter 3		
v	probability of random point mutation per nucleotide site, per division, $(bp)^{-1}d^{-1}$	Eq. (3.4.1)
M	genome size (number of nucleotide pairs in genome), bp	Sect. 3.4
μ	decay rate (number of random mutations per genome per generation), dimensionless	Eq. (3.4.2)
$k_g; k_{wg}; k_{mg}$	number of cell divisions in the germ line; for women; for men, d	Eq. (3.4.2)
n	number of mutations or nucleotide substitutions	Eq. (3.4.3)
N_0	number of normal individuals in the population containing no deleterious substitutions in their genomes	Eq. (3.5.1)
N_n	number of decay individuals containing n decay deleterious substitutions in their genomes	Eq. (3.5.1)
$\dot{N}_n$	time derivative of N_n	Eq. (3.5.1)
$b_n; d_n$	birth rate (fertility); death rate of individual containing n deleterious substitutions in their genome, year^{-1}	Eq. (3.5.1)

Symbol	Definition and Units	First Use
$B_n = b_n e^{-\mu}$	birth rate share of offspring containing no changes in their genomes as compared to the parent genome, year^{-1}	Eq. (3.5.1)
B	B_n in the case when neither birth nor death rate of decay individuals is regulated, year^{-1}	Eq. (3.5.1)
n_L	lethal threshold of the number of deleterious substitutions	Sect. 3.5
δ_{nn_L}	Kronecker symbol	Eq. (3.5.5)
T_s	average lifespan of the species, year^{-1}	Sect. 3.5
β_n	relative birth rate, dimensionless	Eq. (3.5.6)
δ_n	relative death rate, dimensionless	Eq. (3.5.6)
γ_n	noncompetitiveness, dimensionless	Eq. (3.5.10)
W	absolute fitness, year^{-1}	Sect. 3.5
w	relative fitness, dimensionless	Sect. 3.5
s	coefficient of selection, dimensionless	Sect. 3.5
$w_n; s_n$	fitness; coefficient of selection of decay individuals containing n deleterious substitutions	Eq. (3.5.11)
n_c	maximum number of decay (deleterious) substitutions evading detection during competitive interaction of individuals (sensitivity threshold of competitive interaction or threshold of truncating selection in natural conditions). All individuals containing $n < n_c$ have the normal genotype	Sect. 3.6
$r_c \equiv n_c/M$	average permitted density of decay substitutions in the normal genome, dimensionless	Sect. 3.6
$l_c \equiv r_c^{-1}$	average relative length of the normal genome free of decay substitutions, dimensionless	Sect. 3.6
τ_g	time lapse between the two successive cell divisions in germ line, s	Sect. 3.7
n_0	number of neutral sites in which neutral substitutions may arise	Sect. 3.7

Symbol	Definition and Units	First Use
N_u	population number in which a neutral mutation occurs at a probability of unity in each single generation	Sect. 3.7
ν_{12}	probability of transition from state 1 to state 2	Sect. 3.7
$n_{min} > n_c$	minimal number of decay substitutions in the perturbed external conditions	Sect. 3.9
μ_{gen}	decay rate of a single gene (number of mutations per gene per generation)	Sect. 3.11
μ_s	somatic decay rate (number of mutations per genome in somatic line)	Sect. 3.12
k_s	number of divisions in somatic line	Eq. (3.12.1)
H	heterozygosity of diploid genome (including X and Y chromosomes)	Sect. 3.13
μ_{2s}	diploid somatic decay rate	Eq. (3.13.1)
μ_{ns}	n-ploid somatic decay rate	Eq. (3.13.2)
M_n	total length of n-ploid genome (total length of all chromosomes), bp	Sect. 3.13
H_n	heterozygosity of n-ploid genome, dimensionless	Eq. (3.13.3)
H_0	heterozygosity corresponding to X and Y chromosome (X and Y chromosomes to total genome length ratio)	Eq. (3.13.5)
H_c	maximum heterozygosity of normal genotype: individuals of heterozygosity below H_c have equal competitiveness	Eq. (3.13.5)
H_L	lethal threshold of heterozygosity	Eq. (3.13.6)
$\mu^- \equiv \mu$	decay rate of genome, dimensionless	Sect. 3.15
μ^+	generative rate of genome (number of progressive mutations per genome per generation), dimensionless	Eq. (3.15.1)
κ_e	ratio of decay to progressive mutations in eukaryotes	Eq. (3.5.1)

Symbol	Definition and Units	First Use
κ_p	ratio of decay to progressive mutations in prokaryotes	Eq. (3.15.2)
$v^- \equiv v$	probability of a decay mutation per nucleotide site per division, $(bp)^{-1}d^{-1}$	Eq. (3.15.1)
v^+	probability of a progressive mutation per nucleotide site per division, $(bp)^{-1}d^{-1}$	Eq. (3.15.1)
T_e	age of life (complete time of biological evolution), years	Sect. 3.17

Chapter 4

Symbol	Definition and Units	First Use
T	time interval of evolutionary change, that is the order of mean lifespan of species, T_s, year	Sect. 4.2
τ	time of noticeable change of the store of nutrients in the environment of order of residence time, year	Sect. 4.2
$M^\pm$	mass of organic (+) and inorganic (−) nutrients per unit surface area, $kg\ m^{-2}$	Sect. 4.2
$\dot{M}^\pm$	time derivative of $M^\pm$, $kg\ m^{-2}year^{-1}$	Eq. (4.3.1)
$P^\pm$	productivity (+) and destructivity (−) of organic matter, $kg\ m^{-2}\ year^{-1}$	Eq. (4.3.1)
$F^\pm$	net physical flux of organic matter evacuated from (+) and inorganic matter imported into (−) one reservoir, $kg\ m^{-2}\ year^{-1}$	Eq. (4.3.1)
$F_{in}^\pm, F_{out}^\pm$	overall input, output fluxes, $kg\ m^{-2}\ year^{-1}$	Sect. 4.3
κ	breach of biological cycles (relative difference between production and destruction of organic matter), dimensionless	Eq. (4.3.2)
$\nu^\pm; \nu_{in}^\pm$	net; gross openness of a reservoir, dimensionless	Eq. (4.3.3)
$T^\pm$	time of complete restructuring of the environment, years	Eq. (4.3.4)
$\tau^\pm$	residence time of organic (+) and inorganic (−) matter, years	Eq. (4.3.4)
κ_0	equilibrium breach κ	Eq. (4.3.5)

Symbol	Definition and Units	First Use
$\kappa_l; \kappa_s$	breach on land (l); in ocean (s)	Eq. (4.3.7)
$\alpha_l; \alpha_s$	relative land and ocean production, dimensionless	Eq. (4.3.7)
ν_l	openness on land	Sect. 4.3
X	chemical element in either organic or inorganic nutrient	Sect. 4.4
$P_X^\pm$	productivity (+) and destructivity (−) of nutrient X, kg X m^{-2} year^{-1}	Eq. (4.4.1)
$M_X^\pm$	mass of nutrient X in organic (+) and in-organic (−) matter per unit surface area, kg X m^{-2}	Eq. (4.4.1)
$m^\pm$	mass increment, kg X m^{-2}	Eq. (4.4.1)
β_X	slope of scaling relation, dimensionless	Eq. (4.4.1)
k	stability coefficient, year^{-1}	Eq. (4.4.2)
$[X_{in}]$; $[X_{out}]$	concentration of nutrient X inside and outside local ecosystem, kg X m^{-3}	Sect. 4.6
$\Delta[X]$	difference in concentration inside and outside the local ecosystem, kg X m^{-3}	Sect. 4.6
ε	relative change in the concentration X	Sect. 4.6
ε_{min}	sensitivity limit	Sect. 4.6
$\Delta_y[X]$; $\Delta_z[X]$	concentration difference of nutrient X in horizontal (y) and vertical (z) directions, kg X m^{-3}	Sect. 4.6
D	diffusivity, m^2/year	Eq. (4.6.1)
H_e	vertical size of local ecosystem, m	Eq. (4.6.1)
R_e	external resistance to diffusion transport, year/m	Eq. (4.6.1)
R_i	internal resistance to synthesis of organic matter, year/m	Eq. (4.6.3)
R_{iX_k}	internal resistance to synthesis organic nutrient X_k, year/m	Eq. (4.7.2)
$[X_{min}]$	minimum concentration below which life becomes impossible, kg X m^{-3}	Sect. 4.7

Symbol	Definition and Units	First Use
$[X_{max}]$	maximum concentration related to the maximum productivity at a prescribed incoming flux of external energy, kg X m^{-3}	Sect. 4.7
$M_\alpha^+; P_\alpha^\pm;$ $F_{\alpha\,in,out}^\pm$	biomass (population number) ; birth $(+)$ and death $(-)$ rates, $year^{-1}$; immigration (in) and emigration (out), $year^{-1}$, in unit surface area of individuals of unit body mass of the α species	Eq. (4.8.2)
$\nu_{\alpha\,in}^+ \equiv$ $F_{\alpha\,in}^+/P_\alpha^+$	species α openness of the local ecosystem, dimensionless	Eq. (4.8.2)
$[\alpha]$	concentration of individuals of the α species	Eq. (4.8.3)
D_α	horizontal diffusivity of individuals of the α species, m^2/year	Eq. (4.8.3)
L	horizontal size of community (local ecosystem), m	Eq. (4.8.3)
H_α	vertical dimension occupied by the α species in a community, m	Eq. (4.8.3)
$[\Sigma CO_2]$	total surface concentration of dissolved inorganic carbon, mole C/m^3	Eq. (4.9.1)
$[CO_2]$	surface concentration of dissolved CO_2 molecules, mole C/m^3	Eq. (4.9.1)
$[HCO_3^-];$ $[CO_3^{2-}]$	surface concentration of bicarbonate and carbonate ions, mole C/m^3	Eq. (4.9.1)
$\Delta[CO_2];$ $\Delta[\Sigma CO_2]$	$[CO_2]; [\Sigma CO_2]$ increments, mole C/m^3	Eq. (4.9.2)
ζ	buffer (Revelle) factor, dimensionless	Eq. (4.9.2)
$A_C^+; A^+$	carbonate; total (titrate) alkalinity, mole/m^3	Eq. (4.9.3)
$[CO_2]_a$	concentration of atmospheric CO_2, mole C/m^3	Eq. 4.9.7)
ξ	equilibrium atmospheric to total dissolved inorganic carbon concentration ratio, dimensionless	Eq. (4.9.7)
$m_a; m_s^\pm$	increment of carbon mass in atmosphere (a) and ocean (s) in organic ($+$) and inorganic ($-$) forms, Gt C	Eq. (4.9.8)

Symbol	Definition and Units	First Use
$V_a; V_s$	volume of the atmosphere (a) and of the world ocean (s), m^3	Eq. (4.9.8.)
Z	ocean depth, m	Sect. 4.10
$F_X^\pm(Z)$	net flux of nutrient X in organic (+) and inorganic (−) form at depth Z, mole C m^{-2} year^{-1}	Eq. (4.10.1)
$D(Z)$	eddy diffusivity at depth Z, m^2/year	Eq. (4.10.2)
$b(Z)$	difference between the densities of destruction and production of organic matter per unit volume at depth Z, mole C m^{-3} year^{-1}	Eq. (4.10.3)
$P_n^\pm, P_{nX}^\pm$	new productivity (+) and destructivity (−) of organic matter, of nutrient X, mole C m^{-2} year^{-1}	Eqs. (4.10.4) and (4.10.8)
$P_g^\pm, P_{gX}^\pm$	gross (total) and net primary productivity (+) and destructivity (−) of organic matter of nutrient X, and (4.10.10) mole C m^{-2} year^{-1}	Eqs. (4.10.4)
H	depth at which concentration gradients become zero, m	Eq. (4.10.4)
$f = \frac{P_n^+}{P_g^+}$	new to total productivity ratio, dimensionless	Eq. (4.10.4)
$L^\pm$	average depth at which new production is synthesized (+) and destroyed (−), m	Eq. (4.10.5)
$\delta(Z), \vartheta(Z)$	Dirac delta-function, step function	Eq. (4.10.6)
$[X]_s; [X]_d$	surface and deep concentration of inorganic X, mole X/m^3	Eq. (4.10.8)
L_s	depth of the well-mixed surface layer, m	Eq. (4.10.9)
L_e	depth of layer in which the gradient of nutrient concentration is observed, m	Eq. (4.10.9)
D_e	average diffusivity in the layer L_e, m^2/year	Eq. (4.10.9)
R_e	external resistance, year/m	Eq. (4.10.9)
R_{gX}, R_{nX}	internal resistance corresponding to gross, new production of organic nutrient X, year/m	Eq. (4.10.10)
$b \equiv$ $[CO_2]_s/[CO_2]_a$	solubility of CO_2, dimensionless	Eq. (4.10.12)

Symbol	Definition and Units	First Use
$[CO_2]_{max}$, $[CO_2]_{min}$	maximum $(P_n^+ = 0)$, minimum $(P_n^+ = P_g^+)$ atmospheric CO_2 concentration, mole C/m^3	Eqs. (4.10.13) and (4.10.14)
$P^{\pm DOC}$	productivity (+) and destructivity (−) of the dissolved organic carbon, Gt C/year	Eq. (4.11.1)
$P_0^{\pm DOC}$	preindustrial value of $P^{\pm DOC}$, Gt C/year	Eq. (4.11.2)
$\dot{m}_a; \dot{m}_s;$ $\dot{m}_f; \dot{m}_b$	rate of change of carbon mass in the atmosphere (a); ocean (s); fossil fuel (f); land biota (b), Gt C/year	Eq. (4.12.1)
k_s	carbon stability (relaxation) coefficient for the world ocean, year^{-1}	Eq. (4.12.2)
$k_s^{\pm}$	physico-chemical (−) and biological (+) carbon stability coefficient for the world ocean, year^{-1}	Sect. 4.12
$P_s^{\pm}; P_{s0}^{\pm}$	recent and preindustrial ocean gross primary productivity (+) and destructivity (−), kg Cm^{-2} year^{-1}	Eq. (4.12.3)
$\Delta P_s^{\pm} \equiv$ $P_s^{\pm} - P_{s0}^{\pm}$	increment of $P_s^{\pm}$, kg C m^{-2} year^{-1}	Eq. (4.12.3)
β_s^+	slope of the scaling relation for the global carbon change, dimensionless	Eq. (4.12.4)
τ_s^+	turnover time of atmospheric carbon in the oceanic biota, year	Eq. (4.12.4)
M_{a0}	preindustrial (equilibrium) atmospheric carbon mass, Gt C	Eq. (4.12.4)
$k_a; k_s; k_f; k_b$	carbon stability coefficient of the atmosphere (a); ocean (s); fossil fuel (f); land biota (b), year^{-1}	Eq. (4.12.6)

Chapter 5

Symbol	Definition and Units	First Use
$K_C; K$	energy content per unit mass of organic carbon J (kg C)$^{-1}$ and per unit living body mass, J kg^{-1}	Eqs. (5.1.1) and (5.1.2)
ω, T^+	average velocity of all the body's molecules after instant combustion of all their body organics, their absolute temperature	Eqs. (5.1.2) and (5.1.3)
R	gas constant, JK^{-1}mole^{-1}	Eq. (5.1.3)
T_0	average absolute temperature of the Earth's surface, K	Eq. (5.1.3)

Symbol	Definition and Units	First Use
η	maximum efficiency of internal energy expenditure for living individuals, dimensionless	Eq. (5.1.3)
q; $Q \equiv q/K$; $Q_{\mathrm{C}} \equiv q/K_{\mathrm{C}}$	metabolic rate in power units, W; in living mass units, kg year^{-1}; and in carbon units, kg C year^{-1}	Sect. 5.1
$q(T)$	temperature dependence of metabolic rate, W	Sect. 5.1
Q_{10}	ratio $q(T+10°\mathrm{C})/q(T)$, dimensionless	Sect. 5.1
q_0	basal metabolic rate (power), W	Eq. (5.1.4)
A; $\bar{A}$	total activity; mean total existence activity, dimensionless	Eq. (5.1.4)
m; mg	body mass, kg; body weight, N	Eq. (5.2.1)
ρ	water (living body) density, kg/m^3	Sect. 5.2
l; s	effective individual size, m; Earth's surface projection area, m^2	Eq. (5.2.1)
g	acceleration of free fall, m/s^2	Eq. (5.2.2)
j; λ; $\hat{\lambda}$	metabolic rate (power) per unit body projection area, W/m^2; weight, m/s; volume, W/m^3	Eq. (5.2.2)
T_B; s_B	body temperature, K; body surface area, m^2	Sect. 5.2
j_B	metabolic rate per unit body surface area, W/m^2	Sect. 5.2
h_B; l_B	heat conductivity, Wm^{-1}K^{-1}; thickness of the insulating body layer, m	Sect. 5.2
$j_{e\,\mathrm{min}}$; $j_{e\,\mathrm{max}}$	minimum and maximum metabolic rate per unit body projection area for endothermic animal, W/m^2	Sect. 5.2
P_1^+; p_1^+	net primary productivity in units of live mass, kg m^{-2} year^{-1}; in power units, W/m^2	Eqs. (5.3.1) and (5.3.6)
k_T	transpiration coefficient: amount of moisture transpired per unit live mass of plant production, dimensionless	Eq. (5.3.7)
E	total evaporation rate, m/year	Eq. (5.3.7)
α_T	ratio of transpiration to total evaporation	Eq. (5.3.7)
η_T	transpiration efficiency: share of solar energy spent on transpiration, dimensionless	Eq. (5.3.8)

Symbol	Definition and Units	First Use
E_{max}	global average maximum evaporation rate when all the solar energy is spent on evaporation, m/year	Eq. (5.3.8)
L_w	latent heat of evaporation for water, J/kg	Eq. (5.3.9)
η_p	photosynthesis efficiency, dimensionless	Eq. (5.3.9)
N	number of mutually uncorrelated parts of local ecosystem	Eq. (5.4.1)
κ	breach: relative difference of net primary production and organic destruction	Sect. 5.4, see Eq. (4.3.2)
L_c	size of local ecosystem, m	Eq. (5.4.1)
r^+	average correlation radius for plants, m	Eq. (5.4.1)
n^+	number of plant species in the community determining the main part of net primary productivity	Eq. (5.4.2)
β	share of consumption of the net primary production by an animal of a given body size, dimensionless	Eq. (5.5.1)
n	number of equally represented species in the community corresponding to a given body size	Eq. (5.5.1)
β_i	consumption share of net primary production for species i, dimensionless	Eq. (5.6.2)
Δz	relative interval of body size, dimensionless	Eq. (5.6.2)
z	decimal logarithm of body size	Eq. (5.6.2)
$\beta(z)$	community consumption share per unit relative body size interval (destructivity size spectrum), dimensionless	Eq. (5.6.2)
β_l	share of consumption by an individual of body size l averaged over all the species in the community, dimensionless	Sect. 5.6
B	biomass of individual of body size l, averaged over all the species in the community, kg/m^2	Sect. 5.6
L	biomass layer thickness of individual of body size l, averaged over all the species in the community, m	Sect. 5.6
d_0	leaf area index, dimensionless	Table 5.1

Symbol	Definition and Units	First Use
$d \equiv \frac{L}{l}$	projection area index for heterotrophs, dimensionless	Sect. 5.6
u	speed of animal movement, m/s	Eq. (5.7.1)
$q(u);$ $A(u)$	metabolic rate, W; total activity, dimensionless, of an animal moving at speed u	Eq. (5.7.2)
$a; b$	net moving activity and readiness, dimensionless	Eq. (5.7.2)
u_0	speed for movement when $a = 1$, m/s	Eq. (5.7.2)
$t_a; T$	duration of activity state; duration of day, s	Sect. 5.7
x_a	relative duration of activity state for animal, dimensionless	Eq. (5.7.3)
$L_T;$ $L_{T\,max}$	daily travelling distance and its maximum, m	Eq. (5.7.4)
$u_a \approx u_0$	available speed of animal movement, m/s	Eq. (5.7.5)
ρ_c	air density, kg/m^3	Sect. 5.8
$l \equiv \left(\frac{m}{\rho}\right)^{1/3}$	effective body size of mobile animal, m	Eq. (5.8.1)
$\gamma_{tot};$ $\gamma; \gamma_c$	total, ground and air dissipation coefficients, dimensionless	Eqs. (5.8.2) and (5.8.3)
λ_0	basal metabolic rate per unit body weight, m/s	Eq. (5.8.5)
α	efficiency of transformation of metabolic power into the power of mechanical movement, dimensionless	Eq. (5.8.5)
ε	energy cost of moving unit weight through unit distance, dimensionless	Eq. (5.8.6)
u_{max}	maximum speed of running recorded for animal of body size l, m/s	Eq. (5.8.7)
k^2	Froude number for maximum speed of running independent of body size l, dimensionless	Eqs. (5.8.4) and (5.8.7)
$B_1; L_1$	vegetation biomass, kg/m^2; thickness of its layer, m	Sect. 5.9
B_L	part of vegetation biomass consumed by animal of body size l, kg/m^2	Sect. 5.9
$B_{L\,min}$	minimum value of B_L	Eq. (5.9.4)
$\beta_L = \frac{B_L}{B_1}$	share of vegetation biomass consumed by animal of body size l, dimensionless	Eq. (5.9.1)

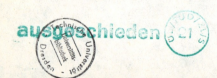

Symbol	Definition and Units	First Use
$\beta_{L\,\text{min}}$	minimum value of β_L	Eq. (5.9.3)
u_n	speed necessary to support the animal's existence, m/s	Eq. (5.9.2)
S	area of animal's feeding ground (home range), m^2	Sect. 5.10
τ_S	time in which the animal makes a round of its feeding ground, years	Eq. (5.10.1)
Λ	metabolic rate per unit body volume in units of living mass, $\text{kg m}^{-3}\ \text{year}^{-1}$	Eq. (5.10.2)

Bibliography

Ajtay G.L., Ketner P. and Duvigneaud P. (1979) Terrestrial primary production and phytomass. In: Bolin B. (Ed.) *The Global Carbon Cycle*, SCOPE, **13**, 129 (Wiley, Chichester)

Ayala F.J. and Kiger J.A. (1984) *Modern Genetics* (Benjamin, London)

Allen C.W. (1955) *Astrophysical Quantities* (Athione Press, London)

Allen J. and Nelson M. (1989) *Space Biospheres* (Synergetic, Arizona)

Altukhov Yu.P. (1991) *Population Genetics. Diversity and Stability* (Harwood Acad., New York)

Alwarez W. and Asaro F. (1990) An extraterrestrial impact. Sci. Am. **263**, 78

Amabile-Cuevas C.F. and Chicurel M.E. (1992) Bacterial Plasmids and Gene Flux. Cell **70**, 189

Andelman S.J. (1987) Evolution of concealed ovulation in vervet monkeys (*Cercopithecus aethiops*). Am. Nat. **129**, 785

Anderson P.W. (1983) Suggested model for prebiotic evolution: The use of chaos. Proc. Natl. Acad. Sci. USA **80**, 3386

Andrijanov A.P. (1954) *Fishes of North Seas of USSR* (Acad., Moscow) (Russian)

Andrijanov B.V. (1978) *Farming of Our Ancestors* (Nauka, Moscow) (Russian)

Arley N. and Buch K.R. (1950) *Introduction to the Theory of Probability and Statistics* (Wiley, New York)

Atkins A.R. and Nicholson J.D. (1963) An accurate constant-work-rate ergometer. J. Appl. Physiol. **18**, 205

Austin C.R. and Short R.V., (1984) *Reproduction in Mammals* (Book 3: Hormonal Control of Reproduction) (Cambridge Univ., London)

Avetisov V.A. and Goldanskii V.I. (1993) Chirality and the equation of "biological big band". Phys. Letters A **172**, 407

Bakker R.T. (1975) Dinosaur renaissance. Sci. Am. **232**, 58

Bärlocher F. (1990) The Gaia hypothesis – a fruitful fallacy? Experientia. March. Review Articles, **46**, 232

Barlow C. (Ed.) (1991) *From Gaia to Selfish Genes: Selected Writings in the Life Sciences* (MIT)

Barnola J.M., Pimienta P., Raynaud D. and Korotkevich Y.S. (1991) CO_2 climate relationship as deduced from Vostok ice core: a reexamination based on new measurements and on re-evolution of the air dating. Tellus **43B**, 83

Barrett S.C.H. (1989) Waterweed invasions. Sci. Am. **261**, 66

Baumgartner H. and Reichel E. (1975) *The World Water Balance: Mean Annual Global Continental and Maritime Precipitation. Evaporation and Runoff* (Elsevier, Amsterdam)

Bazzaz F.A. and Fajer E.D. (1992) Plant life in a CO_2-rich world. Sci. Am. **266**, 18

Begon M., Harper J.L. and Townsend C.R. (1986) *Ecology. Individuals, Populations and Communities* (Blackwell Sci. Publ., London)

Bell G. (1982) *The Masterpiece of Nature: The Evolution and Genetic of Sexuality* (Univ. California, San Francisco)

Berger A.L. (1988) Milankovitch theory and climate. Rev. Geophys. **26**, 624

Berggren W.A. and Van Couverin J.A. (Eds) (1984) *Catastrophes and Earth History. The New Uniformism* (Princeton Univ., New York)

Berman E.R. (1975) *Geothermal Energy* (Neyes Data Co, London)

Bloom F.E., Lazerson A. and Hofstadter L. (1985) *Brain, Mind and Behavior* (N.H.Frieman and Co. Educational Broadcasting Corporation, New York)

Blumenschine R.J. and Cavallo J.A. (1992) Scavenging and human evolution. Sci. Am. **267**, 70

Bogue D.J. (1969) *Principles of Demography* (Wiley, New York)

Bolin B., Björkström A., Holmén K. and Moore B. (1982) The simultaneous use of tracers for ocean circulation studies. Report CM-58, Sept. 1982 (Stockholm Meteorolog. Inst., Stockholm)

Bolin B., Björkström A., Holmén K. and Moore B. (1983) The simultaneous use of tracers for ocean circulation studies. Tellus **35B**, 206

Bormann F.H. and Likens G.E. (1979) *Pattern and Process in a Forested Ecosystem* (Springer, Berlin)

Bouwman A.F. (1989) The role of soil and land use in the greenhouse effect. (International Soil Reference and Information Center (ISRIC), Wageningen. The Netherlands)

Bradbury J.W. and Andersson M.B. (1987) *Sexual Selection Testing the Alternatives* (Wiley, New York)

Brian M.V. (1983) *Social Insects. Ecology and Behavioral Biology* (Chapman and Hall, London)

Brain K. and McNab B.K. (1980) Food habits, energetics, and population biology of mammals. Am. Nat. **116**, 116

Brillouin L. (1956) *Science and Information Theory* (Academic, New York)

Brimhall G. (1991) The genesis of ores. Sci. Am. **264**, 48

Brody S. (1945) *Bioenergetics and Growth* (Reinhold, New York)

Broecker W.S. (1982) Ocean chemistry during glacial time. Geochim. Cosmochim. Acta **46**, 1689

Broecker W.S. and Denton G.H. (1990) What drives glacial cycles? Sci Am. **262**, 49

Broecker W.S. and Peng T.-H. (1974) Gas exchange rates between air and sea. Tellus **26**, 21

Broecker W.S., Takahachi T., Simpson H.J. and Peng T.-H. (1979) Rate of fossil fuel carbon dioxide and the global carbon budget. Science **206**, 409

Broecker W.S., Peteet D.M. and Ring D. (1985a) Does the ocean-atmosphere system have more than one stable mode of operation? Nature **315**, 21

Broecker W.S., Peng T.-H., Ostlund G. and Stuiver M. (1985b) The distribution of bomb radiocarbon in the ocean. J. Geophys. Res. **90**, 6953

Broecker W.S., Ledwell J.R., Takahashi T., et al. (1986) Isotopic versus micrometeorologic ocean CO_2 fluxes: a serious conflict. J. Geophys. Res. **91**, 10517

Bromley Yu.V., Pershitz A.I. and Semenov Yu.I. (Eds) (1983) *History of a Primitive Society* (Nauka, Moscow) (Russian)

Brutsaert W. (1982) *Evaporation into the Atmosphere (Theory, History and Applications)* (D.Riedel Publ., Dorrdecht Holland)

Buckingham R.H. and Grosjean H. (1986) The accuracy of mRNA-tRNA recognition. In: Galas D.J., T.B.L.Kirkwood and R.F.Rosenberger (Eds) *Accuracy in Molecular Processes: its Control and Relevance to Living Systems* (Chapman and Hall, London)

Budyko M.I., Ronov A.B. and Yanshin A.L. (1987) *History of the Earth's Atmosphere* (Springer, Berlin)

Burt A., Bell G and Harvey P.H. (1991) Sex differences in recombination. J. Evol. Biol. **4**, 259

Burwell C.C. (1978) Solar biomass energy: an overview of U.S. potential. Science **199**, 1041

Calder W.A. (1974) Consequences of Body Size for Avian Energetics. In: Paynter R.A.(Ed.) *Avian Energetics* (Publ. Nuttal Ornithological Club, Cambridge), No.15, 41

Calow P. (1983) *Evolutionary Principles* (Blackie, London)

Cann R.L., Stoneking M. and Wilson A.C. (1987) Mitochondrial DNA and human evolution. Nature **325**, 31

Cano M.I. and Santos J.L. (1990) Chiasma frequencies and distributions in gomphocerine grasshoppers: a comparative study between sexes. Heredity **64**, 17

Cavagna G.A. and Kaneko M. (1977) Mechanical work and efficiency in level walking and running. J. Physiol. **268**, 467

Cavalier-Smith T. (1980) How selfish is DNA. Nature **285**, 617

Cess R.D., Potter G.L., Blanchet J.P. et al. (1989) Interpretation of cloud-climate feedback as produced by 14 atmospheric general circulation model. Science **245**, 513

Chahine M.T. (1992) The hydrological cycle and its influence on climate. Nature **359**, 373

Chappellaz J., Barnola J.M., Raynaud D. et al. (1990) Ice-core record of atmospheric methane over the past 160,000 years. Nature **345**, 127

Chen T.-H. and Drake E.T. (1986) Carbon dioxide increase in the atmosphere and oceans and possible effects on climate. Ann. Rev. Earth Planet Sci. **14**, 201

Childs W.H. (1958) *Physical Constants* (Methuel Co, London)

Chislenko L.L. (1981) *Structure of Flora and Fauna as Related to Body Size in Organisms* (Moscow Univ., Moscow) (Russian)

Clark W.C. (1989) Managing planet Earth. Sci. Am. **261**, 46

Clark W.C. and Munn R. (Eds.) (1986) *Sustainable Development of the Biosphere* (Cambridge Univ. Press, Cambridge)

Clutton-Brock T.H. (1974) Primate social organization and ecology. Nature **250**, 539

Clutton-Brock T.H. (1982) Sons and daughters. Nature **298**, 11

Cohn J.P. (1986) Surprising cheetah genetics. Bio Science **36**, 358

Coleman J.D. (1972) The breeding biology of the rook, *Corvus frugilegus L.* in Canterbury. New Zealand – Notornis **19**, 118

Cook E. (1971) The flow of energy in an industrial society. Sci. Am. **224**, 135

Cooke D., Gleckman P., Krebs H. et al. (1990) Sunlight brighter than the Sun. Nature **346**, 802

Courtillot V.E. (1990) Volcanic eruption. Sci. Am. **263**, 85

Coyne J.A. (1992) Genetics and speciation. Nature **355**, 511

Crick F. and Koch C. (1992) The problem of consciousness. Sci. Am. **267**, 153

Crosson P.R. and Rosenberg N.J. (1989) Strategies for agriculture. Sci. Am. **261**, 128

Crow J.F. (1958) Some possibilities for measuring selection intensities in man. Human Biology **30**, 1

Crow J.F. (1970) Genetic loads and the cost of natural selection. In: Kojima K. (Ed.) *Mathematical Topics in Population Genetics* (Springer, Berlin), 128

Crow J.F. and Kimura M. (1965) Evolution in sexual and asexual populations. Am. Natur. **99**, 439

Curtis D. and Bender W. (1991) Gene conversion in Drosophila and the effects of the meiotic mutants mei-9 and mei-218. Genetics **127**, 739

Cushing D.H. (1975) *Marine Ecology and Fisheries* (Cambridge Univ., Cambridge)

Damuth J. (1981a) Population density and body size in mammals. Nature **290**, 699

Damuth J. (1981b) Home range, home range overlap and species energy use among herbivorous mammals. Biol. J. Linneau Soc. **15**, 185

Davis C.D. (1990) Energy for planet Earth. Sci Am. **263**, 55

Dawkins R. (1976) *The Selfish Gene* (Oxford Univ., Oxford)

Dawkins R. (1979) Twelve misunderstandings of kin selection. Z. Tierphysiol. **51**, 184

Dawkins R. (1982) *The Extended Phenotype* (Oxford Univ., Oxford)

Degens E.T., Berendt M., Gotthardt B. and Reppmann E. (1968) Metabolic fractionation of carbon isotopes in marine plankton. Deep-Sea Res. **15**, 11

Degens E.T., Kempe S. and Spitzy A. (1984) Carbon Dioxide: a Biological Portrait. In: Hutziger O. (Ed.) *The Handbook of Environmental Chemistry* (vol. 1, part C) (Springer, Berlin)

De Salle R., Freedman T., Prager E.M. and Wilson A.C. (1987) Tempo and mode of sequence evolution in mitochondrial DNA of Hawaiian Drosophila. J. Mol. Evol. **26**, 157

De Voogs C.G.N. (1979) Primary production in aquatic environments. In: B. Bolin, E.T. Degens, S. Kempe and P. Ketner (Eds.) *The Global Carbon Cycle* (Wiley, New York), 259

Diamond J.M. (1991) Borrowed sexual ornaments. Nature **349**, 105

Dickinson R.E. and Cicerone R.J. (1986) Future global warming from atmospheric trace gases. Nature **319**, 109

Dobzhansky T. (1951) *Genetics and the Origin of Species* 3nd ed. Columbia Univ., New York)

Dogel V.A. (1975) *Zoology of Invertebrates* (Wisshaja Shkola, Moscow) (Russian)

Dolgikh V.O. (1962) Density of populations of the Sibirian aboriginal peoples. Material Presented at the 1st Internat. Conference on the Geography of Population, Moscow, (5), 52 (Russian)

Dolnik V.R. (1975) *Migrations State of Birds* (Nauka, Moscow) (Russian)

Dolnik V.R. (Ed.) (1982) *Population Ecology of the Chaffinch (Fringilla coelebs)* (Nauka, Leningrad) (Russian)

Doolittle W.F. (1981) Is nature really Motherly? CoEvolution Quarterly **29**, 58

Doolittle W.F. and Sapienza C. (1980) Selfish genes, the phenotype paradigm and genome evolution. Nature **284**, 601

Donis-Keller H., Green P., Helms C. et al. (1987) A genetic linkage map of the human genome. Cell **51**, 319

Donnis-Keller H., Guyer M., Cann H. et al. (1992) A comprehensive genetic linkage map of the human genome. Science **258**, 67

Dover G.A. (1987) DNA turnover and molecular clock. J. Mol. Evol. **26**, 47

Dover G.A. (1988) rDNA world falling to pieces. Nature **336**, 623

Drake J.W. (1969) Comparative rates of spontaneous mutation. Nature **221**, 1132

Drake J.W. (1974) The role of mutation in bacteria evolution. Symp. Soc. Gen. Microbiol. **24**, 41

Drake J.W., Allen E.F., Forsberg S.A., Preparata R.-A. and Greening E.O. (1969) Spontaneous mutation. Nature **221**, 1128

Druffel E.R.M. and Benavides L.M. (1986) Input of excess CO_2 to surface ocean based on $^{13}C/^{12}C$ ratios in a banded Jamaican sclerosponge. Nature **321**, 58

Druffel E.R.M. and Suess H.E. (1983) On the radiocarbon record in banded corals: Exchange parameters and net transport of $^{14}CO_2$ between atmosphere and surface ocean. J. Geophys. Res. **88**, 1271

Druffel E.R.M. and Williams P.M. (1990) Identification of a deep marine source of particulate organic carbon using bomb ^{14}C. Nature **347**, 172

Druffel E.R.M., Williams P.M. and Suzuki Y. (1989) Concentrations and radiocarbon signatures of dissolved organic matter in the Pacific ocean. Geophys. Res. Lett. **15**, 991

Dugdale R.C. and Goering J.J. (1967) Uptake of new and regenerated forms of nitrogen in primary productivity. Limnol. Oceanogr. **12**, 196

Dunbrack R.L. (1989) Answer to Kirkpatrick and Jenkins. Nature **342**, 232

Duvigneaud P. (1974) *La Synthese Ecologue* (Doin, Paris)

Eckman J.P. and Ruelle D. (1985) Ergodic theory of chaos and strange attractor. Rev. Mod. Phys. **57**, 617

Edelman G.M. (1990) *The Remembered Present: A Biological Theory of Consciousness* (Basic Books)

Ehrhardt J.P. and Seguin G. (1978) *Le plancton, composition, ecologie, pollution* (Borgas, Paris)

Eigen M. (1971) *Selforganization of Matter and the Evolution of Biological Macromolecules* (Springer, Berlin)

Eisenberg J. (1981) *The Mammalian Radiations: an Analysis of Trends in Evolution, Adaptation and Behavior* (Athlone Press, London)

Elinek Ja. (1982) *Big Illustrated Atlas of Primitive Man* (Artija, Praha) (Russian)

Emlen S.T. and Oring L.W. (1977) Ecology, sexual selection, and the evolution of mating systems. Science **197**, 215

Eppley R.W. and Peterson B.J. (1979) Particulate organic matter flux and planktonic new production in the deep ocean. Nature **282**, 677

Erlich P.R. and Holm R.W. (1963) *The Process of Evolution* (McGraw-Hill Book Co, New York)

Erlich P.R. and Raven P.H. (1969) Differentiation of populations. Science **165**, 1228

Etcheto J., Boutin J. and Merlivat L. (1991) Seasonal variation of the CO_2 exchange coefficient over the global ocean using satellite wind speed measurements. Tellus **43B**, 247

Falkowski P.G. and Wilson C. (1992) Phytoplankton productivity in the North Pacific Ocean since 1900 and implications for absorption of anthropogenic CO_2. Nature **358**, 741

Falkowski P.G. and Woodhead A.D. (Eds.) (1992) *Primary Productivity and Biogeochemical Cycles in the Sea* (Plenum, New York)

Farrar J.F. (1976) The Lichen as an Ecosystem: Observation and Experiment. In: Brown D.H., Hawksworth D.L. and Bayley R.H. (Eds.) *Lichenology: Progress and Problems* (Academic, New York), 385

Fincham J.R.S. (1966) *Genetic Complementation* (Benjamin, New York)

Finegan B. (1984) Forest succession. Nature **312**, 103

Finnegan D.J. (1989) Eucariotic transposable elements and genome evolution. TIG **5**, 103

Fischbach G.D. (1992) Mind and brain. Sci. Am. **267**, 48

Fisher R.A. (1930) *The Genetical Theory of Natural Selection* (Clarendon Press, Oxford)

Fisher R.A. (1958) Polymorphism and natural selection. J. Animal Ecol. **46**, 289

Fogg G.E. (1975) Biochemical pathways in unicellular plants. In: Cooper J.P. (Ed.) *Photosynthesis and Productivity in Different Environments* (Cambridge Univ., Cambridge)

Foley R. (1987) *Another Unique Species. Pattern in Human Evolutionary Ecology* (Longman Group UK Limited, London)

Foote S., Vollrath D., Hilton A. and Page D.C. (1992) The human Y chromosome: overlapping DNA clones spanning the euchromatic region. Science **258**, 60

Foster T.J. (1983) Plasmid-determined resistance to antimicrobial drugs and toxic metal ions in bacteria. Microbiol. Rev. **47**, 361

Freed L.A. (1987) Prospective infanticide and protection of genetic paternity in tropical house wren. Amer. Natur. **130**, 948

Friedli H., Lotscher H., Oeschger H., Siegenthaler U. and Stauffer B. (1986) Ice core record of the $^{13}C/^{12}C$ ratio in atmospheric CO_2 in the past two centuries. Nature **324**, 237

Frisch K. (1977) *(Aus dem Leben der Bienen* (Springer, Berlin)

Frosch R.A. and Gallopoulos N.E. (1989) Strategies for manufacturing. Sci. Am. **261**, 144

Gammon R.H., Komhyr W.D. and Peterson J.T. (1986) The global atmospheric CO_2 distribution 1968-1983: Interpretation of the results of the NOAA/GMCC measurement program. In: Trabalka J.R. and D.F. Reichle (Eds.) *The changing carbon cycle. A global analysis* (Springer, Berlin)

Garland T. (1983) The relation between maximal running speed and body mass in terrestrial mammals. J. Zool. London **199**, 157

Gell-Mann M. and Low F.F. (1954) Quantum electrodynamics at small distances. Phys. Rev. **95**, 1300

Gershon E.S. and Rieder R.O. (1992) Major disorders of mind and brain. Sci. Am. **267**, 126

Geschwind N. (1979) Specializations of the human brain. Sci. Am. **241**, 158

Gessaman J.A. (Ed.) (1973) *Ecological Energetics of Homeotherms* (Utah State Univ., Logan Utah)

Gibbons J.H., Blair P.D. and Gwin H.L. (1989) Strategies for energy use. Sci. Am. **261**, 136

Giller P.S. (1984) *Community Structure and the Niche* (Chapman and Hall, London)

Ginsburg V.L. (1980) *About Physics and Astrophysics* (Nauka, Moscow) (Russian)

Gleckman P., Krebs H., O'Gallagher J., Sagie D. and Winston R. (1990) Sunlight brighter than the Sun. Nature **246**, 802

Gojobori T. and Yokoyama S. (1987) Molecular evolutionary rates of oncogenes. J. Mol. Evol. **26**, 148

Gojobori T., Moriuama E.N. and Kimura M. (1990) Molecular clock of viral evolution, and the neutral theory. Proc. Natl. Acad. Sci. USA **87**, 10015

Goldanskii V.I., Kuz'min V.V. (1989) Spontaneous mirror symmetry breaking in nature and origin of life. Uspekhi Fizicheskikh Nauk, **157**, 3 (Russian) [English Transl.: Sov. Phys. Usp. **32**, 1]

Goldman-Rakic P.S. (1992) Working memory and the mind. Sci. Am. **267**, 110

Golenberg E.M., Giannasi D.E., Clegg M.T. et al., (1990) Chloroplast DNA sequence from a miocene *Magnolia* species. Nature **344**, 656

Golley F.B. (1973) Impact of small mammals on primary production. In: Gessaman J.A. (Ed.) *Ecological Energetics of Homeotherms* (Utah State Univ., Logan Utah), 142

Gorshkov V.G. (1979) On the role of the terrestrial and marine biota in the global carbon budget. Preprint (534) (Leningrad Nuclear Physics Inst., Leningrad)

Gorshkov V.G. (1980a) Energetic fluxes in the biosphere and their consumption by man. Proceeding of All-Union Geograph. Society **112**, 411 (Russian)

Gorshkov V.G. (1980b) Structure of biospheric energy flows. Botanishe J. **65**, 1579 (Russian)

Gorshkov V.G. (1981) The distribution of energy flows among the organisms of different dimensions. J. General Biology **42**, 417 (Russian)

Gorshkov V.G. (1982a) *Energetics of the Biosphere* (Leningrad Polytechnical Inst., Leningrad) (Russian)

Gorshkov V.G. (1982b) Energetics of moving animals. Ecologija, (1), 1 (Russian). [English transl.: Sov. J. Ecol.].

Gorshkov V.G. (1982c) The possible global budget of carbon dioxide. Nuovo Cimento **5C**, 209

Gorshkov V.G. (1983a) The influence of the oceanic biota on atmospheric carbon dioxide. Preprint (831) (Leningrad Nuclear Physics Inst., Leningrad)

Gorshkov V.G. (1983b) Power and rate of locomotion in animals of different sizes. J. General Biology **44**, 661 (Russian)

Gorshkov V.G. (1984a) Possible role of the oceanic biota on the global carbon cycle. Oceanologija **24**, 453 (Russian) [English translation: Oceanology]

Gorshkov V.G. (1984b) *Ecology of Man* (Leningrad Polytechnical Inst., Leningrad) (Russian)

Gorshkov V.G. (1984c) Energetical efficiency of flight and swimming. J. General Biology **45**, 779 (Russian)

Gorshkov V.G. (1985a) Stability of the biogeochemical matter cycle. Ecologija (2), 3 (Russian) [English transl.: Sov. J. Ecol.]

Gorshkov V.G. (1985b) Natural selection of communities and the stability of biogeochemical cycles. In: Mlikovsky J. and V.J.A. Novak (Eds.) *Evolution and Morphogenesis* (Academia, Praha) 787

Gorshkov V.G. (1986a) Biological and physical adjustment of matter cycles. Proceedings of All-Union Geograph. Society **118**, 20 (Russian)

Gorshkov V.G. (1986b) Atmospheric disturbance of the carbon cycle: impact upon the biosphere. Nuovo Cimento **9C**, 937

Gorshkov V.G. (1987a) Variations in the global content of organic carbon in the oceanic and land biota. Nuovo Cimento **10C**, 365

Gorshkov V.G. (1987b) Biosphere and environment: stability limits. Preprint (1336) (Leningrad Nuclear Physics Inst., Leningrad) (Russian). The same in English 1988

Gorshkov V.G. (1989) Stability and evolution of biological species and communities in the biosphere. Preprint (1505), (Leningrad Nuclear Physics Inst., Leningrad)

Gorshkov V.G. (1990) Stability and evolution of biological species and communities of the biosphere. Doklady (Proceedings) of Acad. Sci. USSR **311**, 1512 (Russian)

Gorshkov V.G. (1991a) Ecological and economical cost of virgin nature. Doklady (Proceedings) of Acad. Sci. USSR **318**, 1507 (Russian)

Gorshkov V.G. (1991b) Modern production of dissolved organic carbon in the ocean is about 10 times larger than its preindustrial value. Doklady (Proceedings) of Acad. Sci. USSR **320**, 492 (Russian)

Gorshkov V.G. (1991c) Ecological stability and local adaptation: the admissible limits of anthropogenic perturbation. Preprint (1701) (Leningrad Nuclear Physics Inst., Leningrad) Ecological stability and local adaptation. J. All-Union Chemical Society **36**, 313 (Russian)

Gorshkov V.G. (1991d) Local adaptation and evolution. 3-rd Congress of E.S.E.B. Abstracts. Debrecen, Hungary, 294

Gorshkov V.G. (1991e) Evolution of procariotes and eucariotes. 3-rd Congress of E.S.E.B. Abstracts. Debrecen, Hungary, 152

Gorshkov V.G. (1992a) "Vanished" carbon in the present-day global cycle. Doklady (Proceedings) of Acad. Sci. Russia **322**, 1177 (Russian)

Gorshkov V.G. (1992b) Ecological stability: admissible limits of anthropogenic perturbations. Proceedings of All-Union Geograph. Society, **124**, 399 (Russian)

Gorshkov V.G. (1992c) Ecological stability: local adaptation and evolution. Proceedings of All-Union Geograph. Society, **124**, 498 (Russian)

Gorshkov V.G. (1993a) Rate of DOC accumulation in ocean increase forty times during industrial era. Paper presented to 4th Internat. Conf. CO_2, Carqueiranne, France, 13-17 Sept., 1993, 98

Gorshkov V.G. (1993b) Global carbon cycle change: uncertainty of conclusion about biomass changes based on ^{13}C data. Doklady (Proceedings) of Acad. Sci. Russia **331**, 641 (Russian)

Gorshkov V.G. (1993c) Modern global environmental change and possibility of its suppression. Doklady (Proceedings) of Acad. Sci. Russia **332**, 802 (Russian)

Gorshkov V.G. and Dolnik V.R. (1980) Energetics of the biosphere. Uspekhi Fizicheskikh Nauk **131**, 441 [English transl.: Sov. Phys. Usp. **23**, 386, American Institute of Physics]

Gorshkov V.V. and Gorshkov V.G. (1992) Recovery characteristics for ecosystems. Preprint (1850) (Petersburg Nuclear Physics Inst., St.Petersburg)

Gorshkov V.G. and Kondratiev K.Ya. (1990) Conceptual aspects of ecological studies: the role of energy- and mass-exchange. Geofisika International **29**, 61

Gorshkov V.G. and Sherman S.G. (1986) Atmospheric CO_2 and destructivity of the land biota: Seasonal variation. Nuovo Cimento **9C**, 902

Gorshkov V.G. and Sherman S.G. (1990) Stability of biological species and sexual dimorphism. Preprint (1610) (Leningrad Nuclear Physics Inst., Leningrad) (Russian). The same in English 1991

Gorshkov V.G. and Sherman S.G. (1991) Stability of species and sexual dimorphism. 3-rd Congress of E.S.E.B. Abstracts. Debrecen, Hungary, 278

Gorshkov V.G. and Sherman S.G. (1993) Absorption of atmospheric CO_2 into ocean through air-sea interface: contradiction in empirical data and their possible resolution. Paper presented to 4th Internat. Conf. CO_2, Carqueiranne, France, 13-17 Sept., 1993, 76

Gorshkov V.G., Kondratiev K.Ya. and Sherman S.G. (1989) The Le-Chatellier principle in reaction of biota to perturbation of the global carbon cycle. Extended Abstracts of Papers at the Third Intern. Conf. on Analysis and Evolution at Atmospheric CO_2 Data, W.M.O., Univ. Heidelberg, 110

Gorshkov V.G., Kondratiev K.Ya. and Sherman S.G. (1990) The global carbon cycle change: Le Chatellier principle in the biota. Nuovo Cimento **13C**, 801

Gould J.L. and Marler P. (1987) Learning by instinct. Sci. Am. **256**, 62

Govindjee O. (Ed.) (1982) *Photosynthesis* (Academic, New York)

Grant P.R. (1991a) Speciation and hybridization in Darwin's finches. Plenary lecture. Proceeding of 3rd Congress of E.S.E.B. Debrecen, Hungary

Grant P.R. (1991b) Natural selection and Darvin's finches. Sci. Am. **265**, 60

Grant V. (1977) *Organismic Evolution* (Freeman Co, San Francisco)

Green N.P.O., Stout G.W., Taylor D.J. and Soper R. (1989) *Biological Science* (Cambridge Univ., Cambridge)

Greenwood J.J.D. (1990) Changing migration behaviour. Nature **345**, 209

Grosjean H., Cedergren R.J. and Mc Kay W. (1982) Structure in tRNA data. Biochimie **64**, 387

Gustavson M.R. (1979) Limits to wind power utilization. Science **204**, 13

Hafele W., Barnert H., Messner S., Strubegger M. and Anderer J. (1986) Novel integrated energy systems: the case of zero emission. In: Clark W.C. and R.E.Munn (Eds.) *Sustainable Development Biosphere* (Cambridge Univ., Cambridge)

Haken H. (1982) *Synergetics* (Springer, Berlin)

Haken H. (1984) *Advanced Synergetics* (Springer, Berlin)

Haldane J.B.S. (1954) Measurement of natural selection. Proc. 9th Int. Congress Genet., 480

Haldane J.B.S. (1957) The cost of natural selection. J. Genet. **55**, 511

Hamilton W.D. (1964) The genetical evolution of sexual behaviour. J. Theoret. Biol. **7**, 1

Hamilton W.D., Axelrod R. and Tanese R. (1990) Sexual reproduction as an adaptation to resist parasites: a review. Proc. Natl. Acad. Sci. **87**, 3566

Hansen J.E. and Lacis A.A. (1990) Sun and dust versus greenhouse gases: an assessment of their relative roles in global climate change. Nature **346**, 713

Harestad A.S. and Bunnell F.L. (1979) Home range and body weight – a reevaluation. Ecology **60**, 389

Harlan J.R. (1976) The plants and animals that nourish man. Sci. Am. **235**, 88

Harvey J.G. (1976) *Atmosphere and Ocean* (Artemis Press, Wisbech)

Harvey P.H. (1985) Intra-demic selection and the sex ratio. In: Sibley R.M. and R.H.Smith (Eds.) *Behavioural Ecology: Ecological Consequences of Adaptive Behaviour* (Blackwell, Oxford), 59

Hedfick P.W. and Whittam T.S 1989: Sex in diploids. Nature **342** (16 Nov.), 231

Heglund N.C., Cavagna G.A., Fedak M.A. and Taylor C.R. (1979) Muscle efficiency during locomotion: how does it vary with body size and speed? (Museum of Comp. Zool. Harvard Univ. Cambridge) MA 02138 and Univ. of Milan (FASEB Abstract speed)

Hemmingsen A.M. (1960) Energy metabolism as related to body size and respiratory surfaces, its evolution. Rept. Steno Mem. Hosp. Nord. Insulin Lab. **9**, 7

Henderson-Sellers A. and Cogley J.G. (1982) The Earth's early hydrosphere. Nature **298**, 832

Hesin R.V. (1984) *Nonconstancy of Genom* (Nauka, Moscow) (Russian)

Hill A.V. (1960) Production and absorption of work by muscle. Science **131**, 897

Hinde R.A. (1970) *Animal Behaviour* (Univ. Cambridge, New York)

Hitchcock D.R. and Lovelock J.E. (1966) Life detection by atmospheric analysis. Icarus 7, 149

Ho M.-W. and Saunders R.T. (1984) *Beyond Neo-Darwinism* (Academic, New York)

Hochachka P.W. and Somero G.H. (1973) *Strategies of Biochemical Adaptation* (Saunders Co, Philadelphia)

Hodgkin J. (1990) Sex determination compared in Drosophila and Caenornabditis. Nature 344, 721

Hoffman A. (1991) Testing the Red Queen hypothesis. J. Evol. Biol. 4, 1

Hofker M.H., Skraastad M.I., Bergen A.A.B. et al. (1986) The X chromosome shows less genetic variation at restriction sites than the autosomes. Am. J. Hum. Genet. 39, 438

Hofshi H., Gersani M. and Katzir G. (1987) A case of infanticide among Fvistram's Grackles, *Onychognathus tvistramii*. Ibis 129, 389

Holing K. (Ed.) (1978) *Adaptive Environmental* (Chichester, London)

Holland H.D. (1984) *The Chemical Evolution of the Atmosphere and Oceans* (Princeton Univ., New York)

Holland H.D., Lazar B. and Mc Caffrey M. (1986) Evolution of the atmosphere and oceans. Nature 320, 27

Holland J., Spinder K. and Horodyski F. et al. (1982) Rapid evolution of RNA genomes. Science 215, 1577

Holligan P.M. and de Boois H. (Eds.) (1993) Land-Ocean Interactions in the Coastal Zone. Global Change (IGBP report No.25, Stockholm)

Holling C.S. (1986) The resilience of terrestrial ecosystems: local surprise and global change. In: Clark W.C. and R.E.Munn (Eds.) *Sustainable Development of Biosphere* (Cambridge Univ., Cambridge), 292

Horn H.S. (1975) Forest succession. Sci. Am. 232, 90

Houghton R.A. (1989) The long-term flux of carbon to the atmosphere from changes in land use. Extended Abstracts of Papers Presented at the Third Internat. Conf. on Analysis and Evolution of Atmospheric CO_2 Data. W.M.O. Univ. Heidelberg, 80

Houghton R.A., Hobbie J.E., Melillo J.M. et al. (1983) Changes in the content of terrestrial biota and soils between 1860 and 1980: a net release of CO_2 to the atmosphere. Ecological Monographs 53, 235

Houghton R.A., Boone R.D., Fruci J.R. et al. (1987) The flux of carbon from terrestrial ecosystems to the atmosphere in 1980 due to changes in land use: geographic distribution of the global flux. Tellus 39B, 122

Hubbert M.K. (1971) The energy resources of the Earth. Sci. Am. 225, 61

Hubel D.H. (1979) The brain. Sci. Am. 241, 39

Hutchinson G.E. and MacArthur R.H. (1959) A theoretical ecological model of size distributions among species of animals. Am. Natur. 43, 117

Isaev A.S., Khlebopros R.G., Nedoresov L.V., Kondakov Ju.P. and Kiselev V.V. (1984) *Population Dynamics of the Forest Insects* (SO Nauka, Novosibirsk) (Russian)

Ivanoff A. (1972), (1975) *Introduction a L'Océanigraphie* (Tome 1, 2) (Librarie Vuibert, Paris)

Janick J., Noller C.H. and Rhykerd C.L. (1976) The cycles of plant and animal nutrition. Sci. Am. 235, 74

Jaworowski Z., Sedalstad T.V. and Ono N. (1992) Do glaciers tell a true atmospheric CO_2 story? The Science of the Total Environment 114, 227

Johanson D.C. and Edey M.A. (1981) *Lucy. The Beginning of Humankind* (Warner Books. A Warner Communication Co, New York)

Jones D. (1990) Time twisters. Nature 347, 130

Jones D.H., Sakamoto K., Vorce R.L. and Howard B.H. (1990) DNA mutagenesis and recombination. Nature 344, 793

Joos F. and Siegenthaler U. (1989) Study of the oceanic uptake of anthropogenic CO_2 and ^{14}C using a high-latitude exchange/interior diffusion-advection (HILDA) model.

Extended Abstracts of Papers Presented at the Third Internat. Conf. on Analysis and Evolution of Atmospheric CO_2 Data. W.M.O., Univ. Heidelberg, 203

Jukes T.H. (1987) Transversions and molecular evolutionary clock. J. Mol. Evol. **26**, 87

Kaiser F. (1990) Nonlinear dynamics and deterministic chaos, their relevance for biological function and behaviour. In: Tomassen G.J.M. et al. (Eds.) *Geo-cosmic Relations, the Earth and its Macro-environment* (Pudoc, Wageningen), 315

Kamenir Yu.G. (1991) Comparison of size spectra of living matter of three aquatic ecosystems. Synt. Anal. Model. Stimul. **8**, 72

Kamenir Yu.G. and Khailov K.M. (1987) The metabolism parameters and the world oceanic living matter integral spectra: comparison of size spectra. Oceanologia **27**, 656 (Russian)

Kandel E.R. and Hawkins R.D. (1992) The biological basis of learning and individuality. Sci. Am. **267**, 78

Kanwisher J.W. and Ridgway S.H. (1983) The physiological ecology of whales and porpoises. Sci. Am. **248**, 110

Kasinov V.B. (1968) On the inheritance of the left- and right-handedness in*Lemnaceae*. Genetika **4**, 11 (Russian)

Kauffman S.A. (1991) Antichaos and adaptation. Sci. Am. **265**, 64

Kawai M. (1965) Newly acquired pre-cultural behaviour of natural troops of Japanese monkeys on Koshima Islet. Primates **6**, 1

Keeling C.D. (1973) The carbon dioxide cycle. In: Rasool S. (Ed.) *Chemistry of the Lower Atmosphere* (Plenum Press, New York), 251

Keeling R.F. and Shertz R. (1992) Seasonal and interannual variations in atmospheric oxygen and implications for the global carbon cycle. Nature **358**, 723

Keith L.B. (1963) *Wildlife's Ten-Year Cycle* (Univ. Wisconsin, Madison)

Kellogg W.W. and Schneider S.H. (1974) Climate stabilization: for better of for worse? Science **186**, 1163

Kemp W.B. (1971) The flow of energy in a hunting society. Sci. Am. **224**, 105

Kendeigh S.C. (1974) *Ecology with Special References to Animals and Man* (Englewood Cliffs. Prentice-Hall, New York)

Kendeigh S.C., Dolnik V.R. and Gavrilov V.M. (1977) Avian energetics. In: Pinanski J. and S.C.Kendeigh (Eds.) *Graniverous Birds in Ecosystems* International Biological Program, **12** (Cambridge Univ., Cambridge), 127

Kerr R.A. (1992) SETI faces uncertainty on Earth and in the Stars. Science **258**, 27

Keyfitz N. (1989) The growing human population. Sci. Am. **261**, 118

Khailov K.M. (1971) *Ecological Metabolism in the Sea* (Naukova Dumka, Kiev) (Russian)

Kimura M. (1964) Diffusion models in population genetics. J. Appl. Probab. (1), 177

Kimura M. (1968) Evolutionary rate at the molecular level. Nature **217**, 624

Kimura M. (1983) *The Neutral Theory of Molecular Evolution* (Cambridge Univ., Cambridge)

Kimura M. (1987) Molecular evolutionary clock and neutral theory. J. Mol. Evol. **26**, 24

Kimura M. (1989) The neutral theory of molecular evolution and the world view of neutralists. Genome **31**, 24

Kimura M. and Crow J.F. (1963) The measurement of effective population number. Evol. **17**, 279

Kimura M. and Maruyama T. (1966) The mutational load with epistatic gene interactions in fitness. Genetics **5**, 1337

Kimura M. and Ohta T. (1974) On some principle governing molecular evolution. Proc. Natl. Acad. Sci. USA **71**, 2848

King J.L. and Jukes T.H. (1969) Non-Darwinian evolution. Science **164**, 788

King T. (1974) Seasonal allocation of time and energy resources in birds. In: Paunter R.A. (Ed.) *Avian Energetics* (Publ. Nuttul Ornitholog. Club, Cambridge), (15), 4

Kirchner J.W. (1989) The Gaia hypothesis: can it be tested? Rev. of Geophysics **27**, 223

Kirkpatrick M. and Jenkins C.D. (1989) Genetic segregation and the maintenance of sexual reproduction. Nature **339**, 300

Kisel W.A. (1980) Optical activity and the dissymmetry of biological systems. Yspekhi Fizicheskikh Nauk **131**, 209 (Russian). [English transl.: Sov. Phys. Usp. **23**, (6)]

Kisel W.A. (1985) *Physical causes of dissymmetry of living systems* (Nauka, Moskow) (Russian)

Kleiber M. (1961) *The Fire of Life* (Wiley, New York)

Knox F. and McElroy M.B. (1984) Changes in atmospheric CO_2: Influence of the marine biota at high latitudes. J. Geophys. Res. **89**, 1405

Kohlmaier G.H., Brohl H., Size E.O., Plochl M. and Ravelle R. (1987) Modelling stimulation of plants and ecosystem response to present levels of excess atmospheric CO_2. Tellus **39B**, 155

Kondrashov A.S. (1982) Selection against harmful mutations in large sexual and asexual populations. Genet. Res. Camb. **40**, 325

Kondrashov A.S. (1988) Deleterious mutations and the evolution of sexual reproduction. Nature **336**, 435

Kondrashov A.S. (1992) Species and speciation, Nature **356**, 752

Kondrashov A.S. and Crow J.F. (1991) Haploidy or diploidy: Which is better? Nature **351**, 314

Kordum V.A. (1982) *Evolution and Biosphere* (Naukova Dumka, Kiev) (Russian)

Kump L.R. (1989) Chemical stability of the atmosphere and ocean. Paleogeography, Paleoclimatology, Paleogeology (Global and Planetary Change Section) **75**, 123

Landau L.D. and Lifshitz E.M. (1964) *Theoretical Physics* (Statistical Physics, vol 5) (Nauka, Moscow) (Russian)

Larcher V. (1976) *Ökologie der Pflanzen* (Verlag Eugen Ulmer, Stutgart)

Lehman S.J. and Keigwin L.D. (1992) Sudden changes in North Atlantic ejaculation during the last deglaciation. Nature **356**, 757

Lehninger A. (1982) *Principles of Biochemistry* (Worths Publishers Inc., New York)

Leuenberger M., Siegenthaler U. and Langway C.C. (1992) Carbon isotope composition of atmospheric CO_2 during the last ice age from Antarctic ice core. Nature **357**, 488

Levitus S. (1982) *Climatological Atlas of the World Ocean* NOAA Professional Paper,**13**, Geophysical Fluid Dynamics Lab., (Princeton, New Jersey)

Levitz V.G. (1962) *Handbook of Theoretical Physics* (vol. 1) (Gos. Isd. Phys. Math. Lit., Moscow) (Russian)

Lewin B. (1983) *Genes* (Wiley, New York)

Lewis M.P., Harrison W.G., Oakey N.S., Hebert D. and Platt T. (1986) Vertical nitrate fluxes in the oligotrophic ocean. Science **234**, 870

Lewontin R.C. (1974) *The Genetic Basis of Evolutionary Change* (Columbia Univ., New York)

Lima-de-Faria A. (1988) *Evolution without Selection. Form and Function by Autoevolution* (Elsevier, Amsterdam)

Lisovskii G.M. (Ed.) (1979) *Closed System: Man–Higher Plants* (Nauka, Novosibirsk) (Russian)

Lively C.M., Craddock C. and Vrijenhoek R.C. (1990) Red Queen hypothesis supported by parasitism in sexual and clonal fish. Nature **344**, 864

Livesey P.J. (1986) *Learning and Emotion: A Biological Synthesis* (Evolutionary Processes, vol. 1) (Lawrence Erlbaum)

Loeb L.A. and Kunkel T.A. (1982) Fidelity of DNA synthesis. Ann. Rev. Biochem. **52**, 429

Lorenz K.Z. (1981) *The Foundation of Ethology* (Springer, Berlin)

Lorius C., Jouzel J., Raynaud D., Hansen J. and Le Treut H. (1990) The ice-core record: climate sensitivity and future greenhouse warming. Nature **347**, 139

Lotka A.J. (1925) *Elements of Physical Biology* (Williams Wilking Co., Baltimore)

Lovejoy C.O. (1981) The origin of man. Science **211**, 341

Lovejoy C.O. (1988) Evolution of human walking. Sci. Am. **259**, 82

Lovelock J.E. (1972) *Gaia as Seen through the Atmosphere* Atmospheric Environment, **6**, (Pergamon Press, New York) 579

Lovelock J.E. (1982) *Gaia. A New Look at Life on Earth* (Oxford Univ., New York)

Lovelock J.E. (1986) Geophysiology: a new look at Earth science. Bulletin Am. Meteorol. Soc. **67**, 392

Lovelock J.E. (1988) *The Ages of Gaia. A Biography of our Living Earth* (Oxford Univ., New York)

Lovelock J.E. (1989) Geophysiology, the science of Gaia. Rev. Geophysics **27**, 215

Lovelock J.E. and Margulis L. (1973) Atmospheric homeostasis by and for the biosphere: The Gaia hypothesis. Tellus **26**, 1

Lovins A.B., Lovins L.H., Krause F. and Bach W. (1981) *Cost Energy Solving the CO_2 Problem* (Brick House Pub. Co, Andover Massachusetts)

Lvovitsh M.I. (1974) *World Water Resources and their Future* (Misl, Moscow) (Russian)

MacFadden B.J. and Hubbert R.C.Jr. (1988) Explosive speciation at the base of the adaptive radiation of Miocene grazing horses. Nature **336**, 466

MacNeill J. (1989) Strategies for sustainable economic development. Sci. Am. **261**, 154

Maier-Reimer E. and Hasselmann K. (1987) Transport and storage of CO_2 in the ocean – an inorganic ocean – circulation carbon cycle model. Climate Dynamics **2**, 63

Maksudov G.Ju., Artinshkova V.A. and Troshko E.V. (1988) *Estimation of animal's sperm quality. Conservation of genetical resources* (Puschino Inst. of Biophysics, Puschino) (Russian)

Malingreau J.P. and Tucker C.J. (1988) Southern Amazon based deforestation monitoring using satellite data slide sets. Ambio **17**, 49

Mandel J.-L., Monaco A.P., Nelson D.L., Schlessinger D. and Willard H. (1992) Genome analysis and the human X chromosome. Science **258**, 103

Mandelbrot B.B. (1982) *The Fractal Geometry of Nature* (Freeman, San Francisco)

Manning A. (1979) *An introduction to animal behaviour* (Edward Arnold Ltd, New York)

Margulis L. (1971) Symbiosis and evolution. Sci. Am. **225**, 48

Margulis L. (1975) Symbiosis in cell evolution life and its environment on the yearly Earth. In: Jennigs D.H. and D.L. Lee (Eds.) *Symbiosis* (Cambridge Univ., Cambridge) 21

Marland G. and Rotty R. (1984) Carbon dioxide emission from fossil fuels: a procedure for estimating and results for 1950–1982, Tellus **36B**, 232

Marland G., Boden T.A., Griffin R.C., Huand S.F., Kanciruk P. and Nelson (1988) Estimates of CO_2 emission from fossil fuel burning and cement manufacturing using the United Nations energy statistics and the U.S.Bureau of Mines cement manufacturing data NDPO30, Carbon Dioxide Information Analysis Center, Oak Ridge National Laboratory. Tennessee, Oak Ridge

Martin J.H. and Fitzwater S.E. (1992) Dissolved organic carbon in Atlantic, Southern and Pacific oceans. Nature **256**, 699

Martin J.P. and Fridovich I. (1981) Evidence for a natural gene transfer from the ponyfish to its bioluminiscent bacterial symbiont *Photobacter beioguanthi* J. Biol. Chemistry **256**, 6080

May R.M. (1990) How many species? Phyl. Trans. Roy. Soc. London **330B**, 293

May R.M. (1992) How many species inhabit the Earth? Sci. Am. **267**, 18

Maynard Smith J. (1964) Group selection and kin selection. Nature **201**, 1145

Maynard Smith J. (1974) *Models in Ecology* (Cambridge Univ., Cambridge)

Maynard Smith J. (1978) *The Evolution of Sex* (Cambridge Univ., Cambridge)

Maynard Smith J. (1991) Recipe for bad science? Nature **352**, 206

Mayr E. (1963) *Animal Species and Evolution* (Harvard Univ., Cambridge Mass.)

McElroy M.B. (1986) Change in the natural environment of the Earth: the historical record. In: Clark W.C. and R.E. Munn (Eds.) *Sustainable Development of the Biosphere* (Cambridge Univ., Cambridge)

McFarland D. (1985) *Animal Behaviour. Psychology, Ethology and Evolution* (Pitman, Oxford Univ.Press, London), 106

McNab B.K. (1983) Energetics, body size, and the limits to endothermy. J. Zool. London **199**, 1

McNeill S. and Lawton J.H. (1970) Annual production and respiration in animal populations. Nature **225**, 472

Meadows D.H., Meadows D.L., Randers J. and Behrens W.W.III (1972) *The Limits to Growth* (Potomac, New York)

Meadows D.H., Meadows D.L. and Randers J. (1992) *Beyond the Limits* (Chelsea Green Publ. Co, Post Milles Vermont)

Meadows D.L., Behrens W.W.III, Meadows D.H., Naill R.F., Randers J. and Zahn E.K.O. (1974) *Dynamics of Growth in a Finite World* (Wright Allen Press, New York)

Mesarovic M. and Pestel E. (1974) *Mankind at the Turning Point* (Dutton, New York)

Mettler L.E. and Gregg T. (1969) *Population Genetics and Evolution* (Prentice Hall, New Jersey)

Michod R.E. and Hamilton W.D. (1980) Coefficients of relatedness in sociobiology. Nature **288**, 694

Michod R.E. and Lewin B.R. (1988) *The Evolution of Sex: An Examination of Current Ideas* (Sinauer, Sunderland)

Mitchell J. (1989) The "greenhouse" effect and climate change. Rev. Geophys. **27**, 115

Modi R.I. and Adams J. (1991) Coevolution in bacterial-plasmid populations. Evolution **45**, 656

Modrich P. (1987) DNA mismatch correlation. Ann. Rev. Biochem. **56**, 435

Moller A.P. (1990) Parasites and sexual selection: Current status of the Hamilton and Zuk hypothesis. J. Evol. Biol. **3**, 319

Moody M.E. and Baston C.J. (1990) The evolution of latent genes in subdivided populations. Genetics **124**, 187

Mopper K. and Degens E.T. (1979) Organic carbon in the ocean: nature and cycling. In: Bolin B., E.T. Degens, S. Kempe and P. Ketner (Eds.) *The Global Carbon Cycle* (Wiley, New York), 451

Morneau C. and Payette S. (1989) Postfire lichen - spruce woodland recovery at the limit of the boreal forest in northern Quebec. Can. J. Botany **67**, 2770

Morosov L.L. (1978) Spontaneous braking of mirror symmetry as aspect of biochemical evolutiton. Doklady (Proceedings) of Acad. Sci. Russia **241**, 481 (Russian)

Moses Ph.B. and Chua N.-H. (1988) Light switches for plant genes. Sci. Am. **258**, 64

Muller H.J. (1964) The relation of recombination to mutational advance. Mutation Res. **1**, 2

Murata A.M. (1993) Atmospheric pCO_2 variability over the western North Pacific in the period 1990-1992. Paper presented 4th Internat. Conf. CO_2, Carqueiranne, France, 13-17 Sept., 1993, 11

Najjar R., Sarmiento J.L. and Toggweiler J.R. (1989) Parameter sensitivity of organic matter remineralization using an ocean general circulation model. Extended Abstracts of Papers Presented at the Third Internat. Conf. on Analysis and Evolution of Atmospheric CO_2 Data. W.M.O., Univ. Heidelberg, 116

Neshyba S. (1987) *Oceanography Perspectives on a Fluid Earth* (Wiley, New York)

Newbold G. (1990) The path of drug resistance. Nature **345**, 202

Newkirk G. (1980) Solar variability of time scales of 10^5 years to $10^{9.6}$ years. In: Pepin R.O. and J.A.Eddy (Eds.) Proc. Conf. Ancient Sun USA, 293

Nicolis J.S. (1986) *Dynamics of Hierarchial Systems. An Evolutionary Approach* (Springer, Berlin)

Nicolis J.S. and Prigogine I. (1977) *Self-organization in Nonequilibrium Systems. From Dissipative Structures to Order through Fluctuations* (Wiley, New York)

North G.H., Cahalan R.F. and Cookley J.A. (1981) Energy balance climate models. Rev. Geophys. and Space Physics **19**, 91

Ochman H. and Wilson A.C. (1987) Evolution in bacteria: evidence for a universal substitution rate in cellular genomes. J. Mol. Evol. **26**, 74

Odum E.P. (1983) *Basic Ecology* (Saunders College Pub., New York)

Oeschger H. and Stauffer B. (1986) Review of the history of atmospheric CO_2 recorded in ice cores. In: Trabalka J.R. and D.F. Reichle (Eds.) *The Changing of the Carbon Cycle: A Global Analysis* (Springer, Berlin)

Oeschger H., Siegenthaler U., Schotterer U. and Gugelman A. (1975) A box diffusion model to study the carbon dioxide exchange in nature. Tellus **27**, 168

Ogawa H. and Ogura N. (1992) Comparison of two methods for measuring dissolved organic carbon in sea water. Nature **256**, 696

Ohno S. (1970) *Evolution by Gene Duplication* (Springer, Berlin)

Ohta T. (1987) Very slightly deleterious mutations and the molecular clock. J. Mol. Evol. **26**, 1

Okun L.B. (1988) *Physics of Elementary Particles* (Nauka, Moscow) (Russian)

Orgel L.E. (1992) Molecular replication. Nature **358**, 203

Orgel L.E. and Crick F.H.C. (1980) Selfish DNA: the ultimate parasite. Nature **284**, 604

Orr H.A. (1991) Is single-gene speciation possible? Evolution **45**, 764

Paladino F.V., O'Connor M.P. and Spotila J.R. (1990) Metabolism of leatherback turtles' gigantothermy, and thermoregulation of dinosaurus. Nature **344**, 858

Palmen E. and Newton C.W. (1969) *Atmospheric Circulation Systems* (Academic, New York)

Pankow W., Boller T. and Weimken A. (1991) Structure function and ecology of the mycorrhizal symbiosis. Experientia **47**, 311

Panov E.N. (Ed.) (1983) *Problems of the Ethology of the Terrestrial Vertebrates* (Zool. Vertebrates, vol. 12) (VINITI, Moscow) (Russian)

Pardé J. (1980) Forest biomass. Forestry Abstract Rev. Articles **41**, 343

Parker G.A. and Maynard Smith J. (1990) Optimality theory in evolutionary biology. Nature **348**, 27

Partridge L. and Harvey P. (1986) Contentious issues in sexual selection. Nature **323**, 580

Paune R.B. and Westneat D.F. (1988) A genetic and behavioural analysis of mate choice and song neighborhoods in indigo buntings. Evolution **42**, 935

Peixoto J.P. and Oort A.H. (1984) Physics of climate. Rev. Modern Phys. **56**, 365

Peng C.-K., Buldyrev S.V., Goldberger A.L., Halvin S., Sciortino F., Simons M. and Stanley H.E. (1992) Long-range correlation in nucleotide sequences. Nature **256**, 168

Peng T.-H., Takahachi T., Broecker W.S. and Olafsson J. (1987) Seasonal variability of carbon dioxide, nutrients and oxygen in the northern North Atlantic surface water: observations and a model. Tellus **39B**, 439

Penney T.R. and Bharathan D. (1987) Power from the sea. Sci. Am. **256**, 74

Peters R.H. (1983) *The Ecological Implications of Body Size* (Cambridge Univ., Cambridge)

Pianka R.H. (1970) On r- and K-selection. Am. Natur. **104**, 592

Pipkin F.M. and Ritter R.C. (1983) Precision measurements and fundamental constants. Science **219**, 913

Platt T. and Rao D.V.S. (1975) Primary production of marine microphytes. In: Cooper J.P. (Ed.) *Photosynthesis and Productivity in Different Environments* (Cambridge Univ., London), 249

Platt T., Harrison W.G., Lewis M.R. et al. (1989) Biological production of the oceans: the case for a consensus. Mar. Ecol. Prog. Ser. **52**, 77

Prentice K.C. and Fung I.Y. (1990) The sensitivity of terrestrial carbon storage to climate change. Nature **346**, 48

Prigogine I. (1978) Time, structure and fluctuations. Science **201**, 777

Prigogine I. (1980) *From Being to Becoming: Time and Complexity in Physical Science* (Freeman and Co, San Fransisco)

Prinn R.G. (1982) Origin and evolution of planetary atmospheres: an introduction to the problem. Planet. Space Sci. **30**, 741

Ptashne M. (1986), (1987) *Genetic Switch. Gene Control and Phage* λ (Cell Press and Blackwell Sci.Publ., New York)

Quay P.D., Tilbrook B. and Wong C.S. (1992) Oceanic uptake of fossil fuel CO_2: carbon-13 evidence. Science **256**, 74

Radman M. and Wagner R. (1986) Mismatch repair in Escherichia Coli. Ann. Rev. Genetics **20**, 523

Radman M. and Wagner R. (1988) The high fidelity of DNA duplication. Sci. Am. **259**, 40

Ramanathan V. (1987) The role of Earth radiation budget studies in climate and general circulation research. J. Geophys. Res. **92D**, 4075

Rapoport A. (1986) *General System Theory* (Mass Abacus Press, Cambridge)

Rappaport R.A. (1971) The flow of energy in an agriculture. Sci. Am. **224**, 117

Raval A. and Ramanathan V. (1989) Observational determination of the greenhouse effect. Nature **342**, 758

Raup D.M. and Sepkoski J.J.Jr. (1982) Mass extinction in the marine fossil fuel record. Science **215**, 1501

Raven P.H. and Johnson G.B. (1988) *Understanding Biology* (Times Mirror, Mosby Coll. Pub., St.Louis)

Raynaud D., Jouzel J., Barnola J.M., Chappellaz J., Delmas D.J. and Lorius C. (1993) The ice record of greenhouse gases. Science **259**, 926

Redfield A.C. (1958) The biological control of chemical factors in the environment. Am. Sci. **46**, 205

Redfield A.C., Ketchum B.H. and Richards P.A. (1967) The influence of organisms on the composition of sea water. In: *The Sea* (vol. 2) (Willey, New York), 26

Reid R.A. (1980) Selfish DNA in "petite" mutations. Nature **285**, 620

Rennie J. (1992) Living together. Sci. Am. **266**, 104

Revelle R. (1976) The resources available for agriculture. Sci. Am. **235**, 164

Riviere J.W.M. and Marton-Lefevre J. (1992) United Nation conference on environment and development and global change science. Global Change News Letter (11), September, 1

Robertson J.E. and Watson A.J. (1992) Thermal effect of the surface ocean and its implications for CO_2 uptake. Nature **358**, 738

Robinson A.L. (1984) Computing without dissipating energy. Science **223**, 1164

Rodin L.E., Basilevich N.I. and Rosov N.I. (1974) *Man and Environment* (Geography Soc. Press, Leningrad) (Russian)

Romme W.H. and Despein D.G. (1989) The Yellowstone Fires. Sci. Am. **261**, 37

Ronov A.B. (1976) Volcanism, carbonate accumulation, life (The regulation of the global geochemistry of carbon). Geochimia (8), 1252 (Russian)

Roosen-Runge E.C. (1962) The process of spermatogenesis in mammals. Biol. Rev. **37**, 343

Roosen-Runge E.C. (1977) *The Progress of Spermatogenesis in Animals* (Cambridge Univ., Cambridge)

Rosental I.L. (1980) Physical laws and numerical values of fundamental constants. Uspekni Fisicheskikh Nauk **131**, 239 [English transl.: Sow. Phys. Usp. **23** (2)]

Rosenzweig M.L. (1973) Evolution of predator isocline. Evolution **27**, 84

Ross K.G. (1986) Kin selection and the problem of sperm utilization in social insects. Nature **323**, 798

Rossi V. and Menozzi P. (1990) The clonal ecology. *Heterocypris inconraens (Ostracoda)*. Oikos **57**, 388

Rotty R.M. (1983) Distribution of and changes in industrial carbon dioxide production. J. Geophys. Res. **88**, 1301

Rucang W. and Shenglong Z. (1983) Peking Man. Sci. Am. **248**, 86

Ryther J.H. (1970) Is the World's oxygen supply threatened? Nature **227**, 374

Sachs L. (1972) *Statistische Auswertungmethoden* (Springer, Berlin)

Sager R. (1972) *Cytoplasmic Genes and Organelles* (Academic, New York)

Sandberg A.A. (Ed.) (1985) *The Y-chromosome* Parts A, B (Liss Press, New York)

Sarmiento J.L. and Toggweiler J.R. (1984) A new model for the role of the oceans in determining atmospheric pCO$_2$. Nature **308**, 621

Sarmiento J.L., Toggweiler J.R. and Najjar R. (1988) Ocean carbon-cycle dynamics and atmospheric pCO$_2$. Trans. R. Soc. London **A325**, 3

Sarmiento J.L., Fasham M.J.R., Siengenthaler U., Najjar R. and Toggweiler J.R. (1989) Models of chemical cycling in the oceans: progress report II. Ocean Tracers Lab. Techn. Report

Savin S. (1977) The history of the Earth's surface temperature during the past 160 million years. Ann. Rev. Earth Planetary Sci. **5**, 319

Sawby S.W. (1973) An evolution of radioisotopic methods of measuring free-living metabolism. In: Gasselman J.A. (Ed.) *Ecological Energetics of homeotherms* (Utah State Univ., Logan, Utah), 86

Schlesinger W.H. (1984) Soil organic matter: a source for atmospheric CO$_2$. In: Woodwell G.M. (Ed.) *The role of terrestrial vegetation in the global carbon cycle* (Wiley, New York), 111

Schlesinger W.H. (1986) Changes in soil carbon storage and associated properties with disturbance and recovery. In: Trabalka J.R. and D.E. Reichle (Eds.) *The Changing Carbon Cycle. A Global Analysis* (Springer, Berlin), 194

Schlesinger W.H. (1990) Evidence from chronosequence studies for a low carbon-storage potential of soils. Nature **348**, 232

Schmidt-Nielsen K. (1972) *How animals work* (Cambridge Univ., Cambridge)

Schmidt-Nielsen K. (1984) *Scaling: Why is Animal Size so Important?* (Cambridge Univ., Cambridge)

Schneider S.H. (1976) *The Genesis Strategy* (Plenum Press, New York)

Schneider S.H. (1989a) The greenhouse effect: science and policy. Science **243**, 771

Schneider S.H. (1989b) The changing climate. Sci Am. **261**, 70

Schrimshaw N.S. and Young Y.R. (1976) The requirements of human nutrition. Sci. Am. **235**, 50

Schrödinger E. (1945) *What is life? The physical aspect of the living cell* (Dublin Trinity College, Inst. for Advanced Studies, Dublin)

Schuster H.G. (1984) *Deterministic Chaos* (Physic-Verlag, Weinheim)

Schwartzman D.W. and Volk T. (1989) Biotic enhancement of weathering and habitability of Earth. Nature **340**, 457

Sedov L.I. (1959) *Similarity and Dimensional Methods in Mechanics* (Acad. Press, New York) [Translated from Russian]

Sedov L.I. (1977) *Methods of similarity and dimensions in mechanics* (Nauka, Moscow) (Russian)

Selkoe D.J. (1992) Aging brain, aging mind. Sci. Am. **267**, 134

Selye H. (1974) *Stress without distress* (M.D., New York)

Sheldon R.W., Prakash A. and Sutcliffe W.H.,Jr. (1972) The size distribution of particles in the ocean. Limnol. Oceanogr. **17**, 327

Shklovskii I.S. (1987) *Universe. Life. Mind* (Nauka, Moskow) (Russian)

Shugart G.W. (1988) Uterovaginal sperm storage glands in sixteen species with comments on morphological differences. Auk **105**, 379

Shugart H.H. (1984) *A Theory of Forest Dynamics: The Ecological Implications of Forest Succession Models* (Springer, Berlin)

Shukla J. and Mintz Y. (1982) Influence of land-surface evapotranspiration on the Earth's climate. Science **215**, 1498

Shushkina E.A. and Vinogradov M.E. (1988) The quantitative characteristic of populations of Pacific oceanic pelagial. The planktonic biomass and productive-destructive processes. Oceanologija **28**, 992 (Russian) [English transl.: Oceanology **28**]

Sieburth J.M. (1976) Bacterial substrates and productivity in marine ecosystems. Ann. Rev. Ecol. Syst. **7**, 259

Sieburth J.M. and Davis P.G. (1982) The role of heterotrophic nanoplankton in the grazing and nurturing of planktonic bacteria in the Sargasso and Caribbean Seas. Ann. Inst. Oceanogr. Paris **58**, 285

Siegenthaler U. and Oeschger H. (1978) Predicting future atmospheric carbon dioxide levels. Science **199**, 388

Siegenthaler U. and Oeschger H. (1987) Biospheric CO_2 emission during the past 200 years reconstructed by deconvolution of ice core data. Tellus **39B**, 140

Siegenthaler U. and Wenk T. (1984) Rapid atmospheric CO_2 variations and ocean circulation. Nature **308**, 624

Simon H.A. (1980) The behavioural and social sciences. Science **209**, 72

Simpson G.G. (1944) *Tempo and Mode in Evolution* (Columbia Univ., New York)

Skinner B.J. (1986) *Earth Resources* (Prentice-Hall Inc., New Jersey)

Smirnov B.M. (1986) Fractal clusters. Uspekhi Fizicheskikh Nauk **149**, 177, [Sow. Phys. Usp. **41** (2), American Institute of Physics]

Sokolov L.V. (1991) *Philopatry and Dispersal of Birds* (vol. 230) (USSR Acad. Sci. Proc. Zool. Inst., Leningrad) (Russian)

Sommerfeld A. (1952) *Thermodynamic and Statistik Vorlesungen uber Theoretische Physik* (Band 5) (Dieterich, Wiesbaden)

Staffelbach T., Stauffer B., Sigg A. and Oeschger H. (1991) CO_2 measurements from polar ice cores: more data from different sites. Tellus **43B**, 91

Stahl F.W. (1990) If it smells like a unicorn. Nature **386**, 791

Stahl W.R. (1963) The analysis of biological similarity. Advan. Biol. Med. Phys. **9**, 355

Stanley S.M. (1973) An explanation of Cope's rule. Evolution **27**, 1

Starke L. (Ed) (1987), (1990) *The State of the World 1987, 1990. Worldwotch Inst. Report on Progress toward a Sustainable Society* (Norton and Co, New York)

Starr C. (1971) Energy and power. Sci. Am. **225**, 37

Stebbins G.L. (1971) *Chromosomal Evolution in Higher Plants* (Edward Arnold, London)

Stebbins G.L. (1974) *Flowering plants: evolution above the species level* (Belknap Press, Harvard Univ. Press, Cambridge, MA)

Stent G.S. and Calender R. (1978) *Molecular Genetics. An Introductory Narrative* (Freeman and Co, San Francisco)

Stevens C.F. (1993) Theories on the brain. Nature **361**, 500

Stuiver M. and Pollach H. (1977) Reporting of ^{14}C data. Radiocarbon **19**, 355

Stuiver M. and Quay P.D. (1983) Abyssal water carbon-14 distribution and the age of the World oceans. Science **219**, 849

Sueoka N. (1988) Directional mutation pressure and neutral molecular evolution. Proc. Natl. Acad. Sci. USA **85**, 2653

Sugimura Y. and Suzuki Y. (1988) A high temperature catalytic oxidation method for determination of non-volatile dissolved organic carbon in seawater by direct injection of liquid samples. Mar. Chem. **24**, 105

Summers C.M. (1971) The conversion of energy. Sci. Am. **224**, 149

Sundquist E.T. (1993) The global carbon budget. Science **259**, 934

Syvanen M. (1984) Conserved regions in mammalian β-globins: Could they arise by Cross-species gene exchange? J. Theor. Biol. **107**, 685

Syvanen M. (1987) Molecular clocks and evolutionary relationships: Possible distortions due to horizontal gene flow. J. Mol. Evol. **26**, 16

Syvanen M. (1989) Classical plant taxonomic ambiguities extend to the molecular level. J. Mol. Evol. **28**, 536

Takahashi T., Broecker W.S. and Bainbridge A.E. (1981) Supplement to the alkalinity and total carbon dioxide concentration in the World oceans. In: Bolin B. (Ed.) *Carbon Cycle Modelling*, SCOPE, **16**, (Wiley, Chichester), 159

Takahashi T., Broecker W.S. and Langer S. (1985) Redfield ratio based on chemical data from isopycnal surface. J. Geophys. Res. **90**, 6907

Tans P.P., Fung I.Y. and Takahashi T. (1990) Observational constraints on the global atmospheric CO_2 budget. Science **247**, 1431

Thomas C.D. (1990) Fewer species. Nature **347**, 237

Thorne A.G. amd Wolpoff M.H. (1992) The multiregional evolution of humans. Sci. Am. **266**, 76

Thribus M. and McIrvine E.C. (1971) Energy and information. Sci. Am. **224**, 179

Tinbergen N. (1968) On war and peace in animal and man. Science **160**, 1411

Toggweiler J.R. (1990) Diving into the organic soup. Nature **345**, 203

Townshend J.R.G. (Ed.) (1992) Improved global data for land application: A proposal for new high resolution data set. (Report of Land Cover Working Group of IGBP – DIS. Global change. Rep. (20), Stockholm)

Townshend J.R.G., Justice C.O., Li W., Gurney C. and McManus J. (1991) Global land cover classification by remote sensing: Present capabilities and future possibilities. Remote Sensing of Environment **35**, 243

Trivers R.L. and Hare H. (1976) Haplodipoidy and evolution of the social insects. Science **191**, 249

Trivett N.B.A. (1989) A comparison of seasonal cycles and trends in atmospheric CO_2 concentration as determined from robust and classical regression techniques. Extended Abstracts of Papers Presented at the Third Internat. Conf. on Analysis and Evolution of Atmospheric CO_2 Data. W.M.O., Univ. Heidelberg, 299

Tseitlin V.B. (1985) Distribution of organisms with their body sizes in various ecosystems. Doklady (Proceedings) Acad. Sci. USSR **285**, 1272 (Russian)

Tseitlin V.B. and Byzova Yu.B. (1986) Size distribution of soil organisms in different natural zones. J.General Biology **47**, 193 (Russian)

Tucker C.J., Townshend J.R.G., Goff T.E. and Holben B.N. (1986) Continental and global scale remote sensing of land cover. In: Trabalka J.R. and D.E. Reichle (Eds.) *The Global Carbon Cycle* (Springer, Berlin), 221

Turner II B.L., Moss R.H. and Skole D.L. (1993) Relating Land Use and Global Land-Cover Change: A Proposal for an IGBP-HDP Core Project, Global Change IGBP report (24), HDP report (5). Stockholm

Urlanis B.Ts. (Ed.) (1978) The Population of Countries of the World (Statistika, Moskow) (Russian)

Van Valen L. (1973) A new evolutionary law. Evol. Theory **1**, 1

Van Valen L. (1977) The Red Queen. Amer. Natur. **111**, 809

Van Valen L. (1979) Taxonomic survivorship curves. Evol. Theory **4**, 129

Vernadsky V.I. (1945) The biosphere and noosphere. Sci. Am. **33**, 1

Vinogradov M.E. and Shushkina E.A. (1988) Quantitative Characteristics of the Pacific pelagic community. Production regions and estimates of photosynthetic primary production. Oceanologija **28**, 819 (Russian) [English transl.: Oceanology]

Vitousek P.M. (1988) Diversity and Biological Invasion of Oceanic Islands. In: Wilson E.O. and Peter F.M. (Eds.) *Biodiversity* (Nat. Acad. Press, Washington), 3

Vitousek P.M., Ehrlich P.R., Ehrlich A.H.E. and Matson P.A. (1986) Human appropriation of the products of photosynthesis. Bioscience **36**, 368

Vogel F. and Motulsky A.G. (1979), (1982), (1986) *Human Genetics* (Springer, Berlin)

Vogel F. and Rathenberg R. (1975) Spontaneous mutation in man. Adv. Hum. Genetics **5**, 223

Vollrath D., Foote S., Hilton A. et al. (1992) The human Y chromosome: a 43-interval map based on naturally occuping deletions. Science **258**, 52

Watson A.J., Upstill-Goddard R.C. and Liss P.S. (1991) Air-sea gas exchange in rough and stormy seas measured by a dual-tracer technique. Nature **349**, 145

Watson J.D., Tooze J. and Kurth D.T. (1983) *Recombinant DNA* (Freeman Co., New York)

Watts J.A. (1982) The carbon dioxide question: Data sampler. In: Clark W.C. (Ed.) *Carbon Dioxide Review,* (Clarendon Press, New York)

Weis-Fogh T. (1972) Energetics of hovering flight in hummingbirds and in Drosophila. J. Exp. Biol. **56**, 79

Weiser M. (1991) The computer for the 21st century. Sci. Am. **265**, 94

Wesson R. (1991) *Beyond Natural Selection* (MIT Press)

White M.J.D. (1973) *Animal Cytology and Evolution* (Cambridge Univ., Cambridge)

White R. and Lalouel J.-M. (1988) Chromosome mapping with DNA markers. Sci. Am. **258**, 22

Whittaker R.H. (1975) *Community and Ecosystems* (MacMillan, New York)

Whittaker R.H. and Likens G.E. (1975) The biosphere and man. In: Lieth H. and R. Whittaker (Eds.) *Primary Productivity of the Biosphere* (Springer, Berlin)

Williams G.C. (1975) *Sex and Evolution* (Princeton Univ., New York)

Williams P.M. and Druffel E.R.M. (1987) Radiocarbon in dissolved organic matter in the central North Pacific Ocean. Nature **330**, 246

Willson R.C. (1984) Measurements of solar total irradiance and its variability. Space Sci. Rev. **38**, 203

Wilson A.C. and Cann R.L. (1992) The recent African genesis of humans. Sci. Am. **266**, 68

Wilson D.S. (1980) *The Natural Selection of Population and Communities* (Benjamin Cummings, Meno Park Ca)

Wilson E.O. (1975) *Sociobiology* (Harvard Univ., Cambridge Mass)

Wilson E.O. (Ed.) (1988) *Biodiversity* (Natl. Acad. Press, Washington)

Wilson E.O. (1989) Threats to biodiversity. Sci. Am. **261**, 108

Wilson K.G. and Kogut J. (1974) The renormalization group and the expansion. Physics Report **12C**, 75

Winberg G.G. (1976) Dependence of energetic metabolism on body mass in water ectothermic animals. J. General Biology **37**, 56 (Russian)

Winberg G.G. (Ed.) (1979) *Fundamentals of a study of aquatic ecosystems* (Nauka, Leningrad) (Russian)

Winston R. (1991) Nonimaging optics. Sci. Am. **264**, 52

World Food Problem (1967) U.S.President's Advisory Committee. The World Food Problem Report of the Panel of the World's Food Supply, (vol. 1–3), (Government Printing Office, Washington DC)

World Resources 1988-1989, (1988) **16**. Land Cover Settlements. (Basic Books. Inc., New York), 264

Wortman S. (1976) Food and agriculture. Sci. Am. **235**, 30

Wrangham R.W. (1977) Feeding behaviour of chimpanzees of Gombe National Park, Tanzania. In: Clutton-Brock T. (Ed.) *Primate Ecology* (Academic, London), 504

Wright S. (1931) Evolution in Mendelian population. Genetics **16**, 97

Wright S. (1932) The roles of mutation, inbreeding, crossbreeding, and selection in evolution. Proc. 6th Int. Congr. Genet., vol. 1, 356

Wright S. (1988) Surfaces of selective value revisited. Am. Natur. **131**, 115

Wynne-Edwards V.C. (1962) *Animal Dispersion in Relation to Social Behaviour* (Pergamon Press, Edinburgh)

Wynne-Edwards V.C. (1963) Intergroup selection in the evolution of social systems. Nature **200**, 623

Wynne-Edwards V.C. (1986) *Evolution thorough Group Selection* (Blackwell, Oxford)

Yablokov A.V. (1987) *Population Biology* (Vyschaya shkola, Moskow) (Russian)

Yonge C.M. (1975) Giant clams. Sci. Am. **232**, 96

Yoshimura J. and Clark C.W. (1991) Individual adaptations in stochastic environments. Evol. Ecology **5**, 173

Yuzhakov S.N. (Ed.) (1904) *Russia: Population, Agriculture. Great Encyclopaedia* (vol. 16) (Prosveschenie, S.Petersburg) (Russian)

Zahavi A. (1975) Mate selection – a selection for a handicap. J. Theor. Biol. **53**, 205

Zeki S. (1992) The visual image in mind and brain. Sci. Am. **267**, 68

Zuckerkandl E. (1987) On the molecular evolutionary clock. J. Mol. Evol. **26**, 34

Zuckerkandl E. and Pauling L. (1965) Evolutionary divergence and convergence in proteins. In: Bryson V. and H.J. Vogel (Eds.) *Evolving Genes and Proteins* (Academic, New York), 97

Subject Index